CARDIOLOGY SECRETS

SECRETS

Fourth Edition

Glenn N. Levine, MD, FACC, FAHA
Professor of Medicine
Baylor College of Medicine
Director
Cardiac Care Unit
Michael E. DeBakey VA Medical Center
Houston, Texas

ELSEVIER
SAUNDERS

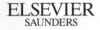

1600 John F. Kennedy Blvd.
Ste 1800
Philadelphia, PA 19103-2899

CARDIOLOGY SECRETS, FOURTH EDITION

ISBN: 978-1-4557-4815-0

Library of Congress Cataloging-in-Publication Data

Cardiology secrets / [edited by] Glenn N. Levine. -- 4th ed.
    p. ; cm. -- (Secrets series)
Includes bibliographical references and index.
ISBN 978-1-4557-4815-0 (pbk.)
I. Levine, Glenn N. II. Series: Secrets series.
[DNLM: 1. Heart Diseases--Examination Questions. WG 18.2]
RC682
616.1'20076--dc23   2013009105

Acquisitions Editor: James Merritt
Developmental Editor: Joanie Milnes
Publishing Services Manager: Anne Altepeter
Project Manager: Jennifer Nemec
Design Manager: Steven Stave

Printed in the United States of America

Last digit is the print number: 9 8 7 6 5 4 3 2 1

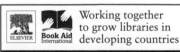

Working together
to grow libraries in
developing countries

www.elsevier.com • www.bookaid.org

CARDIOLOGY SECRETS

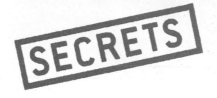

In loving memory of Ginger and Sasha

"Dogs' lives are too short. Their only fault, really."

Agnes Sligh Turnbull

*"You think dogs will not be in heaven?
I tell you, they will be there long before any of us."*

Robert Louis Stevenson

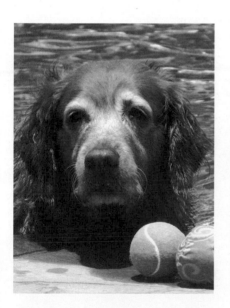
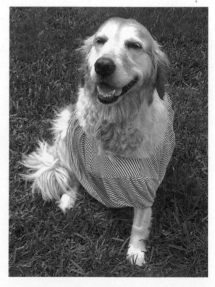

CONTRIBUTORS

Suhny Abbara, MD
Associate Professor, Harvard Medical School; Director, Cardiovascular Imaging Fellowship, Massachusetts General Hospital, Boston, Massachusetts

Anu Elizabeth Abraham, BS, MD
Fellow in Cardiovascular Medicine, Department of Cardiology, Boston Medical Center, Boston, Massachusetts

Anish K. Agarwal, MD, MPH
Research Coordinator, Department of Emergency Medicine, The Hospital of the University of Pennsylvania, Philadelphia, Pennsylvania

Rishi Agrawal, MD
Assistant Professor of Radiology, Thoracic Imaging, Feinberg School of Medicine, Northwestern University, Chicago, Illinois

David Aguilar, MD
Assistant Professor of Medicine, Department of Internal Medicine, Cardiology, Baylor College of Medicine, Houston, Texas

Jameel Ahmed, MD
Assistant Professor of Clinical Medicine, Section of Cardiology, Department of Medicine, Louisiana State University Health Sciences Center – New Orleans, New Orleans, Louisiana

Mahboob Alam, MD, FACC, FSCAI
Assistant Professor, Department of Medicine, Section of Cardiology, Baylor College of Medicine, Houston, Texas

Ashish Aneja, MD
Fellow, Cardiovascular Diagnostic Imaging, The Ohio State University Wexner Medical Center, Columbus, Ohio

Julia Ansari, MD
Cardiology Fellow, Baylor College of Medicine, Houston, Texas

Sameer Ather, MD, PhD
Fellow, Cardiovascular Disease, University of Alabama at Birmingham; Director, National Resident Matching Program, Birmingham, Alabama

Eric H. Awtry, MD
Director of Inpatient Cardiology, Boston Medical Center; Associate Professor of Medicine, Boston University School of Medicine, Boston, Massachusetts

Jose L. Baez-Escudero, MD, FHRS
Staff Cardiac Electrophysiologist, Section of Pacing and Electrophysiology; Robert and Suzanne Tomsich Department of Cardiovascular Medicine, Cleveland Clinic, Weston, Florida

Faisal Bakaeen, MD, FACS
Chief of Cardiothoracic Surgery, Michael E. DeBakey VA Medical Center; Associate Professor of Surgery, Baylor College of Medicine, Houston, Texas

Gary J. Balady, MD
Director, Non Invasive Cardiovascular Labs; Director, Preventive Cardiology, Boston Medical Center; Professor of Medicine, Boston University School of Medicine, Boston, Massachusetts

Luc M. Beauchesne, MD, FACC
Director, Adult Congenital Heart Disease Program, Division of Cardiology, University of Ottawa Heart Institute, Ottawa, Ontario, Canada

Carlos F. Bechara, MD, MS, FACS, RPVI
Assistant Professor of Surgery, Program Director, Vascular Surgery, Baylor College of Medicine, Michael E. DeBakey VA Medical Center, Houston, Texas

Sheilah Bernard, MD, FACC
Associate Program Director, Medicine Residency Program, Department of Medicine, Associate Professor of Medicine, Section of Cardiology, Boston Medical Center, Boston, Massachusetts

Fernando Boccalandro, MD, FACC, FSCAI, CPI
Clinical Assistant Professor, Department of Internal Medicine, Texas Tech University Health Sciences Center, Odessa Heart Institute, Odessa, Texas

Ann Bolger, MD, FAHA, FACC
William Watt Kerr Professor of Medicine, Division of Cardiology, University of California, San Francisco, San Francisco, California

Biykem Bozkurt, MD, PhD, FACC, FAHA
The Mary and Gordon Cain Chair and Professor of Medicine; Director, Winters Center for Heart Failure Research; Associate Director, Cardiovascular Research Institute, Baylor College of Medicine; Chief, Cardiology Section, Michael E. DeBakey VA Medical Center, Houston, Texas

William Ross Brown, MD
Cardiology Fellow, Baylor College of Medicine, Houston, Texas

Blase A. Carabello, MD
The W.A. "Tex" and Deborah Moncrief, Jr., Professor of Medicine, Vice-Chairman, Department of Medicine, Baylor College of Medicine; Medical Care Line Executive, Veterans Affairs Medical Center; Director, Center for Heart Valve Disease, Texas Heart Institute at St. Luke's, Houston, Texas

Christian Castillo, MD
Fellow, Sleep Medicine, Department of Medicine, University of Pittsburgh, Pittsburgh, Pennsylvania

Leslie T. Cooper, Jr., MD
Professor of Medicine, Director, Gonda Vascular Center, Mayo Clinic, Rochester, Minnesota

Lorraine D. Cornwell, MD, FACS
Assistant Professor of Surgery, Baylor College of Medicine; Cardiothoracic Surgery, Michael E. DeBakey VA Medical Center, Houston, Texas

Luke Cunningham, MD
Internal Medicine, Baylor College of Medicine, Houston, Texas

Talal Dahhan, MD
Fellow, Pulmonary Diseases and Critical Care Medicine, Duke University Medical Center, Durham, North Carolina

Maria Elena De Benedetti, MD
Cardiovascular Medicine Fellow, Heart and Vascular Institute, Henry Ford Hospital, Detroit, Michigan

Anita Deswal, MD, MPH
Associate Professor of Medicine, Baylor College of Medicine; Co-Director, Heart Failure Program, Section of Cardiology, Michael E. DeBakey VA Medical Center, Houston, Texas

Vijay G. Divakaran, MD, MPH
Interventional Cardiologist, Scott and White Hospital; Clinical Assistant Professor of Medicine, Texas A&M Health Science Center, Round Rock, Texas

Hisham Dokainish, MD, FRCPC, FACC, FASE
Associate Professor, Division of Cardiology, Department of Medicine, McMaster University, Hamilton, Ontario; Cardiologist, Hamilton Health Sciences

Chantal El Amm, MD
Assistant Professor of Medicine, Division of Cardiovascular Medicine, University Hospitals of Cleveland, Cleveland, Ohio

Michael E. Farkouh, MD, MSc, FACC
Chair and Director, Peter Munk Centre of Excellence in Multinational Clinical Trials, University Health Network; Director, Heart & Stroke Richard Lewar Centre of Excellence in Cardiovascular Research, University of Toronto, Toronto, Canada

G. Michael Felker, MD, MHS, FACC, FAHA
Associate Professor of Medicine, Chief, Heart Failure Section, Division of Cardiology, Duke University School of Medicine; Director, Clinical Research Unit, Duke Heart Center; Director of Heart Failure Research, Duke Clinical Research Institute, Durham, North Carolina

James J. Fenton, MD, FCCP
Clinical Associate Professor, National Jewish Health-South Denver, Englewood, Colorado

Scott D. Flamm, MD, MBA, FACC, FAHA
Head, Cardiovascular Imaging, Imaging Institute, and Heart and Vascular Institute, Cleveland Clinic, Cleveland, Ohio

Lee A. Fleisher, MD, FACC, FAHA
Robert D. Dripps Professor and Chair of Anesthesiology and Critical Care, Professor of Medicine, Perelman School of Medicine; Senior Fellow, Leonard Davis Institute of Health Economics, University of Pennsylvania, Philadelphia, Pennsylvania

Cindy L. Grines, MD, FACC
Corporate Vice Chief of Academic Affairs, Cardiovascular Medicine, William Beaumont Hospital, Royal Oak, Michigan

Gabriel B. Habib, Sr., MS, MD, FACC, FCCP, FAHA
Professor of Medicine (Cardiology), Baylor College of Medicine; Associate Chief and Director of Education, Cardiology Section, Michael E. DeBakey VA Medical Center, Houston, Texas

Stephan M. Hergert, MD
Fellow, Department of Anesthesiology and Intensive Care Medicine, University of Rostock, Rostock, Germany

Ravi S. Hira, MD
Cardiology Fellow, Baylor College of Medicine, Houston, Texas

Brian D. Hoit, MD
Professor of Medicine and Physiology and Biophysics, Case Western Reserve University; Director of Echocardiography, University Hospitals Case Medical Center, Cleveland, Ohio

Hani Jneid, MD, FACC, FAHA, FSCAI
Assistant Professor of Medicine, Director of Interventional Cardiology Research, Division of Cardiology, Baylor College of Medicine, Michael E. DeBakey VA Medical Center, Houston, Texas

Nicole R. Keller, PharmD, BCNSP
Clinical Pharmacy Specialist, Michael E. DeBakey VA Medical Center; Clinical Instructor, Baylor College of Medicine, Adjunct Assistant Professor, University of Texas College of Pharmacy, Houston, Texas

Thomas A. Kent, MD
Professor and Director of Stroke Research and Education, Department of Neurology, Baylor College of Medicine; Chief of Neurology, Michael E. DeBakey VA Medical Center, Houston, Texas

Panos Kougias, MD
Associate Professor of Surgery, Baylor College of Medicine, Houston, Texas

Richard A. Lange, MD
Professor and Executive Vice Chairman, Department of Medicine, Director, Office of Educational Programs, University of Texas Health Science Center at San Antonio, San Antonio, Texas

Rebecca M. LeLeiko, MD
Fellow in Cardiovascular Medicine, Department of Cardiology, Boston Medical Center, Boston, Massachusetts

Glenn N. Levine, MD, FACC, FAHA
Professor of Medicine, Baylor College of Medicine; Director, Cardiac Care Unit, Michael E. DeBakey VA Medical Center, Houston, Texas

Salvatore Mangione, MD
Associate Professor of Medicine, Director of Physical Diagnosis Curriculum, Jefferson Medical College of Thomas Jefferson University, Philadelphia, Pennsylvania

Sharyl R. Martini, MD, PhD
Clinical Instructor, Department of Neurology, University of Cincinnati College of Medicine, Cincinnati, Ohio

Nitin Mathur, MD
Cardiology Clinic of San Antonio – Stone Oak, San Antonio, Texas

James McCord, MD
In-Patient Director, Heart and Vascular Institute, Henry Ford Hospital, Detroit, Michigan

Geno J. Merli, MD, FACP, FHM, FSVM
Professor of Medicine, Jefferson Medical College; Co-Director, Jefferson Vascular Center, Philadelphia, Pennsylvania

Arunima Misra, MD, FACC
Assistant Professor, Director of Nuclear Cardiology, Baylor College of Medicine; Medical Director of the Noninvasive Laboratory, Ben Taub General Hospital, Houston, Texas

Ahmad Munir, MD, FACC
Interventional Cardiologist, Detroit Medical Center, Cardiovascular Institute, Harper University Hospital, Detroit, Michigan

Alejandro Perez, MD, FSVM, RPVI
Assistant Professor of Medicine and Surgery, Department of Surgery, Thomas Jefferson University; Medical Director of Wound Care and Hyperbaric Program, Jefferson Vascular Center, Methodist Hospital, Thomas Jefferson University Hospital, Philadelphia, Pennsylvania

George Philippides, MD, FACC
Associate Professor of Medicine, Boston University School of Medicine; Associate Chair of Clinical Affairs, Cardiovascular Section, Boston Medical Center, Boston, Massachusetts

Vissia S. Pinili, MSN, RN, CPAN, CCRN
Clinical Nurse Educator, Michael E. DeBakey VA Medical Center, Houston, Texas

Andrew Pipe, CM, MD, LLD(Hon), DSc(Hon)
Professor, Faculty of Medicine, University of Ottawa; Chief, Division of Prevention and Rehabilitation, University of Ottawa Heart Institute, Ottawa, Ontario, Canada

Charles V. Pollack, MA, MD, FACEP, FAAEM, FAHA, FCPP
Chairman, Department of Emergency Medicine, Pennsylvania Hospital; Professor, Department of Emergency Medicine, UPHS–Perelman School of Medicine of the University of Pennsylvania, Philadelphia, Pennsylvania

Ourania Preventza, MD, FACS
Attending Cardiothoracic Surgeon, St. Luke's Episcopal Hospital at Texas Heart Institute, Baylor College of Medicine, Houston, Texas

Shawn T. Ragbir, MD
Fellow, Cardiovascular Disease, Ochsner Clinic Foundation, New Orleans, Louisiana

Kumudha Ramasubbu, MD, FACC
Director, Non-Invasive Laboratory, Michael E. DeBakey VA Medical Center; Assistant Professor, Baylor College of Medicine, Houston, Texas

Christopher J. Rees, MD
Attending Physician, Emergency Department, Pennsylvania Hospital; Clinical Instructor in Emergency Medicine, UPHS–Perelman School of Medicine of the University of Pennsylvania, Philadelphia, Pennsylvania

Zeenat Safdar, MD, FCCP, FACP, FPVRI
Associate Professor of Medicine, Co-Director, Baylor Pulmonary Hypertension Center, Baylor College of Medicine, Houston, Texas

Theodore L. Schreiber, MD
Division of Cardiology, Wayne State University Program, Detroit Medical Center, Harper University Hospital, Detroit, Michigan

Paul A. Schurmann, MD
Fellow, Cardiovascular Disease, Baylor College of Medicine, Houston, Texas

Ryan Seutter, MD
Cardiovascular Specialist, Bon Secours Hampton Roads Health System, Suffolk, Virginia

Nishant R. Shah, MD
Fellow, Cardiovascular Disease, Texas Heart Institute, Baylor College of Medicine, Houston, Texas

Sarah A. Spinler, PharmD, FCCP, FCPP, FAHA, FASHP, AACC, BCPS (AQ Cardiology)
Professor of Clinical Pharmacy, Philadelphia College of Pharmacy, University of the Sciences, Philadelphia, Pennsylvania

Luis A. Tamara, MD
Chief of Nuclear Medicine, Nuclear Cardiology and PET/CT Imaging, Michael E. DeBakey VA Medical Center; Associate Professor of Radiology, Baylor College of Medicine, Houston, Texas

Victor F. Tapson, MD, FCCP, FRCP
Professor of Medicine, Director, Center for Pulmonary Vascular Disease, Duke University Medical Center, Durham, North Carolina

Paaladinesh Thavendiranathan, MD, MSc, FRCPC
Assistant Professor of Medicine, Department of Cardiology and Medical Imaging, University Health Network, University of Toronto, Toronto, Ontario, Canada

Miguel Valderrábano, MD, FACC
Associate Professor of Medicine, Weill College of Medicine; Adjunct Associate Professor of Medicine, Baylor College of Medicine; Director, Division of Cardiac Electrophysiology, Department of Cardiology, The Methodist Hospital, Houston, Texas

PREFACE

As with the third edition of *Cardiology Secrets*, my hope with this revised fourth edition is that it will help educate health care providers in a didactic, interactive, interesting, and enjoyable manner on the optimal evaluation and management of patients with cardiovascular disease and, in doing so, will help to ensure that all patients with cardiovascular disease receive optimal preventive, pharmacologic, diagnostic, and device interventions and therapies. For that is, ultimately, why we have all chosen this profession and continue to educate ourselves, is it not?

I would like to acknowledge and thank the many authors who contributed their time, knowledge, and expertise to this edition of *Cardiology Secrets*. It is their willingness to create free time when none exists to write the chapters that makes this book so successful.

I would again like to also acknowledge those who have served as mentors and role models, and have inspired me in my personal and professional life, including Gary Balady, Joseph Vita, Alice Jacobs, Scott Flamm, Doug Mann, and Eddie Matzger.

I welcome comments and suggestions from readers of this book: glevine@bcm.tmc.edu.

Glenn N. Levine, MD, FACC, FAHA

CONTENTS

SECTION V: VALVULAR DISEASE, STRUCTURAL HEART DISEASE, AND ENDOCARDITIS

SECTION VI: ARRHYTHMIAS

SECTION VII: PRIMARY AND SECONDARY PREVENTION

SECTION VIII: MISCELLANEOUS CARDIOVASCULAR SYMPTOMS AND DISEASES

TOP 100 SECRETS

These secrets are 100 of the top board alerts. They summarize the concepts, principles, and most salient details of cardiology.

1. Coronary flow reserve (the increase in coronary blood flow in response to agents that lead to microvascular dilation) begins to decrease when a coronary artery stenosis is 50% or more luminal diameter. However, basal coronary flow does not begin to decrease until the lesion is 80% to 90% luminal diameter.

2. The most commonly used criteria to diagnose left ventricular hypertrophy (LVH) are R wave in V5 or V6 + S wave in V1 or V2 > 35 mm, or R wave in lead I plus S wave in lead III > 25 mm.

3. Causes of ST segment elevation include acute myocardial infarction (MI) as a result of thrombotic occlusion of a coronary artery, Prinzmetal angina, cocaine-induced MI, pericarditis, left ventricular (LV) aneurysm, left bundle branch block (LBBB), LVH with repolarization abnormalities, J point elevation, and severe hyperkalemia.

4. The initial electrocardiogram (ECG) manifestation of hyperkalemia is peaked T waves. As the hyperkalemia becomes more profound, there may be loss of visible P waves, QRS widening, and ST segment elevation. The preterminal finding is a sinusoidal pattern on the ECG.

5. The classic carotid arterial pulse in a patient with aortic stenosis is reduced *(parvus)* and delayed *(tardus)*.

6. The most common ECG finding in pulmonary embolus is sinus tachycardia. Other ECG findings that can occur include right atrial (RA) enlargement *(P pulmonale)*, right axis deviation, T-wave inversions in leads V1 to V2, incomplete right bundle branch block (IRBBB), and a S1Q3T3 pattern (an S wave in lead I, a Q wave in lead III, and an inverted T wave in lead III).

7. The major *risk factors* for coronary artery disease (CAD) are family history of premature CAD (father, mother, brother, or sister who first developed clinical CAD at age younger than 45 to 55 for males and at age younger than 55 to 60 for females), hypercholesterolemia, hypertension, cigarette smoking, and diabetes mellitus.

8. Important causes of chest pain not related to atherosclerotic CAD include aortic dissection, pneumothorax, pulmonary embolism (PE), pneumonia, hypertensive crisis, Prinzmetal angina, cardiac syndrome X, anomalous origin of the coronary artery, pericarditis, esophageal spasm or esophageal rupture (Boerhaave syndrome), and shingles.

9. The Kussmaul sign is the paradoxical increase in jugular venous pressure (JVP) that occurs during inspiration. JVP normally decreases during inspiration because the inspiratory fall in intrathoracic pressure creates a *sucking effect* on venous return. Kussmaul sign is observed when the right side of the heart is unable to accommodate an increased venous return, such as can occur with constrictive pericarditis, severe heart failure, cor pulmonale, restrictive cardiomyopathy, tricuspid stenosis, and right ventricular (RV) infarction.

10. Other causes of elevated cardiac troponin, besides acute coronary syndrome and myocardial infarction, that should be considered in patients with chest pains include PE, aortic dissection, myopericarditis, severe aortic stenosis, and severe chronic kidney disease.

11. Prinzmetal angina, also called *variant angina*, is an unusual angina caused by coronary vasospasm. Patients with Prinzmetal angina are typically younger and often female. Treatment is based primarily on the use of calcium channel blockers and nitrates.

12. Cardiac syndrome X is an entity in which patients describe typical exertional anginal symptoms, yet are found on cardiac catheterization to have nondiseased, *normal* coronary arteries. Although there are likely multiple causes and explanations for cardiac syndrome X, it does appear that, at least in some patients, microvascular coronary artery constriction or dysfunction plays a role.

13. The three primary antianginal medications used for the treatment of chronic stable angina are β-blockers, nitrates, and calcium channel blockers. Ranolazine, a newer antianginal agent, is generally used only as a third-line agent in patients with continued significant angina despite traditional antianginal therapy who have CAD not amenable to revascularization.

14. Findings that suggest a heart murmur is pathologic and requires further evaluation include the presence of symptoms, extra heart sounds, thrills, abnormal ECG or chest radiography, diminished or absent S2, holosystolic (or late systolic) murmur, any diastolic murmur, and all continuous murmurs.

15. The major categories of ischemic stroke are large vessel atherosclerosis (including embolization from carotid to cerebral arteries), small vessel vasculopathy or lacunar type, and cardioembolic.

16. Hemorrhagic strokes are classified by their location: subcortical (associated with uncontrolled hypertension in 60% of cases) versus cortical (more concerning for underlying mass, arteriovenous malformation, or amyloidosis).

17. Common radiographic signs of congestive heart failure include enlarged cardiac silhouette, left atrial (LA) enlargement, hilar fullness, vascular redistribution, linear interstitial opacities (Kerley lines), bilateral alveolar infiltrates, and pleural effusions (right greater than left).

18. Classic ECG criteria for the diagnosis of ST elevation myocardial infarction (STEMI), warranting thrombolytic therapy, are ST segment elevation greater than 0.1 mV in at least two contiguous leads (e.g., leads III and aVF or leads V2 and V3) or new or presumably new LBBB.

19. *Primary percutaneous coronary intervention (PCI)* refers to the strategy of taking a patient who presents with STEMI directly to the cardiac catheterization laboratory to undergo mechanical revascularization using balloon angioplasty, coronary stents, and other measures.

20. The triad of findings suggestive of RV infarction are hypotension, distended neck veins, and clear lungs.

21. Cessation of cerebral blood flow for as short a period as 6 to 8 seconds can precipitate syncope.

22. The most common causes of syncope in pediatric and young patients are neurocardiogenic syncope (vasovagal syncope, vasodepressor syncope), conversion reactions (psychiatric causes), and primary arrhythmic causes (e.g., long QT syndrome, Wolff-Parkinson-White syndrome). In contrast, elderly patients have a higher frequency of syncope caused by obstructions to cardiac output (e.g., aortic stenosis, PE) and by arrhythmias resulting from underlying heart disease.

23. Preexisting renal disease and diabetes are the two major risk factors for the development of contrast nephropathy. Preprocedure and postprocedure hydration is the most established method of reducing the risk of contrast nephropathy.

24. During coronary angiography, flow down the coronary artery is graded using the *TIMI flow grade* (flow grades based on results of the Thrombolysis in Myocardial Infarction trial), in which TIMI grade 3 flow is normal and TIMI grade 0 flow means there is no blood flow down the artery.

25. The National Cholesterol Education Program (NCEP) Adult Treatment Panel III (ATP III) recommends that all adults age 20 years or older should undergo the fasting lipoprotein profile every 5 years. Testing should include total cholesterol, low-density lipoprotein (LDL) cholesterol, high-density lipoprotein (HDL) cholesterol, and triglycerides.

26. Important *secondary* causes of hyperlipidemia include diabetes, hypothyroidism, obstructive liver disease, chronic renal failure or nephrotic syndrome, and certain drugs (progestins, anabolic steroids, corticosteroids).

27. The minimum LDL goal for secondary prevention in patients with established CAD, peripheral vascular disease, or diabetes is an LDL less than 100 mg/dL. A goal of LDL less than 70 mg/dL should be considered in patients with CAD at very high risk, including those with multiple major coronary risk factors (especially diabetes), severe and poorly controlled risk factors (especially continued cigarette smoking), and multiple risk factors of the metabolic syndrome and those with acute coronary syndrome.

28. Factors that make up *metabolic syndrome* include abdominal obesity (waist circumference in men larger than 40 inches/102 cm or in women larger than 35 inches/88 cm); triglycerides 150 mg/dL or higher; low HDL cholesterol (less than 40 mg/dL in men or less than 50 mg/dL in women); blood pressure 135/85 mm Hg or higher; and fasting glucose 110 mg/dL or higher.

29. Although optimal blood pressure is less than 120/80 mm Hg, the goal of blood pressure treatment is to achieve blood pressure levels less than 140/90 mm Hg in most patients with uncomplicated hypertension.

30. Up to 5% of all hypertension cases are *secondary*, meaning that a specific cause can be identified. Causes of secondary hypertension include renal artery stenosis, renal parenchymal disease, primary hyperaldosteronism, pheochromocytoma, Cushing disease, hyperparathyroidism, aortic coarctation, and sleep apnea.

31. Clinical syndromes associated with hypertensive emergency include hypertensive encephalopathy, intracerebral hemorrhage, unstable angina or acute myocardial infarction, pulmonary edema, dissecting aortic aneurysm, or eclampsia.

32. The Seventh Report of the Joint National Committee on Prevention, Detection, Evaluation, and Treatment of High Blood Pressure (JNC-7) recommends that hypertensive emergencies be treated in an intensive care setting with intravenously administered agents, with an initial goal of reducing mean arterial blood pressure by 10% to 15%, but no more than 25%, in the first hour and then, if stable, to a goal of 160/100 to 160/110 mm Hg within the next 2 to 6 hours.

33. Common causes of depressed LV systolic dysfunction and cardiomyopathy include CAD, hypertension, valvular heart disease, and alcohol abuse. Other causes include cocaine abuse, collagen vascular disease, viral infection, myocarditis, peripartum cardiomyopathy, acquired immunodeficiency syndrome (AIDS), tachycardia-induced cardiomyopathy, hypothyroidism, anthracycline toxicity, and Chagas disease.

34. The classic signs and symptoms of patients with heart failure are dyspnea on exertion (DOE), orthopnea, paroxysmal nocturnal dyspnea (PND), and lower extremity edema.

35. Heart failure symptoms are most commonly classified using the New York Heart Association (NYHA) classification system, in which class IV denotes symptoms even at rest and class I denotes the ability to perform ordinary physical activity without symptoms.

36. Patients with depressed ejection fractions (less than 40%) should be treated with agents that block the rennin-angiotensin-aldosterone system, in order to improve symptoms, decrease hospitalizations, and decrease mortality. Angiotensin-converting enzyme (ACE) inhibitors are first-line therapy; alternate or additional agents include angiotensin II receptor blockers (ARBs) and aldosterone receptor blockers.

37. The combination of high-dose hydralazine and high-dose isosorbide dinitrate should be used in patients who cannot be given or cannot tolerate ACE inhibitors or ARBs because of renal function impairment or hyperkalemia.

38. High-risk features in patients hospitalized with acute decompensated heart failure (ADHF) include low systolic blood pressure, elevated blood urea nitrogen (BUN), hyponatremia, history of prior heart failure hospitalization, elevated brain natriuretic peptide (BNP), and elevated troponin I or T.

39. Atrioventricular (AV) node reentry tachycardia (AVNRT) accounts for 65% to 70% of paroxysmal supraventricular tachycardias (SVTs).

40. Implantable cardioverter defibrillators (ICDs) should be considered for primary prevention of sudden cardiac death in patients whose LV ejection fractions remains less than 30% to 35% despite optimal medical therapy or revascularization and who have good-quality life expectancy of at least 1 year.

41. The three primary factors that promote venous thrombosis (known together as *Virchow triad*) are (1) venous blood stasis; (2) injury to the intimal layer of the venous vasculature; and (3) abnormalities in coagulation or fibrinolysis.

42. *Diastolic heart failure* is a clinical syndrome characterized by the signs and symptoms of heart failure, a preserved LV ejection fraction (greater than 45% to 50%), and evidence of diastolic dysfunction.

43. The four conditions identified as having the highest risk of adverse outcome from endocarditis, for which prophylaxis with dental procedures is still recommended by the American Heart Association, are prosthetic cardiac valve, previous infective endocarditis, certain cases of congenital heart disease, and cardiac transplantation recipients who develop cardiac valvulopathy.

44. Findings that should raise the suspicion for endocarditis include bacteremia and/or sepsis of unknown cause, fever, constitutional symptoms, hematuria and/or glomerulonephritis and/or suspected renal infarction, embolic event of unknown origin, new heart murmurs, unexplained new AV nodal conduction abnormality, multifocal or rapid changing pulmonic infiltrates, peripheral abscesses, certain cutaneous lesions (Osler nodes, Janeway lesions), and specific ophthalmic manifestations (Roth spots).

45. Transthoracic echo (TTE) has a sensitivity of 60% to 75% in the detection of native valve endocarditis. In cases where the suspicion of endocarditis is higher, a negative TTE should be followed by a transesophageal echo (TEE), which has a sensitivity of 88% to 100% and a specificity of 91% to 100% for native valves.

46. The most common cause of culture-negative endocarditis is prior use of antibiotics. Other causes include fastidious organisms (*Haemophilus aphrophilus, Actinobacillus actinomycetemcomitans, Cardiobacterium hominis, Eikenella corrodens,* and various species of *Kingella* [HACEK group]; *Legionella; Chlamydia; Brucella;* and certain fungal infections) and noninfectious causes.

47. Indications for surgery in cases of endocarditis include acute aortic insufficiency or mitral regurgitation leading to congestive heart failure, cardiac abscess formation or perivalvular extension, persistence of infection despite adequate antibiotic treatment, recurrent peripheral emboli, cerebral emboli, infection caused by microorganisms with a poor response to antibiotic treatment (e.g., fungi), prosthetic valve endocarditis (particularly if hemodynamic compromise exists), "mitral kissing infection," and large (greater than 10 mm) mobile vegetations.

48. The main echocardiographic criteria for severe mitral stenosis are mean transvalvular gradient greater than 10 mm Hg, mitral valve area less than 1 cm^2, and pulmonary artery (PA) systolic pressure greater than 50 mm Hg.

49. The classic auscultatory findings in mitral valve prolapse (MVP) is a midsystolic click and late systolic murmur, although the click may actually vary somewhat within systole, depending on changes in LV dimension, and there may actually be multiple clicks. The clicks are believed to result from the sudden tensing of the mitral valve apparatus as the leaflets prolapse into the LA (LA) during systole.

50. In patients with pericardial effusions, echocardiography findings that indicate elevated intrapericardial pressure and tamponade physiology include diastolic indentation or collapse of the RV, compression of the RA for more than one third of the cardiac cycle, lack of inferior vena cava (IVC) collapsibility with deep inspiration, 25% or more variation in mitral or aortic Doppler flows, and 50% or greater variation of tricuspid or pulmonic valve flows with inspiration.

51. The causes of pulseless electrical activity (PEA) can be broken down to the *H's and T's* of PEA, which are hypovolemia, hypoxemia, hydrogen ion (acidosis), hyperkalemia or hypokalemia, hypoglycemia, hypothermia, toxins, tamponade (cardiac), tension pneumothorax, thrombosis (coronary and pulmonary), and trauma.

52. Hemodynamically significant atrial septal defects (ASDs) have a shunt ratio greater than 1.5, are usually 10 mm or larger in diameter, and are usually associated with RV enlargement.

53. Findings suggestive of a hemodynamically significant coarctation include small diameter (less than 10 mm or less than 50% of reference normal descending aorta at the diaphragm), presence of collateral blood vessels, and a gradient across the coarctation of more than 20 to 30 mm Hg.

54. Tetralogy of Fallot (TOF) consists of four features: right ventricular outflow tract (RVOT) obstruction, a large ventricular septal defect (VSD), an overriding ascending aorta, and RV hypertrophy.

55. The three *D*s of the Ebstein anomaly are an apically *displaced* tricuspid valve that is *dysplastic*, with a right ventricle that may be *dysfunctional*.

56. Systolic wall stress is described by the law of Laplace, which states that systolic wall stress is equal to:

$$\text{(arterial pressure } (p) \times \text{radius } (r))/2 \times \text{thickness } (h), \text{ or } \sigma = (p \times r)/2h$$

57. Echocardiographic findings suggestive of severe mitral regurgitation include enlarged LA or LV, the color Doppler mitral regurgitation jet occupying a large proportion (more than 40%) of the LA, a regurgitant volume 60 mL or more, a regurgitant fraction 50% or greater, a regurgitant orifice 0.40 cm^2 or greater, and a Doppler vena contracta width 0.7 cm or greater.

58. The seven factors that make up the Thrombolysis in Myocardial Infarction (TIMI) Risk Score are: age greater than 65 years; three or more cardiac risk factors; prior catheterization demonstrating CAD; ST-segment deviation; two or more anginal events within 24 hours; aspirin use within 7 days; and elevated cardiac markers.

59. The components of the Global Registry of Acute Coronary Events (GRACE) Acute Cardiac Syndrome (ACS) Risk Model (at the time of admission) are age; heart rate; systolic blood pressure, creatinine; congestive heart failure (CHF) Killip class, ST-segment deviation; elevated cardiac enzymes and/or markers; and presence or absence of cardiac arrest at admission.

60. Myocarditis is most commonly caused by a viral infection. Other causes include nonviral infections (bacterial, fungal, protozoal, parasitic), cardiac toxins, hypersensitivity reactions, and systemic disease (usually autoimmune). Giant cell myocarditis is an uncommon but often fulminant form of myocarditis characterized by multinucleated giant cells and myocyte destruction.

61. Initial therapy for patients with non–ST segment elevation acute coronary syndrome (NSTE-ACS) should include antiplatelet therapy with aspirin and with either clopidogrel, ticagrelor, or a glycoprotein IIb/IIIa inhibitor, and antithrombin therapy with either unfractionated heparin, enoxaparin, fondaparinux, or bivalirudin (depending on the clinical scenario).

62. Important complications in heart transplant recipients include infection, rejection, vasculopathy (diffuse coronary artery narrowing), arrhythmias, hypertension, renal impairment, malignancy (especially skin cancer and lymphoproliferative disorders), and osteoporosis (caused by steroid use).

63. The classic symptoms of aortic stenosis are angina, syncope, and those of heart failure (dyspnea, orthopnea, paroxysmal nocturnal dyspnea, edema, etc.). Once any of these symptoms occur, the average survival without surgical intervention is 5, 3, or 2 years, respectively.

64. Class I indications for aortic valve replacement (AVR) include (1) development of symptoms in patients with severe aortic stenosis; (2) an LV ejection fraction of less than 50% in the setting of severe aortic stenosis; and (3) the presence of severe aortic stenosis in patients undergoing coronary artery bypass grafting, other heart valve surgery, or thoracic aortic surgery.

65. The major risk factors for venous thromboembolism (VTE) include previous thromboembolism, immobility, cancer and other causes of hypercoagulable state (protein C or S deficiency, factor V Leiden, antithrombin deficiency), advanced age, major surgery, trauma, and acute medical illness.

66. The Wells Score in cases of suspected pulmonary embolism (PE) includes deep vein thrombosis (DVT) symptoms and signs (3 points); PE as likely as or more likely than alternative diagnosis (3 points); heart rate greater 100 beats/min (1.5 points); immobilization or surgery in previous 4 weeks (1.5 points); previous DVT or PE (1.5 points); hemoptysis (1.0 point); and cancer (1 point).

67. The main symptoms of aortic regurgitation (AR) are dyspnea and fatigue. Occasionally patients experience angina because reduced diastolic aortic pressure reduces coronary perfusion pressure, impairing coronary blood flow. Reduced diastolic systemic pressure may also cause syncope or presyncope.

68. The physical findings of AR include widened pulse pressure, a palpable dynamic LV apical beat that is displaced downward and to the left, a diastolic blowing murmur heard best along the left sternal border with the patient sitting upright and leaning forward, and a low-pitched diastolic rumble heard to the LV apex (*Austin Flint* murmur).

69. Class I indications for aortic valve replacement in patients with AR include (1) the presence of symptoms in patients with severe AR, irrespective of LV systolic function; (2) chronic severe AR with LV systolic dysfunction (ejection fraction 50% or less), even if asymptomatic; and (3) chronic, severe AR in patients undergoing coronary artery bypass grafting (CABG), other heart valve surgery, or thoracic aortic surgery.

70. Cardiogenic shock is a state of end-organ hypoperfusion caused by cardiac failure characterized by persistent hypotension with severe reduction in cardiac index (less than 1.8 L/min/m²) in the presence of adequate or elevated filling pressure (LV end-diastolic pressure 18 mm Hg or higher or RV end-diastolic pressure 10 to 15 mm Hg or higher).

71. The rate of ischemic stroke in patients with nonvalvular atrial fibrillation (AF) is about two to seven times that of persons without AF, and the risk increases dramatically as patients age. Both paroxysmal and chronic AF carry the same risk of thromboembolism.

72. In nuclear cardiology stress testing, a *perfusion defect* is an area of reduced radiotracer uptake in the myocardium. If the perfusion defect occurs during stress and improves or normalizes during rest, it is termed *reversible* and usually suggests the presence of inducible ischemia, whereas if the perfusion defect occurs during both stress and rest, it is termed *fixed* and usually suggests the presence of scar (infarct).

73. The main organ systems that need to be monitored with long-term amiodarone therapy are the lungs, the liver, and the thyroid gland. A chest radiograph should be obtained every 6 to 12 months, and liver function tests (LFTs) and thyroid function tests (thyroid-stimulating hormone [TSH] and free T4) should be checked every 6 months.

74. The target international normalized ratio (INR) for warfarin therapy in most cases of cardiovascular disease is 2.5, with a range of 2.0 to 3.0. In certain patients with mechanical heart valves (e.g., older valves, mitral position), the target is 3.0 with a range of 2.5 to 3.5.

75. Lidocaine may cause a variety of central nervous system symptoms including seizures, visual disturbances, tremors, coma, and confusion. Such symptoms are often referred to as *lidocaine toxicity*. The risks of lidocaine toxicity are increased in elderly patients, those with depressed LV function, and those with liver disease.

76. The most important side effect of the antiarrhythmic drug sotalol is QT-segment prolongation leading to torsades de pointes.

77. The major complications of percutaneous coronary intervention (PCI) include periprocedural MI, acute stent thrombosis, coronary artery perforation, contrast nephropathy, access site complications (e.g., retroperitoneal bleed, pseudoaneurysm, arteriovenous fistula), stroke, and a very rare need for emergency CABG.

78. The widely accepted hemodynamic definition of pulmonary arterial hypertension (PAH) is a mean pulmonary arterial pressure of more than 25 mm Hg at rest or more than 30 mm Hg during exercise, with a pulmonary capillary or LA pressure of less than 15 mm Hg.

79. Acute pericarditis is a syndrome of pericardial inflammation characterized by typical chest pain, a pathognomonic pericardial friction rub, and specific electrocardiographic changes (PR depression, diffuse ST-segment elevation).

80. Conditions associated with the highest cardiac risk in noncardiac surgery are unstable coronary syndromes (unstable or severe angina), decompensated heart failure, severe valvular disease (particularly severe aortic stenosis), and severe arrhythmias.

81. General criteria for surgical intervention in cases of thoracic aortic aneurysm are, for the ascending thoracic aorta, aneurysmal diameter of 5.5 cm (5.0 cm in patients with Marfan syndrome), and for the descending thoracic aorta, aneurismal diameter of 6.5 cm (6 cm in patients with Marfan syndrome).

82. Cardiac complications of advanced AIDS in untreated patients include myocarditis and/or cardiomyopathy (systolic and diastolic dysfunction), pericardial effusion/tamponade, marantic (thrombotic) or infectious endocarditis, cardiac tumors (Kaposi sarcoma, lymphoma), and RV dysfunction from pulmonary hypertension or opportunistic infections. Complications with modern antiretroviral therapy (ART) include dyslipidemias, insulin resistance, lipodystrophy, atherosclerosis, and arrhythmias.

83. The radiation dose of a standard cardiac computed tomography (CT) angiography depends on a multitude of factors and can range from 1 mSv to as high as 30 mSv. This compares to an average radiation dose from a nuclear perfusion stress test of 6 to 25 mSv (or as high as more than 40 mSv in thallium stress/rest tests) and an average dose from a simple diagnostic coronary angiogram of approximately 5 mSv.

84. The ankle-brachial index (ABI) is the ankle systolic pressure (as determined by Doppler examination) divided by the brachial systolic pressure. An abnormal index is less than 0.90. The sensitivity is approximately 90% for diagnosis of peripheral arterial disease (PAD). An ABI of 0.41 to 0.90 is interpreted as mild to moderate peripheral arterial disease; an ABI of 0.00 to 0.40 is interpreted as severe PAD.

85. Approximately 90% of cases of renal artery stenosis are due to atherosclerosis. Fibromuscular dysplasia (FMD) is the next most common cause.

86. In very general terms, in cases of carotid artery stenosis, indications for carotid endarterectomy (CEA) are: (1) symptomatic stenosis 50% to 99% diameter if the risk of perioperative stroke or death is less than 6%; and (2) asymptomatic stenosis greater than 60% to 80% diameter if the expected perioperative stroke rate is less than 3%.

87. The most common cardiac complications of systemic lupus erythematosus (SLE) are pericarditis, myocarditis, premature atherosclerosis, and Libman-Sacks endocarditis.

88. Cardiac magnetic resonance imaging (MRI) can be performed in most patients with implanted cardiovascular devices, including most coronary and peripheral stents, prosthetic heart valves, embolization coils, intravenous vena caval filters, cardiac closure devices, and aortic stent grafts. Pacemakers and implantable cardioverter defibrillators are strong relative contraindications to MRI scanning, and scanning of such patients should be done under specific delineated conditions, only at centers with expertise in MRI safety and electrophysiology, and only when MRI imaging in particular is clearly indicated.

89. The clinical manifestations of symptomatic bradycardia include fatigue, lightheadedness, dizziness, presyncope, syncope, manifestations of cerebral ischemia, dyspnea on exertion, decreased exercise tolerance, and congestive heart failure.

90. Second-degree heart block is divided into two types: *Mobitz type I (Wenckebach)* exhibits progressive prolongation of the PR interval before an atrial impulse (P wave) is not conducted, whereas *Mobitz type II* exhibits no prolongation of the PR interval before an atrial impulse is not conducted.

91. Temporary or permanent pacing is indicated in the setting of acute MI, with or without symptoms, for (1) complete third-degree block or advanced second-degree block that is associated with block in the His-Purkinje system (wide complex ventricular rhythm) and (2) transient advanced (second-degree or third-degree) AV block with a new bundle branch block.

92. *Cardiac resynchronization therapy (CRT)* refers to simultaneous pacing of both ventricles (biventricular, or Bi-V, pacing). CRT is indicated in patients with advanced heart failure (usually NYHA class III or IV), severe systolic dysfunction (LV ejection fraction 35% or less), and intraventricular conduction delay (QRS less than 120 ms) who are in sinus rhythm and have been on optimal medical therapy.

93. Whereas the left internal mammary artery (LIMA), when anastomosed to the left anterior descending artery (LAD), has a 90% patency at 10 years, for saphenous vein grafts (SVGs), early graft stenosis or occlusion of up to 15% can occur by 1 year, with 10-year patency traditionally cited at only 50% to 60%.

94. Myocardial contusion is a common, reversible injury that is the consequence of a nonpenetrating trauma to the myocardium. It is detected by elevations of specific cardiac enzymes with no evidence of coronary occlusion and by reversible wall motion abnormalities detected by echocardiography.

95. Causes of restrictive cardiomyopathy include infiltrative diseases (amyloidosis, sarcoidosis, Gaucher disease, Hurler disease), storage diseases (hemochromatosis, glycogen storage disease, Fabry disease), and endomyocardial involvement from endomyocardial fibrosis, radiation, or anthracycline treatment.

96. Classical signs for cardiac tamponade include the Beck triad of (1) hypotension caused by decreased stroke volume, (2) jugulovenous distension caused by impaired venous return to the heart, and (3) muffled heart sounds caused by fluid inside the pericardial sac, as well as pulsus paradoxus and general signs of shock, such as tachycardia, tachypnea, and decreasing level of consciousness.

97. The most common tumors that spread to the heart are lung (bronchogenic) cancer, breast cancer, melanoma, thyroid cancer, esophageal cancer, lymphoma, and leukemia.

98. Primary cardiac tumors are extremely rare, occurring in one autopsy series in less than 0.1% of subjects. Benign primary tumors are more common than malignant primary tumors, occurring approximately three times as often as malignant tumors.

99. The Westermark sign is the finding in pulmonary embolism of oligemia of the lung beyond the occluded vessel. If pulmonary infarction results, a wedge-shaped infiltrate *(Hampton's hump)* may be visible.

100. Patients with cocaine-induced chest pain should be treated with intravenous benzodiazepines, which can have beneficial hemodynamic effects and relieve chest pain, and aspirin therapy, as well as nitrate therapy if the patient remains hypertensive. β-blockers (including labetalol) should not be administered in the acute setting of cocaine-induced chest pain.

CARDIOVASCULAR PHYSICAL EXAMINATION

Salvatore Mangione, MD

Editor's Note to Readers: For an excellent and more detailed discussion of the cardiovascular physical examination, read *Physical Diagnosis Secrets,* ed 2, by Salvatore Mangione.

1. **What is the meaning of a slow rate of rise of the carotid arterial pulse?**
   A carotid arterial pulse that is reduced *(parvus)* and delayed *(tardus)* argues for *aortic valvular stenosis.* Occasionally this also may be accompanied by a palpable thrill. If ventricular function is good, a slower upstroke correlates with a higher transvalvular gradient. In left ventricular failure, however, parvus and tardus may occur even with mild aortic stenosis (AS).

2. **What is the significance of a brisk carotid arterial upstroke?**
   It depends on whether it is associated with *normal* or *widened* pulse pressure. If associated with *normal pulse pressure,* a brisk carotid upstroke usually indicates two conditions:
   - **Simultaneous emptying of the left ventricle into a high-pressure bed (the aorta) and a lower pressure bed:** The latter can be the right ventricle (in patients with ventricular septal defect [VSD]) or the left atrium (in patients with mitral regurgitation [MR]). Both will allow a rapid left ventricular emptying, which, in turn, generates a brisk arterial upstroke. The pulse pressure, however, remains normal.
   - **Hypertrophic cardiomyopathy (HCM):** Despite its association with left ventricular obstruction, this disease is characterized by a brisk and bifid pulse, due to the hypertrophic ventricle and its delayed obstruction.

   If associated with *widened pulse pressure,* a brisk upstroke usually indicates aortic regurgitation (AR). In contrast to MR, VSD, or HCM, the AR pulse has rapid upstroke *and* collapse.

3. **In addition to aortic regurgitation, which other processes cause rapid upstroke and widened pulse pressure?**
   The most common are the hyperkinetic heart syndromes (high output states). These include anemia, fever, exercise, thyrotoxicosis, pregnancy, cirrhosis, beriberi, Paget disease, arteriovenous fistulas, patent ductus arteriosus, aortic regurgitation, and anxiety—all typically associated with rapid ventricular contraction and low peripheral vascular resistance.

4. **What is pulsus paradoxus?**
   Pulsus paradoxus is an exaggerated fall in systolic blood pressure during quiet inspiration. In contrast to evaluation of arterial contour and amplitude, it is best detected in a peripheral vessel, such as the radial artery. Although palpable at times, optimal detection of the pulsus paradoxus usually requires a sphygmomanometer. Pulsus paradoxus can occur in cardiac tamponade and other conditions.

5. **What is pulsus alternans?**
   Pulsus alternans is the alternation of strong and weak arterial pulses despite *regular rate and rhythm.* First described by Ludwig Traube in 1872, pulsus alternans is often associated with alternation of strong and feeble heart sounds (auscultatory alternans). Both indicate severe left ventricular dysfunction (from ischemia, hypertension, or valvular cardiomyopathy), with worse ejection fraction and higher pulmonary capillary pressure. Hence, they are often associated with an S_3 gallop.

6. What is the Duroziez double murmur?

The *Duroziez murmur* is a to-and-fro double murmur over a large central artery—usually the femoral, but also the brachial. It is elicited by applying gradual but *firm* compression with the stethoscope's diaphragm. This produces not only a systolic murmur (which is normal) but also a *diastolic* one (which is pathologic and typical of AR). The Duroziez murmur has 58% to 100% sensitivity *and* specificity for AR.

7. What is the carotid shudder?

Carotid shudder is a palpable thrill felt at the peak of the carotid pulse in patients with AS, AR, or both. It represents the transmission of the murmur to the artery and is a relatively specific but rather insensitive sign of aortic valvular disease.

8. What is the Corrigan pulse?

The *Corrigan pulse* is one of the various names for the bounding and quickly collapsing pulse of aortic regurgitation, which is both visible *and* palpable. Other common terms for this condition include *water hammer, cannonball, collapsing,* or *pistol-shot pulse.* It is best felt for by elevating the patient's arm while at the same time feeling the radial artery at the *wrist.* Raising the arm higher than the heart reduces the intraradial diastolic pressure, collapses the vessel, and thus facilitates the palpability of the subsequent systolic thrust.

9. How do you auscultate for carotid bruits?

To auscultate for *carotid bruits,* place your bell on the neck in a quiet room and with a relaxed patient. Auscultate from just behind the upper end of the thyroid cartilage to immediately below the angle of the jaw.

10. What is the correlation between symptomatic carotid bruit and high-grade stenosis?

It's high. In fact, bruits presenting with transient ischemic attacks (TIAs) or minor strokes in the anterior circulation should be evaluated aggressively for the presence of high-grade (70%-99%) carotid stenosis, because endarterectomy markedly decreases mortality and stroke rates. Still, although presence of a bruit significantly increases the likelihood of high-grade carotid stenosis, its absence doesn't exclude disease. Moreover, a bruit heard over the bifurcation may reflect a narrowed *external* carotid artery and thus occur in angiographically normal or completely occluded *internal* carotids. Hence, surgical decisions should *not* be based on physical examination alone; imaging is mandatory.

11. What is central venous pressure (CVP)?

Central venous pressure is the pressure within the right atrium–superior vena cava system (i.e., the right ventricular filling pressure). As pulmonary capillary wedge pressure reflects left ventricular end-diastolic pressure (in the absence of mitral stenosis), so CVP reflects right ventricular end-diastolic pressure (in the absence of tricuspid stenosis).

12. Which veins should be evaluated for assessing venous pulse and CVP?

Central veins, as much in direct communication with the right atrium as possible. The ideal one is therefore the internal jugular. Ideally, the right internal jugular vein should be inspected, because it is in a more direct line with the right atrium and thus better suited to function as both a manometer for venous pressure and a conduit for atrial pulsations. Moreover, CVP may be spuriously higher on the left as compared with the right because of the left innominate vein's compression between the aortic arch and the sternum.

13. Can the external jugulars be used for evaluating central venous pressure?

Theoretically not, practically yes. *Not* because:

- While going through the various fascial planes of the neck, they often become compressed.
- In patients with increased sympathetic vascular tone, they may become so constricted as to be barely visible.

- They are farther from the right atrium and thus in a less straight line with it. Yet, both internal *and* external jugular veins can actually be used for estimating CVP because they yield comparable estimates.

 Hence, if the only visible vein is the external jugular, do what Yogi Berra recommends you should do when coming to a fork in the road: take it.

14. What is a "cannon" A wave?

A *cannon A wave* is the hallmark of atrioventricular dissociation (i.e., the atrium contracts against a closed tricuspid valve). It is different from the other prominent outward wave (i.e., the presystolic giant A wave) insofar as it begins just after S_1, because it represents atrial contraction against a closed tricuspid valve.

15. How do you estimate the CVP?

- By positioning the patient so that you can get a good view of the internal jugular vein and its oscillations. Although it is wise to start at 45 degrees, it doesn't really matter which angle you will eventually use to raise the patient's head, as long as it can adequately reveal the vein. In the absence of a visible internal jugular, the external jugular may suffice.
- By identifying the highest point of jugular pulsation that is transmitted to the skin (i.e., the meniscus). This usually occurs during exhalation and coincides with the peak of A or V waves. It serves as a bedside pulsation manometer.
- By finding the sternal angle of Louis (the junction of the manubrium with the body of the sternum). This provides the standard zero for jugular venous pressure (JVP). (The standard zero for CVP is instead the center of the right atrium.)
- By measuring in centimeters the vertical height from the sternal angle to the top of the jugular pulsation. To do so, place two rulers at a 90-degree angle: one horizontal (and parallel to the meniscus) and the other vertical to it and touching the sternal angle (Fig. 1-1). The extrapolated height between the sternal angle and meniscus represents the JVP.

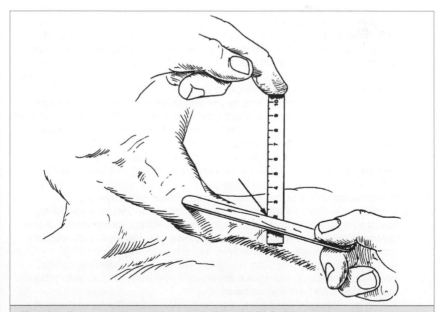

Figure 1-1. Measurement of jugular venous pressure. (From Adair OV: *Cardiology secrets,* ed 2, Philadelphia, 2001, Hanley & Belfus.)

■ By adding 5 to convert jugular venous pressure into central venous pressure. This method relies on the fact that the zero point of the entire right-sided manometer (i.e., the point where CVP is, by convention, zero) is the center of the right atrium. This is vertically situated at 5 cm below the sternal angle, a relationship that is present in subjects of normal size and shape, regardless of their body position. Thus, using the sternal angle as the external reference point, the vertical distance (in centimeters) to the top of the column of blood in the jugular vein will provide the JVP. Adding 5 to the JVP will yield the CVP.

16. **What is the significance of leg swelling without increased CVP?**
It reflects either bilateral venous insufficiency or noncardiac edema (usually hepatic or renal). This is because any cardiac (or pulmonary) disease resulting in right ventricular failure would manifest itself through an increase in CVP. Leg edema *plus ascites* in the absence of increased CVP argues in favor of a hepatic or renal cause (patients with cirrhosis do *not* have high CVP). Conversely, a high CVP in patients with ascites and edema argues in favor of an underlying cardiac etiology.

17. **What is the Kussmaul sign?**
The *Kussmaul sign* is the paradoxical increase in JVP that occurs during inspiration. JVP normally *decreases* during inspiration because the inspiratory fall in intrathoracic pressure creates a "sucking effect" on venous return. Thus, the Kussmaul sign is a true physiologic paradox. This can be explained by the inability of the right side of the heart to handle an increased venous return.
   Disease processes associated with a positive Kussmaul sign are those that interfere with venous return and right ventricular filling. The original description was in a patient with constrictive pericarditis. (The Kussmaul sign is still seen in one third of patients with severe and advanced cases, in whom it is often associated with a positive abdominojugular reflux.) Nowadays, however, the most common cause is severe heart failure, independent of etiology. Other causes include cor pulmonale (acute or chronic), constrictive pericarditis, restrictive cardiomyopathy (such as sarcoidosis, hemochromatosis, and amyloidosis), tricuspid stenosis, and right ventricular infarction.

18. **What is the "venous hum"?**
Venous hum is a *functional* murmur produced by turbulent flow in the internal jugular vein. It is *continuous* (albeit louder in diastole) and at times strong enough to be associated with a palpable thrill. It is best heard on the right side of the neck, just above the clavicle, but sometimes it can become audible over the sternal and/or parasternal areas, both right and left. This may lead to misdiagnoses of carotid disease, patent ductus arteriosus, AR, or AS. The mechanism of the venous hum is a mild compression of the internal jugular vein by the transverse process of the atlas, in subjects with strong cardiac output and increased venous flow. Hence, it is common in young adults or patients with a high output state. A venous hum can be heard in 31% to 66% of normal children and 25% of young adults. It also is encountered in 2.3% to 27% of adult outpatients. It is especially common in situations of arteriovenous fistula, being present in 56% to 88% of patients undergoing dialysis and 34% of those *between* sessions.

19. **Which characteristics of the apical impulse should be analyzed?**
■ **Location:** Normally over the fifth left interspace midclavicular line, which usually (but not always) corresponds to the area just below the nipple. *Volume loads* to the left ventricle (such as aortic or mitral regurgitation) tend to displace the apical impulse downward and laterally. Conversely, *pressure loads* (such as aortic stenosis or hypertension) tend to displace the impulse more upward and medially—at least initially. Still, a failing and decompensated ventricle, independent of its etiology, will typically present with a downward and lateral shift in point of maximal impulse (PMI). Although not too sensitive, this finding is very specific for cardiomegaly, low ejection fraction, and high pulmonary capillary wedge pressure. Correlation of the PMI with anatomic landmarks (such as the left anterior axillary line) can be used to better characterize the displaced impulse.

- **Size:** As measured in left lateral decubitus, the normal apical impulse is the size of a dime. Anything larger (nickel, quarter, or an old Eisenhower silver dollar) should be considered pathologic. A diameter greater than 4 cm is quite specific for cardiomegaly.
- **Duration and timing:** This is probably one of the most important characteristics. A normal apical duration is brief and never passes midsystole. Thus, a *sustained impulse* (i.e., one that continues into S_2 and beyond—often referred to as a "heave") should be considered pathologic until proven otherwise and is usually indicative of pressure load, volume load, or cardiomyopathy.
- **Amplitude:** This is not the length of the impulse, but its *force*. A *hyperdynamic* impulse (often referred to as a "thrust") that is forceful enough to lift the examiner's finger can be encountered in situations of volume overload and increased output (such as AR and VSD), but may also be felt in normal subjects with very thin chests. Similarly, a *hypodynamic* impulse can be due to simple obesity but also to congestive cardiomyopathy. In addition to being hypodynamic, the precordial impulse of these patients is large, somewhat sustained, and displaced downward and/or laterally.
- **Contour:** A normal apical impulse is single. Double or triple impulses are clearly pathologic. Hence, a normal apical impulse consists of a single, dime-sized, brief (barely beyond S_1), early systolic, and nonsustained impulse, localized over the fifth interspace midclavicular line.

20. **What is a thrill?**

A palpable vibration associated with an audible murmur. A thrill automatically qualifies the murmur as being more than 4/6 in intensity and thus pathologic.

BIBLIOGRAPHY, SUGGESTED READINGS, AND WEBSITES

1. Geisel School of Medicine at Dartmouth: *On doctoring: physical examination movies.* Available at: http://dms.dartmouth.edu/ed_programs/course_resources/ondoctoring_yr2/. Accessed March 26, 2013.
2. Basta LL, Bettinger JJ: The cardiac impulse, *Am Heart J* 197:96–111, 1979.
3. Constant J: Using internal jugular pulsations as a manometer for right atrial pressure measurements, *Cardology* 93:26–30, 2000.
4. Cook DJ, Simel N: Does this patient have abnormal central venous pressure? *JAMA* 275:630–634, 1996.
5. Davison R, Cannon R: Estimation of central venous pressure by examination of the jugular veins, *Am Heart J* 87:279–282, 1974.
6. Drazner MH, Rame JE, Stevenson LW, et al: Prognostic importance of elevated jugular venous pressure and a third heart sound in patients with heart failure, *N Engl J Med* 345:574–581, 2001.
7. Ellen SD, Crawford MH, O'Rourke RA: Accuracy of precordial palpation for detecting increased left ventricular volume, *Ann Intern Med* 99:628–630, 1983.
8. Mangione S: *Physical diagnosis secrets*, ed 2, Philadelphia, 2008, Mosby.
9. McGee SR: Physical examination of venous pressure: a critical review, *Am Heart J* 136:10–18, 1998.
10. O'Neill TW, Barry M, Smith M, et al: Diagnostic value of the apex beat, *Lancet* 1:410–411, 1989.
11. Sauve JS, Laupacis A, Ostbye T, et al: The rational clinical examination. Does this patient have a clinically important carotid bruit? *JAMA* 270:2843–2845, 1993.

CHAPTER 2

HEART MURMURS

Salvatore Mangione, MD

Editor's Note to Readers: For an excellent and more detailed discussion of heart murmurs, read *Physical Diagnosis Secrets*, ed 2, by Salvatore Mangione.

1. **What are the auscultatory areas of murmurs?**

   Auscultation typically starts in the aortic area, continuing in clockwise fashion: first over the pulmonic, then the mitral (or apical), and finally the tricuspid areas (Fig. 2-1). Because murmurs may radiate widely, they often become audible in areas outside those historically assigned to them. Hence, "inching" the stethoscope (i.e., slowly dragging it from site to site) can be the best way to avoid missing important findings.

2. **What is the Levine system for grading the intensity of murmurs?**

   The intensity or loudness of a murmur is traditionally graded by the Levine system (no relation to this book's editor) from 1/6 to 6/6. Everything else being equal, increased intensity usually reflects increased flow turbulence. Thus, a louder murmur is more likely to be pathologic and severe.

   - **1/6:** a murmur so soft as to be heard only intermittently, never immediately, and always with concentration and effort
   - **2/6:** a murmur that is soft but nonetheless audible immediately and on every beat
   - **3/6:** a murmur that is easily audible and relatively loud
   - **4/6:** a murmur that is relatively loud and associated with a palpable thrill (always pathologic)
   - **5/6:** a murmur loud enough that it can be heard even by placing the edge of the stethoscope's diaphragm over the patient's chest
   - **6/6:** a murmur so loud that it can be heard even when the stethoscope is not in contact with the chest, but held slightly above its surface

3. **What are the causes of a systolic murmur?**

   - **Ejection:** increased "forward" flow over the aortic or pulmonic valve. This can be:
     - **Physiologic:** normal valve, but flow high enough to cause turbulence (anemia, exercise, fever, and other hyperkinetic heart syndromes)
     - **Pathologic:** abnormal valve, with or without outflow obstruction (i.e., aortic stenosis versus aortic sclerosis)
   - **Regurgitation:** "backward" flow from a high- into a low-pressure bed. Although this is usually due to incompetent atrioventricular (AV) valves (mitral or tricuspid), it also can be due to ventricular septal defect.

4. **What are functional murmurs?**

   They are benign findings caused by turbulent ejection into the great vessels. Functional murmurs have no clinical relevance, other than getting into the differential diagnosis of a systolic murmur.

5. **What is the most common systolic ejection murmur of the elderly?**

   The murmur of aortic sclerosis is common in the elderly. This early peaking systolic murmur is extremely age related, affecting 21% to 26% of persons older than 65, and 55% to 75% of octogenarians. (Conversely, the prevalence of aortic stenosis [AS] in these age groups is 2% and 2.6%, respectively.) The murmur of aortic sclerosis may be due to either a degenerative change of the aortic valve or abnormalities of the aortic root. Senile degeneration of the aortic valve includes thickening, fibrosis, and

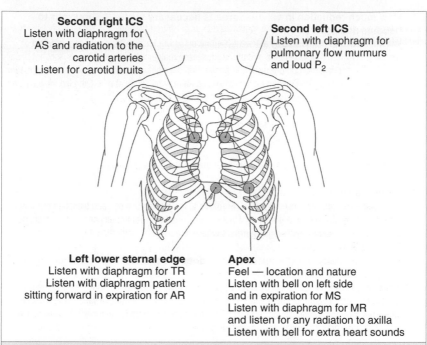

Second right ICS
Listen with diaphragm for
AS and radiation to the
carotid arteries
Listen for carotid bruits

Second left ICS
Listen with diaphragm for
pulmonary flow murmurs
and loud P₂

Left lower sternal edge
Listen with diaphragm for TR
Listen with diaphragm patient
sitting forward in expiration for AR

Apex
Feel — location and nature
Listen with bell on left side
and in expiration for MS
Listen with diaphragm for MR
and listen for any radiation to axilla
Listen with bell for extra heart sounds

Figure 2-1. Sequence of auscultation of the heart. *AR*, Aortic regurgitation; *AS*, aortic stenosis; *ICS*, intercostal space; *MR*, mitral regurgitation; *MS*, mitral stenosis; *TR*, tricuspid regurgitation. (From Baliga R: *Crash course cardiology*, St Louis, 2005, Mosby.)

occasionally calcification. This can stiffen the valve and yet not cause a transvalvular pressure gradient. In fact, commissural fusion is typically absent in aortic sclerosis. Abnormalities of the aortic root may be diffuse (such as a tortuous and dilated aorta) or localized (like a calcific spur or an atherosclerotic plaque that protrudes into the lumen, creating a turbulent bloodstream).

6. **How can physical examination help differentiate functional from pathologic murmurs?**
   There are two golden and three silver rules:
   - The first golden rule is to always judge (systolic) murmurs like people: by the company they keep. Hence, murmurs that keep bad company (like symptoms; extra sounds; thrill; and abnormal arterial or venous pulse, electrocardiogram, or chest radiograph) should be considered pathologic until proven otherwise. These murmurs should receive extensive evaluation, including technology-based assessment.
   - The second golden rule is that a diminished or absent S₂ usually indicates a poorly moving and abnormal semilunar (aortic or pulmonic) valve. This is the hallmark of pathology. As a flip side, functional systolic murmurs are always accompanied by a well-preserved S₂, with normal split.

   The three silver rules are:
   - All holosystolic (or late systolic) murmurs are pathologic.
   - All diastolic murmurs are pathologic.
   - All continuous murmurs are pathologic.

   Thus, functional murmurs should be systolic, short, soft (typically less than 3/6), early peaking (never passing mid-systole), predominantly circumscribed to the base, and associated with a well-preserved and normally split-second sound. They should have an otherwise normal cardiovascular examination and often disappear with sitting, standing, or straining (as, for example, following a Valsalva maneuver).

7. **How much reduction in valvular area is necessary for the AS murmur to become audible?**
Valvular area must be reduced by at least 50% (the minimum for creating a pressure gradient at rest) for the AS murmur to become audible. Mild disease may produce loud murmurs, too, but usually significant hemodynamic compromise (and symptoms) does not occur until a 60% to 70% reduction in valvular area exists. This means that early to mild AS may be subtle at rest. Exercise, however, may intensify the murmur by increasing the output and gradient.

8. **What factors may suggest severe AS?**
- Murmur intensity and timing (the louder and later peaking the murmur, the worse the disease)
- A single S_2
- Delayed upstroke and reduced amplitude of the carotid pulse (pulsus parvus and tardus)

9. **What is a thrill?**
It is a palpable vibratory sensation, often compared to the purring of a cat, and typical of murmurs caused by very high pressure gradients. These, in turn, lead to great turbulence and loudness. Hence, thrills are only present in pathologic murmurs whose intensity is greater than 4/6.

10. **What is isometric hand grip, and what does it do to AS and mitral regurgitation (MR) murmurs?**
Isometric hand grip is carried out by asking the patient to lock the cupped fingers of both hands into a grip and then trying to pull them apart. The resulting increase in peripheral vascular resistance intensifies MR (and ventricular septal defect) while softening instead AS (and aortic sclerosis). Hence, a positive hand grip argues strongly in favor of MR.

11. **What is the Gallavardin phenomenon?**
The Gallavardin phenomenon is noticed in some patients with AS, who may exhibit a dissociation of their systolic murmur into two components:
- A typical AS-like murmur (medium to low pitched, harsh, right parasternal, typically radiated to the neck, and caused by high-velocity jets into the ascending aorta)
- A murmur that instead mimics MR (high pitched, musical, and best heard at the apex)
This phenomenon reflects the different transmission of AS: its medium frequencies to the base and its higher frequencies to the apex. The latter may become so prominent as to be misinterpreted as a separate apical "cooing" of MR.

12. **Where is the murmur of hypertrophic cardiomyopathy (HCM) best heard?**
It depends. When septal hypertrophy obstructs not only left but also right ventricular outflow, the murmur may be louder at the left lower sternal border. More commonly, however, the HCM murmur is louder at the apex. This may often cause a differential diagnosis dilemma with the murmur of MR.

13. **What are the characteristics of a ventricular septal defect (VSD) murmur?**
VSD murmurs may be holosystolic, crescendo-decrescendo, crescendo, or decrescendo. A crescendo-decrescendo murmur usually indicates a defect in the muscular part of the septum. Ventricular contraction closes the hole toward the end of systole, thus causing the decrescendo phase of the murmur. Conversely, a defect in the membranous septum will enjoy no systolic reduction in flow and thus produce a murmur that remains constant and holosystolic. VSD murmurs are best heard along the left lower sternal border, often radiating left to right across the chest. VSD murmurs always start immediately after S_1.

14. **What is a systolic regurgitant murmur?**
One characterized by a pressure gradient that causes a retrograde blood flow across an abnormal opening. This can be (1) a ventricular septal defect, (2) an incompetent mitral valve, (3) an incompetent tricuspid valve, or (4) fistulous communication between a high-pressure and a low-pressure vascular bed (such as a patent ductus arteriosus).

15. **What are the auscultatory characteristics of systolic regurgitant murmurs?**
   They tend to start immediately after S_1, often extending into S_2. They also may have a musical quality, variously described as "honk" or "whoop." This is usually caused by vibrating vegetations (endocarditis) or chordae tendineae (MVP, dilated cardiomyopathy) and may help separate the more musical murmurs of AV valve regurgitation from the harsher sounds of semilunar stenosis. Note that in contrast to systolic ejection murmurs like AS or VSD, systolic regurgitant murmurs do not increase in intensity after a long diastole.

16. **What are the characteristics of the MR murmur?**
   It is loudest at the apex, radiated to the left axilla or interscapular area, high pitched, plateau, and extending all the way into S_2 (holosystolic). S_2 is normal in intensity but often widely split. If the gradient is high (and the flow is low), the MR murmur is high pitched. Conversely, if the gradient is low (and the flow is high) the murmur is low pitched. In general, the louder (and longer) the MR murmur, the worse the regurgitation.

17. **What are the characteristics of the acute MR murmur?**
   The acute MR murmur tends to be very short, and even absent, because the left atrium and ventricle often behave like a common chamber, with no pressure gradient between them. Hence, in contrast to that of chronic MR (which is either holosystolic or late systolic), the acute MR murmur is often early systolic (exclusively so in 40% of cases) and is associated with an S_4 in 80% of the patients.

18. **What are the characteristics of the mitral valve prolapse (MVP) murmur?**
   It is an MR murmur—hence, loudest at the apex, mid to late systolic in onset (immediately following the click), and usually extending all the way into the second sound (A_2). In fact, it often has a crescendo shape that peaks at S_2. It is usually not too loud (never greater than 3/6), with some musical features that have been variously described as whoops or honks (as in the honking of a goose). Indeed, musical murmurs of this kind are almost always due to MVP.

19. **How are diastolic murmurs classified?**
   Diastolic murmurs are classified by their timing. Hence, the most important division is between murmurs that start just after S_2 (i.e., early diastolic—reflecting aortic or pulmonic regurgitation) versus those that start a little later (i.e., mid to late diastolic, often with a presystolic accentuation—reflecting mitral or tricuspid valve stenosis) (Fig. 2-2).

20. **What is the best strategy to detect the mitral stenosis (MS) murmur?**
   The best strategy consists of listening over the apex, with the patient in the left lateral decubitus position, at the end of exhalation, and after a short exercise. Finally, applying the bell with very light pressure also may help. (Strong pressure will instead completely eliminate the low frequencies of MS.)

21. **What are the typical auscultatory findings of aortic regurgitation (AR)?**
   Depending on severity, there may be up to three murmurs (one in systole and two in diastole) plus an ejection click. Of course, the typical auscultatory finding is the diastolic tapering murmur, which, together with the brisk pulse and the enlarged and/or displaced point of maximal impulse (PMI), constitutes the bedside diagnostic triad of AR. The diastolic tapering murmur is usually best heard over the Erb point (third or fourth interspace, left parasternal line) but at times also over the aortic area, especially when a tortuous and dilated root pushes the ascending aorta anteriorly and to the right. The decrescendo diastolic murmur of AR is best heard by having the patient sit up and lean forward while holding breath in exhalation. Using the diaphragm and pressing hard on the stethoscope also may help because this murmur is rich in high frequencies. Finally, increasing peripheral vascular resistances (by having the patient squat) will also intensify the murmur. A typical, characteristic early diastolic murmur argues very strongly in favor of the diagnosis of AR.
   An accompanying systolic murmur may be due to concomitant AS but most commonly indicates severe regurgitation, followed by an increased systolic flow across the valve. Hence, this accompanying

systolic murmur is often referred to as *comitans* (Latin for "companion"). It provides an important clue to the severity of regurgitation. A second diastolic murmur can be due to the rumbling diastolic murmur of Austin Flint (i.e., functional MS). The Austin Flint murmur is a mitral stenosis–like diastolic rumble, best heard at the apex, and results from the regurgitant aortic stream preventing full opening of the anterior mitral leaflet.

Phonocardiogram (inspiration unless noted)   Description

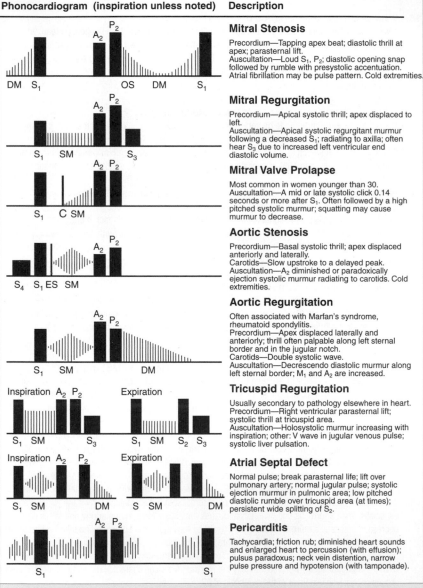

Mitral Stenosis

Precordium—Tapping apex beat; diastolic thrill at apex; parasternal lift.
Auscultation—Loud S_1, P_2; diastolic opening snap followed by rumble with presystolic accentuation. Atrial fibrillation may be pulse pattern. Cold extremities.

Mitral Regurgitation

Precordium—Apical systolic thrill; apex displaced to left.
Auscultation—Apical systolic regurgitant murmur following a decreased S_1; radiating to axilla; often hear S_3 due to increased left ventricular end diastolic volume.

Mitral Valve Prolapse

Most common in women younger than 30.
Auscultation—A mid or late systolic click 0.14 seconds or more after S_1. Often followed by a high pitched systolic murmur; squatting may cause murmur to decrease.

Aortic Stenosis

Precordium—Basal systolic thrill; apex displaced anteriorly and laterally.
Carotids—Slow upstroke to a delayed peak.
Auscultation—A_2 diminished or paradoxically ejection systolic murmur radiating to carotids. Cold extremities.

Aortic Regurgitation

Often associated with Marfan's syndrome, rheumatoid spondylitis.
Precordium—Apex displaced laterally and anteriorly; thrill often palpable along left sternal border and in the jugular notch.
Carotids—Double systolic wave.
Auscultation—Decrescendo diastolic murmur along left sternal border; M_1 and A_2 are increased.

Tricuspid Regurgitation

Usually secondary to pathology elsewhere in heart.
Precordium—Right ventricular parasternal lift; systolic thrill at tricuspid area.
Auscultation—Holosystolic murmur increasing with inspiration; other: V wave in jugular venous pulse; systolic liver pulsation.

Atrial Septal Defect

Normal pulse; break parasternal life; lift over pulmonary artery; normal jugular pulse; systolic ejection murmur in pulmonic area; low pitched diastolic rumble over tricuspid area (at times); persistent wide splitting of S_2.

Pericarditis

Tachycardia; friction rub; diminished heart sounds and enlarged heart to percussion (with effusion); pulsus paradoxus; neck vein distention, narrow pulse pressure and hypotension (with tamponade).

Figure 2-2. Phonocardiographic description of pathologic cardiac murmurs. (From James EC, Corry RJ, Perry JF: *Principles of basic surgical practice,* Philadelphia, 1987, Hanley & Belfus.)

22. What is a mammary soufflé?

A mammary soufflé is not a fancy French dish, but a systolic-diastolic murmur heard over one or both breasts in late pregnancy and typically disappearing at the end of lactation. It is caused by increased flow along the mammary arteries, which explains why its systolic component starts just a little after S_1. It can be obliterated by pressing (with finger or stethoscope) over the area of maximal intensity.

BIBLIOGRAPHY, SUGGESTED READINGS, AND WEBSITES

1. Blaufuss Medical Multimedia Laboratories: *Heart sounds and cardiac arrhythmias, an excellent audiovisual tutorial on heart sounds.* Available at: http://www.blaufuss.org/. Accessed January 14, 2013.

2. Constant J, Lippschutz EJ: Diagramming and grading heart sounds and murmurs, *Am Heart J* 70:326–332, 1965.

3. Danielsen R, Nordrehaug JE, Vik-Mo H: Clinical and haemodynamic features in relation to severity of aortic stenosis in adults, *Eur Heart J* 12:791–795, 1991.

4. Etchells E, Bell C, Robb K: Does this patient have an abnormal systolic murmur? *JAMA* 277:564–571, 1997.

5. Mangione S: *Physical diagnosis secrets*, ed 2, Philadelphia, 2008, Mosby.

6. University of Washington Department of Medicine: *Examination for heart sounds and murmurs.* Available at: http://depts.washington.edu/physdx/heart/index.html. Accessed January 14, 2013.

CHAPTER 3

ELECTROCARDIOGRAM

Glenn N. Levine, MD, FACC, FAHA

1. **What are the most commonly used criteria to diagnose left ventricular hypertrophy (LVH)?**
   - R wave in V5-V6 + S wave in V1-V2 > 35 mm
   - R wave in lead I + S wave in lead III > 25 mm

2. **What are the most commonly used criteria to diagnose right ventricular hypertrophy (RVH)?**
   - R wave in V1 ≥ 7 mm
   - R/S wave ratio in V1 > 1

3. **What criteria are used to diagnose left atrial enlargement (LAE)?**
   - P wave total width of > 0.12 sec (3 small boxes) in the inferior leads, usually with a double-peaked P wave
   - Terminal portion of the P wave in lead V1 ≥ 0.04 sec (1 small box) wide and ≥ 1 mm (1 small box) deep

4. **What electrocardiogram (ECG) finding suggests right atrial enlargement (RAE)?**
   - P-wave height in the inferior leads (II, III, and aVF) ≥ 2.5 to 3 mm (2.5 to 3 small boxes) (Fig. 3-1)

5. **What is the normal rate of a junctional rhythm?**
   The normal rate is 40 to 60 beats/min. Rates of 61 to 100 beats/min are referred to as *accelerated junctional rhythm,* and rates of >100 beats/min or higher are referred to as *junctional tachycardia.*

6. **How can one distinguish a junctional escape rhythm from a ventricular escape rhythm in a patient with complete heart block?**
   Junctional escape rhythms usually occur at a rate of 40 to 60 beats/min and will usually be narrow complex (unless the patient has a baseline bundle branch block), whereas ventricular escape rhythms will usually occur at a rate of 30 to 40 beats/min and will be wide complex.

7. **Describe the three types of heart block.**
   - **First-degree heart block:** The PR interval is a fixed duration of more than 0.20 seconds.
   - **Second-degree heart block:** In Mobitz type I (Wenckebach) block, the PR interval increases until a P wave is nonconducted (Fig. 3-2). The cycle then resets and starts again. Mobitz type I second-degree heart block is sometimes due to increased vagal tone and is usually a relatively benign finding. In Mobitz type II block, the PR interval is fixed and occasional P waves are nonconducted. Mobitz type II second-degree heart block usually indicates structural disease in the atrioventricular (AV) node or His-Purkinje system and is an indication for pacemaker implantation.
   - **Third-degree heart block:** All P waves are nonconducted, and there is either a junctional or ventricular escape rhythm. To call a rhythm third-degree or complete heart block, the atrial rate (as evidenced by the P waves) should be faster than the ventricular escape rate (the QRS complexes). Third-degree heart block is almost always an indication for a permanent pacemaker.

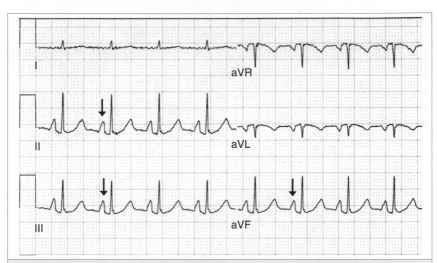

Figure 3-1. Right atrial enlargement. The tall P waves in the inferior leads (II, III, and aVF) are more than 2.5 to 3 mm high.

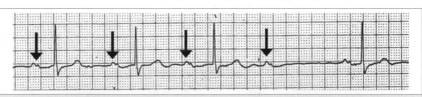

Figure 3-2. Wenckebach block (Mobitz type I second-degree AV block). The PR interval progressively increases until there is a nonconducted P wave.

8. **What are the causes of ST segment elevation?**
   - Acute myocardial infarction (MI) due to thrombotic occlusion of a coronary artery
   - Prinzmetal angina (variant angina), in which there is vasospasm of a coronary artery
   - Cocaine-induced MI, in which there is vasospasm of a coronary artery, with or without additional thrombotic occlusion
   - Pericarditis, in which there is usually diffuse ST segment elevation
   - Left ventricular aneurysm
   - Left bundle branch block (LBBB)
   - Left ventricular hypertrophy with repolarization abnormalities
   - J point elevation, a condition classically seen in young African American patients but that can be seen in any patient, which is thought to be due to "early repolarization"
   - Severe hyperkalemia

9. **What are the electrocardiographic findings of hyperkalemia?**
   Initially, a "peaking" of the T waves is seen (Fig. 3-3). As the hyperkalemia becomes more profound, "loss" of the P waves, QRS widening, and ST segment elevation may occur. The preterminal finding is a sinusoidal pattern on the ECG (Fig. 3-4).

10. **What are the ECG findings in pericarditis?**
    The first findings are thought to be PR segment depression (Fig 3-5, A), possibly caused by repolarization abnormalities of the atria. This may be fairly transient and is often not present by the time the patient

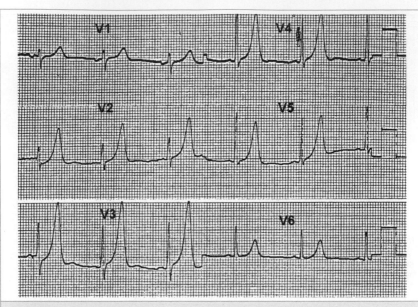

Figure 3-3. Hyperkalemia. Peaked T waves are seen in many of the precordial leads. (Adapted with permission from Levine GN, Podrid PJ: *The ECG workbook: a review and discussion of ECG findings and abnormalities,* New York, 1995, Futura Publishing Company, p 405.)

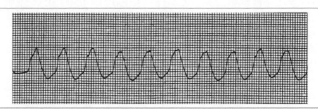

Figure 3-4. Severe hyperkalemia. The rhythm strip demonstrates the preterminal rhythm sinusoidal wave seen in cases of severe hyperkalemia. (Adapted with permission from Levine GN, Podrid PJ: *The ECG workbook: a review and discussion of ECG findings and abnormalities,* New York, 1995, Futura Publishing Company, p 503.)

is seen for evaluation. Either concurrent with PR segment depression or shortly following PR segment depression, diffuse ST segment elevation occurs (Fig. 3-5, *B*). At a later time, diffuse T-wave inversions may develop.

11. **What is electrical alternans?**
    In the presence of large pericardial effusions, the heart may "swing" within the large pericardial effusion, resulting in an alteration of the amplitude of the QRS complex (Fig. 3-6).

12. **What is the main ECG finding in hypercalcemia and hypocalcemia?**
    With hypercalcemia, the QT interval shortens. With hypocalcemia, prolongation of the QT interval occurs as a result of delayed repolarization (Fig. 3-7).

13. **What ECG findings may be present in pulmonary embolus?**
    - Sinus tachycardia (the most common ECG finding)
    - Right atrial enlargement (P pulmonale)—tall P waves in the inferior leads

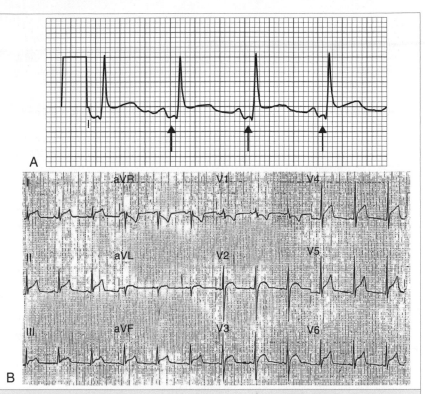

Figure 3-5. **A,** PR depression seen early in pericarditis. **B,** Diffuse ST elevation in pericarditis.

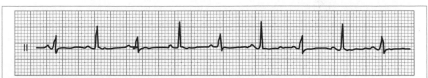

Figure 3-6. Electrical alternans in a patient with a large pericardial effusion. Note the alternating amplitude of the QRS complexes. (From Manning WJ: Pericardial disease. In Goldman L, editor: *Cecil medicine,* ed 23, Philadelphia, 2008, Saunders.)

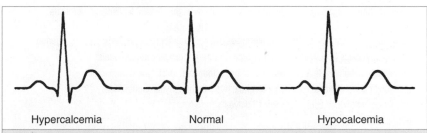

Figure 3-7. Electrocardiographic findings of hypercalcemia and hypocalcemia. With hypercalcemia, the QT interval shortens. With hypocalcemia there is prolongation of the QT interval due to delayed repolarization. (From Park MK, Guntheroth WG: *How to read pediatric ECGs,* ed 4, Philadelphia, 2006, Mosby.)

- Right axis deviation
- T wave inversions in leads V1-V2
- Incomplete right bundle branch block (IRBBB)
- S1Q3T3 pattern—an S wave in lead I, a Q wave in lead III, and an inverted T wave in lead III. Although this is only occasionally seen with pulmonary embolus, it is quite suggestive that a pulmonary embolus has occurred.

14. **How is the QT interval calculated and what are the causes of short QT and long QT intervals?**
    The QT interval is measured from the beginning of the QRS complex to the end of the T wave. The corrected QT interval (QTc) takes into account the heart rate, as the QT interval increases at slower heart rates. The formula is:

    $$QTc = \frac{Measured\ QT}{\sqrt{RR\ interval}}$$

    Causes of short QT interval include hypercalcemia, congenital short QT syndrome, and digoxin therapy. Numerous drugs, metabolic abnormalities, and other conditions can cause a prolonged QT interval (Table 3-1). QTc values greater than 440 to 460 milliseconds are considered prolonged, though the risk of arrhythmia is generally ascribed to be more common at QTc values greater than 500 milliseconds.

15. **What is torsades de pointes?**
    Torsades de pointes is a ventricular arrhythmia that occurs in the setting of QT prolongation, usually when drugs that prolong the QT interval have been administered. It may also occur in the setting of congenital prolonged QT syndrome and other conditions. The term was reported coined by Dessertenne to describe the arrhythmia, in which the QRS axis appears to twist around the isoelectric line (Fig. 3-8). It is usually a hemodynamically unstable rhythm that can further degenerate and lead to hemodynamic collapse.

16. **What are cerebral T waves?**
    Cerebral T waves are strikingly deep and inverted T waves, most prominently seen in the precordial leads, that occur with central nervous system diseases, most notably subarachnoid and intracerebral hemorrhages. They are thought to be due to prolonged and abnormal repolarization of the left ventricle, presumably as a result of autonomic imbalance. They should not be mistaken for evidence of active cardiac ischemia (Fig. 3-9).

TABLE 3-1. CAUSES OF PROLONGED QT INTERVAL

Antiarrhythmic drugs (e.g., Amiodarone, sotalol, quinidine, procainamide, ibutilide, dofetilide, flecainide)

Psychiatric medications, particularly overdoses (tricyclic antidepressants, antipsychotic agents)

Certain antibiotics (e.g., Macrolides, fluoroquinolones, antifungals, antimalarials)

Certain antihistamines (e.g., Diphenhydramine, astemizole, loratadine, terfenadine)

Electrolyte abnormalities (e.g., Hypocalcemia, hypokalemia, hypomagnesemia)

Raised intracranial pressure ("cerebral T waves")

Hypothermia

Hypothyroidism

Congenital long QT syndrome

17. What are Osborne waves?

Osborne waves are upward deflections that occur at the J point of the QRS complex, which occur in the setting of hypothermia (Fig. 3-10). They are thought to result from hypothermia-induced repolarization abnormalities of the ventricle.

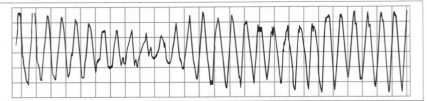

Figure 3-8. Torsades de pointes, in which the QRS axis seems to rotate about the isoelectric point. (From Olgin JE, Zipes DP: Specific arrhythmias: diagnosis and treatment. In Libby P, Bonow R, Mann D, et al, editors: *Braunwald's heart disease: a textbook of cardiovascular medicine,* ed 8, Philadelphia, 2008, Saunders.)

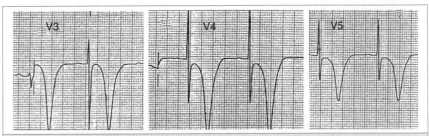

Figure 3-9. Cerebral T waves. The markedly deep and inverted T waves are seen with central nervous system disease, particularly subarachnoid and intracerebral hemorrhages. (Reproduced with permission from Levine GN, Podrid PJ: *The ECG workbook: a review and discussion of ECG findings and abnormalities,* New York, 1995, Futura Publishing Company, p 437.)

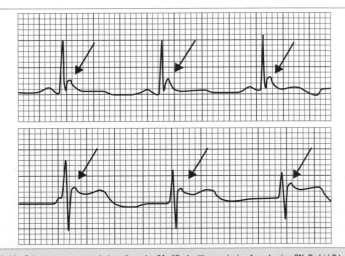

Figure 3-10. Osborne waves seen in hypothermia. (Modified with permission from Levine GN, Podrid PJ: *The ECG workbook: a review and discussion of ECG findings and abnormalities,* New York, 1995, Futura Publishing Company, p 417.)

BIBLIOGRAPHY, SUGGESTED READINGS, AND WEBSITES

1. Dublin D: *Rapid interpretation of EKGs*, Tampa, Fla, 2000, Cover Publishing.
2. Jenkins D, Gerred S: *ECG library*. Available at: http://www.ecglibrary.com/ecghome.html. Accessed September 6, 2009.
3. Levine GN: *Diagnosing (and treating) arrhythmias made easy*, St Louis, 1998, Quality Medical Publishers.
4. Levine GN, Podrid PJ: *The ECG workbook*, Armonk, NY, 1995, Futura Publishing.
5. Mason JW, Hancock EW, Gettes LS: Recommendations for the standardization and interpretation of the electrocardiogram: part II: electrocardiography diagnostic statement list, a scientific statement from the American Heart Association Electrocardiography and Arrhythmias Committee, Council on Clinical Cardiology; the American College of Cardiology Foundation; and the Heart Rhythm Society endorsed by the International Society for Computerized Electrocardiology, *J Am Coll Cardiol* 49(10):1128–1135, 2007.
6. Segal A: *Electrocardiography: an on-line tutorial in lead II ECG interpretation*. Available at: http://www.drsegal.com/medstud/ecg/. Accessed September 6, 2009.
7. Wagner GS: *Marriot's practical electrocardiography*, Philadelphia, 2008, Lippincott Williams & Wilkins.
8. Wolters Kluwer Health Clinical Solutions: *ECG tutorial*. In Basow, DS, editor: UpToDate, Waltham, MA, 2013, UpToDate. Available at: http://www.uptodate.com/contents/ecg-tutorial. Accessed March 26, 2013.
9. Wartak J: *Electrocardiogram rhythm tutor*. Available at: http://www.coldbacon.com/mdtruth/more/ekg.html. Accessed September 7, 2009.

CHAPTER 4

CHEST RADIOGRAPHS

James J. Fenton, MD, FCCP, Glenn N. Levine, MD, FACC, FAHA

1. **Describe a systematic approach to interpreting a chest radiograph (chest x-ray [CXR]) (Fig. 4-1).**
   Common recommendations are to:
   1. Begin with general characteristics such as the age, gender, size, and position of the patient.
   2. Next, examine the periphery of the film, including the bones, soft tissue, and pleura. Look for rib fractures, rib notching, bony metastases, shoulder dislocation, soft tissue masses, and pleural thickening.
   3. Then, evaluate the lung, looking for infiltrates, pulmonary nodules, and pleural effusions.
   4. Finally, concentrate on the heart size and contour, mediastinal structures, hilum, and great vessels. Also note the presence of pacemakers and sternal wires.

2. **Identify the major cardiovascular structures that form the silhouette of the mediastinum (Fig. 4-2)**
   - **Right side:** Ascending aorta, right pulmonary artery, right atrium, right ventricle
   - **Left side:** Aortic knob, left pulmonary artery, left atrial appendage, left ventricle

3. **How is heart size measured on a chest radiograph?**
   Identification of cardiomegaly on a CXR is subjective, but if the heart size is equal to or greater than twice the size of the hemithorax, then it is enlarged. Remember that a film taken during expiration, in a supine position, or by a portable anteroposterior (AP) technique will make the heart appear larger.

4. **What factors can affect heart size on the chest radiograph?**
   - **Size of the patient:** Obesity decreases lung volumes and enlarges the appearance of the heart.
   - **Degree of inspiration:** Poor inspiration can make the heart appear larger.
   - **Emphysema:** Hyperinflation changes the configuration of the heart, making it appear smaller.
   - **Contractility:** Systole or diastole can make up to a 1.5-cm difference in heart size. In addition, low heart rate and increased cardiac output lead to increased ventricular filling.
   - **Chest configuration:** Pectus excavatum can compress the heart and make it appear larger.
   - **Patient positioning:** The heart appears larger if the film is taken in a supine position.
   - **Type of examination:** On an AP projection, the heart is farther away from the film and closer to the camera. This creates greater beam divergence and the appearance of an increased heart size.

5. **What additional items should be reviewed when examining a chest radiograph from the intensive care unit (ICU)?**
   On portable coronary care unit (CCU) and ICU radiographs, particular attention should be paid to:
   - Placement of the endotracheal tube
   - Central lines
   - Pulmonary arterial catheter
   - Pacing wires
   - Defibrillator pads
   - Intraaortic balloon pump

- Feeding tubes
- Chest tubes

A careful inspection should be made for pneumothorax (Fig. 4-3), subcutaneous emphysema, and other factors that may be related to instrumentation and mechanical ventilation.

6. **How can one determine which cardiac chambers are enlarged?**
   - **Ventricular enlargement:** usually displaces the lower heart border to the left and posteriorly. Distinguishing right ventricular (RV) from left ventricular (LV) enlargement requires evaluation of

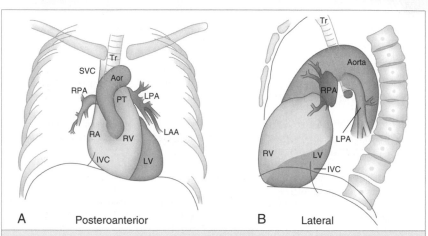

Figure 4-1. Diagrammatic representations of the anatomy of the chest radiograph. **A,** *Aor,* Aorta; *IVC,* inferior vena cava; *LAA,* left atrial appendage; *LPA,* left pulmonary artery; *LV,* left ventricle; *PT,* pulmonary trunk; *RA,* right atrium; *RPA,* right pulmonary artery; *RV,* right ventricle; *SVC,* superior vena cava; *Tr,* trachea. **B,** *IVC,* inferior vena cava; *LPA,* left pulmonary artery; *LV,* left ventricle; *RPA,* right pulmonary artery; *RV,* right ventricle; *Tr,* trachea. (From Inaba AS: Cardiac disorders. In Marx J, Hockberger R, Walls R, editors: *Rosen's emergency medicine: concepts and clinical practice,* ed 6, Philadelphia, 2006, Mosby.)

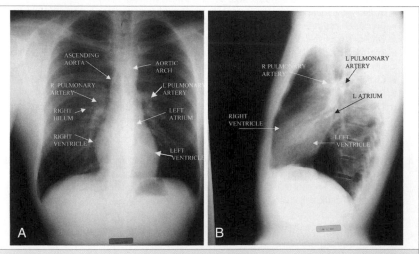

Figure 4-2. Major cardiovascular structures evident on chest radiograph.

the outflow tracts. In RV enlargement, the pulmonary arteries are often prominent and the aorta is diminutive. In LV enlargement, the aorta is prominent and the pulmonary arteries are normal.

- **Left atrial (LA) enlargement:** creates a convexity between the left pulmonary artery and the left ventricle on the frontal view. Also, a *double density* may be seen inferior to the carina. On the lateral view, LA enlargement displaces the descending left lower lobe bronchus posteriorly.
- **Right atrial enlargement:** causes the lower right heart border to bulge outward to the right.

7. **What are some of the common causes of chest pain that can be identified on a chest radiograph?**
   - Aortic dissection
   - Pneumonia
   - Pneumothorax
   - Pulmonary embolism
   - Subcutaneous emphysema
   - Pericarditis (if a large pericardial effusion is suggested by the radiograph)
   - Esophageal rupture
   - Hiatal hernia

   All patients with chest pain should undergo a CXR even if the cause of the chest pain is suspected myocardial ischemia.

8. **What are the causes of a widened mediastinum?**
   There are multiple potential causes of a widened mediastinum (Fig. 4-4). Some of the most concerning causes of mediastinal widening include aortic dissection and/or rupture and mediastinal bleeding from chest trauma or misplaced central venous catheters. One of the most common causes of mediastinal widening is thoracic lipomatosis in an obese patient. Tumors should also be considered as a cause of a widened mediastinum—especially germ cell tumors, lymphoma, and thymomas. The mediastinum may also appear wider on a portable AP film compared with a standard posteroanterior/lateral chest radiograph.

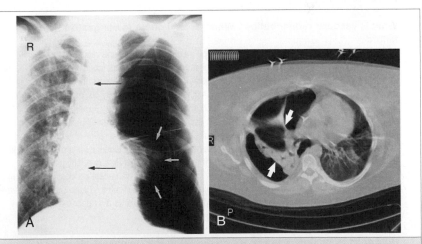

Figure 4-3. Tension pneumothorax. On a posteroanterior chest radiograph **(A)** the left hemithorax is very dark or lucent because the left lung has collapsed completely *(white arrows)*. The tension pneumothorax can be identified because the mediastinal contents, including the heart, are shifted toward the right *(black arrows)* and the left hemidiaphragm is flattened and depressed. **B,** A computed tomography scan done on a different patient with a tension pneumothorax shows a completely collapsed right lung *(arrows)* and shift of the mediastinal contents to the left. (From Mettler: *Essentials of radiology,* ed 2, Philadelphia, 2005, Saunders.)

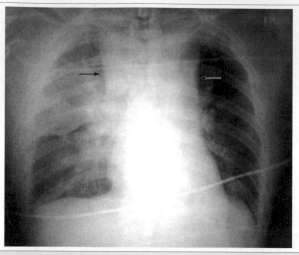

Figure 4-4. Widened mediastinum *(arrows)*. (From Marx J, Hockberger R, Walls R, editors: *Rosen's emergency medicine: concepts and clinical practice,* ed 6, Philadelphia, 2006, Mosby.)

9. **What are the common radiographic signs of congestive heart failure?**
   - Enlarged cardiac silhouette
   - Left atrial enlargement
   - Hilar fullness
   - Vascular redistribution
   - Linear interstitial opacities (Kerley lines)
   - Bilateral alveolar infiltrates
   - Pleural effusions (right greater than left)

10. **What is vascular redistribution? When does it occur in congestive heart failure?**
    Vascular redistribution occurs when the upper-lobe pulmonary arteries and veins become larger than the vessels in the lower lobes. The sign is most accurate if the upper lobe vessels are increased in diameter greater than 3 mm in the first intercostal interspace. It usually occurs at a pulmonary capillary occlusion pressure of 12 to 19 mm Hg. As the pulmonary capillary occlusion pressure rises above 19 mm Hg, interstitial edema develops with bronchial cuffing, Kerley B lines, and thickening of the lung fissures. Vascular redistribution to the upper lobes is probably most consistently seen in patients with chronic pulmonary venous hypertension (e.g., mitral valve disease or left ventricular dysfunction) because of the body's attempt to maintain more normal blood flow and oxygenation in this area. Some authors think that vascular redistribution is a cardinal feature of congestive heart failure, but it may be a particularly unhelpful sign in the ICU patient with acute congestive failure. In these patients, all the pulmonary arteries look enlarged, making it difficult to assess upper and lower vessel size. In addition, the film is often taken supine, which can enlarge the upper lobe pulmonary vessels because of stasis of blood flow and not true redistribution.

11. **How does LV dysfunction and RV dysfunction lead to pleural effusions?**
    - LV dysfunction causes increased hydrostatic pressures, which lead to interstitial edema and pleural effusions. Right pleural effusions are more common than left pleural effusions, but the majority are bilateral.
    - RV dysfunction leads to system venous hypertension, which inhibits normal reabsorption of pleural fluid into the parietal pleural lymphatics.

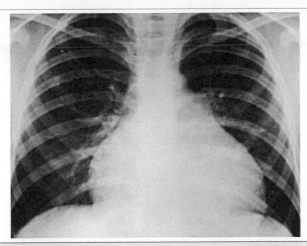

Figure 4-5. The *water bottle* configuration that can be seen with a large pericardial effusion. (From Kliegman RM, Behrman RE, Jenson HB, et al: *Nelson textbook of pediatrics,* ed 18, Philadelphia, 2007, Saunders.)

12. **How helpful is the chest radiograph at identifying and characterizing a pericardial effusion?**
The CXR is not sensitive for the detection of a pericardial effusion, and it may not be helpful in determining the extent of an effusion. Smaller pericardial effusions are difficult to detect on a CXR but can still cause tamponade physiology if fluid accumulation is rapid. A large *"water bottle"* cardiac silhouette (Fig. 4-5), however, may suggest a large pericardial effusion. Distinguishing pericardial fluid from chamber enlargement is often difficult.

13. **What are the characteristic radiographic findings of significant pulmonary hypertension?**
Enlargement of the central pulmonary arteries with rapid tapering of the vessels is a characteristic finding in patients with pulmonary hypertension (Fig. 4-6). If the right descending pulmonary artery is greater than 17 mm in transverse diameter, it is considered enlarged. Other findings of pulmonary hypertension include cardiac enlargement (particularly the right ventricle) and calcification of the pulmonary arteries. Pulmonary arterial calcification follows atheroma formation in the artery and represents a rare but specific radiographic finding of severe pulmonary hypertension.

14. **What is the Westermark sign and a Hampton hump?**
The Westermark sign is seen in patients with pulmonary embolism and represents an area of oligemia beyond the occluded pulmonary vessel. If pulmonary infarction results, a wedge-shaped infiltrate (a "Hampton hump") may be visible (Fig. 4-7).

15. **What is rib notching?**
Rib notching is erosion of the inferior aspects of the ribs (Fig. 4-8). It can be seen in some patients with coarctation of the aorta and results from a compensatory enlargement of the intercostal arteries as a means of increasing distal circulation. It is most commonly seen between the fourth and eighth ribs. It is important to recognize this life-saving finding because aortic coarctation is treatable with percutaneous or open surgical intervention.

16. **What does the finding in Figure 4-9 suggest?**
The important finding in this figure is pericardial calcification. This can occur in diseases that affect the pericardium, such as tuberculosis. In a patient with signs and symptoms of heart failure, this finding would be highly suggestive of the diagnosis of constrictive pericarditis.

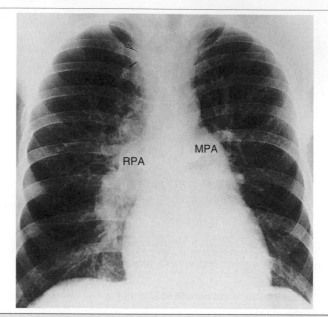

Figure 4-6. Pulmonary arterial hypertension. Marked dilation of the main pulmonary artery *(MPA)* and right pulmonary artery *(RPA)* is noted. Rapid tapering of the arteries as they proceed peripherally is suggestive of pulmonary hypertension and is sometimes referred to as *pruning.* (From Mettler FA: *Essentials of radiology,* ed 2, Philadelphia, 2005, Saunders.)

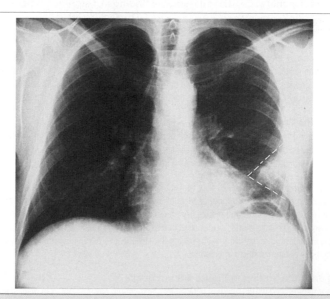

Figure 4-7. A peripheral wedge-shaped infiltrate *(white dashed lines)* seen after a pulmonary embolism has led to infarction. This finding is sometimes called a "Hampton hump." (From Mettler FA: *Essentials of radiology,* ed 2, Philadelphia, 2005, Saunders.)

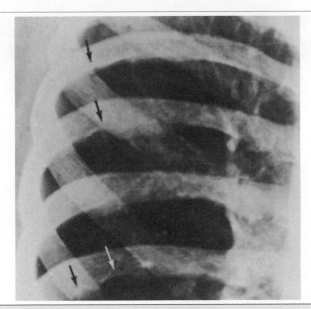

Figure 4-8. Rib notching in a patient with coarctation of the aorta. (From Park MK: *Pediatric cardiology for practitioners,* ed 5, Philadelphia, 2008, Mosby.)

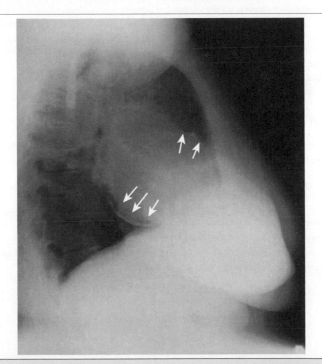

Figure 4-9. Pericardial calcification *(arrows).* In a patient with signs and symptoms of heart failure, this finding would strongly suggest the diagnosis of constrictive pericarditis. (From Libby P, Bonow RO, Mann DL, et al: *Braunwald's heart disease,* ed 8, Philadelphia, 2008, Saunders.)

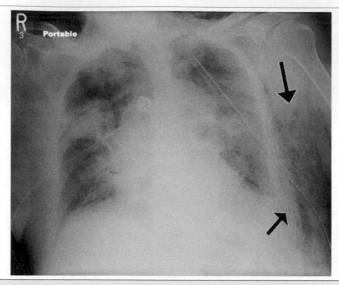

Figure 4-10. Subcutaneous emphysema *(arrows).*

17. What is subcutaneous emphysema?

Subcutaneous emphysema is the accumulation of air in the subcutaneous tissue, often tracking along tissue plains. Subcutaneous emphysema in the chest can be caused by numerous conditions, including pneumothorax, ruptured bronchus, ruptured esophagus, blunt trauma, stabbing or gunshot wound, or invasive procedure (e.g., endoscopy, bronchoscopy, central line placement, or intubation). The finding of subcutaneous emphysema almost always is associated with a serious medical condition or complication. The example of subcutaneous emphysema in Figure 4-10 emphasizes the importance of examining the entire chest x-ray.

BIBLIOGRAPHY, SUGGESTED READINGS, AND WEBSITES

1. Baron MG: Plain film diagnosis of common cardiac anomalies in the adult, *Radiol Clin North Am* 37:401–420, 1999.

2. Chandraskhar AJ: *Chest X-ray atlas.* Available at, http://www.meddean.luc.edu/lumen/MedEd/medicine/pulmonar/cxr/atlas/cxratlas_f.htm. Accessed March 8, 2012.

3. Hollander JE, Chase M: *Evaluation of chest pain in the emergency department.* Available at, http://www.uptodate.com/contents/evaluation-of-chest-pain-in-the-emergency-department. Accessed January 14, 2013.

4. MacDonald SLS, Padley S: The mediastinum, including the pericardium. In Adam A, Dixon AK, editors: *Grainger & Allsion's diagnostic radiology*, ed 5, Philadelphia, 2008, Churchill Livingstone.

5. Meholic A: *Fundamentals of chest radiology*, Philadelphia, 1996, Saunders.

6. Mettler FA: Cardiovascular system. In Mettler FA, editor: *Essentials of radiology*, ed 2, Philadelphia, 2005, Saunders.

7. Newell J: Diseases of the thoracic aorta: a symposium, *J Thorac Imag* 5:1–48, 1990.

CHAPTER 5

ECHOCARDIOGRAPHY

Hisham Dokainish, MD, FACC, FASE, and Glenn N. Levine, MD, FACC, FAHA

1. **How does echocardiography work?**

   Echocardiography uses transthoracic and transesophageal probes that emit ultrasound directed at cardiac structures. Returning ultrasound signals are received by the probe, and the computer in the ultrasound machine uses algorithms to reconstruct images of the heart. The time it takes for the ultrasound to return to the probe determines the depth of the structures relative to the probe because the speed of sound in soft tissue is relatively constant (1540 m/sec). The amplitude (intensity) of the returning signal determines the density and size of the structures with which the ultrasound comes in contact.

   The probes also perform Doppler ultrasonography, which measures the frequency shift of the returning ultrasound signal to determine the speed and direction of moving blood through heart structures (e.g., through the aortic valve) or in the myocardium itself (tissue Doppler imaging).

   Appropriateness criteria for obtaining an echocardiogram are given in Box 5-1.

2. **What is the difference between echocardiography and Doppler?**

   Echocardiography usually refers to two-dimensional (2-D) ultrasound interrogation of the heart in which the brightness mode is used to image cardiac structures based on their density and location relative to the chest wall. Two-dimensional echocardiography is particularly useful for identifying cardiac anatomy and morphology, such as identifying a pericardial effusion, left ventricular aneurysm, or cardiac mass.

   Doppler refers to interrogation of the movement of blood in and around the heart, based on the shift in frequency *(Doppler shift)* that ultrasound undergoes when it comes in contact with a moving object (usually red blood cells). Doppler has three modes:
   - Pulsed Doppler (Fig. 5-1, *A*), which can localize the site of flow acceleration but is prone to aliasing
   - Continuous-wave Doppler (Fig. 5-1, *B*), which cannot localize the level of flow acceleration but can identify very high velocities without aliasing
   - Color Doppler (Fig. 5-2), which uses different colors (usually red and blue) to identify flow toward and away from the transducer, respectively, and identify flow acceleration qualitatively by showing a mix of color to represent high velocity or aliased flow

   Doppler is particularly useful for assessing the hemodynamic significance of cardiac structural disease, such as the severity of aortic stenosis (see Fig. 5-1), degree of mitral regurgitation (see Fig. 5-2), flow velocity across a ventricular septal defect, or severity of pulmonary hypertension. The great majority of echocardiograms are ordered as *echocardiography with Doppler* to answer cardiac morphologic and hemodynamic questions in one study (e.g., a mitral stenosis murmur); 2-D echo to identify the restricted, thickened, and calcified mitral valve (Fig. 5-3); and Doppler to analyze its severity based on transvalvular flow velocities and gradients.

3. **How is systolic function assessed using echocardiography?**

   The most commonly used measurement of left ventricular (LV) systolic function is left ventricular ejection fraction (LVEF), which is defined by:

   $$\text{LVEF} = \frac{(\text{End-diastolic volume} - \text{End-systolic volume})}{\text{End-diastolic volume}}$$

Box 5-1 APPROPRIATENESS CRITERIA FOR ECHOCARDIOGRAPHY

Appropriate indications include, but are not limited to:

- Symptoms possibly related to cardiac etiology, such as dyspnea, shortness of breath, lightheadedness, syncope, cerebrovascular events
- Initial evaluation of left-sided ventricular function after acute myocardial infarction
- Evaluation of cardiac murmur in suspected valve disease
- Sustained ventricular tachycardia or supraventricular tachycardia
- Evaluation of suspected pulmonary artery hypertension
- Evaluation of acute chest pain with nondiagnostic laboratory markers and electrocardiogram
- Evaluation of known native or prosthetic valve disease in a patient with change of clinical status

Uncertain indications for echocardiography:

- Cardiovascular source of embolic event in a patient who has normal transthoracic echocardiogram (TTE) and electrocardiogram findings and no history of atrial fibrillation or flutter

Inappropriate indications for echocardiography:

- Routine monitoring of known conditions, such as heart failure, mild valvular disease, hypertensive cardiomyopathy, repair of congenital heart disease, or monitoring of an artificial valve, when the patient is clinically stable
- Echocardiography is also not the test of choice in the initial evaluation for pulmonary embolus and should not be routinely used to screen asymptomatic hypertensive patients for heart disease.

Appropriate indications for transesophageal echocardiography (TEE) as the initial test instead of TTE:

- Evaluation of suspected aortic pathology, including dissection
- Guidance during percutaneous cardiac procedures, including ablation and mitral valvuloplasty
- To determine the mechanism of regurgitation and suitability of valve repair
- Diagnose or manage endocarditis in patients with moderate to high probability of endocarditis
- Persistent fever in a patient with an intracardiac device
- TEE is *not* appropriate in evaluation for a left atrial thrombus in the setting of atrial fibrillation when it has already been decided to treat the patient with anticoagulant drugs.

Modified from Douglas PS, Khanderia B, Stainback RF, et al: ACCF/ASE/ACEP/ASNC/SCAI/SCCT/SCMR 2007 appropriateness criteria for transthoracic and transesophageal echocardiography. *J Am Coll Cardiol* 50:187-204, 2007.

- The Simpson method (method of discs) in which the LV endocardial border of multiple "slices" of the left ventricle is traced in systole and diastole, and the end-diastolic and end-systolic volumes are computed from these tracings, is one of the most common methods of calculating LVEF.
- The Teicholz method, in which the shortening fraction:

    (LV end-diastolic dimension − LV end-systolic dimension)/LV end-diastolic dimension

    is multiplied by 1.7, can also be used to estimate LVEF (although this method is inaccurate in patients with regional wall motion abnormalities).
- Visual estimation of LVEF by expert echocardiography readers is also commonly used.
- Increasingly, state-of-the-art full volume acquisition using 3-dimensional (3-D) echocardiography can be used to provide accurate LVEF.
- Systolic dysfunction in the presence of preserved LVEF (more than 50%-55%)—such as is found in patients with hypertrophic hearts, ischemic heart disease, or infiltrative cardiomyopathies—can be identified by depressed systolic tissue Doppler velocities.

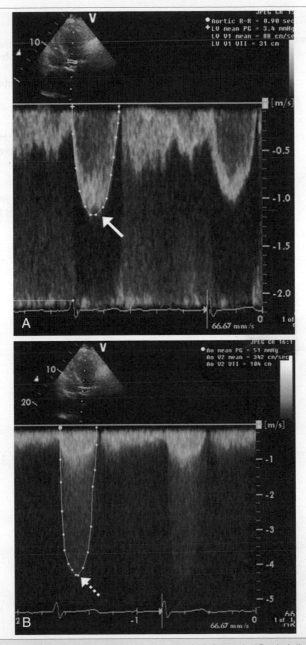

Figure 5-1. Doppler assessment used in patients with aortic stenosis. **A** shows pulsed Doppler in the left ventricular outflow tract in a patient with aortic stenosis. The peak velocity of the spectral tracing *(arrow)* is 1.2 msec, indicating normal flow velocity proximal to the aortic valve. **B** shows continuous Doppler across the aortic valve revealing a peak velocity of 4.5 msec *(dashed arrow)*. Therefore, the blood-flow velocity nearly quadrupled across the stenotic aortic valve, consistent with severe aortic stenosis.

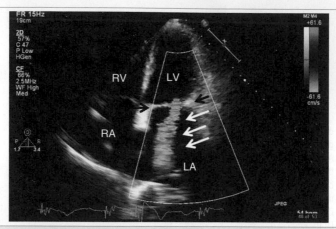

Figure 5-2. Mitral regurgitation. Apical four-chamber view with color Doppler revealing severe mitral regurgitation *(white arrows). Black arrows* point to the mitral valve. Note that in actuality, the regurgitant jet is displayed in color, corresponding to the flow of blood. *LA,* Left atrium; *LV,* left ventricle; *RA,* right atrium; *RV,* right ventricle.

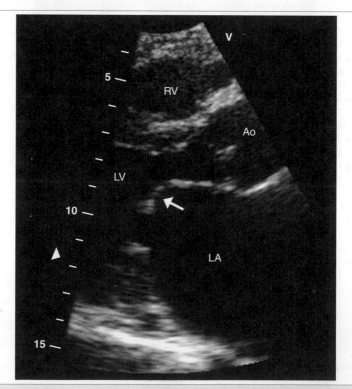

Figure 5-3. Parasternal long-axis view showing typical *hockey stick* appearance of the mitral valve *(arrow)* in rheumatic mitral stenosis. *Ao,* Aortic valve; *LA,* left atrium; *LV,* left ventricle; *RV,* right ventricle.

4. **What is an echocardiographic diastolic assessment? What information can it provide?**

A diastolic assessment does two things: identifies LV relaxation and estimates LV filling pressures. LV relaxation is described as the time it takes for the LV to relax in diastole to accept blood from the left atrium (LA) through an open mitral valve. A normal heart is very elastic *(lusitropic)* and readily accepts blood during LV filling. When relaxation is impaired, the LV cannot easily accept increased volume, and this increased LV preload results in increases in LA pressure, which in turn results in pulmonary edema.

- LV relaxation is usually best determined using tissue Doppler imaging, which assesses early diastolic filling velocity (Ea) of the LV myocardium. Normal hearts have Ea of 10 cm/sec or greater; impaired relaxation is present when Ea is less than 10 cm/sec.
- An indicator of LV preload is peak transmitral early diastolic filling velocity (E), which measures the velocity of blood flow across the mitral valve. An estimate of the LV filling pressure can be made using the ratio of blood flow velocity across the mitral valve (E) to the velocity of myocardial tissue during early diastole (Ea). A high ratio (e.g., E/Ea $\geq$ 15) indicates elevated LV filling pressure (LA pressure $\geq$ 15 mm Hg); a lower ratio (e.g., E/Ea $\leq$ 10) indicates normal LV filling pressure (LA pressure < 15 mm Hg).

5. **How can echocardiography with Doppler be used to answer cardiac hemodynamic questions?**

- Stroke volume and cardiac output can be obtained with measurements of the LV outflow tract and time-velocity integral (TVI) of blood through the LV outflow tract.
- Doppler evaluation of right ventricular outflow tract diameter and TVI similarly allow measurement of right ventricular output.
- Tricuspid regurgitation peak gradient can be added to estimate of right atrial pressure to in turn estimate pulmonary artery systolic pressure.
- Mitral inflow velocities, deceleration time, pulmonary venous parameters, and tissue Doppler imaging of the mitral annulus can give accurate assessment of LV diastolic function, including LV filling pressures.
- Measurement of TVI and valve annular diameters can be used to assess intracardiac shunts (Qp/Qs) and regurgitant flow volumes, where Qp is flow out the right ventricular outflow tract and Qs is flow out the left ventricular outflow tract.
- Pressure gradients across native and prosthetic valves and across cardiac shunts can be used to assess hemodynamic severity of valve stenosis, regurgitation, or shunt severity, respectively.
- Respiratory variation in valvular flow can aid in the diagnosis of cardiac tamponade or constrictive pericarditis.

6. **How is echocardiography used to evaluate valvular disease?**

- Two-dimensional echocardiography can provide accurate visualization of valve structure to assess morphologic abnormalities (calcification, prolapse, flail, rheumatic disease, endocarditis). Figure 5-3 demonstrates the restricted movement of the mitral valve in a patient with mitral stenosis.
- Color Doppler can provide semiquantitative assessment of the degree of valve regurgitation (mild, moderate, severe) in any position (aortic, mitral, pulmonic, tricuspid).
- Pulsed Doppler can help pinpoint the location of a valvular abnormality (e.g., subaortic vs aortic vs supraaortic stenosis). Pulsed Doppler can also be used to quantitate regurgitant volumes and fractions using the continuity equation.
- Continuous-wave Doppler is useful for determining the hemodynamic severity of stenotic lesions, such as aortic or mitral stenosis.

7. **How can echocardiography help diagnose and manage patients with suspected pericardial disease?**

- Echocardiography can diagnose pericardial effusions (Fig. 5-4) because fluid in the pericardial space readily transmits ultrasound (appears black on echo).

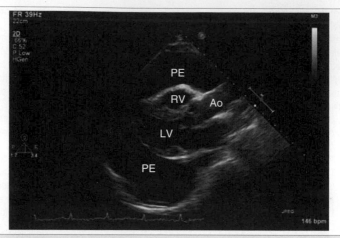

Figure 5-4. Parasternal long-axis view showing a large pericardial effusion *(PE)* surrounding the heart. *Ao,* Aorta; *LV,* left ventricle; *RV,* right ventricle. (From Kabbani SS, LeWinter M: Cardiac constriction and restriction. In Crawford MH, DiMarco JP, editors: *Cardiology,* St Louis, 2001, Mosby.)

- Two-dimensional echocardiography and Doppler are pivotal in determining the hemodynamic impact of pericardial fluid; that is, whether the patient has elevated intrapericardial pressure or frank cardiac tamponade.
- The following are indicators of elevated intrapericardial pressure in the setting of pericardial effusion:
  - ○ Diastolic indentation or collapse of the right ventricle (RV)
  - ○ Compression of the right atrium (RA) for more than one-third of the cardiac cycle
  - ○ Lack of inferior vena cava (IVC) collapsibility with deep inspiration
  - ○ 25% or greater variation in mitral or aortic Doppler flows
  - ○ 50% or greater variation of tricuspid or pulmonic valves flows with inspiration
- Echocardiographic signs of constrictive pericarditis include thickened or calcified pericardium, diastolic *bounce* of the interventricular septum, restrictive mitral filling pattern with 25% or greater respiratory variation in peak velocities, and lack of inspiratory collapsibility of the inferior vena cava.
- Echocardiography is additionally useful for guiding percutaneous needle pericardiocentesis by identifying the transthoracic or subcostal window with the largest fluid *cushion,* monitoring decrease of fluid during pericardiocentesis, and in follow-up studies, assessing for reaccumulation of fluid.

8. **What is the role of echocardiography in patients with ischemic stroke?**
   The following are echocardiographic findings that may be associated with a cardiac embolic cause in patients with stroke:
   - Depressed LV ejection fraction, generally less than 40%
   - Left ventricular or left atrial clot (Fig. 5-5)
   - Intracardiac mass such as tumor or endocarditis
   - Mitral stenosis (especially with a history of atrial fibrillation)
   - Prosthetic valve in the mitral or aortic position
   - Significant atherosclerotic disease in the aortic root, ascending aorta, or aortic arch
   - Saline contrast study indicating a significant right-to-left intracardiac shunt, such as atrial septal defect

   Note: A normal transthoracic echocardiogram in a patient without atrial fibrillation generally excludes a cardiac embolic source of clot and generally obviates the need for transesophageal echocardiography (TEE).

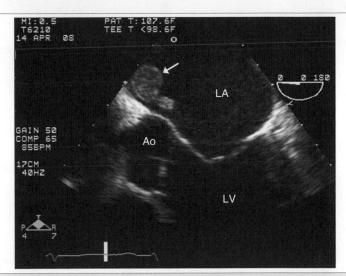

Figure 5-5. Transesophageal echocardiography showing a left atrial thrombus *(arrow)*. *Ao*, Aortic valve; *LA*, left atrium; *LV*, left ventricle.

9. **What are the echocardiographic findings in hypertrophic cardiomyopathy (HCM)?**
   - Septal, concentric, or apical hypertrophy (walls greater than 1.5 cm in diameter)
   - The presence of systolic anterior motion (SAM) of the mitral valve in some cases of obstructive hypertrophic cardiomyopathy (Fig. 5-6)
   - Dynamic left ventricular outflow tract (LVOT) gradients caused by SAM, midcavitary obliteration, or apical obliteration

10. **What are the common indications for transesophageal echocardiography?**
    - Significant clinical suspicion of endocarditis in patients with suboptimal transthoracic windows
    - Significant clinical suspicion of endocarditis in patients with prosthetic heart valve
    - Suspected aortic dissection (Fig. 5-7)
    - Suspected atrial septal defect (ASD) or patent foramen ovale in patients with cryptogenic embolic stroke
    - Embolic stroke with nondiagnostic transthoracic echo
    - Endocarditis with suspected valvular complications (abscess, fistula, pseudoaneurysm)
    - Evaluation of the mitral valve in cases of possible surgical mitral valve
    - Intracardiac shunt in which the location is not well seen on transthoracic echocardiography
    - Assessment of the left atria and left atrial appendage for the presence of thrombus (clot) (see Fig. 5-5) prior to planned cardioversion

11. **What is contrast echocardiography?**
    Contrast echocardiography involves injection of either saline contrast agent or synthetic microbubbles (perflutren bubbles) into a systemic vein, then imaging the heart using ultrasound. Saline contrast agent, because of its relatively large size, does not cross the pulmonary capillary bed, and it consequently is confined to the right heart. Therefore, rapid appearance of saline contrast in the left heart indicates an intracardiac shunt.

    Because synthetic microbubbles are smaller than saline bubbles, they cross the pulmonary capillaries and are used to image left heart structures. Most commonly, synthetic microbubbles are used to achieve better endocardial border definition in patients with suboptimal echocardiographic

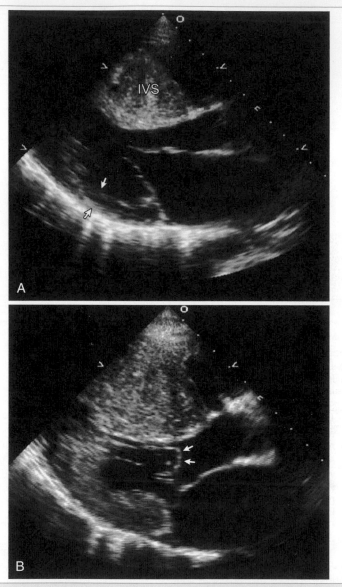

Figure 5-6. Echocardiographic findings in hypertrophic cardiomyopathy. **A,** Parasternal long axis image during diastole demonstrating massive thickening of the interventricular septum *(IVS)* when compared to the thickness of the posterior wall *(arrows)*. **B,** During systole, echocardiography demonstrates systolic anterior motion (SAM) of the mitral valve, with the leaflets actually bowing in to the left ventricular outflow tract *(arrows)*.

windows. Contrast echocardiography is also used to better visualize structures such as possible LV clots or other masses.

Both synthetic and saline contrast agents can be used to augment Doppler signals, for example, in patients with pulmonary hypertension in whom a tricuspid regurgitation jet is needed to estimate pulmonary artery pressure.

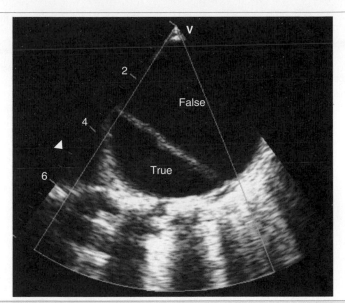

Figure 5-7. Transesophageal echocardiography revealing dissection of the descending thoracic aorta. The true aortic lumen *(True)* is seen separated from the false lumen *(False)* by the dissection.

12. What is stress echocardiography?

Stress echocardiography involves imaging the heart first at rest and subsequently during either exercise (treadmill or bike) or pharmacologic (usually dobutamine) stress to identify left ventricular (LV) wall motion abnormalities resulting from the presence of flow-limiting coronary artery disease.

Other uses of stress echocardiography include:

- Assessment of mitral or aortic valve disease in patients who have moderate disease at rest but significant symptoms with exercise
- Assessment of patients with suspected exercise-induced diastolic dysfunction
- Assessment of viability in patients with depressed ejection fractions. Improvement in left ventricular function with infusion of low-dose dobutamine (less than 10 μg/kg/min) suggests viable myocardium.
- Distinguishing between true aortic stenosis and *pseudo* aortic stenosis in patients with mild-to-moderate aortic stenosis at rest and depressed ejection fraction with low cardiac output

BIBLIOGRAPHY, SUGGESTED READINGS, AND WEBSITES

1. Abraham TP, Dimaano VL, Liang HY: Role of tissue Doppler and strain echocardiography in current clinical practice, *Circulation* 116:2597–2609, 2007.
2. Armstrong WF, Zoghbi WA: Stress echocardiography: current methodology and clinical applications, *J Am Coll Cardiol* 45:1739–1747, 2005.
3. Douglas PS, Khandheria B, Stainback RF, et al: ACCF/ASE/ACEP/ASNC/SCAI/SCCT/SCMR 2007 appropriateness criteria for transthoracic and transesophageal echocardiography, *J Am Coll Cardiol* 50:187–204, 2007.
4. Evangelista A, Gonzalez-Alujas MT: Echocardiography in infective endocarditis, *Heart* 90:614–617, 2004.
5. Grayburn PA: How to measure severity of mitral regurgitation: valvular heart disease, *Heart* 94:376–383, 2008.
6. Kirkpatrick JN, Vannan MA, Narula J, et al: Echocardiography in heart failure: applications, utility, and new horizons, *J Am Coll Cardiol* 50:381–396, 2007.
7. Lang RM, Mor-Avi V, Sugeng L, et al: Three-dimensional echocardiography: the benefits of the additional dimension, *J Am Coll Cardiol* 48:2053–2069, 2006.

8. Lester SJ, Tajik AJ, Nishimura RA, et al: Unlocking the mysteries of diastolic function: deciphering the Rosetta Stone 10 years later, *J Am Coll Cardiol* 51:679–689, 2008.

9. Otto CM: Valvular aortic stenosis: disease severity and timing of intervention, *J Am Coll Cardiol* 47:2141–2151, 2006.

10. Peterson GE, Brickner ME, Reimold SC: Transesophageal echocardiography: clinical indications and applications, *Circulation* 107:2398–2402, 2003.

11. Stewart MJ: Contrast echocardiography, *Heart* 89:342–348, 2003.

CHAPTER 6

EXERCISE STRESS TESTING

Fernando Boccalandro, MD, FACC, FSCAI

1. **What is the purpose of exercise stress testing (EST) and how can a patient exercise during stress testing?**

   EST using electrocardiography (ECG) is routinely performed to diagnose myocardial ischemia, estimate prognosis, evaluate the outcome of therapy, and assess cardiopulmonary reserve. Exercise is used as a physiological stress to detect cardiac abnormalities that are not present at rest. They are accomplished with a treadmill, bicycle ergometer, or, rarely, with an arm ergometer, and may involve ventilatory gas analysis (the latter is called a cardiopulmonary stress test). Different protocols of progressive cardiovascular workload have been developed specifically for EST (e.g., Bruce, Cornell, Balke-Ware, ACIP, mAICP, Naughton, Weber). Bicycle ergometers are less expensive and smaller than treadmills and produce less motion of the upper body, but early fatigue of the lower extremities is a common problem that limits reaching maximal exercise capacity. As a result, treadmills are more commonly used in the United States for EST. Much of the reported data are based on the multistage Bruce Protocol, which is performed on a treadmill and has become the most commonly used protocol in clinical practice. ESTs may involve only ECG monitoring or may be combined with other imaging modalities (i.e., nuclear imaging, echocardiography).

2. **What is the difference between a maximal and submaximal EST?**

   - *Maximal EST or symptoms-limited EST* is the preferred means to perform an EST and attempts to achieve the maximal tolerated exercise capacity of the patient. It is terminated based on patient symptoms (e.g., fatigue, angina, shortness of breath); an abnormal ECG (e.g., significant ST depression or elevation, arrhythmias); or an abnormal hemodynamic response (e.g., abnormal blood pressure response). A goal of maximal EST is to achieve a heart rate response of at least 85% of the maximal predicted heart rate (see Question 9).
   - *Submaximal EST* is performed when the goal is lower than the individual maximal exercise capacity. Reasonable targets are 70% of the maximal predicted heart rate, 120 beats per minute, or 5 to 6 metabolic equivalents (METs) of exercise capacity (see Question 12). Submaximal EST is used early after myocardial infarction (see Question 8).

3. **How helpful is an EST in the diagnosis of coronary artery disease?**

   Multiple studies have been reported comparing the accuracy of EST with coronary angiography. However, different criteria have been used to define a significant coronary stenosis, and this lack of standardization, in addition to a variable prevalence of coronary artery disease in different populations, complicates the interpretation of the available data. A meta-analysis of 24,074 patients reported a mean sensitivity of 68% and a mean specificity of 77%. The sensitivity increases to 81% and the specificity decreases to 66% for multivessel disease, and to 86% and 53%, respectively, for left main disease or three-vessel coronary artery disease. The diagnostic accuracy of EST can be improved by combining other imaging techniques with EST such as echocardiography or myocardial perfusion imaging.

4. **What are the risks associated with EST?**

   When supervised by an adequately trained physician, the risks are very low. In the general population, the morbidity is less than 0.05% and the mortality is less than 0.01%. A survey of 151,944 patients 4 weeks after a myocardial infarction showed slight increased mortality and morbidity of 0.03%

> ### Box 6-1 INDICATIONS FOR EXERCISE STRESS TESTING
>
> - When diagnosing suspected obstructive coronary artery disease (CAD) based on age, gender, and clinical presentation, including those with right bundle branch block and less than 1 mm of resting ST depression
> - For risk stratification, functional class assessment, and prognosis in patients with suspected or known CAD based on age, gender, and clinical presentation
> - When evaluating patients with known CAD who witnessed a significant change in their clinical status
> - To evaluate patients with vasospastic angina
> - To evaluate patients with low- or intermediate-risk unstable angina after they had been stabilized and who had been free of active ischemic symptoms or heart failure
> - After myocardial infarction for prognosis assessment, physical activity prescription, or evaluation of current medical treatment; before discharge with a submaximal stress test 4 to 6 days after myocardial infarction, or after discharge with a symptoms-limited EST at least 14 to 21 days after myocardial infarction
> - To detect myocardial ischemia in patients considered for revascularization
> - After discharge for physical activity prescription and counseling after revascularization, as part of a cardiac rehabilitation program
> - In patients with chronic aortic regurgitation, to assess the functional capacity and symptomatic responses in those with a history of equivocal symptoms
> - When evaluating the proper settings in patients who received rate-responsive pacemakers
> - When investigating patients with known or suspected exercise-induced arrhythmias

and 0.09%, respectively. According to the national survey of EST facilities, myocardial infarction and death can be expected in 1 per 2,500 tests.

5. **What are the indications for EST?**
   The most common indications for EST, according to the current American College of Cardiology (ACC) and American Heart Association (AHA) guidelines, are summarized in Box 6-1. When considering ordering an EST, three fundamental factors need to be considered to have an optimal diagnostic test: a normal baseline ECG, a patient who is able to exercise to complete the exercise protocol planned, and an appropriate indication for EST.

6. **Should asymptomatic patients undergo ESTs?**
   In general, asymptomatic patients should be discouraged from undergoing EST because the pretest probability of coronary artery disease in this population is low, leading to a significant number of false-positive results, requiring unnecessary follow-up tests and expenses without a well-documented benefit. There are no data from randomized studies that support the use of routine screening EST in asymptomatic patients to reduce the risk of cardiovascular events. Nevertheless, selected asymptomatic patients may be considered for EST under specific clinical circumstances if clinically appropriate (e.g., diabetic patients planning to enroll in a vigorous exercise program, certain high-risk occupations, positive calcium score, family history).

7. **What are contraindications for EST?**
   The contraindications for EST according to the current ACC/AHA guidelines are summarized in Box 6-2.

8. **What parameters are monitored during an EST?**
   During EST, three parameters are monitored and reported: the clinical response of the patient to exercise (e.g., shortness of breath, dizziness, chest pain, angina pectoris, Borg Scale score), the hemodynamic response (e.g., heart rate, blood pressure response), and the ECG changes that occur during exercise and the recovery phase of EST.

Box 6-2 CONTRAINDICATIONS FOR EXERCISE STRESS TESTING

Absolute Contraindications
Acute myocardial infarction within 2 days
High-risk unstable angina
Uncontrolled cardiac arrhythmias causing symptoms or hemodynamic compromise
Advanced atrioventricular block
Severe, hypertrophic obstructive cardiomyopathy
Severe, symptomatic aortic stenosis
Acute aortic dissection
Acute pulmonary embolism or infarction
Decompensated heart failure
Acute myocarditis or pericarditis

Relative Contraindications
Left main coronary stenosis
Moderate aortic stenosis
Electrolyte abnormalities
Uncontrolled hypertension
Arrhythmias
Moderate hypertrophic cardiomyopathy and other forms of left ventricular outflow obstruction
Mental or physical impairment leading to inability to exercise adequately

---

9. **What is an adequate heart rate to elicit an ischemic response?**
   It is accepted that a heart rate of 85% of the maximal predicted heart rate for the age of the patient is usually sufficient to elicit an ischemic response in the presence of a hemodynamic significant coronary stenosis, and is considered an adequate heart rate for a diagnostic EST.

10. **How do I calculate the predicted maximal heart rate?**
    The maximal predicted heart rate can be estimated with the following formula:

    $$Maximal\ predicted\ heart\ rate = 220 - Age$$

11. **What is the Borg scale?**
    The Borg Scale is a numeric scale of perceived patient exertion commonly used during EST. Values of 7 to 9 reflect light work and 13 to 17 hard work; a value above 18 is close to the maximal exercise capacity. Readings of 14 to 16 reach the anaerobic threshold. The Borg Scale is particularly useful when evaluating the patient functional capacity during EST.

12. **What is a metabolic equivalent (MET)?**
    METs are defined as the caloric consumption of an active individual compared with their resting basal metabolic rate. They are used during EST as an estimate of functional capacity. One MET is defined as 1 kilocalorie per kilogram per hour and is the caloric consumption of a person while at complete rest (i.e., 2 METs will correspond to an activity that is twice the resting metabolic rate). Activities of 2 to 4 METs (light walking, doing household chores, etc.) are considered light, whereas running or climbing can yield 10 or more METs. A functional capacity below 5 METs during treadmill EST is associated with a worse prognosis, whereas higher METs during exercise are associated with better outcomes. Patients who can perform more than 10 METs during EST usually have a good prognosis regardless of their coronary anatomy.

13. **What is considered a hypertensive response to exercise?**

The current ACC/AHA guidelines for EST suggest a hypertensive response to exercise is one in which systolic blood pressure rises to more than 250 mm Hg or diastolic blood pressure rises to more than 115 mm Hg. This is considered a relative indication to terminate an EST.

14. **Can I order an EST in a patient taking beta-blockers?**

An EST in patients taking beta-blockers may have reduced diagnostic and prognostic value because of inadequate heart rate response. Nonetheless, according to the current ACC/AHA guidelines for exercise testing, stopping beta-blockers before EST is discouraged to avoid "rebound" hypertension or anginal symptoms.

15. **What baseline ECG findings interfere with the interpretation of an EST?**

Patients with left bundle branch block (LBBB), ventricular pacing, baseline ST depressions (such as with "LVH with strain"), and those with preexcitation syndromes (Wolf-Parkinson-White syndrome) should be considered for imaging stress testing because their baseline ECG abnormalities prevent an adequate ECG interpretation during exercise. Right bundle branch block does not reduce significantly the accuracy of the EST for the diagnosis of ischemia. Digoxin may also cause false-positive ST depressions during exercise and is also an indication for imaging during stress testing.

16. **When can an EST be performed after an acute myocardial infarction?**

Submaximal EST is occasionally recommended after myocardial infarction as early as 4 days after the acute event. This can be followed by later (3 to 6 weeks) symptom-limited EST. EST in this circumstance assists in formulating a prognosis, determining activity levels, assessing medical therapy, and planning cardiac rehabilitation. It is unclear if asymptomatic patients who had an acute myocardial infarction (MI) with a consequent revascularization procedure benefit from follow-up EST after myocardial infarction, although it is not generally recommended if the patient is clinically stable.

17. **Are the patient's sex and age considerations for EST?**

Women have more false-positive ST-segment depression during EST than do men, which may limit the sensitivity of EST for the detection of coronary artery disease in this population. This problem reflects differences in exercise and coronary physiology with a higher sympathetic activation, which could lead to coronary vasospasm, a cyclic hormonal milieu, different body habitus, different ECG response to exercise, and a lower prevalence of coronary artery disease compared with men. Despite these limitations, EST should be considered as the initial diagnostic test in the evaluation of women with a normal baseline ECG when ischemic heart disease is suspected, because functional capacity and hemodynamic response are robust predictors of cardiovascular events independent of the ECG findings. The use of imaging EST (i.e., nuclear or echocardiography EST) needs to be considered for women with abnormal baseline ECG or poor exercise tolerance. Age is not an important consideration for EST if the patient is fit to complete an exercise protocol adequately.

18. **When is an EST interpreted as *positive*?**

It is important for the physician supervising the test to consider the individual pretest probability of the patient undergoing EST to have underlying coronary artery disease while interpreting the results, and to consider not only the ECG response but all the information provided by the test, including functional capacity, hemodynamic response, and symptoms during exercise. ECG changes consisting of greater than or equal to 1 mm of horizontal or down-sloping ST-segment depression or elevation at least 60 to 80 msec after the end of the QRS complex during EST in three consecutive beats are considered a positive ECG response for myocardial ischemia (Fig. 6-1). Also, the occurrence of angina is important, particularly if it forces early termination of the test. Abnormalities in exercise capacity, blood pressure, and heart rate response to exercise are also important to be considered when reporting the results of EST.

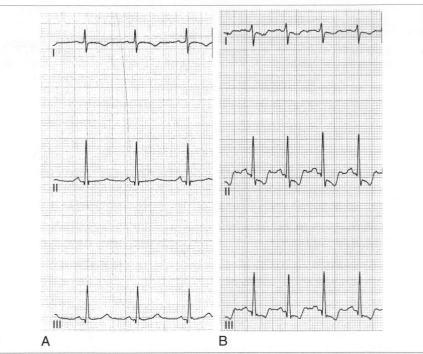

Figure 6-1. Abnormal electrocardiographic (ECG) response to exercise in a patient found to have a severe stenosis of the right coronary artery. **A,** Normal baseline ECG. **B,** Abnormal ECG response at peak exercise with marked downsloping ST depression and T-wave inversion.

19. **What are the indications to terminate an EST?**

The *absolute indications* to stop EST according to the current ACC/AHA guidelines include a drop of more than 10 mm Hg in the systolic blood pressure despite an increased workload in addition to other signs of ischemia (i.e., angina, ventricular arrhythmias), ST elevation of more than 1 mm in leads without diagnostic Q waves (other than V1 and aVR), moderate to severe angina, increased autonomic nervous system symptoms (i.e., ataxia, dizziness, near syncope), signs of poor perfusion (i.e., cyanosis or pallor), difficulties monitoring the ECG or blood pressure, the patient requests to stop the test, and sustained ventricular tachycardia.

Relative indications include a drop of more than 10 mm Hg in the systolic blood pressure despite an increased workload in the absence of other evidence of ischemia; excessive ST depression (more than 2 mm of horizontal or downsloping ST depression) or marked QRS axis shift; arrhythmias other than sustained ventricular tachycardia; fatigue, shortness of breath, wheezing, leg cramps, or claudication; development of bundle branch block or intraventricular conduction delay that cannot be distinguished from ventricular tachycardia; hypertensive response to exercise; and increasing nonanginal chest pain.

20. **What is a cardiopulmonary EST and what are the indications of this diagnostic test?**

During a cardiopulmonary EST, the patient's ventilatory gas exchange is monitored in a closed circuit and measurements of gas exchange are obtained during exercise (i.e., oxygen uptake, carbon dioxide output, anaerobic threshold), in addition to the information provided during routine EST. Cardiopulmonary EST is indicated to differentiate cardiac versus pulmonary causes of exercise-induced dyspnea or impaired exercise capacity. It is also used in the follow-up of patients with heart failure or who are being considered for heart transplantation.

21. **Can I localize which coronary artery is affected using the ECG during EST?**
The ability of an ECG to localize an ischemic coronary territory during EST depends on the type of ST segment change noted during exercise. Exercise-induced ST depression is a nonspecific ischemic change, and cannot be used to localize any given coronary territory. Conversely, ST elevation in a lead with no prior Q waves in a patient with no history of prior myocardial infarction is consistent with transmural ischemia, and can be used to localize the coronary territory affected.

22. **Can one obtain a stress test if a patient cannot exercise?**
If the patient is unable to exercise, pharmacologic methods can detect ischemia employing imaging modalities such as echocardiography, myocardial nuclear perfusion imaging, computed tomography, or magnetic resonance imaging. Imaging methods can increase the accuracy for detection of coronary artery disease at a higher cost compared with EST alone, but cannot predict functional capacity.

23. **How often should an EST be repeated?**
Repeating an EST without a specific clinical indication at any interval has not been shown to improve risk stratification or prognosis in patients with or without known coronary artery disease, and is discouraged. An EST can be repeated when a significant change in the patient's cardiovascular status is suspected, or according to the appropriate indications as noted in Box 6-1. In patients who had prior revascularization, stress imaging studies are preferred because they provide better information regarding the coronary distribution and severity of myocardial ischemia when compared with EST.

24. **Can I use the ECG tracings from the stress test to interpret my patient's 12-lead ECG?**
To avoid motion during exercise, the conventional 12-lead ECG positions require that the extremity electrodes move close to the torso. This alternate lead positioning is called the Mason-Likar modification and requires placing the arm electrodes in the lateral aspect of the infraclavicular fossa, and the leg electrodes between the iliac crest and below the rib cage. This lead change causes a right axis deviation and increased voltage in the inferior leads, which can obscure inferior Q waves and create new Q waves in aVL. Thus the ECG tracing obtained during an EST should not be used to interpret a diagnostic 12-lead ECG.

25. **What is the Duke treadmill score?**
This is a validated ECG treadmill score that was created at Duke University based on data from 2,758 patients who had chest pain and underwent EST and coronary angiography. The goal of the Duke treadmill score was to more effectively estimate the prognosis after EST. This treadmill score used three exercise-derived parameters:

$$
\text{Duke Treadmill Score} = \text{Exercise time in minutes (Bruce Protocol)} - 5 \times (\text{max ST segment deviation [mm]}) - 4 \times (\text{angina index } [0 = \text{none}, 1 = \text{nonlimiting}, 2 = \text{exercise limiting}])
$$

Patients can be stratified: a low risk score is +5 or greater, moderate risk scores range from +4 to −10, and a high risk score is −11 or less.

The treadmill score adds independent prognostic information to that provided by clinical information, left ventricular function, or coronary anatomy, and it can be used to identify patients in the moderate to high-risk group that may benefit from further risk stratification.

BIBLIOGRAPHY, SUGGESTED READINGS, AND WEBSITES

1. Gibbons RJ, Balady GJ, Bricker JT, et al: ACC/AHA 2002 guideline update for exercise testing. Summary article. A report of the American College of Cardiology/American Heart Association Task Force on Practice Guidelines, *Circulation* 106:1883–1892, 2002. Available at: http://circ.ahajournals.org/content/106/14/1883.full. Accessed March 26, 2013.

2. Lauer M, Froelicher ES, Williams M, Kligfield P: *AHA Scientific Statement: Exercise Testing in Asymptomatic Adults*, 2005. Available at: http://circ.ahajournals.org/content/112/5/771.full. Accessed March 26, 2013.

3. Hendel RC, Berman DS, Di Carli MF, et al: ACCF/ASNC/ACR/AHA/ASE/SCCT/SCMR/SNM 2009 Appropriate use criteria for cardiac radionuclide imaging. *J Am Coll Cardiol* 53(23):2201–2229, 2009.

4. Chou R, Arora B, Dana T, Fu R, Walker M, Humphrey L: Screening asymptomatic adults with resting or exercise electrocardiography: a review of the evidence for the U.S. Preventive Services Task Force. *Ann Intern Med* 155:375–385, 2011.

5. Miller TD: Stress Testing: the case for the standard treadmill test. *Curr Opin Cardiol* 26:363–369, 2011.

6. Lee TH, Boucher CH: Noninvasive tests in patients with stable coronary artery disease, *N Engl J Med* 344:1840–1845, 2001.

7. Arena R, Sietsema KE: Cardiopulmonary exercise testing in the clinical evaluation of patients with heart and lung disease. *Circulation* 123:668–680, 2011.

8. Chaitman BR: *Exercise stress testing*. In Bonow R, Mann DL, Zipes D, Libby P, editors: *Braunwald's heart disease: A textbook of cardiovascular medicine*, ed 9, Philadelphia, 2011, Saunders, pp 168–192.

9. Mayo Clinic Cardiovascular Working Group on Stress Testing: Cardiovascular stress testing: a description of the various types of stress tests and indications for their use. *Mayo Clinic Proc* 71:43–52, 1996.

CHAPTER 7

NUCLEAR CARDIOLOGY

Arunima Misra, MD, FACC

1. What is nuclear cardiology?

Nuclear cardiology is a field of cardiology that encompasses cardiac radionuclide imaging, which uses radioisotopes to assess myocardial perfusion or myocardial function in different clinical settings, as well as radionuclide angiography, metabolic and receptor imaging, and positron emission tomography.

2. What is myocardial perfusion imaging (MPI)?

MPI is a noninvasive method that uses radioisotopes to assess regional myocardial blood flow, function, and viability. The basis for MPI rests on the ability of this technique to demonstrate inhomogeneity of blood flow during stress compared with rest, thereby identifying ischemic or infarcted regions.

During the *stress* portion of the test, exercise or a pharmacologic agent is used to produce vasodilation in the coronary vascular bed. Whereas a normal vessel can vasodilate and increase coronary blood flow up to four times basal blood flow, a significantly diseased or stenosed vessel cannot increase blood flow. Because radiotracer uptake into the myocardium is dependent on blood flow, the areas that are supplied by normal vessels in which there is maximally increased blood flow will take up more radiotracer than areas supplied by the stenosed vessel with relatively less blood flow. Therefore, there will be heterogeneous radiotracer uptake, which will be seen as a perfusion defect.

3. Define a perfusion defect and differentiate between a reversible and fixed defect.

A *perfusion defect* is an area of reduced radiotracer uptake in the myocardium.

If the perfusion defect occurs during stress and improves or normalizes during rest, it is termed *reversible* (Fig. 7-1). Generally, a reversible perfusion defect suggests the presence of ischemia.

If the perfusion defect occurs during both stress and rest, it is termed a *fixed* defect. Generally, a fixed defect suggests the presence of scar. However, in certain settings a fixed defect may not be scar. Instead, a fixed defect may represent viable tissue that is hibernating due to chronic significant or severe stenosis. Hibernating myocardium alters its metabolism in order to conserve energy. Therefore, it appears underperfused and has hypokinetic or akinetic function.

4. What are the different uses of MPI?

- MPI is used to diagnose coronary artery disease (CAD) in patients with intermediate risk for CAD who present with chest pain or its equivalent.
- MPI can be used to localize and quantify perfusion abnormalities or physiologic ischemia in patients with known CAD.
- MPI can be used to assess the presence of viability in areas of fixed defects using rest and redistribution studies with thallium.
- MPI can also be used for risk assessment and determination of prognosis with regard to cardiovascular events. It can be used as a prognostic tool in post–myocardial infarction patients, including patients with and without ST elevation, to identify further areas of myocardium at risk.
- MPI can also be used in the preoperative assessment to identify perioperative or postoperative cardiovascular risk. The extent and severity of perfusion defects are proportional to the risk of perioperative cardiac events.

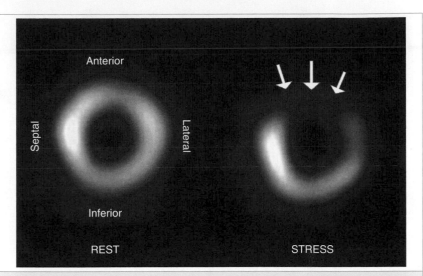

Figure 7-1. Nuclear stress testing short-axis view demonstrating a reversible perfusion defect. Normal myocardial perfusion occurred during resting images *(left panel)*, but a large anterior wall perfusion defect *(arrows)* was seen during previous stress imaging *(right panel)*. (Modified from Texas Heart Institute Website: Nuclear stress test. Available at http://www.texasheartinstitute.org/HIC/Topics/Diag/dinuc.cfm. Accessed March 22, 2013.)

5. **Is MPI the most sensitive and specific test for diagnosing CAD?**

   The ischemic cascade suggests that MPI would be a more sensitive test to detect ischemia because in the setting of ischemia, a perfusion abnormality occurs before a wall motion abnormality. The sensitivity of MPI is slightly better than stress echocardiography (85% versus 75%, respectively) and the specificity slightly worse (79% versus 88%). This results in similar accuracy for both types of stress tests. Both modalities are more sensitive and specific than treadmill or exercise electrocardiography testing, although according to the American Heart Association/American College of Cardiology (AHA/ACC) guidelines, the latter should be the first-line test for the diagnosis of CAD in someone who can exercise and has a relatively normal electrocardiogram (ECG).

6. **List the different perfusion agents used in MPI.**

   For an agent to be an effective radiopharmaceutical, its distribution has to be proportional to regional blood flow, have a high level of extraction by the organ of interest, and have rapid clearance from the blood. The two most important physiologic factors that affect myocardial uptake of a radiotracer are variations in regional blood flow and the myocardial extraction of the radiotracer. In other words, there will be more uptake of a radiotracer in areas of increased blood flow and less in areas supplied by diseased or stenosed vessels. Importantly, because myocardial extraction is an active process with regard to thallium-201 and a mitochondrial-dependent process with regard to the technetium-99m agents, it can only occur if the cells in that region are viable. The relative advantages and disadvantages of thallium-201 and technitium-99 are summarized in Table 7-1.

   - **Thallium-201** (TI-201) is a potassium analog used for MPI. It is the oldest and best studied of the present-day agents. Thallium distribution is dependent on blood flow and tracer extraction by the myocardium. It enters the myocardium by active transport of membrane-bound Na^+,K^+-ATPase. One of the most important characteristics of TI-201 is its myocardial redistribution. A dynamic quality to the uptake of TI-201 gives it the ability to redistribute over time. There is continued influx of TI-201 over time from the blood-pool activity and a clearance or washout from the myocardium. This phenomenon results in normalization or reversibility in areas that are ischemic, and over additional time, improvement or normalization can occur in areas that are viable but appeared as scar during the first rest imaging.

TABLE 7-1. RELATIVE ADVANTAGES OF TC-99M AND TL-201 IN NUCLEAR CARDIOLOGY STRESS TESTING

Advantages of Tc-99m Compared with Tl-201	Advantages of Tl-201 Compared with Tc-99m
■ Shorter half-life allows for higher dose, resulting in better count statistics ■ Less radiation exposure ■ Less attenuation effects ■ Higher energy level allows for improved resolution with gamma camera, especially in gated SPECT studies ■ Faster imaging protocols due to reinjection	■ Redistribution allows for single-injection studies and viability assessment ■ Less expensive ■ Less abdominal and hepatic uptake during exercise ■ Diagnostic and prognostic value of lung uptake of Tl-201

SPECT, Single-photon emission computed tomography.

■ **Technetium-99m** (Tc-99m) comprises many radiotracers. Some agents include Tc-99m sestamibi, Tc-99m teboroxime (not used clinically at present), Tc-99m tetrofosmin, and Tc-99m N-NOET.

■ **Tc-99m sestamibi** or Tc-99m MIBI (Cardiolite) is the third of the isonitriles to be developed but the first of the Tc-99m agents to be approved for commercial use. It contains a hydrophilic cation and the isonitrile hydrophobic portion that allows for the necessary interactions with the cell membrane for uptake into the myocardium. The uptake of MIBI is dependent on mitochondrial-derived membrane electrochemical gradient, cellular pH, and intact energy production. Unlike Tl-201, Tc-99m MIBI does not possess a strong redistribution quality. The reason for this is that the clearance of MIBI is slow even though continued uptake occurs during the rest phase of a study. Therefore, there may be some improvement in 2 to 3 hours between stress and rest, but the degree of redistribution is slower and less complete than Tl-201. Importantly, however, only viable tissue can extract and uptake MIBI.

■ **Tc-99m tetrofosmin** (Myoview) is the newest of the Tc-99m agents to be approved for clinical use. Its properties are similar to Tc-99m MIBI, although the mechanism by which myocardial uptake occurs is not well elucidated; however, uptake is dependent on intact mitochondrial potentials (i.e., viable cells). Studies show similar characteristics to MIBI, with a more rapid clearance from the liver allowing for faster imaging times.

■ **Tc-99m furifosmin** is similar to Tc-99m tetrofosmin but is not currently approved for clinical use.

■ **Tc-99m N-NOET** is an investigational agent that has similar physical and imaging properties to that of other Tc-99m agents but also favorable redistribution qualities similar to Tl-201. For reasons that are unclear, it was never approved for use.

7. **How is stress produced for MPI in the evaluation of CAD?**
   Stress can be produced in different ways. The goal of MPI is to produce vasodilation in order to assess the presence of diseased or stenosed vessels, which will vasodilate to a lesser extent than healthy, non-stenosed vessels. Forms of stress are either exercise or pharmacologic (Table 7-2).
   ■ Exercise can include treadmill, supine or erect bicycle, dynamic arm, or isometric handgrip. In general, because of its diagnostic and prognostic value, the treadmill is used most often. Functional capacity can also be determined during treadmill exercise testing. In addition, prognosis for cardiac events can be determined using the Duke treadmill score when using the Bruce protocol. Exercise increases myocardial blood flow and metabolic demand.

TABLE 7-2. THE STRESS AGENTS USED FOR MYOCARDIAL PERFUSION IMAGING, AND THEIR INDICATIONS, CONTRAINDICATIONS, ADVANTAGES AND DISADVANTAGES

STRESS AGENTS FOR MPI

	Indications	Contraindications	Pros	Cons
Exercise	Diagnose CAD, assess risk for those who can exercise, but whose ECG is abnormal	Can't exercise, have LBBB on ECG, or comorbid condition such as severe AS, CHF (see guidelines)	Assess functional status (FS) as well as diagnosis and prognosis for CAD	None
Adenosine	Diagnose CAD, assess risk for those who can't exercise	Bronchospastic COPD or asthma, heart block, hypotension	Produces excellent vasodilation greater to that of exercise	Cannot assess FS
Dipyridamole	Diagnose CAD, assess risk for those who can't exercise	Bronchospastic COPD or asthma, heart block, hypotension	Produces excellent vasodilation greater to that of exercise	Cannot assess FS
Regadenoson	Diagnose CAD, assess risk for those who can't exercise	Bronchospastic COPD or asthma, heart block, hypotension	Produces excellent vasodilation equal to that of exercise	Cannot assess FS
Dobutamine	Diagnose CAD, assess risk for those who can't exercise	Tachyarrhythmias, uncontrolled hypertension, AS (similar to those for exercise)	Reserved for those who need pharmacologic MPI but who have bronchospastic disease	Does not produce good vasodilation and cannot assess FS

AS, Aortic stenosis; *CAD*, coronary artery disease; *CHF*, congestive heart failure; *COPD*, chromic obstructive pulmonary disease; *ECG*, electrocardiogram; *FS*, functional status; *LBBB*, left bundle branch block; *MPI*, myocardial perfusion imaging.

- Pharmacologic agents include dobutamine, dipyridamole, adenosine, and regadenoson. Dobutamine is a β_1-adrenoceptor agonist that increases heart rate and contractility and thereby produces an indirect increase in myocardial blood flow as a result of increased metabolic demand. This agent is used for nuclear stress MPI when vasodilators are contraindicated, such as in bronchospastic lung disease or bradycardia and heart block.
- Dipyridamole, adenosine, and regadenoson are all vasodilators. They purely produce vasodilation by acting on the adenosine receptors. Dipyridamole does this by increasing the endogenous levels of adenosine by preventing its breakdown, whereas adenosine and regadenoson are given exogenously to increase levels. The differences between adenosine and regadenoson are multiple but the biggest difference is that the regadenoson is a specific A_{2A} adenosine receptor agent rather than a nonspecific agent like adenosine. They do not affect myocardial metabolic demand.

TABLE 7-3. RADIATION EXPOSURE FROM VARIOUS STUDIES	
PA chest film	0.02 mSv
Background radiation	3 mSv
Coronary catheterization	5 mSv
CT angiography	10-14 mSv
CT coronary angiography 64 slice	17 mSv
CT of the body	20-40 mSv
Tc-99m MIBI (10 mCi [rest]/27.5 mCi [stress])	14.6 mSv
Tl-201 (3.5 mCi)	29 mSv
Calcium scoring	2.6 mSv

CT, Computed tomography, *mCi,* millicurie; *MIBI,* methoxyisobutylisonitrile; *mSv,* millisievert; *PA,* posteroanterior.

8. **How much radiation exposure does a patient get from a typical MPI study? How does it compare to other cardiac studies?**
   It depends on the radiotracer used and the protocol. Exposure can vary from about 10 mSv to upwards of 30 mSv. Table 7-3 summarizes radiation exposure from various tests.

9. **Is it possible to assess both myocardial perfusion and left ventricular (LV) function with one study?**
   Yes. Both Tc-99m agents and Tl-201 have been validated in assessing LV volumes and left ventricular ejection fraction (LVEF) using gated single-photon emission computed tomography (SPECT) imaging. Thus, one can gate stress and rest portions of the MPI when using gated SPECT technology. Gating is a method of stopping cardiac motion that allows for the assessment of the different phases of the cardiac cycle. This triggering of the imaging camera at the onset of the R wave over multiple cardiac cycles provides an 8- or 16-frame average of multiple cardiac beats, which are needed to accurately assess wall motion and thickening. Gated studies improve specificity by helping to differentiate fixed defects caused by attenuation versus scar.

10. **Functional assessment of cardiac performance is determined using which nuclear cardiology techniques?**
    The term *radionuclide angiography* encompasses both the first-pass bolus technique and gated equilibrium blood pool imaging, both of which can be used to assess LV function.
    - First-pass radionuclide angiography (FPRNA) uses a bolus technique and rapid acquisition to track the tracer bolus through the right atrium, right ventricle, pulmonary arteries, lungs, left atrium, left ventricle, and finally aorta. The first-pass technique can be used to assess both left and right ventricular ejection fraction, regional wall motion, and cardiopulmonary shunts. FPRNA can be done both at rest and during exercise.
    - Gated equilibrium blood pool imaging or multiple gated acquisition (MUGA) can also be used to assess left ventricular function and ejection fraction. The right ventricle is not easily assessed with this technique because of overlap of cardiac structures but can be done if care is taken in imaging. The technique is performed after a sample of the patient's red blood cells is labeled with Tc-99m sodium pertechnetate and then reinjected for planar imaging in three different views. The gating is done similarly to SPECT gating; however, instead of a standard number of frames per cardiac cycle, there can be a variable number, depending on the R-to-R cycle length or heart rate. The cardiac images are then compiled into summed images. They are then processed and displayed as a continuous cinematic loop. From the cinematic loop, one can assess wall motion

in the different views, including left anterior oblique (LAO), lateral, and anterior. The data from the LAO view is also displayed as still images so that the counts in the region of interest (the left ventricle) at end-systole and end-diastole can be used to calculate the end-diastolic volume (EDV) and end-systolic volume (ESV) and subsequently the ejection fraction.

$$LVEF = \frac{(EDV - \text{background counts}) - (EDV - \text{background counts})}{(EDV - \text{background counts})}$$

Importantly, this technique can be done both at rest and during stress to give accurate volumetric information for comparison.

11. Why should one use radionuclide angiography to assess LVEF?

- It is a precise and accurate measure of LVEF that is more reproducible than standard two-dimensional echocardiography, especially when doing serial studies to look for changes in LVEF caused by cardiotoxic agents, valvular heart disease, and new therapeutic agents in clinical trials.
- It is less expensive and more feasible than magnetic resonance imaging for evaluation of LVEF.
- On a more practical level, radionuclide angiography can be used to assess LVEF when other methods are not possible because of poor images as a result of body habitus, lung disease, or chest wall deformities.
- LVEF is an independent predictor of cardiac events and thus serves as a valid prognostic index in many clinical settings.

BIBLIOGRAPHY, SUGGESTED READINGS, AND WEBSITES

1. Baghdasarian SB, Heller GV: The role of myocardial perfusion imaging in the diagnosis of patients with coronary artery disease: developments over the past year, *Curr Opin Cardiol* 20:369–374, 2005.

2. Berman DS, Shaw LJ, Hachamovitch R, et al: Comparative use of radionuclide stress testing, coronary artery calcium scanning, and noninvasive coronary angiography for diagnostic and prognostic cardiac assessment, *Semin Nucl Med* 37:2–16, 2007.

3. Bourque JM, Velasquez EJ, Tuttle RJ, et al: Mortality risk associated with ejection fraction differs across resting nuclear perfusion findings, *J Nucl Cardiol* 14:165–173, 2007.

4. Brindis RG, Douglas PS, Hendel RC, et al: ACCF/ASNC appropriateness criteria for single-photon emission computed tomography myocardial perfusion imaging (SPECT MPI), *J Am Cardiol* 51:1127–1147, 2005.

5. Hachamovitch R, Berman DS: The use of nuclear cardiology in clinical decision making, *Semin Nucl Med* 35:62–72, 2005.

6. Hachamovitch R, Hayes SW, Friedman JD, et al: Comparison of the short-term survival benefit associated with revascularization compared with medical therapy in patients with no prior coronary artery disease undergoing stress myocardial perfusion single photon emission computed tomography, *Circulation* 107:2900–2906, 2003.

7. Iskanderian AE, Verani MS: *Nuclear cardiac imaging principles and applications*, ed 3, New York, 2003, Oxford University Press.

8. Klocke FJ, Baird MG, Bateman TM, et al: ACC/AHA/ASNC guidelines for the clinical use of cardiac radionuclide imaging, *J Am Cardiol* 42:1318–1333, 2003.

9. Metz LD, Beattie M, Hom R, et al: The prognostic value of normal exercise myocardial perfusion imaging and exercise echocardiography, *J Am Coll Cardiol* 49:227–237, 2007.

10. Miller TD, Redberg RF, Wackers FJT: Screening asymptomatic diabetic patients for coronary artery disease, why not, *J Am Coll Cardiol* 48:761–764, 2006.

11. Shaw LJ, Berman DS, Maron DJ, et al: Optimal medical therapy with or without percutaneous coronary intervention to reduce ischemic burden: results from the Clinical Outcomes Utilizing Revascularization and Aggressive Drug Evaluation (COURAGE) trial nuclear substudy, *Circulation* 117:1283–1291, 2008.

12. Travin MI, Bergman SR: Assessment of myocardial viability, *Semin Nucl Med* 35:2–16, 2005.

CHAPTER 8

HOLTER MONITORS, EVENT MONITORS, AMBULATORY MONITORS, AND IMPLANTABLE LOOP RECORDERS

Nitin Mathur, MD, Ryan Seutter, MD and Glenn N. Levine, MD, FACC, FAHA

1. **What are the major indications for ambulatory electrocardiography (AECG) monitoring?**
   AECG monitoring allows the noninvasive evaluation of a suspected arrhythmia during normal daily activities. It aids in the diagnosis, documentation of frequency, severity, and correlation of an arrhythmia with symptoms such as palpitations, lightheadedness, or overt syncope. AECG monitoring can be extremely helpful in excluding an arrhythmia as a cause for a patient's symptoms if there is no associated event during monitoring. AECG can also be used to assess antiarrhythmic drug response in patients with defined arrhythmias. Occasionally AECG is also used in other situations. The current major indications for AECG monitoring, from the American College of Cardiology/American Heart Association (ACC/AHA), are given in Box 8-1.

Box 8-1. SUMMARY OF THE AMERICAN COLLEGE OF CARDIOLOGY/AMERICAN HEART ASSOCIATION GUIDELINES FOR AMBULATORY ELECTROCARDIOGRAPHY

Class I (Recommended)
- Patients with unexplained syncope, near syncope, or episodic dizziness in whom the cause is not obvious
- Patients with unexplained recurrent palpitations
- To assess antiarrhythmic drug response in individuals with well-characterized arrhythmias
- To aid in the evaluation of pacemaker and implantable cardioverter defibrillator (ICD) function and guide pharmacologic therapy in patients receiving frequent ICD therapy

Class IIa (Weight of Evidence/Opinion Is in Favor of Usefulness/Efficacy)
- To detect proarrhythmic responses in patients receiving antiarrhythmic therapy
- Patients with suspected variant angina

Class IIb (Usefulness/Efficacy Is Less Well Established by Evidence/Opinion)
- Patients with episodic shortness of breath, chest pain, or fatigue that is not otherwise explained
- Patients with symptoms such as syncope, near syncope, episodic dizziness, or palpitation in whom a probable cause other than an arrhythmia has been identified but in whom symptoms persist despite treatment
- To assess rate control during atrial fibrillation
- Evaluation of patients with chest pain who cannot exercise
- Preoperative evaluation for vascular surgery of patients who cannot exercise
- Patients with known coronary artery disease and atypical chest pain syndrome
- To assess risk in asymptomatic patients who have heart failure or idiopathic hypertrophic cardiomyopathy or in post–myocardial infarction patients with ejection fraction less than 40%
- Patients with neurologic events, when transient atrial fibrillation or flutter is suspected

---

2. What are the different types of AECG monitoring available?

The major types of AECG monitoring include Holter monitors, event monitors, ambulatory telemetry, and implantable loop recorders (ILRs). The type and duration of monitoring is dependent on the frequency and severity of symptoms. Most modern devices have the capability for telephonic transmission of electrocardiography (ECG) data during or after a detected arrhythmia. Each system has advantages and disadvantages; selection must be tailored to the individual. With any system, however, patients must record in some fashion (e.g., diary, electronically) symptoms and activities during the monitored period.

- A *Holter monitor* constantly monitors and records two to three channels of ECG data for 24 to 48 hours. It is ideal for patients with episodes that occur daily.
- An *event monitor* constantly monitors two to three channels of ECG data for 30 to 60 days. However, it will only record events when the patient experiences a symptom and presses a button that triggers the event monitor to store ECG data 1 to 4 minutes before and 1 to 2 minutes after the event. Some event monitors will also store arrhythmias that are detected by the monitor itself, based on preprogrammed parameters. An event monitor is appropriate for patients with episodes that occur weekly or monthly.
- *Ambulatory real-time cardiac monitoring* has various monikers. it has been termed *ambulatory telemetry*, *real-time continuous cardiac monitoring*, or *mobile cardiac outpatient telemetry* (MCOT). Ambulatory telemetry is a monitoring system that continuously records a 1- to 3-lead strip for 14 to 30 days. Depending on the vendor, the ECG data is either stored for offline

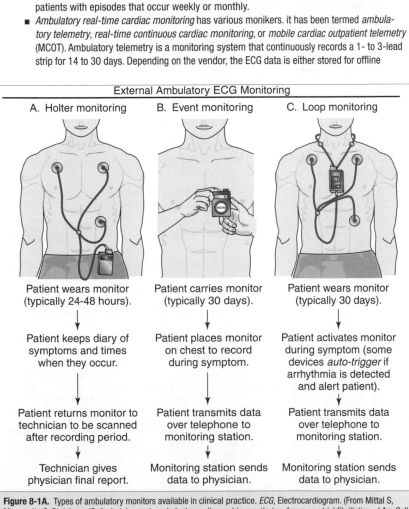

External Ambulatory ECG Monitoring

A. Holter monitoring	B. Event monitoring	C. Loop monitoring

Patient wears monitor (typically 24-48 hours). → Patient carries monitor (typically 30 days). → Patient wears monitor (typically 30 days).

Patient keeps diary of symptoms and times when they occur. → Patient places monitor on chest to record during symptom. → Patient activates monitor during symptom (some devices *auto-trigger* if arrhythmia is detected and alert patient).

Patient returns monitor to technician to be scanned after recording period. → Patient transmits data over telephone to monitoring station. → Patient transmits data over telephone to monitoring station.

Technician gives physician final report. → Monitoring station sends data to physician. → Monitoring station sends data to physician.

Figure 8-1A. Types of ambulatory monitors available in clinical practice. *ECG,* Electrocardiogram. (From Mittal S, Movsowitz C, Steinberg JS: Ambulatory external electrocardiographic monitoring: focus on atrial fibrillation, *J Am Coll Cardiol* 58:1741-1749, 2011.)

interpretation or instantaneously transmitted for interpretation by a monitoring technician. In cases where the rhythm is monitored by a technician in real time, the patient or physician can be contacted immediately after an arrhythmia has been detected, to minimize delays in treatment. No patient action is necessary for an arrhythmia to be stored, and patient compliance can easily be assessed. These features facilitate the detection of silent or asymptomatic arrhythmias.

■ An *implantable loop recorder* (ILR) is an invasive monitoring device allowing long-term monitoring and recording of a single ECG channel for over a year. It records events similarly to an event monitor, based on patient's symptoms or automatically based on heart rate. It is best reserved for patients with more infrequent episodes occurring greater than 1 month apart from each other.

3. **How does an ILR work?**

An ILR is surgically placed subcutaneously below the left shoulder. As discussed earlier, it can continuously monitor bipolar ECG signals for more than 1 year. The patient may use a magnetic activator held over the device to signal an event at the time of symptoms. In addition, the device automatically records episodes of bradycardia and tachycardia (Figs. 8-1A and 8-1B). The device is

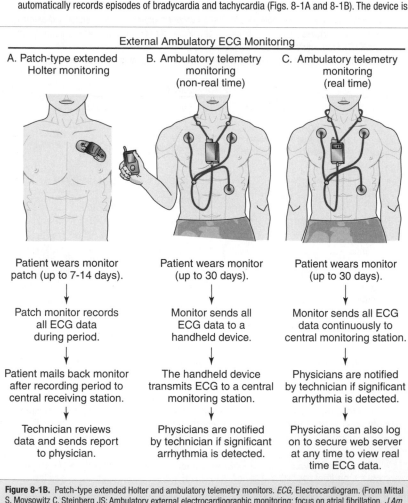

External Ambulatory ECG Monitoring

A. Patch-type extended Holter monitoring	B. Ambulatory telemetry monitoring (non-real time)	C. Ambulatory telemetry monitoring (real time)
Patient wears monitor patch (up to 7-14 days).	Patient wears monitor (up to 30 days).	Patient wears monitor (up to 30 days).
↓	↓	↓
Patch monitor records all ECG data during period.	Monitor sends all ECG data to a handheld device.	Monitor sends all ECG data continuously to central monitoring station.
↓	↓	↓
Patient mails back monitor after recording period to central receiving station.	The handheld device transmits ECG to a central monitoring station.	Physicians are notified by technician if significant arrhythmia is detected.
↓	↓	↓
Technician reviews data and sends report to physician.	Physicians are notified by technician if significant arrhythmia is detected.	Physicians can also log on to secure web server at any time to view real time ECG data.

Figure 8-1B. Patch-type extended Holter and ambulatory telemetry monitors. *ECG,* Electrocardiogram. (From Mittal S, Movsowitz C, Steinberg JS: Ambulatory external electrocardiographic monitoring: focus on atrial fibrillation, *J Am Coll Cardiol* 58:1741-1749, 2011.)

then interrogated with an external programmer, and recorded events are reviewed (Fig. 8-2) as with a permanent pacemaker. After a diagnosis is obtained, the device is surgically extracted. In patients with unexplained syncope, an ILR yields a diagnosis in more than 90% of patients after 1 year.

4. **Do patients with a pacemaker or implantable cardioverter-defibrillators (ICDs) require Holter monitors for detecting atrial arrhythmias?**
   In certain situations, a pacemaker or ICD can be programmed to detect and store arrhythmia data. The number and type of arrhythmias detected depends on the number of leads, device type and programming, as well as manufacturing specifications. In most cases, dual-chamber pacemakers and ICDs can be programmed to continuously monitor and record supraventricular arrhythmias. Detected arrhythmias can be reviewed upon device interrogation.

5. **Is every "abnormality" detected during monitoring a cause for concern?**
   It is not uncommon to identify several arrhythmias that are not necessarily pathological during AECG monitoring. These include sinus bradycardia during rest or sleep, sinus arrhythmia with pauses less than 3 seconds, sinoatrial exit block, Wenckebach atrioventricular (AV) block (type I second-degree AV block), wandering atrial pacemaker, junctional escape complexes, and premature atrial or ventricular complexes.

   In contrast, often of concern are frequent and complex atrial and ventricular rhythm disturbances that are less commonly observed in normal subjects, including second-degree AV block type II, third-degree AV block, sinus pauses longer than 3 seconds, marked bradycardia during waking hours, and tachyarrhythmias (Fig. 8-3). One of the most important factors for any documented arrhythmia is the correlation with symptoms. In some situations, even some "benign" rhythms may warrant treatment if there are associated symptoms.

6. **What is the diagnostic yield of Holter monitors, event monitors, and ILRs in palpitations and syncope?**
   Choosing a Holter monitor, an event monitor, or an ILR depends on the frequency of symptoms. In patients with palpitations, the highest diagnostic yield occurred in the first week, with 80% of patients receiving a diagnosis. During the next 3 weeks, only an additional 3.4% of patients receive a diagnosis. In patients with recurrent but infrequent palpitations (less than one episode per month lasting less than 1 minute), ILR resulted in a diagnosis in 73% of patients. In contrast to palpitations, syncope usually requires a longer monitoring period to achieve a diagnosis, with the highest yield coming from the implantation of an ILR (Fig. 8-4).

7. **How often are ventricular arrhythmias identified in apparently healthy subjects during AECG monitoring?**
   Ventricular arrhythmias are found in 40% to 75% of normal persons as assessed by 24- to 48-hour Holter monitors. The incidence and frequency of ventricular ectopy increases with age, but this has no impact on long-term prognosis in apparently healthy subjects.

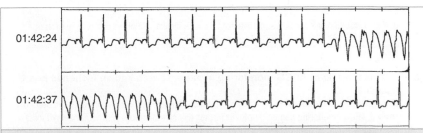

01:42:24

01:42:37

Figure 8-2. Representative printout from an implantable loop recorder demonstrating a run of nonsustained ventricular tachycardia.

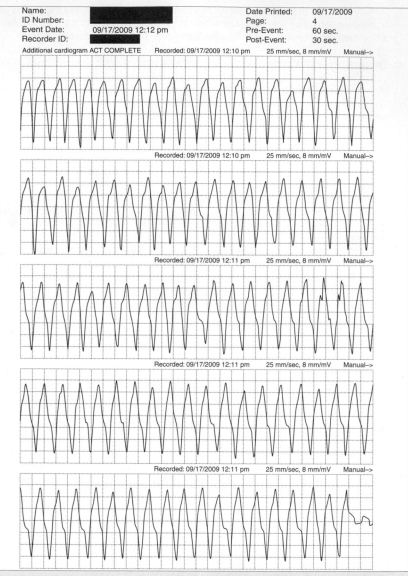

Name:		Date Printed:	09/17/2009
ID Number:		Page:	4
Event Date:	09/17/2009 12:12 pm	Pre-Event:	60 sec.
Recorder ID:		Post-Event:	30 sec.

Additional cardiogram ACT COMPLETE   Recorded: 09/17/2009 12:10 pm   25 mm/sec, 8 mm/mV   Manual–>

Recorded: 09/17/2009 12:10 pm   25 mm/sec, 8 mm/mV   Manual–>

Recorded: 09/17/2009 12:11 pm   25 mm/sec, 8 mm/mV   Manual–>

Recorded: 09/17/2009 12:11 pm   25 mm/sec, 8 mm/mV   Manual–>

Recorded: 09/17/2009 12:11 pm   25 mm/sec, 8 mm/mV   Manual–>

Figure 8-3. Sustained ventricular tachycardia detected by a Holter monitor in a patient with daily episodes of palpitations and lightheadedness.

8. **What is the role of AECG monitoring in patients with known ischemic heart disease?**

Although ejection fraction after myocardial infarction (MI) is one of the strongest predictors of survival, AECG monitoring can be helpful in further risk stratification. Ventricular arrhythmias occur in 2% to 5% of patients after transmural infarction in long-term follow-up. In the post-MI patient, the occurrence of frequent premature ventricular contractions (PVCs) (more than 10 per hour) and nonsustained ventricular tachycardia (VT) by 24-hour monitoring is associated with a

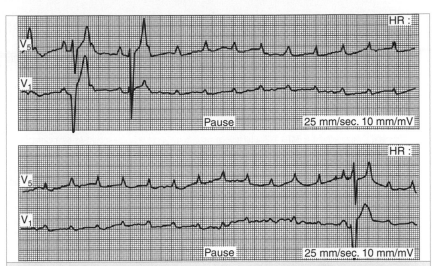

Figure 8-4. Ambulatory monitor tracing in an elderly patient with intermittent syncope. The tracing shows complete heart block with a 9-second pause. (From Jaeger FJ: Cardiac arrhythmias. In: Cleveland Clinic: *Current clinical medicine*, ed 2, Philadelphia, 2010, Saunders, Philadelphia, pp 114-128.)

1.5- to 2.0-fold increase in death during the 2- to 5-year follow-up, independent of left ventricular (LV) function.

9. **Can Holter monitors assist in the diagnosis of suspected ischemic heart disease?**
   Yes. Transient ST-segment depressions 0.1 mV or greater for more than 30 seconds are rare in normal subjects and correlate strongly with myocardial perfusion scans that show regional ischemia.

10. **What have Holter monitors demonstrated about angina and its pattern of occurrence?**
    Holter monitoring has shown that the majority of ischemic episodes that occur during normal daily activities are silent (asymptomatic) and that symptomatic and silent episodes of ST-segment depression exhibit a circadian rhythm, with ischemic ST changes more common in the morning. Studies also have shown that nocturnal ST-segment changes are a strong indicator of significant coronary artery disease.

11. **What is a signal-averaged ECG?**
    A *signal-averaged ECG* (SAECG) is a unique type of ECG initially developed to identify patients at risk for sudden cardiac death and complex ventricular arrhythmias. In patients susceptible to VT and ventricular fibrillation (VF), there can be slowing of electrical potentials through diseased myocardium, resulting in small, delayed electrical signals (late potentials) not easily visible on a normal ECG. Through the use of amplification and computerized signal averaging, these microvolt late potentials can be visualized on a SAECG and potentially assist in risk-stratifying patients susceptible to certain arrhythmias.

12. **When should a signal-averaged ECG be considered?**
    The use of SAECG to identify late potentials and those post-MI patients at greatest risk for sudden death has been extensively evaluated. Although an association exists between late potentials and increased risk of ventricular arrhythmias after MI, the positive predictive value of SAECG is low. In the Coronary Artery Bypass Graft (CABG) Patch Trial, patients with an abnormal SAECG and depressed

ejection fraction who were to undergo cardiac surgery were randomized to ICD implantation or no implantation and then followed for an average of 32 months. The study could detect no benefit for ICD implantation in this patient population with abnormal SAECGs. A study of SAECG use in patients treated with reperfusion, mainly primary percutaneous coronary intervention (PCI), did not find SAECG to be a useful risk stratification tool in this patient population. In current practice, the test is rarely used for risk stratification.

13. **What is microvolt T-wave alternans and does it predict outcomes in certain patients?**
Microvolt T-wave alternans (MTWA) is a technique used to measure very small beat-to-beat variability in T-wave voltage not generally detectable on a standard ECG. Significant MTWA changes are associated with increased risk of sudden cardiac death and complex ventricular arrhythmias. The benefit of MTWA for risk stratification is greatest in patients with a history of coronary artery disease and reduced ejection fraction. A positive MTWA test predicts nearly a fourfold risk of ventricular arrhythmias compared with MTWA-negative patients. The ACC/AHA/European Society of Cardiology (ESC) guidelines on ventricular arrhythmias and prevention of sudden cardiac death state that it is reasonable to use T-wave alternans for improving the diagnosis and risk stratification of patients with ventricular arrhythmias or who are at risk for developing life-threatening ventricular arrhythmias (class IIa; level of evidence A).

14. **Does heart-rate variability have predictive value in certain patients?**
Diminished heart-rate variability is an independent predictor of increased mortality after MI and results from decreased beat-to-beat vagal modulation of heart rate. The predictive value of heart-rate variability is low after MI. It is recommend by the ACC as a class IIb recommendation to assess risk for future events in asymptomatic patients who:
- Are post-MI with LV dysfunction
- Have heart failure
- Have idiopathic hypertrophic cardiomyopathy

15. **What is the role of ambulatory monitoring in stroke?**
Approximately 25% of stroke remains unexplained after a thorough clinical evaluation and is labeled as cryptogenic. Asymptomatic paroxysmal atrial fibrillation may not occur during telemetry monitoring during hospitalization. Occult atrial fibrillation is identified by ambulatory monitoring in approximately 6% to 8% of patients with cryptogenic stroke in whom atrial fibrillation is not detected during their hospitalization.

BIBLIOGRAPHY, SUGGESTED READINGS, AND WEBSITES

1. American College of Cardiology: Signal-averaged electrocardiography: ACC Expert Consensus Document, *J Am Coll Cardiol* 27:238–249, 1996.

2. Assar MD, Krahn AD, Klein GJ, et al: Optimal duration of monitoring in patients with unexplained syncope, *Am J Cardiol* 92:1231–1233, 2003.

3. Bass EB, Curtiss EI, Arena VC, et al: The duration of Holter monitoring in patients with syncope: is 24 hours enough? *Arch Intern Med* 50:1073–1078, 1990.

4. Bigger TJ Jr: Prophylactic use of implanted cardiac defibrillators in patients at high risk for ventricular arrhythmias after coronary-artery bypass graft surgery. Coronary Artery Bypass Graft (CABG) Patch Trial investigators, *N Engl J Med* 337:1569–1575, 1997.

5. Chow T, Kereiakes DJ, Bartone C, et al: Microvolt T-wave alternans identifies patients with ischemic cardiomyopathy who benefit from implantable cardioverter-defibrillator therapy, *J Am Coll Cardiol* 49:50–58, 2007.

6. Crawford MH, Bernstein SJ, Deedwania PC, et al: ACC/AHA guidelines for ambulatory electrocardiography: executive summary and recommendations: a report of the American College of Cardiology/American Heart Association Task Force on Practice Guidelines (Committee to Revise the Guidelines for Ambulatory Electrocardiography), *J Am Coll Cardiol* 34:912–948, 1999.

7. Dixit S, Marchlinski FE: Role of continuous monitoring for optimizing management strategies in patients with early arrhythmia recurrences after atrial fibrillation ablation, *Circ Arrhythm Electrophysiol* 4:791–793, 2011.

8. Epstein AE, Hallstrom AP, Rogers WJ, et al: Mortality following ventricular arrhythmia suppression by encainide, flecainide, and moricizine after myocardial infarction. The original design concept of the Cardiac Arrhythmia Suppression Trial (CAST), *JAMA* 270(20):2451–2455, 1993.

9. Kadish AH, Reiffel JA, Clauser J, et al: Frequency of serious arrhythmias detected with ambulatory cardiac telemetry, *Am J Cardiol* 105(9):1313–1316, 2010.

10. Kennedy HL, Whitlock JA, Sprague MK, et al: Long-term follow-up of asymptomatic healthy subjects with frequent and complex ventricular ectopy, *N Engl J Med* 312:193–197, 1985.

11. Maggioni AP, Zuanetti G, Franzosi MG, et al: Prevalence and prognostic significance of ventricular arrhythmias after acute myocardial infarction in the fibrinolytic era. GISSI-2 results, *Circulation* 87:312–322, 1993.

12. Mittal S, Movsowitz C, Steinberg JS: Ambulatory external electrocardiographic monitoring: focus on atrial fibrillation, *J Am Coll Cardiol* 58:1741–1749, 2011.

13. Narayan SM: T-Wave (Repolarization) Alternans: Clinical Aspects. In Basow, DS, editor: UpToDate, Waltham, MA, 2013, UpToDate. Available at: http://www.uptodate.com/contents/t-wave-repolarization-alternans-clinical-aspects. Accessed March 26, 2013.

14. Narayan SM, Cain ME: Clinical Applications of the Signal-Averaged Electrocardiogram: Overview. In Basow, DS, editor: UpToDate, Waltham, MA, 2013, UpToDate. Available at: http://www.uptodate.com/contents/clinical-applications-of-the-signal-averaged-electrocardiogram-overview. Accessed March 26, 2013.

15. Zeldis SM, Levine BJ, Michaelson EL, et al: Cardiovascular complaint. Correlation with cardiac arrhythmias on 24 hour electrocardiographic monitoring, *Chest* 78:456–461, 1980.

16. Zimetbaum P, Goldman A: Ambulatory arrhythmia monitoring: choosing the right device, *Circulation* 122:1629–1636, 2010.

17. Zipes DP, Camm AJ, Borggrefe M, et al: ACC/AHA/ESC 2006 guidelines for management of patients with ventricular arrhythmias and the prevention of sudden cardiac death, *J Am Coll Cardiol* 48:1064–1108, 2006.

CHAPTER 9

CARDIAC CT ANGIOGRAPHY

Rishi Agrawal, MD, and Suhny Abbara, MD

1. **What are the contraindications for cardiac computed tomography (CT)?**
   An inability to remain still, breath-hold, or follow instructions are contraindications to coronary computed tomographic angiography (CTA). Anaphylactic reaction to intravenous iodinated contrast agents is considered an absolute contraindication, though less severe allergic reactions may be acceptable if the patient has been adequately premedicated, usually with a combination of intravenous or oral diphenhydramine and corticosteroids.

2. **What is the difference between prospective triggering and retrospective gating?**
   Prospective triggering is an axial (step-and-shoot) image technique that acquires images of the heart in a predetermined phase of the cardiac cycle, for example 60% to 80% of the R-R interval. During the remainder of the cardiac cycle, the CT tube current is turned off. This is in contrast to retrospective gating, which is a spiral acquisition where the CT tube current remains on during the entire R-R interval. To reduce radiation, the tube current may be decreased during systole (electrocardiography [ECG] tube current modulation). However, there is a significant reduction in radiation dose when using prospective triggering (Fig. 9-1).

3. **When might retrospective gating be used rather than prospective triggering?**
   Retrospective gating is needed when cardiac function measurements are needed. Because images are acquired throughout the cardiac cycle, volume measurements of the right and left ventricles can

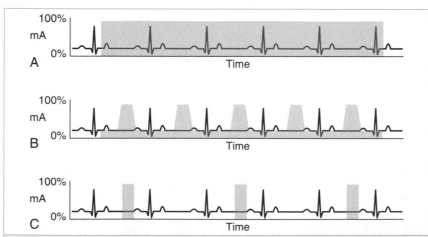

Figure 9-1. Schematic drawings of retrospective gating **(A, B)** and prospective triggering **(C)** techniques. Retrospective gating without tube current modulation **(A)** uses full tube current throughout the duration of the cardiac cycle. With tube current modulation applied **(B)**, the full current is only delivered during a specified portion of the R-R interval (usually late diastole). In this case, the remainder of the cardiac cycle receives only 20% of the full tube current. Prospective triggering **(C)** only uses full tube current through a specified portion of the R-R interval. Every other heartbeat is imaged in prospective triggering to allow time for table movement.

be obtained in end-systole and end-diastole, allowing the calculation of stroke volume, ejection fraction, and cardiac output. Retrospective gating is also helpful in patients with irregular heart rhythm to help ensure diagnostic images of the coronary arteries are acquired. In contrast to prospective triggering, retrospective gating allows the user to employ ECG editing to remove artifacts related to premature ventricular contractions or dropped beats.

4. **What is the radiation dose of a standard cardiac CT examination?**
The radiation dose of a standard cardiac CTA depends on a multitude of factors and can range from less than 1 mSv to as high as 30 mSv with older high dose techniques and scanners. The median dose in an older registry study showed the cardiac CT dose to be just less than 10 mSv; however, since that time, there has been development of several new scanners and associated hardware, as well as new dose reduction strategies. At several hospitals (such as Massachusetts General Hospital), the median reported dose ranges from 3 to 5 mSv. To put things in perspective, the average dose from a nuclear perfusion stress test is 6 to 25 mSv (or as high as 40 mSv or more in thallium stress/rest tests), and the average dose from a simple diagnostic coronary angiogram is 5 to 7 mSv. Factors affecting the radiation dose of a cardiac CT include the type of scanner (single-source versus dual-source), the number of detectors (z-axis coverage), the body habitus of the patient, the selection of kilovolt peak (kVp) and milliampere seconds (mAs), and the scan mode (prospective triggering versus retrospective gating with or with or without tube current modulation, high pitch [FLASH] acquisitions). General measures to reduce the radiation dose to the patient should be used whenever possible, according to the "as low as reasonably achievable" (ALARA) principle. Tube modulation routinely should be applied if retrospective gating is selected, unless a specific reason prohibits its use (Fig. 9-2).

5. **What is blooming and what techniques can be done to reduce it?**
Blooming is an artifact created when material with very high attenuation is being imaged. The borders of a high-attenuation material will "bleed" into adjacent structures. In the case of coronary CTA, blooming from calcified plaque can lead to overestimation of the degree of coronary stenosis. For this reason, a very high calcium score (generally greater than 1000) may yield nonevaluable coronary artery segments. Using a higher current (mA) and/or tube potential (kVp) can reduce blooming artifact. Using a sharp reconstruction kernel and thin slices can help in postprocessing and interpretation (Fig. 9-3).

6. **Are β-blockers necessary for coronary CTA?**
The ability of a scanner to "freeze" cardiac motion is dependent on the speed of rotation of the gantry, technique used, and the patient's heart rate. Most currently available 64-slice scanners have gantry rotation speeds in the range of 150 to 210 ms for a half-gantry rotation (only a 180-degree rotation is needed to reconstruct an image). With these scanners, a target heart rate of 60 beats per minute or less is required for optimal image quality free of motion artifact. A slower heart rate and regular rhythm are also generally required for prospective triggering, which allows a significant reduction in the radiation dose. Newer scanners such as the 256-slice Brilliance iCT (Philips Healthcare, Andover, Mass.) have half-gantry rotation speeds as fast as 135 ms. Second-generation dual source CT (Somatom Definition FLASH; Siemens Healthcare, Forchheim, Germany) has two x-ray tubes oriented 90° apart, housed within the same gantry. Rather than a 180° gantry rotation, only 90° is required to generate an image, resulting in a temporal resolution of approximately 73 ms. This allows images to be acquired without the use of β-blockers in a greater proportion of patients.

7. **A 66-year-old man with diabetes and smoking history comes to your clinic because he wants to check his calcium score. He states he read in a magazine that it is a good screening test for coronary artery disease (CAD). What is your response?**
A calcium score is a specialized cardiac CT without contrast that is processed with software to quantify the amount of coronary calcium. This number, the Agatston score, is used as a surrogate for the total amount of coronary plaque and is correlated with patients of the same age and gender. It

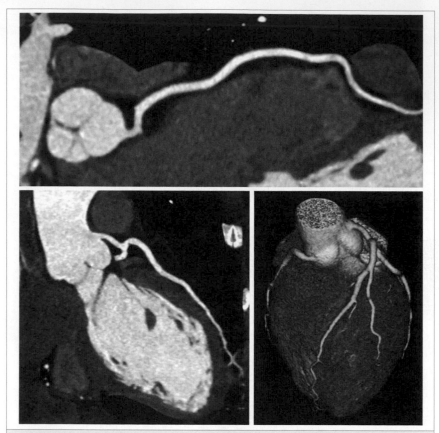

Figure 9-2. Curved multiplanar reconstructions of the right coronary artery *(top)* and left anterior descending coronary artery *(bottom left)* and volume-rendered three-dimensional reconstruction *(bottom right)* show absence of coronary plaque or stenosis. A negative computed tomography scan with good image quality has a very high negative predictive value and may spare the patient a diagnostic invasive angiogram. This study was done with a total radiation dose of 2.4 mSv.

is most useful in patients with unclear or intermediate CAD risk, to guide decision-making. Whether this patient in question has a high or low calcium score, he is already considered high risk (ATP III/ Framingham) and should be treated accordingly.

8. **What is the value of a negative calcium score in a patient with low risk to intermediate risk?**
   A negative calcium score in a low-risk patient is associated with very low likelihood of coronary events. The "warranty period" for patients with 0 calcium score and low CAD risk is approximately 4 years. For patients with a 0 calcium score and low to intermediate risk, the negative predictive value for detecting obstructive CAD is between 95% and 99%. However, calcium scoring is not recommended in the acute chest pain setting, whereas coronary CTA may be a consideration (Fig. 9-4).

9. **Is calcium scoring an appropriate test in a patient of low CAD risk but with a family history of premature CAD?**
   Patients with a family history of premature CAD have been shown to have detectable coronary artery calcium despite a low Framingham risk estimation. Thus, calcium scoring is an appropriate test to evaluate for subclinical coronary atherosclerosis in this population.

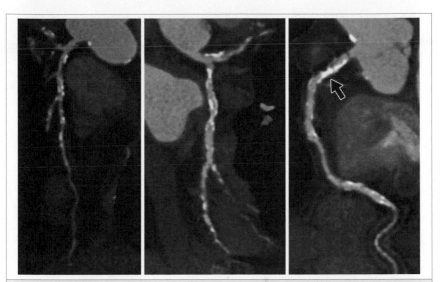

Figure 9-3. Curved multiplanar reconstructions of the left anterior descending coronary artery *(left)*, left circumflex coronary artery *(middle)*, and right coronary artery *(right)* demonstrate substantial calcification with blooming artifact. Evaluation of the degree of stenosis is limited in areas of extensive calcification, for example in the proximal right coronary artery *(arrow)*. This patient had a calcium score of 867.

10. **Summarize the current consensus of indications for coronary CTA in the management of CAD in patients with nonacute and acute symptoms without known heart disease.**
    Coronary CTA is appropriate in patients with nonacute symptoms potentially representing an ischemic equivalent and low or intermediate pretest probability of CAD. It is also appropriate in patients presenting acutely with suspected acute coronary syndrome (ACS) who have low or intermediate pretest probability of CAD and normal, nondiagnostic, or uninterpretable ECG or cardiac biomarkers (see Fig. 9-4).

11. **A 49-year-old man with severe osteoarthritis presents with nonacute chest pain. You determine he has an intermediate pretest probability of CAD. Would cardiac CT be an appropriate first test to evaluate for CAD?**
    Coronary CTA is an appropriate first test in patients who are unable to exercise and who have either a low or intermediate probability of CAD. Coronary CTA has been shown to be a highly sensitive test for the detection of CAD with negative predictive values approaching 97% to 99%. Patients who are able to exercise with intermediate pretest probability are also appropriate candidates for coronary CTA.

12. **A 59-year-old woman with low to intermediate pretest probability of CAD presents with acute chest pain. Despite negative ECG and cardiac biomarkers, you are still suspicious for ACS. Is coronary CTA an appropriate test to evaluate for CAD?**
    Yes, patients with low to intermediate pretest probability of CAD and normal and/or equivocal ECG and biomarkers are appropriate for evaluation by coronary CTA. The Rule Out Myocardial Infarction Using Computer Assisted Tomography (ROMICAT) trials demonstrated that patients with no evidence of CAD by coronary CTA have essentially 0% chance of a major adverse cardiovascular event for at least two years, and subsequent trials have confirmed a close to zero event rate in this setting. Additionally, coronary CTA was shown to reduce the length of hospital stay compared with a standard in-hospital workup (Fig. 9-5).

13. **A 61-year-old woman presents to your office with nonacute chest pain. She has a history of prior stent placement in the right coronary artery (RCA). The stent is 2.5 mm in diameter. Is coronary CTA a useful test for detecting in-stent restenosis in this patient?**

Accurate assessment of in-stent restenosis is based on a number of factors, including the diameter of the stent, material used, and size of the struts, as well as the capabilities of the CT scanner. Based on

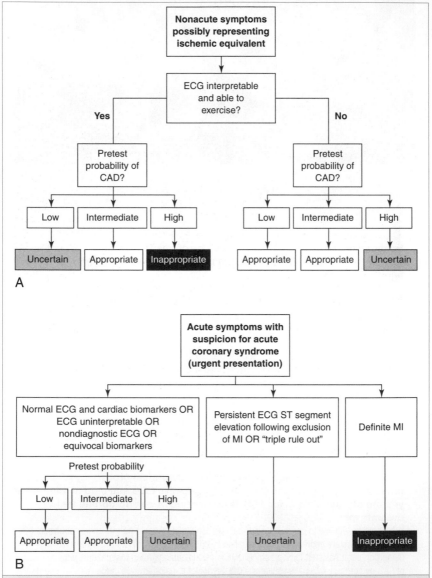

Figure 9-4. Flowcharts of suggested diagnostic imaging workup for patients with no known coronary artery disease *(CAD)* presenting with nonacute **(A)** and acute **(B)** symptoms suggestive of coronary ischemia. *ECG*, electrocardiogram; *MI*, myocardial infarction. (From Taylor AJ, Cerqueira M, Hodgson JM, et al: ACCF/SCCT/ACR/AHA/ASE/ASNC/NASCI/SCAI/SCMR 2010 Appropriate use criteria for cardiac computed tomography, *J Cardiovasc Comput Tomogr* 4:407.e1-33, 2010.)

recent appropriateness criteria, stents less than 3 mm in diameter are not appropriate for evaluation by coronary CTA. A stent is considered occluded if the lumen is unopacified and there is absent distal runoff. The presence of distal contrast opacification alone is not an adequate sign of stent patency because of the potential for retrograde filling from collateral vessels. Figure 9-6 demonstrates a patent stent in a different patient with a larger stent.

14. **A 69-year-old man with history of prior coronary artery bypass graft (CABG) presents with nonacute chest pain. Is coronary CTA useful for detecting graft stenosis in this patient?**
Coronary CTA is indicated for symptomatic patients with prior CABG to evaluate for graft patency. It is also an excellent method for evaluating graft thrombosis, malposition, aneurysms, and pseudoaneurysms.

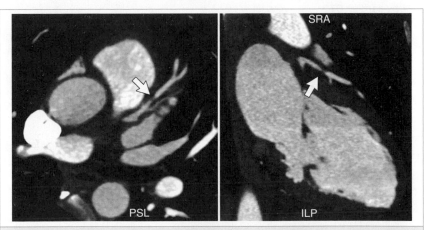

Figure 9-5. Multiplanar reformatted images demonstrate focal, severe stenosis of the mid left anterior descending (LAD) coronary artery *(arrow)*. This patient was experiencing symptoms of acute chest pain. Conventional cardiac catheterization showed 85% stenosis in the mid LAD. Angioplasty and stenting were performed.

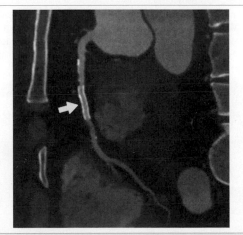

Figure 9-6. Curved multiplanar reconstruction of the right coronary artery (RCA) showing a patent stent in the mid RCA *(arrow)*. Note contrast opacification within the stent and distal to the stent. A sharp reconstruction kernel and thin slices were used for reconstructions. This particular stent measured 3.5 mm in diameter.

Inclusion of the entire chest is helpful in the postoperative period for evaluating pericardial or pleural effusions, mediastinal or wound infection, and the integrity of the sternotomy (Fig. 9-7).

15. **What is the role of cardiac CT in patients presenting for noncoronary cardiac surgery?**

Coronary CTA in this setting is useful for the assessment of coronary arteries for obstructive disease in young and middle-aged patients presenting for noncoronary cardiac surgery such as valve repair, resection of cardiac masses, and aortic surgery. Older patients, however, tend to have a higher calcium score, and up to 10% to 25% of studies in octogenarians may not allow definitive exclusion of obstructive coronary artery disease because of one or more nonevaluable segments.

16. **What is the diagnostic accuracy and clinical utility of plaque characterization by cardiac CT?**

Cardiac CT is excellent for detection and quantification of calcified portions of coronary plaque (Agatston score) and for differentiation of calcified, mixed, and noncalcified plaques. However, when compared with the gold standard of intravascular ultrasound (IVUS), CT is only modestly accurate in the detection and quantification of the volume of noncalcified plaques (stable fibrous or potentially vulnerable lipid rich), and differentiation of the two subtypes is not reliably possible, although emerging data suggest that high risk features (including positive remodeling and low attenuation) do correlate with future events. However, plaque characterization remains a work in progress, and currently there is no demonstrable utility of plaque characterization for directing medical or interventional therapy.

17. **Is cardiac CT safe and useful in patients presenting with newly diagnosed heart failure? What is the objective in this patient population?**

Coronary CTA is an appropriate test for patients with low or intermediate pretest probability of CAD and new-onset or newly diagnosed clinical heart failure with reduced left ventricular ejection fraction. The objective is to exclude coronary artery disease as a cause of heart failure. In patients with heart failure with normal left ventricular ejection fraction and diastolic dysfunction, coronary CTA can be performed, although the level of evidence supporting its use in this circumstance is not as robust.

18. **Can cardiac CT be used to differentiate between a subacute and an old myocardial infarction (MI)?**

Characteristic morphologic changes in the myocardium can be detected in patients who have a remote history of MI. Patients usually develop wall thinning in relation to normal, adjacent myocardium. In some instances, fatty metaplasia or calcification may develop. If retrospective gating is used, a regional wall motion abnormality is usually seen. Delayed enhancement imaging reveals an area of

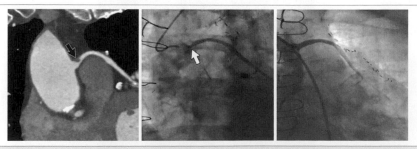

Figure 9-7. Curved multiplanar reconstruction *(left image)* of a saphenous vein graft demonstrates focal, proximal stenosis of the graft *(black arrow)*. Conventional angiogram *(middle image)* confirms the high-grade stenosis *(white arrow)*. After intervention with balloon angioplasty, the vessel is widely patent *(right image)*.

hyperenhancement in the appropriate coronary territory. In contrast, an acute myocardial infarct will appear as a hypoperfused, akinetic area of myocardium with normal wall thickness (Fig. 9-8).

19. **Should noncoronary structures be reviewed and reported on during cardiac CT examination?**

The current consensus and standard of care is to include in the final report all significant findings noted in the acquired data set, using a wide field of view. Everything that is part of the originally acquired data set should be reviewed and reported on if potentially significant.

20. **Summarize the appropriate uses of cardiac CT in regard to evaluation of cardiac structure and function.**

Cardiac CT is an excellent test for evaluation of coronary anomalies and assessment of adult congenital heart disease. It is appropriate for evaluating left ventricular function after MI or in patients with congestive heart failure (CHF) when other imaging modalities are inadequate, and it is

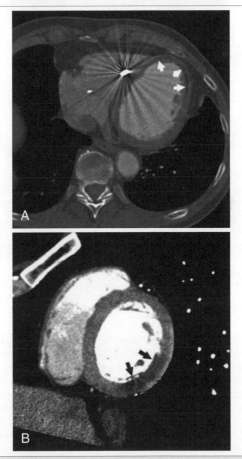

Figure 9-8. A, Cardiac-gated axial computed tomography (CT) shows apical myocardial thinning and deposition of subendocardial low-attenuation material *(arrows)* measuring −15 Hounsfield units (HU), indicating fatty metaplasia in a patient with remote left anterior descending myocardial infarction. **B,** Cardiac-gated CT in left ventricular short axis shows inferolateral subendocardial hypoenhancement that measures 35 HU *(arrows)* and normal myocardial wall thickness, representing a perfusion defect in a patient with acute left circumflex myocardial infarction.

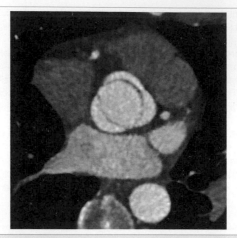

Figure 9-9. Systolic frame of retrospectively gated cardiac computed tomography in short-axis plane of the aortic valve shows an open, bicuspid aortic valve. There is congenital fusion of the right and left coronary cusps.

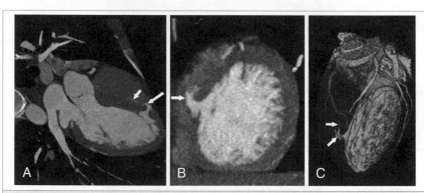

Figure 9-10. Cardiac gated computed tomographic angiogram in **(A)** left ventricle (LV) long-axis and **(B)** short-axis views shows a defect in the ventricular septum with contrast spilling from the opacified LV cavity across the septum into the otherwise unopacified right ventricle *(arrows)*. **C,** The volume-rendered image shows the contrast within the LV cavity and the small shunt volume *(arrows)* crossing into the unopacified right ventricle.

useful for evaluating the right ventricular morphology and function, including in cases of suspected arrhythmogenic right ventricular dysplasia (ARVD). When other imaging modalities are inadequate or incomplete, it is useful for evaluating native or prosthetic cardiac valves in the setting of valvular dysfunction and for evaluating cardiac masses. Prior to invasive procedures, cardiac CT is useful for pulmonary vein mapping, coronary vein mapping, and for localizing bypass grafts and other retrosternal anatomy. Finally, cardiac CT is an appropriate test for evaluation of the pericardium.

21. **Would cardiac CT be an appropriate first modality in the assessment of a 29-year-old woman with suspected Turner's syndrome presenting with symptoms of dyspnea, murmur, and hypertension?**
    Patients with suspected Turner's syndrome may have multiple congenital anomalies, including a bicuspid aortic valve, coarctation of the aorta, elongation of the transverse aortic arch, atrial or ventricular septal defect, and partial anomalous pulmonary venous return. Cardiac CT is a reasonable choice as the first modality in assessing all of these congenital anomalies in a single study (Figs. 9-9 and 9-10).

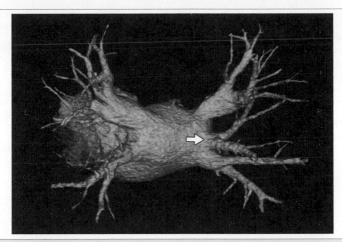

Figure 9-11. Volume-rendered computed tomographic angiogram; a three-dimensional reconstruction of the left atrium and pulmonary veins. Note the right middle pulmonary vein *(arrow)*. The study was done for pulmonary vein mapping prior to pulmonary vein isolation.

22. **A 22-year-old female is being evaluated for syncope. Echocardiography was not able to demonstrate a normal origin of the RCA. Is coronary CTA an appropriate next test?**

Coronary CTA is an excellent test for the evaluation of anomalous coronary arteries. Cardiac gating allows accurate assessment of the aortic root, sinuses of Valsalva, and coronary arteries. In cases of anomalous coronary arteries, both the origin and course of the vessel may be abnormal. Accurate delineation of the course of the artery is necessary to determine whether surgical correction is necessary. A comprehensive cardiac CT examination is capable of identifying many additional congenital anomalies with a single study.

23. **A 45-year-old female is having a CT of the pulmonary veins prior to radiofrequency ablation for atrial fibrillation. What is the purpose of pulmonary vein mapping? What is the most common anatomic variant of the pulmonary veins?**

Intraoperative pulmonary vein mapping with conventional angiography can be time consuming, and significant time-savings can be realized by mapping the pulmonary veins with CT. Digital Imaging and Communications in Medicine (DICOM) image datasets can be uploaded into cardiac imaging software for direct correlation and fusion with electroanatomic maps during the pulmonary vein isolation procedure. Preoperative mapping is also useful for detecting variant anatomy, which can be fairly common; the most common anatomic variant is a separate ostium for the right middle pulmonary vein. Measurement of the pulmonary vein ostia may be important for the proper catheter selection and for future comparison if there is a question of pulmonary vein stenosis (Fig. 9-11).

BIBLIOGRAPHY, SUGGESTED READINGS, AND WEBSITES

1. Abbara S, Walker TG: *Diagnostic imaging: cardiovascular*, ed 1, Salt Lake City, 2008, Amirsys.
2. Achenbach S, Cardiac CT: State of the art for the detection of coronary arterial stenosis, *J Cardiovasc Comput Tomogr* 1:3–20, 2007.
3. Budoff M, Achenbach S, Narula J: *Atlas of cardiovascular computed tomography*, Philadelphia, 2007, Current Medicine.
4. Cronin P, Sneider MB, Kazerooni EA, et al: MDCT of the Left Atrium and Pulmonary Veins in Planning Radiofrequency Ablation for Atrial Fibrillation: A How-To Guide, *Am J Roentgenol* 183:767–778, 2004.

5. Hoffmann U, Bamberg F, Chae CU, et al: Coronary Computed Tomography Angiography for Early Triage of Patients With Acute Chest Pain - The ROMICAT (Rule Out Myocardial Infarction Using Computer Assisted Tomography) Trial, *J Am Coll Cardiol* 53:1642–1650, 2009.

6. Lu M, Chen JJ, Awan O, et al: Evaluation of Bypass Grafts and Stents, *Radiol Clin N Am* 48:757–770, 2010.

7. Schoepf UJ: *CT of the heart: principles and applications*, ed 2, Totowa, NJ, 2008, Humana Press.

8. Taylor AJ, Cerqueira M, Hodgson J, et al: ACCF/SCCT/ACR/AHA/ASE/ASNC/NASCI/SCAI/SCMR 2010 Appropriate Use Criteria for Cardiac Computed Tomography: A Report of the American College of Cardiology Foundation Appropriate Use Criteria Task Force, the Society of Cardiovascular Computed Tomography, the American College of Radiology, the American Heart Association, the American Society of Echocardiography, the American Society of Nuclear Cardiology, the North American Society for Cardiovascular Imaging, the Society for Cardiovascular Angiography and Interventions, and the Society for Cardiovascular Magnetic Resonance, *J Am Coll Cardiol* 56:1864–1894, 2010.

9. Zadeh AA, Miller JM, Rochitte CE, et al: Diagnostic Accuracy of Computed Tomography Coronary Angiography According to Pre-Test Probability of Coronary Artery Disease and Severity of Coronary Arterial Calcification - The CORE-64 International Multicenter Study, *J Am Coll Cardiol* 59:379–387, 2012.

CHAPTER 10

CARDIAC MAGNETIC RESONANCE IMAGING

Paaladinesh Thavendiranathan, MD, MSc, FRCPC,
and Scott D. Flamm, MD, MBA, FACC, FAHA

1. **How does cardiac magnetic resonance imaging (CMR) produce images?**
   CMR uses a strong magnet (1.5 to 3.0 Tesla; equivalent to 30,000 to 60,000 times the strength of the earth's magnetic field), radiofrequency pulses, and gradient magnetic fields to obtain images of the heart. When placed in the bore of a magnet, positively charged protons, mainly from water, are aligned in the direction of the magnetic field, creating a net magnetization. Radiofrequency pulses are used to tilt these protons away from their alignment, shifting them to a higher energy state. These protons then return to their equilibrium state through the process of relaxation and emit a signal. The relaxation consists of two components: *T1 and T2 relaxation*. Magnetic gradients are applied across the tissue of interest to localize these signals. The signals are then collected using a receiver coil and placed in a data space referred to as *k-space*, which is then used to create an image. CMR uses differences in relaxation properties between different tissues, fluids, and blood, and changes that occur due to pathological processes to create contrast in the image.

2. **What is unique about CMR?**
   Similar to echocardiography, CMR allows the generation of images of the heart without exposure to ionizing radiation. Although the spatial resolution of CMR is comparable to echocardiography (approximately 1 mm), the contrast-to-noise and signal-to-noise ratios are far superior (Fig. 10-1). The latter allows easier delineation of borders between tissues and between blood pool and tissue. The contrast between blood pool and myocardium (see Fig. 10-1) is generated using differences in signal properties of the different tissues without the use of contrast agents. CMR is also not limited by "acoustic windows" that may hinder echocardiography, and images can be obtained in any tomographic plane. Finally, CMR can provide information about tissue characteristics using differences in T1 and T2 signals, and with addition of contrast agents.

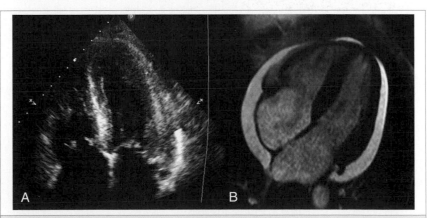

Figure 10-1. Comparison of **(A)** an echocardiographic and **(B)** cardiac MRI (CMR) cine image of a four-chamber view of the same patient. The superior contrast-to-noise and signal-to-noise ratios are clearly evident in the CMR image, with clear delineation of the endocardial and epicardial borders of both ventricles.

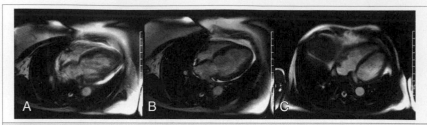

Figure 10-2. A, Four-chamber view in a patient with difficulty holding their breath (blurry). **B,** The same patient who was able to breath-hold after the acquisition period was shortened. **C,** Another patient with a real-time acquisition while breathing freely.

3. What are the limitations of CMR?

The major limitation of CMR is availability. Given the cost, the special construction necessary to host a CMR system, and the technical expertise and support necessary, CMR is not widely available at all centers. CMR is limited with respect to portability, unlike echocardiography where imaging can be performed at the patient's bedside. There is also a set of contraindications (listed later) that limits the use of this technology in selected patient populations. Image acquisition can be challenging in patients with an irregular cardiac rhythm or difficulty holding their breath, though newer real-time techniques provide an opportunity to overcome these barriers (Fig. 10-2). Finally, because patients have to lie still in a long hollow tube for up to an hour during imaging, claustrophobia may become an important limiting factor.

4. What are the common imaging pulse sequences used in CMR?

Pulse sequences are orchestrated actions of turning on and off various coils, gradients, and radio-frequency pulses to produce a CMR image. In very simple terms, the pulse sequences are based on either gradient echo or spin echo sequences. The most common sequences used are bright blood sequences (where the blood pool is bright); dark blood sequences (where the blood pool is dark); steady state free precession sequences (most commonly used for function or cine images); and inversion recovery sequences (e.g., delayed enhancement imaging used to assess myocardial scar).

5. What are the appropriate uses of CMR?

Although echocardiography is usually the first-line imaging modality for questions of left ventricular (LV) function and assessment of valvular disease, CMR still has many important indications. The following questions and answers pertain to the appropriate use of CMR in the clinical setting, as recommended in the multisociety appropriateness criteria published in 2006.

6. What is delayed enhancement (DE) CMR imaging?

One of the unique aspects of CMR is the ability to identify myocardial scar and/or fibrosis. This is most commonly performed using DE imaging. Gadolinium-based contrast agents are first administered, then after waiting approximately 10 minutes and allowing time for the contrast to distribute into areas of scar and fibrosis, an inversion recovery sequence is performed. This sequence nulls (makes it black) normal myocardium and anything that is bright within the myocardium is most likely myocardial scar or fibrosis (Fig. 10-3).

7. Does CMR have a role in the evaluation of chest pain?

In patients with chest pain syndrome, CMR stress testing can be performed to assess flow-limiting coronary stenosis. This is most appropriate in patients with intermediate pretest probability of CAD with uninterpretable ECG or who are unable to exercise. The two stress methods used are vasodilator perfusion CMR or dobutamine stress function CMR. Vasodilator stress testing is performed identically to nuclear stress testing with the use of adenosine. With peak coronary vasodilation, gadolinium contrast agent is administered and perfusion of the myocardium during the first pass of the contrast

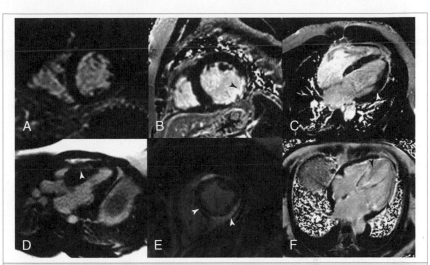

Figure 10-3. Delayed enhancement (DE) patterns. **A,** A normal short-axis DE image. **B,** A transmural scar in the circumflex territory. **C,** Cardiomyopathy secondary to sarcoidosis. **D,** Hypertrophic obstruction cardiomyopathy with basal anterior septal midmyocardial DE. **E,** Myocarditis with both midmyocardial and epicardial DE. **F,** Cardiac amyloidosis with diffuse enhancement of the entire left ventricle.

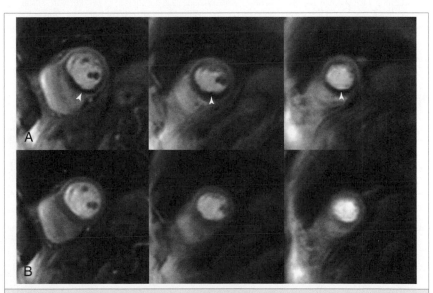

Figure 10-4. Adenosine perfusion imaging. **A,** Peak stress short-axis and four-chamber perfusion images showing ischemia *(arrows)* in the basal to apical inferior and inferior septal segments, consistent with ischemia in the right coronary artery territory. **B,** Rest images illustrate normal perfusion.

agent is captured. Areas of perfusion abnormality can be detected as dark areas (Fig. 10-4). Resting perfusion is also commonly performed, mainly to differentiate imaging artifacts from a true perfusion defect. This is then followed by DE imaging to assess for myocardial scar. Alternatively, graded doses of dobutamine can be administered to provide a sympathetic stress with cine imaging to identify regions of wall motion abnormality, in a manner similar to echocardiography.

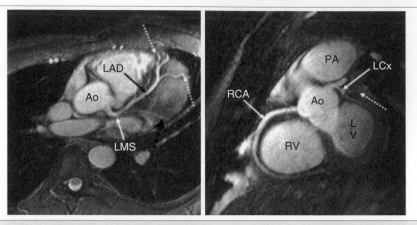

Figure 10-5. Cardiovascular magnetic resonance angiography at 3 Tesla. *Left panel,* Left coronary artery and branches *(dotted arrows). Right panel,* Right coronary artery *(RCA). Ao,* Aorta; *LAD,* left anterior descending artery; *LCx,* left circumflex artery; *LMS,* left main stem; *LV,* left ventricle; *PA,* pulmonary artery; *RV,* right ventricle. (From Stuber M, Botnar RM, Fischer SE, et al: Preliminary report on in vivo coronary MRA at 3 Tesla in humans, *Magn Reson Med* 48:425-429, 2002. Reprinted with permission of Wiley-Liss, Inc., a subsidiary of John Wiley & Sons, Inc.)

8. **Can CMR coronary angiography be used to assess chest pain?**
   Coronary angiography for assessment of coronary stenosis is not commonly performed in clinical settings. However, it is appropriate to use coronary magnetic resonance angiography (MRA) to assess the origin, branching pattern, and proximal course of the coronary arteries to assess for coronary anomalies (Fig. 10-5). This can be performed without the use of contrast agents. However, the acquisition may require a substantial amount of time and is susceptible to artifacts. The use of this technique may be particularly important, however, in young patients, thereby avoiding radiation exposure from invasive coronary angiography or coronary CT angiography.

9. **What is the role of CMR in the assessment of ventricular function?**
   CMR is considered the reference standard for the assessment of ventricular volumes, ejection fraction, and ventricular mass of both the left and right ventricles, as a result of the excellent accuracy and reproducibility of this technique for these measurements. The most appropriate use of CMR is in the evaluation of LV function after myocardial infarction or in heart failure patients with technically limited echocardiographic images. In other patient populations, CMR can be used to assess LV function when there is discordant information from prior tests.

10. **Does CMR have a role in the assessment of cardiomyopathies?**
    CMR has an important role in the evaluation of specific cardiomyopathies, particularly in the infiltrative diseases (e.g., amyloidosis and sarcoidosis), hypertrophic cardiomyopathy, and cardiomyopathies due to cardiotoxic therapies. Although CMR-based ventricular morphology and functional images can provide certain clues to the etiology of the underlying cardiomyopathy, the most important CMR technique in the assessment of cardiomyopathies is DE imaging. Certain DE patterns have been associated with particular cardiomyopathies and can be easily identified by experienced readers (see Fig. 10-3). Another specific cardiomyopathy that can be assessed by CMR is arrhythmogenic right ventricular cardiomyopathy (ARVC). CMR may be specifically used in patients presenting with syncope or ventricular arrhythmias to provide excellent assessment of right ventricular (RV) function, RV dilation, focal aneurysms, and also myocardial scar using DE imaging both in the LV and RV.

11. **What is the role of CMR in myocardial infarction?**
    After an acute myocardial infarction, CMR can be used to assess the extent of myocardial necrosis (see Fig. 10-3, *B*) and areas of microvascular obstruction ("no reflow regions") (Fig. 10-6) using

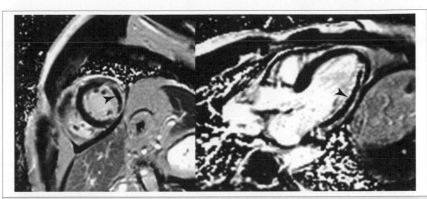

Figure 10-6. Microvascular obstruction post infarction. A short-axis *(left)* and long-axis *(right)* image of microvascular obstruction *(arrows)* seen on delayed enhancement imaging. Both images are from the same patient.

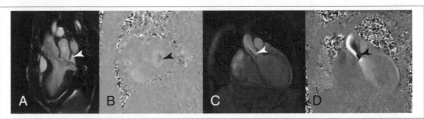

Figure 10-7. Valvular disease assessment. **A,** Three-chamber steady-state free precession (SSFP) image showing bileaflet mitral valve prolapse and a jet of mitral regurgitation *(arrow).* **B,** Short-axis phase-contrast image of the mitral valve during systole showing the mitral regurgitant orifice *(arrow).* **C, D,** Magnitude and phase contrast images, respectively, of the aortic valve showing flow acceleration at and beyond the aortic valve of aortic stenosis *(arrows).*

DE imaging. Both the extent of necrosis and the presence of microvascular obstruction have been shown to have prognostic value. In addition, DE imaging can be used to determine the likelihood of recovery of function with revascularization (surgical or percutaneous) or medical therapy. Segments of myocardium with more than 50% transmural scar are less likely to recover with revascularization. Another important use of CMR is in patients who present with a positive troponin test but have normal coronary angiography. CMR can help identify myocarditis (see Fig. 10-3, *E*), Tako-tsubo syndrome, or even myocardial infarction with recanalized coronary artery.

12. **Can valvular disease by assessed by CMR?**
    Echocardiography remains the most commonly used method for assessment of stenotic and regurgitant lesions of both native and prosthetic valves. The role of CMR is mainly in patients with technically limited images from echocardiography. CMR can be used to assess the significance of the valve lesions using several techniques. First, an en face image of the valvular lesion can be obtained for visual assessment and planimetry of the stenotic or regurgitant orifices. However, the most useful CMR techniques are the quantitative assessment of valvular stenosis obtained by transvalvular gradients, or of regurgitant lesions obtained by volumes and flow measurements. The latter is often obtained using a combination of stroke volumes by planimetry of the ventricles and phase-contrast imaging (analogous to Doppler imaging in echocardiography) (Fig. 10-7).

13. **Can CMR be used in the assessment of congenital heart disease?**
    Among imaging tests, CMR is likely one of the best modalities for the assessment of congenital heart disease. The ability to assess the heart and its relationship to the arterial and venous circulation in

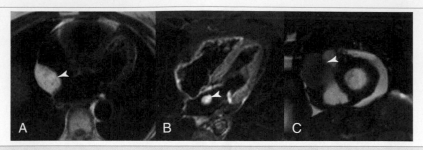

Figure 10-8. Cardiac masses. Three cardiac masses *(arrows)* are illustrated using three different cardiac magnetic resonance imaging sequences. **A,** Lipoma; **B,** left atrial myxoma; and **C,** metastatic melanoma.

three-dimensional space and obtain hemodynamic data in the same study is unique to CMR. Images can be obtained in any preferred plane, often essential in patients with complex congenital heart disease or with complex repairs. Also, important parameters, such as LV and RV volumes and function, that are used to make important clinical decisions, can be measured in an accurate and reproducible manner. Furthermore, as these patients are young and typically require multiple imaging studies throughout their lives, CMR provides excellent assessment without ionizing radiation exposure. The major limitation of CMR in this population is the susceptibility to artifacts from previous surgeries involving surgical clips, valves, and coils.

14. **Can CMR be used to assess cardiac masses?**
CMR is a good modality for the assessment of tumors (Fig. 10-8) as tissue characterization using various sequences may provide insights into the differential diagnosis of an identified mass. However, the initial hopes that CMR could definitively characterize tumor tissue (e.g., a *noninvasive biopsy*) have not quite come to fruition. Nevertheless, CMR can still help narrow the differential diagnosis and provide information about whether the tumor has characteristics suggestive of malignancy. However, small tumors and those with high frequency motion may not be appropriately assessed using CMR.

15. **What are some of the other clinical uses of CMR?**
Some of the other appropriate uses of CMR includes the assessment of pericardial conditions such as pericardial mass and constrictive pericarditis. Specifically, in constrictive pericarditis, CMR can provide assessment of the thickness of the pericardium, the presence of pericardial enhancement suggestive of recent pericardial inflammation or neovascularization, and assessment of some of the physiological changes seen.

CMR can also be used to assess the pulmonary vein anatomy prior to ablation for atrial fibrillation. The number, size, and orientation of the pulmonary veins can be assessed, and also information about the left atrium can be provided.

CMR is also used for the assessment of aortic dissection. However, given the length of the examination and difficulty monitoring the patient closely during the examination, CMR is generally not considered the first modality for dissection assessment in the acute setting.

16. **What are the contraindications to CMR?**
All devices should be checked for magnetic resonance imaging (MRI) compatibility prior to taking the patient into the MRI room. A good reference website to check the compatibility of a device is www.mrisafety.com. Alternatively, the manufacturer of the device should be contacted to check for compatibility. Some of the most common contraindications to CMR are provided in the list that follows.
- Ocular foreign body (e.g., metal in eye)
- Central nervous system aneurysm clips
- Implanted neural stimulator
- Cochlear implant

- Implanted cardiac pacemaker or defibrillator
- Other implanted medical devices (e.g., drug infusion ports, insulin pump)
- Swan-Ganz catheters
- Metal shrapnel or bullet
- Pregnancy

17. **Can CMR be performed in patients with implanted cardiovascular devices?**
Most implanted cardiovascular devices are not ferromagnetic or only weakly ferromagnetic. This includes most commonly used coronary stents, peripheral vascular stents, inferior vena cava (IVC) filters, prosthetic heart valves, cardiac closure devices, aortic stent grafts, and embolization coils. A statement on the safety of scanning patients with cardiovascular devices was published by the American Heart Association, giving guidelines of the timing and safety of device scanning.

Pacemakers and implantable cardioverter defibrillators are strong relative contraindications to MRI scanning, and scanning of such patients should be done only under specific conditions in centers with expertise in performing these studies. However, given the widespread use of pacemakers, concerns about not being able to perform MRI for even noncardiac indications have encouraged manufactures to make MRI-safe pacemakers. One such device is the Revo MRI SureScan system (Medtronic, Minneapolis), which was approved by the U.S. Food and Drug Administration (FDA) in 2011 for use as an MRI-conditional device. The conditional designation still necessitates specific patient and MRI protocols to be followed to ensure safety. Although this will make it possible to perform noncardiac MRI imaging, the artifacts that result from an implanted pacemaker and its leads will still make CMR challenging.

18. **What is nephrogenic systemic fibrosis?**
Nephrogenic systemic fibrosis (NSF) is a fibrosing condition involving skin, joints, muscles (including cardiac myocytes), and other internal organs. Although first identified in 1997, the association of this entity with gadolinium-based contrast agents (GBCA) was only described in 2006. The most important risk factors for development of NSF after use of GBCA are advanced renal disease, recent vascular surgical procedures, dialysis, acute renal failure, and higher doses of contrast agent (more than 0.1 mmol/kg). On average, the time interval between administration of GBCA and NSF is 60 to 90 days. As a consequence of the concern of NSF, the FDA has issued a black-box warning on the use of GBCA, making its use in cardiac applications an "off label" use. However, since this black box warning was issued, centers have adopted methods to carefully screen patients for risk factors prior to GBCA administration. This has resulted in virtually no new cases of NSF reported over the past 3 to 4 years.

In patients with advanced renal disease (glomerular filtration rate below 30 mL/min), the risks and benefits of gadolinium-enhanced MRI scans should be carefully weighed and alternate imaging modalities should first be considered. If a contrast-based CMR study is absolutely necessary, then the risks, benefits, and methods to avoid NSF should be discussed with imaging staff, nephrology service, and the patient prior to the study, and the patient should be carefully monitored after the CMR.

BIBLIOGRAPHY, SUGGESTED READINGS, AND WEBSITES

1. IMAIOS SAS: *MRI step-by-step, interactive course on magnetic resonance imaging.* Available at: www.imaios.com/en/e-Courses/e-MRI. Accessed January 25, 2013.
2. Shellock FG: *Website for* MRIsafety.com. Available at: www.mrisafety.com. Accessed January 25, 2013.
3. Society for Cardiovascular Magnetic Resonance: *Website for SCMR.* Available at: www.scmr.org. Accessed January 25, 2013.
4. U.S. Food and Drug Administration Information for Healthcare Professionals: Gadolinium-based contrast agents for magnetic resonance imaging (Marketed as Magnevist, MultiHance, Omniscan, OptiMARK, ProHance). Available at: http://www.fda.gov/Drugs/DrugSafety/PostmarketDrugSafetyInformationforPatientsandProviders/ucm142884.htm. Accessed January 25, 2013.
5. ACCF/ACR/SCCT/SCMR/ASNC/NASCI/SCAI/SIR: 2006 Appropriateness criteria for cardiac computed tomography and cardiac magnetic resonance imaging, *J Am Coll Radiol* 48:1476–1497, 2006.

6. Cummings KW, Bhalla S, Javidan-Nejad C, et al: A pattern-based approach to assessment of delayed enhancement in non-ischemic cardiomyopathy at MR imaging, *Radiographics* 29:89–103, 2009.

7. Kanal E, Broome DR, Martin DR, et al: Response to the FDA's May 23, 2007, nephrogenic systemic fibrosis update, *Radiology* 246:11–14, 2008.

8. Kim RJ, Wu E, Rafael A, et al: The use of contrast-enhanced magnetic resonance imaging to identify reversible myocardial dysfunction, *N Engl J Med* 343:1445–1453, 2000.

9. Levine GN, Gomes AS, Arai AE, et al: Safety of magnetic resonance imaging in patients with cardiovascular devices: an American Heart Association scientific statement from the Committee on Diagnostic and Interventional Cardiac Catheterization, Council on Clinical Cardiology, and the Council on Cardiovascular Radiology and Intervention: endorsed by the American College of Cardiology Foundation, the North American Society for Cardiac Imaging, and the Society for Cardiovascular Magnetic Resonance, *Circulation* 116:2878–2891, 2007.

10. Lin D, Kramer C: Late gadolinium-enhanced cardiac magnetic resonance, *Curr Cardiol Rep* 10:72–78, 2008.

11. Shinbane JS, Colletti PM, Shellock FG, et al: Magnetic resonance imaging in patients with cardiac pacemakers: era of "MR Conditional" designs, *J Cardiovasc Magn Reson* 2011(13):63, 2011.

12. Zou Z, Zhang HL, Roditi GH, et al: Nephrogenic systemic fibrosis review of 370 biopsy-confirmed cases, *JACC Cardiovasc Imaging* 4:206–216, 2011.

CARDIAC POSITRON EMISSION TOMOGRAPHY

Luis A. Tamara, MD

CHAPTER 11

1. **What is positron emission tomography (PET)?**
   A positron, as its name implies, is a positively charged particle that is ejected from the nucleus of an unstable atom. It is identical in mass to an electron. Strictly speaking, it is "antimatter" and very shortly after leaving the nucleus it collides with an electron in what is called an annihilation reaction. This reaction generates two 511 keV gamma photons that are emitted almost diametrically opposite from each other. The energy of these photons is captured by a special (PET) scanner and through a sophisticated network of electronics as well as computer software and hardware, it is transformed into an image.

2. **Which are the two most common PET radiopharmaceuticals used for myocardial perfusion imaging (MPI)?**
   Rubidium-82 (Rb-82) and nitrogen-13 (N-13) ammonia.

3. **What are the characteristics of Rb-82?**
   Rb-82 is a monovalent cation analog of potassium. It is commercially available as a strontium-82 generator. Its physical half-life is 75 seconds. It is extracted with high efficiency by myocardial cells through the Na^+,K^+-ATPase pump. The adult radiation dose from a Rb-82 MPI varies from 1.75 to 7.5 mSv (Fig. 11-1).

4. **What are the characteristics of N-13 ammonia?**
   N-13 Ammonia is an extractable myocardial perfusion tracer which, due to its 10 minute half-life, requires an on-site cyclotron. It is retained in myocardial tissue as N-13 glutamine by the action of glutamine synthetase. The adult radiation dose from an N-13 ammonia MPI is approximately 1.4 mSv.

5. **What are the advantages of PET MPI over single-photon emission computed tomography (SPECT)?**
   - It is more sensitive and specific (93% and 92%, respectively).
   - It is cost effective. This is primarily due to a reduction in unnecessary coronary angiographies.
   - It results in lower radiation dose to the patient.
   - It allows for absolute quantification in myocardial blood flow, expressed as mL/min/g of tissue.

6. **My patient's PET myocardial perfusion study was reported as demonstrating severe ischemia, but the coronary angiogram showed only nonobstructive coronary artery disease (CAD). How can this be?**
   This can happen because the correlation between stenosis severity and coronary flow reserve (CFR) is weak and non-linear. Therefore, angiographically mild stenoses can cause severe derangement of CFR whereas severe coronary atherosclerosis can result in little to no alteration in myocardial perfusion.

7. **What is the radiopharmaceutical used in cardiac PET for the assessment of myocardial viability?**
   Fluorine-18 (F-18) fluorodeoxyglucose (FDG).

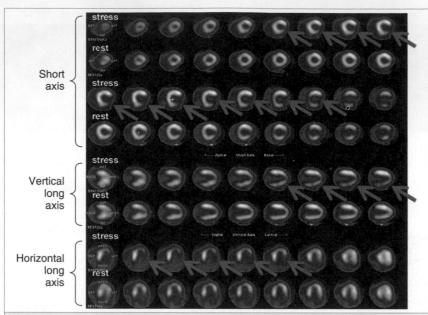

Figure 11-1. Abnormal Rb-82 myocardial perfusion imaging demonstrating inducible ischemia of left circumflex vascular territory. The figure shows stress and rest images displayed in three planes: short axis (apex to base), vertical long axis (septum to lateral wall), and horizontal long axis (from inferior to anterior). The rest images demonstrate good perfusion throughout the left ventricle. The stress images demonstrate decreased tracer in the lateral wall *(arrows)*. (Modified with permission from Branch KR, Caldwell JH, Soine LS, et al: Vascular [humoral] cardiac allograft rejection manifesting as inducible myocardial ischemia on nuclear perfusion imaging, *J Nucl Cardiol.* 12(1):123-124, 2005.)

8. **What is meant by "glucose loading" when a viability F-18 FDG cardiac PET is being performed?**
   Under fasting nonischemic conditions, the myocardium preferentially oxidizes fatty acids. Under ischemic conditions, the myocardium switches to oxidation of glucose, as it can do this with a lower oxygen requirement. In order to promote accumulation of F-18 FDG (a glucose analog) within viable myocardial tissue, an oral or intravenous "glucose load" is administered to the patient prior to the injection of F-18 FDG. Under fasting conditions, the relative abundance of circulating glucose will cause the myocardium to switch to glucose oxidation and thus enhance the uptake of F-18 FDG into viable hibernating myocardial tissue.

9. **What is meant by perfusion-metabolism (P-M) "match" or "mismatch" on cardiac PET viability imaging?**
   A P-M match is present when there is markedly decreased FDG uptake that corresponds to the area of decreased perfusion. This finding would be consistent with a myocardial scar.
   A P-M mismatch would be present if the area of decreased perfusion demonstrates normal or increased FDG uptake (Fig. 11-2). This finding would be consistent with an area of viable hibernating myocardium.

10. **Are there any other tracers that can be used for PET cardiac imaging?**
    Yes. There are many other useful radiopharmaceuticals that can be used to interrogate different aspects of myocardial metabolism, innervation, ATP generation, etc. Some of these include:
    - Carbon-11 (C-11) acetate (Krebs cycle)
    - C-11 Palmitate (fatty acid metabolism)

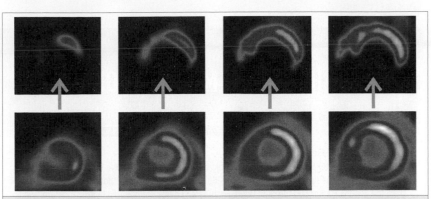

Figure 11-2. Viability study showing four short-axis slices of the left ventricle. The top row of images display perfusion with Rb-82, demonstrating markedly decreased perfusion of the inferior wall *(arrows)*. The bottom row of images display F-18 fluorodeoxyglucose (FDG) uptake in the inferior wall, indicating that the poorly perfused inferior wall still consists of viable, hibernating myocardium. (Modified with permission from Taegtmeyer H, Dilsizian V: Imaging myocardial metabolism and ischemic memory. *Nat Clin Pract Cardiovasc Med.* Suppl 2:S42-8, 2008.)

- C-11 Lactate (myocardial lactate utilization)
- C-11 Phenylephrine (presynaptic catecholamine uptake and metabolism)
- F-18 Fluorodopamine (presynaptic sympathetic function)

Additionally, there are several tracers currently under development for imaging of α- and β-adrenergic cardiac receptors.

BIBLIOGRAPHY, SUGGESTED READINGS, AND WEBSITES

1. Bengel F, Schwaiger M: PET metabolism, innervations and receptors. In Dilsizian V, Pohost GM, editors: *Cardiac CT, PET and MR*, ed 1, Malden, MA, 2006, Blackwell Futura.

2. Di Carli: PET assessment of myocardial perfusion. In Dilsizian V, Pohost GM, editors: *Cardiac CT, PET and MR*, ed 1, Malden, MA, 2006, Blackwell Futura.

3. Machac J: Cardiac positron emission tomography imaging, *Semin Nucl Med* 35(1):17–36, 2005.

4. Dilsizian V, Bacharach SL, Beanlands RS, et al: ASNC Imaging guidelines for nuclear cardiology procedures: PET myocardial perfusion and metabolism clinical imaging. Available at: http://asnc.org/imageuploads/ ImagingGuidelinesPETJuly2009.pdf. Accessed March 27, 2013.

CHAPTER 12

BEDSIDE HEMODYNAMIC MONITORING

Jameel Ahmed, MD and George Philippides, MD

1. **What is a Swan-Ganz catheter?**

   A Swan-Ganz catheter is a relatively soft, flexible catheter with an inflatable balloon at its tip that is used in right heart catheterization. The balloon-tip allows the catheter to "float" with the flow of blood from the great veins through the right heart chambers and into the pulmonary artery, before "wedging" in a distal branch of the pulmonary artery.

2. **How is a Swan-Ganz catheter constructed?**

   The basic Swan-Ganz catheter in current clinical use has four lumens. One is connected to the distal port of the catheter, allowing for measurement of the pulmonary artery pressure when the balloon is deflated, and the pulmonary artery wedge pressure (PAWP) when the balloon is inflated. The second lumen is attached to a temperature-sensing thermocouple 5 cm proximal to the catheter tip and is used for measurement of cardiac output (CO) by thermodilution. The third lumen is connected to a port 15 cm proximal to the catheter tip, allowing for measurement of pressure in the right atrium and for infusion of drugs or fluids into the central circulation. The fourth lumen is used to inflate the balloon with air when initially floating the catheter into position and later to reinflate the balloon for intermittent measurement of PAWP. Many catheters contain an additional proximal port for infusion of fluids and drugs. Some catheters have an additional lumen through which a temporary pacing electrode can be passed into the apex of the right ventricle for internal cardiac pacing.

3. **What information can be gained from a Swan-Ganz catheter?**

   Direct measurements obtained from the catheter include vascular pressures and oxygen saturations within the cardiac chambers, cardiac output, and systemic venous oxygen saturation (Svo_2). These hemodynamic measurements can be used to calculate other hemodynamic parameters, such as systemic vascular resistance and pulmonary vascular resistance.

4. **How is a Swan-Ganz catheter inserted?**

   At the bedside, venous access is usually obtained by introducing an 8.5 French sheath into the internal jugular or subclavian vein using the Seldinger technique. The right internal jugular or left subclavian veins are preferred sites as the natural curve of the catheter will allow easier flotation into the pulmonary artery. Less commonly, the antecubital or femoral veins are used.

   Next, a 7.5 French Swan-Ganz catheter is passed through the introducer sheath and advanced approximately 15 cm to exit the sheath into the central vein. The balloon is then inflated with 1.5 mL of air, and the catheter is advanced slowly, allowing the balloon to float through the right atrium, right ventricle, and pulmonary artery, and finally achieving a wedge position in a distal branch of the pulmonary artery that is smaller in diameter than the balloon itself. The wedge position is usually achieved when the catheter has advanced a total of 35 to 55 cm, depending on which central vein is cannulated.

5. **Describe the normal pressure waveforms along the path of an advancing Swan-Ganz catheter.**

   The *a wave* is produced by atrial contraction and follows the electrical *P wave* of an electrocardiogram (ECG). The *x descent* reflects atrial relaxation. The *c wave* is produced at the beginning of ventricular systole as the closed tricuspid valve bulges into the right atrium. The *x′ descent* is

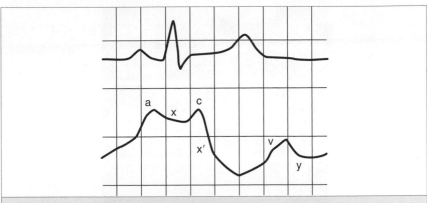

Figure 12-1. Atrial pressure tracing. See text for label descriptions.

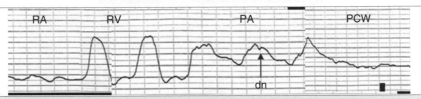

Figure 12-2. Pressure tracings as a catheter is advanced through the right-sided chambers. As the catheter moves from the right atrium to the right ventricle, a ventricular wave form is seen representing isovolumic contraction, ejection, and diastole. When the catheter passes into the pulmonary artery, the diastolic pressure rises. The dicrotic notch *(dn)*, is produced by the closure of the pulmonic valve. If the catheter is advanced further, it attains the wedge position. *PA,* Pulmonary artery; *PCW,* pulmonary capillary wedge; *RA,* right atrium; *RV,* right ventricle.

thought to be the result of the descent of the atrioventricular ring during ventricular contraction as well as continued atrial relaxation. The *v wave* is caused by venous filling of the atrium during ventricular systole, when the tricuspid valve is closed. This should correspond with the electrical *T wave.* However, at the bedside, due to a lag in pressure transmission, the a wave will align with the QRS complex and the v wave will follow the T wave. Finally, the *y descent* is produced by rapid atrial emptying, when the tricuspid valve opens at the onset of diastole (Fig. 12-1).

6. **How is the location of the catheter determined?**
   At the bedside, continuous monitoring of pressure tracings from the distal port and simultaneous ECG tracings allow the operator to determine the catheter's position and to detect any arrhythmias caused by the catheter, as it passes through the right ventricle. Fluoroscopy can be used in the cardiac catheterization lab to guide placement. The use of fluoroscopy should especially be considered if a Swan-Ganz catheter is placed via the femoral or brachial veins or in patients with dilated right ventricles.

7. **How do we know that the catheter is in the true wedge position?**
   There are three ways to confirm that the catheter is in the wedge position (Figures 12-1 and 12-2). At the bedside, an atrial tracing (reflecting left atrial pressure) will be seen when the catheter is in the wedge position. Secondly, if the catheter is withdrawn from the wedge position, the mean arterial pressure should be observed to rise from the wedge pressure (reflecting a physiologic gradient between the mean pulmonary artery and mean wedge pressure). Gentle aspiration of blood from the distal port should reveal high-oxygenated blood if the catheter is truly wedged. Additionally, in the catheterization lab, fluoroscopy can be used to determine that the catheter is in a distal pulmonary arteriole, immobile in the wedge position.

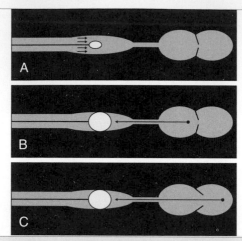

Figure 12-3. A, With the balloon tip deflated, the pressure transducer at the catheter tip sees blood flow from the proximal pulmonary artery. **B,** With the balloon tip inflated, proximal blood flow is occluded and a static column of blood is created between the catheter tip and the distal cardiac chamber. With the mitral valve closed, left atrial pressure is approximated. **C,** With the mitral valve open at end diastole, left ventricular end diastolic pressure can be measured, assuming there is no significant mitral stenosis.

8. **What does the PAWP signify?**

When the catheter is in the wedge position (Fig. 12-3, *B*), proximal blood flow is occluded and a static column of blood is created between the catheter tip and the distal cardiac chambers. With the balloon shielding the catheter tip from the pressure in the pulmonary artery proximally, the pressure trans-ducer measures pressure distally in the pulmonary arterioles. This pressure closely approximates left atrial pressure. When the mitral valve is open at end diastole, left ventricular (LV) end diastolic pressure is measured (Fig. 12-3, *C*), assuming that there is no obstruction between the catheter tip and the LV (i.e., mitral stenosis). The PAWP can be used to approximate LV preload.

9. **How is cardiac output determined?**

Cardiac output can be determined either by the measured thermodilution method or the calculated Fick method.

With *thermodilution*, 5 to 10 mL of normal saline is injected rapidly via the proximal port into the right atrium. The injectate mixes completely with blood and causes a drop in temperature that is measured continuously by a thermocouple near the catheter tip. The area under the curve is calcu-lated and is inversely related to cardiac output (Fig. 12-4). This method of measurement is not reli-able in patients with low cardiac output or significant tricuspid regurgitation. In a low cardiac output state, blood is rewarmed by the walls of the cardiac chambers and surrounding tissue, resulting in an overestimation of cardiac output.

Alternatively, the *Fick method* can be used to calculate cardiac output.

$$CO = \frac{\text{Oxygen consumption(mL/min)}}{\text{Arterial-venous O}_2 \text{ difference} \times \text{Blood O}_2 \text{ capacity}}$$
$$= \frac{\text{Measured O}_2 \text{ consumption(mL/min)}}{\text{A-V difference} \times \text{Hb(gm \%)} \times 1.36(\text{mL O}_2/\text{gm of Hb}) \times 10}$$

This method is based on the principle that the consumption of a substance (oxygen) by any organ is determined by the arterial-venous (A-V) difference of the substance and the blood flow (CO) to that organ. The consumption of oxygen by a patient can be measured using a covered hood in the cardiac catheterization lab and the arterial-venous difference can be measured by obtaining blood samples from the right atrium and pulmonary artery. This method is more accurate in patients with atrial

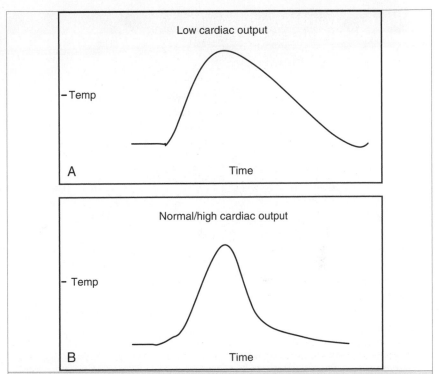

Figure 12-4. Area under the curve (AUC) is inversely proportional to cardiac output. The illustration depicts a larger AUC in a patient with low cardiac output **(A)**. **B,** Temperature equilibrates faster in a patient with a higher cardiac output, resulting in a smaller AUC.

fibrillation, tricuspid regurgitation, and low cardiac output. Common sources of error include improper collection of blood samples.

At the bedside, use of a covered hood can be cumbersome and impractical. For this reason, some laboratories assume that resting oxygen consumption is 125 mL/m^2 and calculate cardiac output based on an assumed Fick equation. However, studies have shown that there is wide variability in resting oxygen consumption among patients, particularly in those patients who are critically ill. As expected, use of an assumed Fick calculation can introduce significant error into the estimation of cardiac output.

10. **What are normal values for intravascular pressures and hemodynamic parameters?**
    The normal values for intravascular pressures and hemodynamic measurements are given in Table 12-1.

11. **Why are cardiac output and LV preload important?**
    In certain clinical situations, the knowledge of cardiac output and PAWP (surrogate of LV preload, see Question 8) can help to make diagnoses and/or guide management (see Question 12). PAWP can be applied to the Starling curve and help to predict whether cardiac output may improve if filling pressures are altered.

12. **When is placing a Swan-Ganz catheter clinically indicated and do all patients derive clinical benefit?**
    The data derived from placement a Swan-Ganz catheter can be useful in the following clinical situations.

TABLE 12-1. NORMAL HEMODYNAMIC MEASUREMENTS		
	Normal Value	Units
Measured Intravascular Pressures		
Right atrium	0-4	mm Hg
Right ventricle	15-30/0-4	mm Hg
Pulmonary artery	15-30/6-12	mm Hg
Pulmonary artery mean	10-18	mm Hg
Pulmonary artery wedge	6-12	mm Hg
	Normal Value	**Units**
Derived Hemodynamic Parameters		
Cardiac index	2-4	L/min/m^2
Stroke volume index	36-48	mL/beat/m^2
RV stroke work index	7-10	g-m/m^2
LV stroke work index	44-56	g-m/m^2
Pulmonary vascular resistance index	80-240	dyne-sec/cm^5/m^2
Systemic vascular resistance index	1200-2500	dyne-sec/cm^5/m^2
Oxygen delivery	500-600	mL/min/m^2
Oxygen uptake	110-160	mL/min/m^2
Oxygen extraction ratio	22-32	—

LV, Left ventricle; *RV,* right ventricle.

HEART FAILURE/SHOCK

- To differentiate between cardiogenic and noncardiogenic pulmonary edema when a trial of diuretic and/or vasodilator therapy has failed
  - *Not* indicated for the routine management of pulmonary edema
- To differentiate causes of shock and to guide management when a trial of intravascular volume expansion has failed (see Question 15)
- Determination of whether pericardial tamponade is present when clinical assessment is inconclusive and echocardiography is unavailable
- Assessment of valvular heart disease
- Determination of reversibility of pulmonary vasoconstriction in patients being considered for heart transplantation
- Management of congestive heart failure refractory to standard medical therapy, especially in the setting of acute myocardial infarction (MI)
  - Of note, a major, randomized trial (ESCAPE) showed no significant difference in endpoints of mortality and days out of hospital at six months in this category of patients.

ACUTE MYOCARDIAL INFARCTION

American College of Cardiology/American Heart Association (ACC/AHA) guidelines state that Swan-Ganz catheters should be used in those patients who have progressive hypotension unresponsive to fluids and in patients with suspected mechanical complications of ST elevation MI if an echocardiogram has not been performed (class I). However, mortality benefit has not been demonstrated in a randomized trial.

The use of Swan-Ganz catheters can also be considered in the following situations:

- Diagnosis of mechanical complications of MI (i.e., mitral regurgitation, ventricular septal defect)
- Diagnosis of intracardiac shunts and to establish their severity before surgical correction (see Question 16)
- Guidance of management of cardiogenic shock with pharmacologic and/or mechanical support
- Guidance of management of right ventricular infarction with hypotension and/or signs of low cardiac output not responding to intravascular volume expansion and/or low doses of inotropic drugs
- Short-term guidance of pharmacologic and/or mechanical management of acute mitral regurgitation before surgical correction

PERIOPERATIVE USE

A 2003 randomized trial in high-risk surgical patients showed no significant difference in mortality with the use of Swan-Ganz catheters. Though the routine use of Swan-Ganz catheters perioperatively remains of unclear benefit, it should be considered in the following situations:

- In patients undergoing cardiac surgery, to differentiate between causes of low cardiac output or to differentiate between right and left ventricular dysfunction, when clinical assessment and echocardiography is inadequate
- Guidance of perioperative management in selected patients with decompensated heart failure, undergoing intermediate- or high-risk noncardiac surgery

PULMONARY HYPERTENSION

- Exclusion of postcapillary causes of pulmonary hypertension (i.e., elevated PAWP)
- To establish diagnosis and assess severity of primary pulmonary hypertension (normal PAWP)
- Selection and establishment of safety and efficacy of long-term vasodilator therapy based on acute hemodynamic response

USE IN INTENSIVE CARE UNITS

- Many studies have shown that clinical data predict PAWP and cardiac output poorly, and that insertion of the catheter frequently changes patient management. However, despite widespread use of these devices in intensive care units, only a few observational studies have shown their use to decrease mortality. A 2005 meta-analysis of several randomized trials showed that the use of Swan-Ganz catheters was associated with neither benefit nor increased mortality. Current thinking is reflected in a 1997 pulmonary artery consensus statement, recommending that the decision to insert a Swan-Ganz catheter be made on an individual basis, such that the potential risks and benefits are considered in each case.

13. **What are absolute and relative contraindications to placement of a Swan-Ganz catheter?**

ABSOLUTE CONTRAINDICATIONS

- Right-sided endocarditis
- Mechanical tricuspid or pulmonic valve prosthesis
- Presence of thrombus or tumor in a right-sided heart chamber

RELATIVE CONTRAINDICATIONS

- Coagulopathy
- Recent implantation of a permanent pacemaker or cardioverter-defibrillator
- Left bundle branch block
- Bioprosthetic tricuspid or pulmonic valve

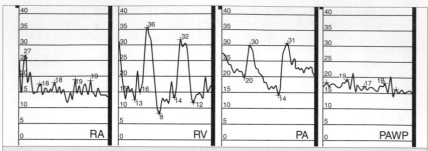

Figure 12-5. Pressure tracings in cardiac tamponade. *PA,* Pulmonary artery; *PAWP,* pulmonary artery wedge pressure; *RA,* right atrium; *RV,* right ventricle. There is equalization of all diastolic pressures across all chambers.

14. What diagnoses can the catheter help make?

The characteristic waveform of the Swan-Ganz catheter is altered in several disease states.

- In pericardial tamponade, equalization of diastolic pressures across all chambers is seen (Fig. 12-5).
- In atrial fibrillation, the a wave disappears from the right atrial pressure tracing, while in atrial flutter, mechanical flutter waves occur at a rate of 300 per minute.
- "Cannon" a waves occur when the atria contract against closed valves due to atrioventricular dissociation. Irregular cannon a waves during a wide-complex tachycardia strongly suggest ventricular tachycardia.
- Complications of MI can be detected on the PAWP tracing, such as giant v waves seen with acute mitral insufficiency, and the "dip and plateau" pattern of the RV pressure tracing seen with RV infarction.

15. How can etiologies of shock be differentiated by Swan-Ganz catheterization?

Table 12-2 presents the hemodynamic parameters in different etiologies of shock.

16. How can left-to-right intracardiac shunts be diagnosed by Swan-Ganz catheterization?

An intracardiac shunt results in flow of blood from left-sided to right-sided cardiac chambers or vice-versa. Left-to-right shunts results in flow from the left-sided chambers to right-sided chambers. With ventricular septal defects, flow is often left-to-right due to higher left-sided pressures. Atrial septal defects can result in a shunt in either direction. Due to the flow of oxygenated blood into right-sided chambers, a sudden increase in oxygen saturation in right-sided chambers is observed. A step-up in mean oxygen saturation of 7% between the caval chambers and the right atrium is diagnostic of an atrial septal defect. A step-up of 5% between the right atrium and right ventricle is diagnostic for a ventricular septal defect.

17. What complications are associated with use of a Swan-Ganz catheter?

- All complications of central venous cannulation including bleeding and infection.
  - ○ Local infection rates range from 18% to 63% in patients with catheter in place for an average of 3 days.
  - ○ Bloodstream infections have been reported in up to 5% of patients.
- Transient right bundle branch block
- Complete heart block (especially in patients with preexisting left bundle branch block)
- Ventricular tachyarrhythmias
  - ○ Clinically insignificant ventricular arrhythmias can occur in up to 30% to 60% of patients.
  - ○ Sustained arrhythmias usually occur in patients with myocardial ischemia or infarction.
- Pulmonary infarction (incidence 0-1.3%)

TABLE 12-2.	HEMODYNAMIC PARAMETERS IN DIFFERENT ETIOLOGIES OF SHOCK					
Etiology	RA	RV	PA	PCWP	CO	SVR
Hypovolemic	↓	↓	↓	↓	↓	↑
Cardiogenic	↑↑	↑↑	↑↑	↑↑	↓	↑
Septic	↔	↔	↔	↔	↑	↓

CO, Cardiac output; *PA*, pulmonary artery; *PCWP*, pulmonary capillary wedge pressure; *RA*, right atrium; *RV*, right ventricle; *SVR*, systemic vascular resistance.

- Pulmonary artery rupture
  ○ Risk factors include pulmonary hypertension and recent cardiopulmonary bypass.
- Thrombophlebitis
- Venous or intracardiac thrombus formation
- Endocarditis
- Catheter knotting

18. **How can complications be minimized?**
    - The use of fluoroscopy should be considered for placement of the catheter, particularly if access is obtained from a nontraditional site, or if the patient has a dilated right ventricle.
    - Consideration should be given to removing the catheter after the first set of data is obtained.
    - The duration the catheter is kept in place should be minimized, as infectious and thrombotic complications increase significantly after 3 to 4 days.
    - Use of the introducer side arm for infusion of medications should be minimized.
    - Manipulation of the catheter should only be performed by trained personnel.

19. **The wedge tracing is abnormal. What do I do?**
    - Check a chest radiogram for proper catheter position. The tip should lie in lung zone 3, below the level of the left atrium.
    - Aspirate and flush the catheter to remove clots and bubbles.
    - Check all connecting lines and stopcocks.
    - Confirm that the pressure transducers are zeroed to the level of the right atrium.
    - Check that the balloon is not overinflated; try letting out the air and refilling it slowly.
    - Consider the possibility that the tracing really is a wedge tracing with a giant v wave, as is seen in acute mitral insufficiency and several other conditions.

20. **The cardiac output doesn't make sense. What is wrong?**
    - Check that at least three values were averaged and that the range of these values is no greater than 20% of the mean.
    - Check the chest radiogram: is the distal tip of the catheter in the pulmonary artery and the proximal port in the right atrium?
    - Check to see if the computer is calibrated to the proper temperatures.
    - If the computer can display the time versus temperature curve, check that the curve is shaped properly.

BIBLIOGRAPHY, SUGGESTED READINGS, AND WEBSITES

1. Baim DS, editor: *Grossman's Cardiac Catheterization, Angiography, and Intervention*, Philadelphia, 2006, Lippincott Williams & Wilkins.
2. Binanay C, Califf RM, Hasselblad V, et al: Evaluation study of congestive heart failure and pulmonary artery catheterization effectiveness: the ESCAPE trial, *JAMA* 294:1625–1633, 2005.

3. Leatherman JW, Marini JJ: Clinical use of the pulmonary artery catheter. In Hall JB, Schmidt GA, Wood LDH, editors: *Principles of Critical Care*, ed 2, New York, 1998, McGraw-Hill, pp 155–177.

4. Mueller HS, Chatterjee K, Davis KB, et al: American College of Cardiology consensus statement. Present use of bedside right heart catheterization in patients with cardiac disease, *J Am Coll Cardiol* 32:840–864, 1998.

5. Pulmonary Artery Catheter Consensus Conference Participants: Pulmonary artery catheter consensus conference: Consensus statement, *Crit Care Med* 25(6):910–925, 1997.

6. Robin ED: The cult of the Swan-Ganz catheter, *Ann Intern Med* 103:445–449, 1985.

7. Sandham JD, Hull RD, Brant RF, et al: A randomized, controlled trial of the use of pulmonary-artery catheters in high-risk surgical patients, *N Engl J Med* 348:5–14, 2003.

8. Shah MR, Hasselblad V, Stevenson LW, et al: Impact of the pulmonary artery catheter in critically ill patients: meta-analysis of randomized clinical trials, *JAMA* 294:1664–1670, 2005.

9. Sharkey SW: Beyond the wedge: Clinical physiology and the Swan Ganz catheter, *Am J Med* 83:111–122, 1987.

10. Sise MJ, Hollingsworth P, Brimm JE, et al: Complications of the flow-directed pulmonary-artery catheter: A prospective analysis of 219 patients, *Crit Care Med* 9:315–318, 1981.

11. Walston A, Kendall ME: Comparison of pulmonary wedge and left atrial pressure in man, *Am Heart J* 86:159–164, 1973.

12. Zipes DP, Libby P, Bonow RO, Braunwald E, editors: *Braunwald's Heart Disease*, Philadelphia, 2005, Elsevier Saunders.

CHAPTER 13

°ENDOMYOCARDIAL BIOPSY

Chantal El Amm, MD, and Leslie T. Cooper Jr., MD

1. Why is an endomyocardial biopsy (EMB) performed?

A few cardiovascular disorders can only or most accurately be diagnosed by examination of heart tissue. These disorders include giant cell myocarditis, amyloidosis, and allograft rejection. In each case, the unique information gained from EMB can inform prognosis and/or guide treatment. The information gained from EMB can also help diagnose certain restrictive cardiomyopathies and cardiac masses.

2. How is an EMB performed?

A bioptome is shown in Figure 13-1. The Stanford-Caves-Schultz and the King bioptomes access the right ventricle through the right internal jugular vein. A modified Cordis bioptome (B-18110, Wolfgang Meiners Medizintechnik, Monheim, Germany) has been used for access from the right femoral vein. The subclavian and left femoral veins are used less frequently.

The femoral artery may be used as a percutaneous access site for left ventricular biopsy.

The right ventricular septum is the preferred site for EMB, to minimize the risk of perforation. Fluoroscopy and/or echocardiography guidance are essential to localize the site of biopsy. Endocardial voltage mapping has been used to identify biopsy sites in suspected arrhythmogenic right ventricular cardiomyopathy/dysplasia (ARVC/D) and cardiac sarcoidosis. Six to eight samples are generally obtained using the Stanford-Caves device. Up to ten samples are obtained by investigators who use the smaller Meiners Medizintechnik bioptome.

The sample must be handled carefully to minimize crush artifacts. The biopsy specimen should be transferred from the bioptome to fixative by use of a sterile needle and not with forceps.

3. What are the risks associated with an EMB?

Risks correlated with EMB are summarized in Table 13-1. EMB is associated with a serious acute complication rate of less than 1% using the current flexible bioptomes, and the overall rate of complication is reported as less than 6% in most case series. Complications include access-site hematoma, transient right bundle branch block (RBBB), transient arrhythmias, tricuspid regurgitation, and, rarely, pulmonary embolism. Life-threatening complications occur far less frequently. Right ventricular perforation was reported in less than 1% of patients. Following cardiac transplant, the risk is especially low. The risks of EMB depend on the clinical state of the patient, the experience of the operator, and site procedural volume.

4. How is the EMB tissue analyzed?

Specimen preparation depends on the clinical question to be answered.

Standard histological preparation for light microscopy can be used in the diagnosis of transplant rejection and myocarditis, and involves formalin fixation and paraffin wax embedding. Transmission electron microscopy requires glutaraldehyde fixation and can be helpful is the assessment of anthracycline drug toxicity and metabolic and storage disorders. Polymerase chain reaction for viral DNA amplification is best performed on unfixed samples. An RNase inhibitor is often used to prevent degradation of RNA virus genomes. Molecular typing of amyloidosis (e.g., AL, ATTR, and familial) is best performed with tandem mass spectroscopy.

5. When should EMB be performed?

EMB is not commonly indicated in the evaluation of heart disease and should only be performed in specific clinical circumstances in which EMB results may meaningfully modify prognosis or guide treatment. In 2007, an American Heart Association, American College of Cardiology, and European Society of Cardiology (AHA/ACC/ESC) scientific statement recommended that EMB be used selectively in a limited set of clinical scenarios described in the answers to Questions 6 through 8. Since that statement, reports suggest that EMB may also have a role in the evaluation of idiopathic heart block for possible cardiac sarcoidosis or giant cell myocarditis.

6. **What are the class I recommendations to perform an EMB?**
   - **Clinical scenario 1:** Unexplained new-onset heart failure (HF) of less than 2 weeks duration associated with a normal size or dilated cardiomyopathy in addition to hemodynamic compromise
   - **Clinical scenario 2:** Unexplained new-onset HF of 2 weeks to 3 months duration associated with a dilated left ventricle and new ventricular arrhythmias, Mobitz type II second-degree atrioventricular (AV) block, third-degree AV block, or failure to respond to usual care within 1 to 2 weeks

7. **When is it reasonable to perform an EMB (class IIa recommendation)?**
   - **Clinical scenario 3:** Unexplained HF of more than 3 months duration associated with a dilated left ventricle and new ventricular arrhythmias, Mobitz type II second-degree AV block, third-degree AV block, or failure to respond to usual care within 1 to 2 weeks

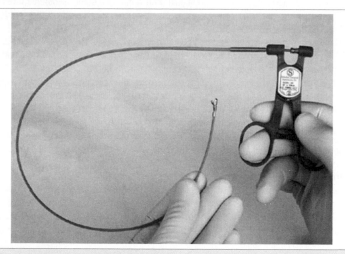

Figure 13-1. An example of a bioptome used for endomyocardial biopsy.

TABLE 13-1.   ADVERSE EVENTS WHICH CAN OCCUR WITH ENDOMYOCARDIAL BIOPSY

- Atrial or ventricular arrhythmia
- Complete heart block (transient)
- RBBB or IVCD
- Tricuspid valve damage
- Myocardial perforation
- Access site complication (bleeding, hematoma, arterial puncture, infection)

IVCD, Intraventricular conduction delay; *RBBB,* right bundle branch block.

- **Clinical Scenario 4:** Unexplained HF with a dilated cardiomyopathy of any duration associated with a suspected allergic reaction in addition to eosinophilia
- **Clinical Scenario 5:** Unexplained HF associated with suspected anthracycline cardiomyopathy
- **Clinical Scenario 6:** HF associated with restrictive cardiomyopathy
- **Clinical Scenario 7:** Suspected cardiac tumors, with the exception of typical myxomas
- **Clinical Scenario 8:** Unexplained cardiomyopathy in children
- **Clinical Scenario 9:** Unexplained new-onset HF of 2 weeks to 3 months duration associated with a dilated cardiomyopathy without new ventricular arrhythmias or AV block
- **Clinical scenario 10:** Unexplained HF of more than 3 months duration associated with a dilated cardiomyopathy without new ventricular arrhythmias or AV block that responds to usual care within 1 to 2 weeks

8. **When can you consider EMB (class IIb recommendation)?**
   - **Clinical Scenario 11:** HF associated with unexplained hypertrophic cardiomyopathy
   - **Clinical Scenario 12:** Suspected arrhythmogenic right ventricular cardiomyopathy
   - **Clinical Scenario 13:** Unexplained ventricular arrhythmias

9. **What are some of the findings on pathology in different cardiac conditions?**
   - Lymphocytic myocarditis: diagnosis of myocarditis is made when there is inflammatory infiltrate with associated myocyte damage
   - Idiopathic giant cell myocarditis: myocyte necrosis, poorly formed granulomas and eosinophils
   - Sarcoidosis: well-formed nonnecrotizing granulomas (Fig. 13-2, *A*)

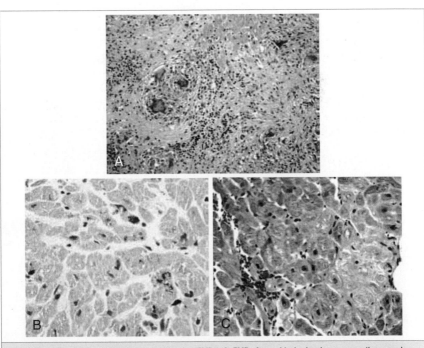

Figure 13-2. Examples of endomyocardial biopsies (EMBs). **A,** EMB of sarcoidosis showing noncaseating granulomas. **B,** EMB of hemochromatosis showing iron deposition in the myocytes. **C,** EMB of amyloid showing pericellular deposition of amyloid. (From Narula N, Narula J, Dec GW: Endomyocardial biopsy for non-transplant related disorders. *Am J Clin Pathol* 123(suppl):S106-S118, 2005.)

- Dilated cardiomyopathy: commonly associated with end-stage hypertensive, ischemic, valvular disease. The most common finding in dilated cardiomyopathy is myocyte hypertrophy and interstitial fibrosis.
- Hemochromatosis: iron is demonstrated (Fig. 13-2, *B*)
- Amyloidosis: a Congo red stain shows apple-green birefringence under polarized light (Fig. 13-2, *C*)

CHAPTER 14

CARDIAC CATHETERIZATION, ANGIOGRAPHY, IVUS, AND FFR

Vijay G. Divakaran, MD, MPH, and Glenn N. Levine, MD

1. What are generally accepted indications for cardiac catheterization?

Although recommendations are consistently evolving, those listed here are generally accepted as reasonable indications for cardiac catheterization. Cardiac catheterization is a relatively safe procedure; however, life-threatening complications can rarely occur (see later), so there needs to be a clearly thought out and documented indication for catheterization and a plan for how to use the information obtained during catheterization for patient management.

- Class III-IV angina despite medical treatment or intolerance of medical therapy
- High-risk results on noninvasive stress testing
- Sustained (more than 30 seconds) monomorphic ventricular tachycardia or nonsustained (less than 30 seconds) polymorphic ventricular tachycardia
- Sudden cardiac death survivors
- Most patients with non–ST-segment elevation acute coronary syndrome (NSTE-ACS) who have high-risk features and no contraindications to early cardiac catheterization and revascularization
- Systolic dysfunction and stress testing results suggesting multivessel disease and potential benefit from revascularization
- Recurrent typical angina within 9 months of percutaneous coronary revascularization
- For assessment of valvular dysfunction or other hemodynamic assessment when the results of echocardiography are indeterminate
- As part of primary percutaneous coronary intervention (PCI) for ST-segment elevation myocardial infarction (STEMI)
- Patients post-STEMI (with or without thrombolytic therapy) with high-risk features, depressed ejection fraction, or high-risk results on subsequent stress testing
- Within 36 hours of STEMI in appropriate patients who develop cardiogenic shock
- In select patients who are to undergo valve replacement or repair
- In assessment and management of patients with congenital heart disease and cardiac transplant recipients

2. What are the risks of cardiac catheterization?

The risks of cardiac catheterization will depend to some extent on the individual patient. For "all comers," the risk of death is approximately 1 in 1000, with the risk of myocardial infarction or stroke rarer than 1 in 1000. The risk of any major complication in "all comers" is less than 1%. These risks are summarized in Table 14-1.

3. How are coronary lesions assessed?

Coronary lesions are most commonly assessed in day-to-day practice based on subjective visual impression (Fig. 14-1). Lesions are subjectively given a percent stenosis, ideally based on ocular assessment of at least two orthogonal images of the lesion. Studies have shown interobserver and intraobserver variability in judging coronary stenosis from as little as 7% to as much as 50%. Quantitative coronary angiography (QCA) more objectively assesses the lesion severity than does "ocular judgment," but is not commonly used in day-to-day practice. QCA generally grades lesions as less severe than does subjective ocular judgment of a lesion's severity. Intravascular ultrasound (IVUS) can more accurately assess the total plaque burden and severity of a lesion than can ocular judgment or QCA. Fractional flow reserve (FFR) is increasingly being used to measure the severity of a lesion from a physiologic standpoint (see later).

4. **What is considered a "significant" stenosis?**
   The classification of significant stenosis depends on the clinical context and what one considers "significant." Coronary flow reserve (the increase in coronary blood flow in response to agents that

TABLE 14-1. RISKS OF CARDIAC CATHETERIZATION AND CORONARY ANGIOGRAPHY	
Complication	Risk (%)
Mortality	0.11
Myocardial infarction	0.05
Cerebrovascular accident	0.07
Arrhythmia	0.38
Vascular complications	0.43
Contrast reaction	0.37
Hemodynamic complications	0.26
Perforation of heart chamber	0.03
Other complications	0.28
Total of major complications	1.70

Reproduced from David CJ, Bonow RO: Cardiac Catheterization. In Libby P, Bonow RO, Mann DL, Zipes DP, editors: *Braunwald's heart disease: a textbook of cardiovascular medicine,* ed 8, Philadelphia, 2007, Saunders, p 461.

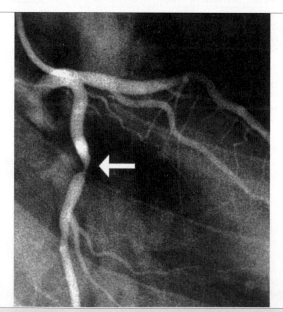

Figure 14-1. Coronary angiography of the left coronary artery demonstrates an approximate 90% lesion *(arrow)* in the left coronary artery.

lead to microvascular dilation) begins to decrease when a coronary artery stenosis is 50% or more of the luminal diameter. However, basal coronary flow does not begin to decrease until the lesion is 80% to 90% of the luminal diameter.

5. **What is fractional flow reserve (FFR)?**
    Physiologic assessment of blood flow through a stenotic lesion can be safely and reliably performed in the catheterization laboratory using a coronary wire with a pressure sensor at its tip. The wire is advanced across the lesion of interest, and the ratio of distal coronary pressure to proximal aortic pressure is assessed after maximal hyperemia is achieved (Fig 14-2). This ratio is called FFR. Normal

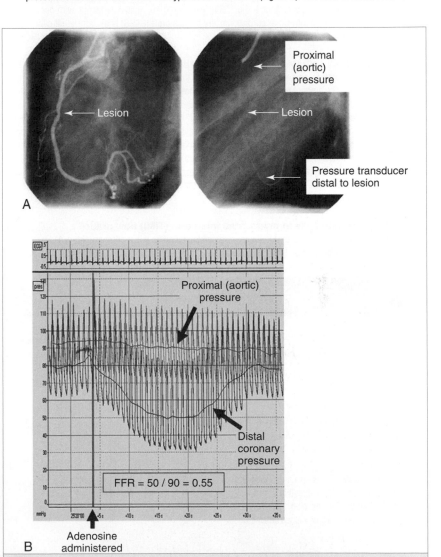

Figure 14-2. Fractional flow reserve. **A,** An intermediate lesion in the right coronary artery. The pressure wire is advanced distal to the lesion. **B,** Pressure tracings proximal to and distal to the lesion. There is a notable fall in distal perfusion pressure after administration of adenosine, indicating a hemodynamically significant lesion.

values are close to 1, and a ratio less than 0.75 to 0.80 is taken as indicating a "physiologically significant stenosis." Adenosine is typically used as a pharmacologic agent to achieve maximal hyperemia.

6. **How is FFR used to guide coronary stenting?**
In patients with angina, if the "culprit" lesion is visually estimated to be intermediate (50% to 70% stenosis) in severity, FFR may be used to guide management in determining if the lesion is physiologically significant. When evaluating whether a lesion warrants revascularization, use of FFR has been shown to be a clinically useful tool. Revascularization may be safely deferred for lesions with FFR greater than 0.75 to 0.80. If the FFR is less than 0.75, revascularization with percutaneous coronary intervention (PCI) or coronary artery bypass graft (CABG) is appropriate if clinically indicated.

7. **During cardiac catheterization, how is aortic or mitral regurgitation graded?**
For aortic regurgitation, an aortogram is performed in the ascending thoracic aorta above the aortic valve and the amount of contrast that regurgitates into the left ventricle is noted. For mitral regurgitation, a left ventriculogram is performed and the amount of contrast that regurgitates into the left atrium is noted. The systems used to grade the degree of regurgitation are similar for the two valvular abnormalities, and based on a 1+ to 4+ system, where 1+ is little if any regurgitation and 4+ is profound or severe regurgitation. Regurgitation of 3+ or 4+ is often considered "surgical" regurgitation, although the criteria for surgery are more complex than this (see Chapters 30 and 31 on aortic valve disease and on mitral valve disease, respectively). Table 14-2 summarizes the grading of regurgitant lesions as assessed by cardiac catheterization and "ballpark" regurgitant fractions for each degree of regurgitation.

8. **What is thrombolysis in myocardial infarction (TIMI) flow grade?**
TIMI flow grade is a system for qualitatively describing blood flow in a coronary artery. It was originally derived to describe blood flow down the infarct-related artery in patients with STEMI.

TABLE 14-2.   VISUAL ASSESSMENT OF VALVULAR REGURGITATION AND APPROXIMATE CORRESPONDING REGURGITANT FRACTION*

Visual Appearance of Regurgitation	Designated Grading (Severity) of Valvular Regurgitation	Approximate Corresponding Regurgitant Fraction
Minimal regurgitant jet seen. Clears rapidly from proximal chamber with each beat.	1+	<20%
Moderate opacification of proximal chamber, clearing with subsequent beats.	2+	21% to 40%
Intense opacification of proximal chamber, becoming equal to that of the distal chamber.	3+	41% to 60%
Intense opacification of proximal chamber, becoming more dense than that of the distal chamber. Opacification often persists over the entire series of images obtained.	4+	>60%

*These regurgitant fraction values are dependent on numerous factors and should be taken only as rough estimates.
Modified from David CJ, Bonow RO: Cardiac Catheterization. In Libby P, Bonow RO, Mann DL, Zipes DP, editors: *Braunwald's heart disease: a textbook of cardiovascular medicine*, ed 8, Philadelphia, 2007, Saunders, p 458.

Reportedly, it was originally written down on a napkin or the back of an envelope during an airplane flight. The grades are based on observing contrast flow down the coronary artery after injection of the contrast agent, and are as follows:

- TIMI grade 3: normal contrast (blood) flows down the entire artery
- TIMI grade 2: contrast (blood) flows through the entire artery but at a delayed rate compared with flow in a normal (TIMI grade 3 flow) artery
- TIMI grade 1: contrast (blood) flows beyond the area of vessel occlusion but without perfusion of the distal coronary artery and coronary bed
- TIMI grade 0: complete occlusion of the infarct-related artery

9. **What is IVUS?**

IVUS is the direct assessment of coronary arterial wall using a flexible catheter with a miniature ultrasound probe at its tip. Upon insertion into the coronary artery, IVUS provides true cross-sectional images of the vessel, delineating the three layers of the vessel wall (Fig 14-3). IVUS may aid in the assessment of coronary stenosis, plaque morphology, and optimal stent expansion when angiographic imaging is inadequate or indeterminate.

10. **What are the different methods of describing the aortic transvalvular gradient in a patient undergoing cardiac catheterization for the evaluation of aortic stenosis?**

Three terms used to describe the gradient are illustrated in Figure 14-4 and are:

- Peak instantaneous gradient: the maximal pressure difference between the left ventricular pressure and aortic pressure assessed at the exact same time
- Peak-to-peak gradient: the difference between the maximal left ventricular pressure and the maximal aortic pressure
- Mean gradient: the integral of the pressure difference between the left ventricle and the aorta during systole

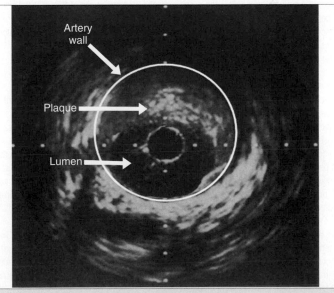

Artery wall

Plaque

Lumen

Figure 14-3. Intravascular ultrasound (IVUS) demonstrating plaque occluding greater than 60% of the arterial lumen. Coronary angiography had demonstrated only mild narrowing in this segment of coronary artery.

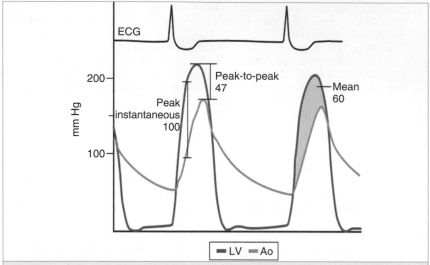

Figure 14-4. Various methods of describing the aortic transvalvular gradient. *Ao,* Aorta; *ECG,* electrocardiogram; *LV,* left ventricle. (From Bashore TM: *Invasive cardiology: principles and techniques,* Philadelphia, 1990, BC Decker, p 258.)

11. **Which patients should be premedicated to prevent allergic reactions to iodine-based contrast agents?**
    In patients with a history of prior true allergic reaction (e.g., hives, urticaria, or bronchoconstriction) to iodine-based contrast agents, the risk of repeat anaphylactoid reaction to contrast agents is reported to be 17% to 35%. Such patients should be premedicated before angiography. The standard regimen is 50 mg of prednisone orally (PO), 13 hours, 7 hours, and 1 hour before the procedure, and 50 mg PO of diphenhydramine 1 hour before the procedure, although a regimen of 60 mg PO of prednisone the night before and morning of the procedue, along with 50 mg PO of diphenhydramine the morning of the procedure, is also used by some. The 2011 American College of Cardiology Foundation/American Heart Association/Society for Cardiovascular Angiography and Interventions (ACCF/AHA/SCAI) guidelines do not consider allergy to fish or shellfish an indication for steroid pretreatment.

12. **What are the major risk factors for contrast nephropathy?**
    Preexisting renal disease and diabetes are the two major risk factors for the development of contrast nephropathy. The risk of contrast nephropathy is also related to the amount of iodine-based contrast used during the catheterization procedure. Preprocedure and postprocedure hydration is the most established method of reducing the risk of contrast nephropathy. The 2011 ACCF/AHA/SCAI PCI guidelines suggest a regimen of isotonic crystalloid (e.g., normal saline) 1.0 to 1.5 ml/kg/hr for 3 to 12 hours before the procedure and continuing for 6 to 24 hours after the procedure. Those same guidelines conclude that treatment with *N*-acetylcysteine does not reduce the risk of contrast nephropathy and is not indicated. Measures of other treatments to decrease the risk of contrast nephropathy, such as sodium bicarbonate infusion or ultrafiltration, have produced heterogeneous and conflicting data.

13. **What are the major vascular complications with cardiac catheterization?**
    In general, major vascular complications are uncommon with diagnostic cardiac catheterization and more common with PCI, which may require larger sheath placement, venous sheath placement, and more intense or prolonged anticoagulation. Nevertheless, practitioners and patients should be aware of the following potential vascular complications:
    - Retroperitoneal hematoma: This should be suspected in cases of flank, abdominal, or back pain, with unexplained hypotension, or with a marked decrease in hematocrit. Diagnosis is by computed tomography (CT) scan.

- Pseudoaneurysm: A pseudoaneurysm results from the failure of the puncture site to seal properly. Pseudoaneurysm is a communication between the femoral artery and the overlying fibromuscular tissue, resulting in a blood-filled cavity. Pseudoaneurysm is suggested by the finding of groin tenderness, palpable pulsatile mass, or new bruit in the groin area. Pseudoaneurysm is diagnosed by Doppler flow imaging.

- Arteriovenous (AV) fistula: An AV fistula can result from sheath-mediated communication between the femoral artery and the femoral vein. AV fistula is suggested by the presence of a systolic and diastolic bruit in the groin area. Diagnosis is confirmed by Doppler ultrasound.

- Stroke: Periprocedural stroke is a rare but morbid complication of cardiac catheterization, and is often associated with unfavorable neurologic outcome. A proportion of strokes may be due to disruption and embolization of atherosclerotic material from the aorta during the procedure.

- Cholesterol emboli syndrome: This is a rare and potentially catastrophic complication that results from plaque disruption in the aorta, with distal embolization into the kidneys, lower extremities, and other organs.

14. **What are vascular closure devices?**
   Vascular closure devices are hemostatic devices that obviate the need for prolonged compression at the arterial access site following angiography. These devices decrease the duration of bed rest and afford earlier mobility after the procedure. Vascular closure devices have not been convincingly demonstrated to decrease the risk of vascular complications, including bleeding.

15. **What is the difference between radial and femoral access in cardiac catheterization?**
   Left heart catheterization and coronary angiography are commonly performed using catheters inserted through either the femoral or radial arteries. Radial access is associated with a lower incidence of vascular complications such as bleeding.

16. **What is intracardiac echo (ICE)?**
   ICE is the direct imaging of cardiac structures via transvenous insertion of a miniaturized echo probe. Most commonly, the device is inserted via the femoral vein and threaded up to the right atrium. ICE is used to visualize the interatrial septum and fossa ovalis, aiding with transseptal puncture, percutaneous treatment of atrial septal defect (ASD) or patent foramen ovale (PFO), and during electrophysiologic procedures, and imaging the fossa ovalis and pulmonary veins.

BIBLIOGRAPHY, SUGGESTED READINGS, AND WEBSITES

1. Boudi FB: Coronary artery atherosclerosis. Available at: www.emedicine.medscape.com. Accessed November 30, 2012.

2. Carrozza JP: Complications of diagnostic cardiac catheterization. In Basow DS, editor: UpToDate, Waltham, MA, 2013, UpToDate. Available at: www.uptodate.com. Accessed March 26, 2013.

3. Levine GN, (chair), Bates ER, Blankenship JC, et al: 2011 ACCF/AHA/SCAI Guideline for Percutaneous Coronary Intervention. 2011 ACCF/AHA/SCAI Guideline for percutaneous coronary intervention: executive summary: a report of the American College of Cardiology Foundation/American Heart Association Task Force on Practice Guidelines and the Society for Cardiovascular Angiography and Interventions, *Circulation* 124:2574–2609, 2011.

4. Levine GN, Kern MJ, Berger PB, et al: Management of patients undergoing percutaneous coronary revascularization, *Ann Intern Med* 139:123–136, 2003.

5. Kern MJ: *The cardiac catheterization handbook*, ed 4, St. Louis, 2011, Mosby.

6. Scanlon PJ, Faxon DP, Audet AM, et al: ACC/AHA guidelines for coronary angiography, *J Am Coll Cardiol* 33:1756–1824, 1999.

CHAPTER 15

CHEST PAINS AND ANGINA

William Ross Brown, MD, and Glenn N. Levine, MD, FACC, FAHA

1. **Are most emergency room (ER) visits for chest pain caused by acute coronary syndromes (ACS)?**
   No. ACS (e.g., unstable angina, myocardial infarction) account for only a small percentage of ER visits for chest pain. Depending on the study, only a small percentage of patients (1% to 11%) will be diagnosed as having chest pains caused by coronary artery disease (CAD) or ACS. *ACS* is the term used to describe the continuum of syndromes that include *unstable angina* and *myocardial infarction* (MI).

2. **What are the other important causes of chest pains besides chronic stable angina and ACS?**
   The differential diagnosis for chest pains include the following:
   - Aortic dissection
   - Severe aortic stenosis
   - Hypertrophic cardiomyopathy
   - Coronary artery spasm (Prinzmetal angina, cocaine abuse)
   - Cardiac syndrome X
   - Hypertensive crisis
   - Musculoskeletal pain and cervical radiculopathies (costochondritis)
   - Pleurisy
   - Pericarditis
   - Pneumonia
   - Pneumothorax
   - Pulmonary embolism
   - Gastrointestinal (GI) causes (reflux, esophagitis, esophageal spasm, peptic ulcer disease, gallbladder disease, and esophageal rupture [Boerhaave syndrome])
   - Dermatologic (such as shingles)

   It is important not to assume that all chest pains are due to angina or ACS, even if someone else has made such a preliminary diagnosis. This is particularly important, as time-to-diagnosis is critical for aortic dissection, where the mortality rate increases by approximately 1% every hour from presentation to diagnosis and treatment. Additionally, the treatment of aortic dissection is dramatically different from the treatment of ACS, as anticoagulation is contraindicated with aortic dissection.

3. **Does an elevated troponin level make the diagnosis ACS?**
   Not necessarily. Although troponin elevations are fairly sensitive and specific for myocardial necrosis, it is well known that other conditions can also be associated with elevations in cardiac troponins. Importantly, troponin elevation can occur with pulmonary embolus and is in fact associated with a worse prognosis in cases of pulmonary embolus in which the troponin levels are elevated. Myopericarditis (inflammation of the myocardium and pericardium) may also cause elevated troponin levels. In addition, aortic dissection that involves the right coronary artery may lead to secondary MI. Further, troponins may be modestly chronically elevated in patients with severe chronic kidney disease. Troponin elevation has also been noted in patients with acute stroke. Studies to delineate the etiology of this are ongoing.

4. **What is angina?**

   Angina is the term used to denote the discomfort associated with myocardial ischemia or MI. Angina occurs when myocardial oxygen demand exceeds myocardial oxygen supply, usually as a result of a severely stenotic or occluded coronary artery. Patients with angina most commonly describe a *chest pain*, *chest pressure*, or *chest tightness* sensation. They may also use words such as *heaviness*, *discomfort*, *squeezing*, or *suffocating*. The discomfort is more commonly over a fist or larger sized wregion than just a pinpoint (though this distinction in itself is not enough to confidently distinguish anginal from nonanginal pain). The discomfort classically occurs over the left precordium but may manifest as right-sided chest discomfort, retrosternal discomfort, or discomfort in other areas of the chest. Some persons may experience the discomfort only in the upper back, in the arm or arms, or in the neck or jaw. Angina is typically further classified into *stable* and *unstable*. Stable angina refers to angina that occurs during situations of increased myocardial oxygen demand. Unstable angina can occur at any time and falls within the spectrum of ACSs.

5. **What are the associated symptoms that persons with angina may experience in addition to chest discomfort?**

   Patients with angina may experience one or more of the following symptoms. Some patients do not experience classic chest discomfort, but instead manifest only one or more of these associated symptoms.
   - Shortness of breath
   - Diaphoresis
   - Nausea
   - Radiating pains. Patients may describe pains or discomfort that *radiate* to the back (typically midscapula), the neck, the jaw, or down one or both arms. They may also describe a *numbness*-type sensation in the arm.

6. **What are the major risk factors for CAD?**
   - Age
   - Sex. Males are at higher risk of developing CAD, particularly earlier in life.
   - Family history of premature CAD. This is traditionally defined as a father, mother, brother, or sister who first developed clinical CAD at age younger than 45 to 55 years for men and at age younger than 55 to 60 years for women.
   - Hypercholesterolemia
   - Hypertension
   - Cigarette smoking
   - Diabetes mellitus

   Other factors that have been associated with an increased risk of CAD include inactivity (lack of regular exercise), elevated C-reactive protein, and obesity (specifically, large abdominal girth).

7. **What symptoms and findings make it more (or less) likely that the patient's chest pains are due to angina (or that the patient has ACS)?**

   The answer to this question is given in Tables 15-1 and 15-2, which are taken from an excellent review article on this subject in the *Journal of the American Medical Association (JAMA)*. The tables summarize many of the relevant questions and the value of the chest pain characteristics in distinguishing angina and ACS-MI pain from other causes. It is important to remember, no single element of chest pain history is a powerful enough predictor to use alone to rule out ACS.
   - **Quality and characteristics of chest discomfort:** Patients who describe a chest *tightness* or *pressure* are more likely to have angina. Pain that is stabbing, pleuritic, positional, or reproducible is less likely to be angina and is often categorized as *atypical chest pain*, although the presence of such symptoms does not 100% rule out that the pain may be due to CAD. Although it is generally accepted that a more diffuse area of discomfort is suggestive of angina, whereas a coin-sized, very focal area of discomfort is more likely to be noncardiac, this distinction in itself is not enough to confidently dismiss very focal pain as noncardiac.

TABLE 15-1. SPECIFIC DETAILS OF THE CHEST PAIN HISTORY HELPFUL IN DISTINGUISHING ANGINAL CHEST PAIN IN PATIENTS WITH MYOCARDIAL INFARCTION FROM NONCARDIAC CAUSES

Element	Question	Comments
Chest Pain Characteristics		
Quality	In your own words, how would you describe the pain? What adjectives would you use?	Pay attention to language and cultural considerations; use interpreter if necessary.
Location	Point with your finger to where you are feeling the pain.	Can elicit size of chest pain area with the same question.
Radiation	If the pain moves out of your chest, trace where it travels with your finger.	Patient may need to point to examiner's scapula or back.
Size of area or distribution	With your finger, trace the area on your chest where the pain occurs.	Focus on distinguishing between a small coin-sized area and a larger distribution.
Severity	If 10 is the most severe pain you have ever had, on this 10-point scale, how severe was this pain?	Patient may need to be coached in this: pain of fetal delivery, kidney stone, bony fracture are good references for 10.
Time of onset and is it continuing	Is the pain still present? Has it gotten better or worse since it began? When did it begin?	Ongoing pain a concern: it is worthwhile to obtain an initial ECG while pain is present.
Duration	Does the pain typically last seconds, minutes, or hours? Roughly, how long is a typical episode?	Focus on the most recent (especially if ongoing) and the most severe episode; be precise: if the patient says "seconds," tap out 4 seconds.
First occurrence	When is the first time you ever had this pain?	Interest should focus on this recent episode, that is, the last few days or weeks.
Frequency	How many times per hour or per day has it been occurring?	Relevant only for recurring pain: a single index episode is not uncommon.
Similar to previous cardiac ischemic episodes	If you have had a heart attack or angina in the past, is this pain similar to the pain you had then? Is it more or less severe?	Follow-up questions elicit how the diagnosis of CAD was confirmed and whether any intervention occurred.
Precipitating or Aggravating Factors		
Pleuritic	Is the pain worse if you take a deep breath or cough?	Distinguish between whether these maneuvers only partially or completely reproduce the pain and if it reproduces the pain only some or all of the time.
Positional	Is the pain made better or worse by your changing body position? If so, what position makes the pain better or worse?	Distinguish between whether these maneuvers only partially or completely reproduce the pain: on physical examination, turn the chest wall, shoulder, and back.
Palpable	If I press on your chest wall, does that reproduce the pain?	Distinguish between whether these maneuvers only partially or completely reproduce the pain: ask the patient to lead you to the area of pain; then palpate.
Exercise	Does the pain come back or get worse if you walk quickly, climb stairs, or exert yourself?	Helpful to quantify a change in pattern (e.g., the number of stairs or distance walked before the pain began).

Continued

TABLE 15-1. SPECIFIC DETAILS OF THE CHEST PAIN HISTORY HELPFUL IN DISTINGUISHING ANGINAL CHEST PAIN IN PATIENTS WITH MYOCARDIAL INFARCTION FROM NONCARDIAC CAUSES—cont'd

Element	Question	Comments
Emotional stress	Does becoming upset affect the pain?	Are there other stress-related symptoms (e.g., acroparesthesias)?
Relieving factors	Are there any things that you can do to relieve the pain, once it has begun?	In particular, ask about response to nitrates, antacids, ceasing strenuous activity.
Associated symptoms	Do you typically get other symptoms when you get this chest pain?	After asking question in open-ended way, ask specifically about nausea or vomiting and about sweating.

CAD, Coronary artery disease; *ECG*, electrocardiogram.
Modified from Swap CJ, Nagurney JT: Value and limitations of chest pain history in the evaluation of patients with suspected acute coronary syndromes, *JAMA* 294:2623-2629, 2005.

TABLE 15-2. VALUE OF SPECIFIC COMPONENTS OF THE CHEST PAIN HISTORY FOR THE DIAGNOSIS OF ACUTE MYOCARDIAL INFARCTION (AMI)

Pain Descriptor	Positive Likelihood Ratio (95% CI)
Increased Likelihood of AMI	
Radiation to right arm or shoulder	4.7 (1.9-12)
Radiation to both arms or shoulders	4.1 (2.5-6.5)
Associated with exertion	2.4 (1.5-3.8)
Radiation to left arm	2.3 (1.7-3.1)
Associated with diaphoresis	2.0 (1.9-2.2)
Associated with nausea or vomiting	1.9 (1.7-2.3)
Worse than previous angina or similar to previous MI	1.8 (1.6-2.0)
Described as pressure	1.3 (1.2-1.5)
Decreased Likelihood of AMI	
Described as pleuritic	0.2 (0.1-0.3)
Described as positional	0.3 (0.2-0.5)
Described as sharp	0.3 (0.2-0.5)
Reproducible with palpation	0.3 (0.2-0.4)
Inframammary location	0.8 (0.7-0.9)
Not associated with exertion	0.8 (0.6-0.9)

AMI, Acute myocardial infarction; *CI*, confidence interval.
Modified from Swap CJ, Nagurney JT: Value and limitations of chest pain history in the evaluation of patients with suspected acute coronary syndromes, *JAMA* 294:2623-2629, 2005.

The severity of the pain or discomfort is not helpful in distinguishing angina from other causes of chest pain. Chest pain that is sudden in onset and maximal intensity at onset is suggestive of aortic dissection. Patients with aortic dissection may describe the pain as *tearing* or *ripping* and may describe pain radiating to the back. The Levine sign (pronounced "la vine," and no relationship to this book's editor) is when the patient spontaneously clenches his or her fist and puts it over the chest while describing the chest discomfort.

- **Duration of the discomfort:** Angina usually lasts on the order of minutes, not seconds or hours (unless the patient is suffering an MI) or days. Typically, patients will describe stable anginal pain as lasting approximately 2 to 10 minutes. Unstable angina pain may last 10 to 30 minutes. Pain that truly lasts just several seconds or greater than 30 minutes is usually not angina, unless the patient is having an acute MI. One has to be careful because some patients will initially describe the pain as lasting seconds when on further questioning it becomes clear it has really lasted minutes. Pain that lasts continuously (not off and on) for a day or days is usually not angina.
- **Precipitating factors:** Because angina results from a mismatch between myocardial oxygen demand and supply, activities that increase myocardial oxygen demand or decrease supply may cause angina. Discomfort that is brought on by exercise or exertion is highly suggestive of angina. Mental stress or anger may not only increase heart rate and blood pressure, but may also lead to coronary artery vasoconstriction, precipitating angina. One has to be careful in not ruling out angina as the cause of the chest discomfort in patients who experience chest discomfort at rest, without precipitation, however, as this may be due to ACS, where the problem is primarily thrombus formation in the coronary artery, leading to decreased myocardial oxygen supply.
- **Relief with sublingual nitroglycerin (SL NTG) or rest:** NTG is a coronary artery vasodilator. While there are some recent studies to the contrary, typically patients who report partial or complete relief of their chest discomfort within 2 to 5 minutes of taking SL NTG are more likely to be experiencing angina as the cause of their chest discomfort. One has to question patients carefully because some will report that the SL NTG decreased their discomfort, but on further questioning one learns that the discomfort only decreased 30 to 60 minutes after taking the SL NTG. Because SL NTG exerts its effect within minutes, this does not necessarily imply that the chest discomfort was *relieved* by the SL NTG. However, in patients experiencing MI caused by an occluded coronary artery, the fact that the chest discomfort is not relieved with SL NTG does not necessarily make it less likely that the pain is due to CAD. Patients who experience the chest discomfort, but then sit or rest for minutes and the chest discomfort gradually resolves, are more likely to have angina.
- **Probability of having CAD:** In patients with multiple risk factors for CAD or with known CAD, the occurrence of chest pains is more likely to be due to angina.
- **Associated symptoms:** The presence of one or more associated symptoms, such as shortness of breathe, diaphoresis, nausea, or radiating pain, increase the likelihood that the discomfort is due to angina.
- **Electrocardiogram (ECG) abnormalities:** ST-segment depressions or elevations, or T-wave inversions, increase the likelihood that the discomfort is due to angina. However, the lack of these findings should not rule out angina as a cause of the chest discomfort. The initial ECG has a sensitivity of only 20% to 60% for MI, let alone merely the presence of CAD.
- **Troponin elevation:** The finding of an elevated troponin level significantly increases the likelihood that the discomfort is due to angina and CAD. However, the lack of an elevated troponin does not rule out angina and CAD as a cause of the discomfort. Further, as discussed earlier, other conditions besides angina can cause an elevated troponin.

8. **If one is still in doubt as to the diagnosis of CAD, should a stress test be obtained?**
   Yes. Stress testing for diagnostic purposes is best in patients who, after initial evaluation, have an intermediate probability of having CAD. For example, in a patient with a pretest probability of having

CAD of 50%, a *positive* exercise stress test makes the posttest probability of CAD 85%, whereas a *negative* exercise stress test makes the posttest probability of CAD just 15%. Stress testing may also be used for prognostic purposes. Stress testing is discussed in greater detail in the chapters on exercise stress testing (Chapter 6), nuclear cardiology (Chapter 7), echocardiography (Chapter 5), and magnetic resonance imaging (Chapter 10). Coronary computed tomography (CT) angiography is an emerging alternate form of diagnosis and is discussed in Chapter 9.

9. **Are there exceptions to the classic presentations of anginal pain?**
   Yes. It is well known that women often do not present with *typical* anginal symptoms (e.g., substernal, exertional pain relieved by rest or NTG). In fact, women are often misdiagnosed because of a lower suspicion by doctors that they have CAD and the fact that they often experience discomfort that is not *classic* for angina. Older patients may have difficulty in remembering or describing their chest discomfort and so also may not describe *classic* anginal symptoms. Some diabetic patients appear to have an impaired sensation of chest discomfort when the heart experiences myocardial ischemia. Thus, some diabetic patients may not report chest discomfort but rather only one or more associated symptoms, such as shortness of breath or diaphoresis. Cardiac transplant patients do not experience ischemic chest pain due to denervation of the transplanted heart.

10. **Who first described angina, and when?**
    The association between chest pain (angina pectoris) and heart disease was first described by Heberden in 1772. He described this as a *strangling sensation in the chest* in his manuscript entitled, "Some Account of a Disorder of the Breast."

11. **What is Prinzmetal angina?**
    Prinzmetal angina, also called *variant angina*, is an uncommon type of angina caused by coronary vasospasm. The coronary artery is believed to spasm, severely reducing myocardial oxygen supply to the affected myocardium. Although the spasm can occur in either a *normal* or a diseased coronary artery, it most commonly occurs within 1 cm of an atherosclerotic plaque. Prinzmetal angina usually does not occur with physical exertion or stress but occurs during rest, most typically between midnight and 8 AM. The pain can be severe, and if an ECG is obtained during an episode, it may demonstrate ST-segment elevations. Patients with Prinzmetal angina are typically younger, often female. Treatment is based primarily on the use of calcium channel blockers, as well as nitrates.

12. **What is cardiac syndrome X?**
    Cardiac syndrome X is an entity in which patients describe exertional anginal symptoms, yet are found on cardiac catheterization to have nondiseased *normal* coronary arteries. They may also have ST-segment depressions on exercise stress testing and even perfusion defects with nuclear stress testing. Unlike Prinzmetal angina, they do not have spontaneous coronary spasm and do not have provokable coronary spasm. Although there are likely multiple causes and explanations for cardiac syndrome X, it does appear that, at least in some patients, microvascular coronary artery constriction or dysfunction plays a role. Treatment is usually individually tailored to the patient and sometimes includes cognitive behavioral therapy and imipramine, which is used in chronic pain syndromes. No one standardized recipe has been established.

BIBLIOGRAPHY, SUGGESTED READINGS, AND WEBSITES

1. Alaeddini J, Angina Pectoris. Available at: http://www.emedicine.com.
2. Cohn JK, Cohn PF: Chest pain, *Circulation* 106:530–531, 2002.
3. Delehanty JM, Cardiac syndrome X: angina pectoris with normal coronary arteries. Available at: http://www.utdol.com.
4. Delehanty JM, Variant Angina. Available at: http://www.utdol.com.
5. Haro LH, Decker WW, Boie ET, et al: Initial approach to the patient who has chest pain, *Cardiol Clin* 24:1–17, 2006.

6. Higginson LAJ: Chest pain. In Porter RS, Kaplan JL, editors: *The Merck Manual Online*, Whitehouse Station, N.J., 2012, Merck Sharp & Dohme Corp. Available at http://www.merck.com/mmpe. Accessed March 27, 2013.

7. Lanza GA: Cardiac syndrome X: a critical overview and future perspectives, *Heart* 93:159–166, 2007.

8. Mayer S, Hillis LD: Prinzmetal variant angina, *Clin Cardiol* 21:243–246, 1998.

9. Meisel JL, Diagnostic Approach to Chest Pains in Adults. Available at: http://www.utdol.com.

10. Ringstrom E, Freedman J: Approach to undifferentiated chest pain in the emergency department: a review of recent medical literature and published practice guidelines, *Mt Sinai J Med* 73:499–505, 2006.

11. Swap CJ, Nagurney JT: Value and limitations of chest pain history in the evaluation of patients with suspected acute coronary syndromes, *JAMA* 294:2623–2629, 2005.

12. Tanser PH: Approach to the cardiac patient. In Porter RS, Kaplan JL, editors: *The Merck Manual Online*, Whitehouse Station, NJ, 2012, Merck Sharp & Dohme Corp. Available at: http://www.merck.com/mmpe. Accessed March 27, 2013.

13. Warnica JW: Angina Pectoris. In Porter RS, Kaplan JL, editors: *The Merck Manual Online*, Whitehouse Station, NJ, 2012, Merck Sharp & Dohme Corp. Available at: http://www.merck.com/mmpe. Accessed March 27, 2013.

CHAPTER 16

CHRONIC STABLE ANGINA

Richard A. Lange, MD, MBA

1. **Can a patient with new-onset chest pain have chronic stable angina?**

   The term "chronic stable angina" refers to angina that has been stable in frequency and severity for at least 2 months and with which the episodes are provoked by exertion or stress of similar intensity. Chronic stable angina is the initial manifestation of coronary artery disease (CAD) in about half of patients; the other half initially experience unstable angina, myocardial infarction (MI), or sudden death.

2. **What causes chronic stable angina?**

   Angina occurs when myocardial oxygen supply is inadequate to meet the metabolic demands of the heart, thereby causing myocardial ischemia. This is usually caused by increased oxygen demands (i.e., increase in heart rate, blood pressure, or myocardial contractility) that cannot be met by a concomitant increase in coronary arterial blood flow, due to narrowing or occlusion of one or more coronary arteries.

3. **How is chronic stable angina classified or graded?**

   The most commonly used system is the Canadian Cardiovascular Society system, in which angina is graded on a scale of I to IV. These grades and this system are described in Table 16-1. This grading system is useful for evaluating functional limitation, treatment efficacy, and stability of symptoms over time.

4. **What tests should be obtained in the patient with newly diagnosed angina?**

   After a careful history and physical examination, the laboratory tests for the patient with suspected angina should include a measurement of hemoglobin, hemoglobin A1c, fasting lipids (i.e., serum concentrations of total cholesterol, high-density lipoprotein (HDL) cholesterol, triglycerides, and calculated low-density lipoprotein (LDL) cholesterol), and a 12-lead electrocardiogram (ECG).

5. **What are the goals of treatment in the patient with chronic stable angina?**
   - Ameliorate angina
   - Prevent major cardiovascular (CV) events, such as heart attack or cardiac death
   - Identify "high risk" patients who would benefit from revascularization

6. **What therapies improve symptoms?**
   - Beta-adrenergic blocking agents (β-blockers)
   - Nitrates
   - Calcium channel blockers
   - Ranolazine

7. **What is the initial approach to the patient with chronic stable angina?**

   The initial approach should be focused on eliminating unhealthy behaviors such as smoking and effectively promoting lifestyle changes that reduce CV risk, such as maintaining a healthy weight, engaging in physical activity, and adopting a healthy diet. In addition, annual influenza vaccination reduces mortality (by approximately 35%) and morbidity in patients with underlying CAD. Tight glycemic control was thought to be important in the diabetic, but this approach actually increases the risk of CV death and complications.

TABLE 16-1. GRADING OF ANGINA BY THE CANADIAN CARDIOVASCULAR SOCIETY CLASSIFICATION SYSTEM

Class I

- Ordinary physical activity, such as walking and climbing stairs, does not cause angina
- Angina occurs with strenuous, rapid, or prolonged exertion at work or recreation.

Class II

- Slight limitation of ordinary activity
- Angina occurs while walking or climbing stairs rapidly; while walking uphill; while walking or climbing stairs after meals in cold or in wind; while under emotional stress; or only during the first several hours after waking.
- Angina occurs while walking > 2 blocks on level grade and climbing > 1 flight of ordinary stairs at a normal pace and in normal conditions.

Class III

- Marked limitations of ordinary physical activity
- Angina occurs while walking 1 or 2 blocks on level grade and climbing 1 flight of stairs in normal conditions and at a normal pace

Class IV

- Inability to engage in any physical activity without discomfort
- Angina may be present at rest

8. **What is first-line drug therapy for the treatment of stable angina?**
When considering medications, β-blockers decrease myocardial oxygen demands by reducing heart rate, myocardial contractility, and blood pressure. They are first-line therapy in the treatment of chronic CAD, as they delay the onset of angina and increase exercise capacity in subjects with stable angina.

9. **Is any β-blocker better than the others?**
Although the various β-blockers have different properties (i.e., cardioselectivity, vasodilating actions, concomitant α-adrenergic inhibition, and partial β-agonist activity [Table 16-2]), they appear to have similar efficacy in patients with chronic stable angina. β-blockers prevent reinfarction and improve survival in survivors of MI, but such benefits have not been demonstrated in patients with chronic CAD without previous MI.

10. **What is the proper dose of β-blocker?**
The dose of β-blocker is titrated to achieve a resting heart rate of 55 to 60 beats per minute and an increase in heart rate during exercise that does not exceed 75% of the heart rate response associated with the onset of ischemia. β-blockers are contraindicated in the presence of severe bradycardia, high-degree atrioventricular block, sinus node dysfunction, and uncompensated heart failure. They are also contraindicated in the patient with vasospastic angina, in whom they may worsen angina as a result of unopposed α-adrenergic stimulation; calcium channel blockers are preferred in these patients.

11. **Calcium channel blocker versus β-blocker: is one more effective than the other?**
Calcium channel blockers and β-blockers are similarly effective at relieving angina and improving exercise time to the onset of angina or ischemia. Calcium channel blockers can be used as monotherapy in patients with chronic stable angina, although combination therapy with a β-blocker or nitrate relieves angina more effectively than does their use alone. In this regard, β-blockers may be particularly useful in blunting the reflex tachycardia that occurs with dihydropyridine calcium channel blocker use.

TABLE 16-2. PROPERTIES OF β-BLOCKERS USED FOR THE TREATMENT OF ANGINA

β BLOCKER	SELECTIVITY	PARTIAL AGONIST ACTIVITY	USUAL DOSE FOR ANGINA
Propranolol	None	No	20-80 mg twice daily
Metoprolol	β_1	No	50-200 mg twice daily
Atenolol	β_1	No	50-200 mg/day
Nadolol	None	No	40-80 mg/day
Timolol	None	No	10 mg twice daily
Acebutolol	β_1	Yes	200-600 mg twice daily
Betaxolol	β_1	No	10-20 mg/day
Bisoprolol	β_1	No	10-20 mg/day
Esmolol (intravenous)	β_1	No	50-300 mcg/kg/min
Labetalol*	None	Yes	200-600 mg twice daily
Pindolol	None	Yes	2.5-7.5 mg 3 times daily

*Labetalol is a combined α- and β-blocker

12. **When should a peripherally acting calcium channel blocker (i.e., a dihydropyridine, such as amlodipine or felodipine) be used versus one that has effects on both the heart and the periphery (e.g., verapamil, diltiazem)?**
Amlodipine and felodipine are used primarily as second- or third-line antianginal agents in patients already on β-blockers (and often, also long-acting nitrates). They act mainly as vasodilators, lowering blood pressure and likely having some coronary vasodilating effects. Verapamil and diltiazem, in addition to having vasodilating effects, have negative chronotropic and inotropic effects. Thus, they are used in patients with contraindications or intolerance to β-blockers. They are usually avoided in the patient with an ejection fraction below 40% or who is on a β-blocker, because of their negative inotropic effects.

13. **Should sublingual nitroglycerin (NTG) or NTG spray be prescribed to all chronic stable angina patients?**
Yes. This is the standard of care. Patients should be instructed on how to use sublingual NTG— generally one pill every 5 minutes, up to a maximum of three tablets. They should be instructed to call 911 and seek immediate medical attention if their angina is not relieved after three pills or 15 minutes.

14. **When is a long-acting nitrate prescribed?**
Long-acting nitrates are often prescribed along with β-blockers or nondihydropyridine calcium channel blocker (i.e., verapamil or diltiazem) as the initial treatments in patients with chronic stable angina (Table 16-3). Continuous exposure to NTG can result in tolerance to its vasodilating effects. Nitrate tolerance can be avoided by providing the patient with a "nitrate-free" period for 4 to 6 hours per day.

15. **When is ranolazine added?**
It's use is reserved for individuals with angina that is refractory to maximal doses of other antianginal medications. Ranolazine targets the underlying derangements in sodium and calcium that occur during myocardial ischemia; it does not affect resting heart rate or blood pressure. Its antianginal efficacy is not related to its effect on heart rate, the hemodynamic state, the inotropic state, or coronary blood flow, as with other currently available agents.

In randomized trials, ranolazine increased exercise tolerance, decreased anginal frequency, and decreased sublingual NTG use, when used as monotherapy or in combination with β-blockers or calcium channel blockers in subjects with chronic stable angina. Randomized long-term trials evaluating its impact on mortality in stable CAD have not been performed.

Because ranolazine prolongs the QTc interval, it should not be used in patients with baseline QT prolongation or those on other medications that can prolong the QT interval. Furthermore, patients initiated on this drug should have their QT duration monitored periodically with 12-lead ECGs.

16. **What medications prevent MI or death in patients with stable chronic angina?**
    - Antiplatelet agents
    - Angiotensin-converting enzyme (ACE) inhibitors (in selected patients)
    - Lipid-lowering therapy

17. **What's the proper dose of aspirin?**
    An aspirin dose of 75 to 162 mg daily is equally as effective as 325 mg, but with a lower risk of bleeding. Doses less than 75 mg have less proven benefit. In patients with chronic CAD, aspirin

TABLE 16-3. ANTIANGINAL CLASSES, EFFECTS, SIDE EFFECTS, AND CONTRAINDICATIONS

CLASS	EFFECTS	SIDE EFFECTS	CONTRAINDICATIONS
β Blockers	■ Negative chronotropy ■ Negative inotropy	■ Extreme bradycardia ■ AV node block and PR prolongation ■ Exacerbation of acute heart failure ■ Bronchospasm ■ Blood pressure reduction	■ Resting bradycardia ■ Prolonged PR internal (>220-240 ms) ■ Acute decompensated heart failure ■ Severe reactive airway disease ■ Baseline hypotension
Long-acting nitrates	■ Coronary vasodilation ■ Venodilation	■ Headache ■ Venous pooling	■ Use of erectile dysfunction medications
Calcium-channel blockers: verapamil and diltiazem	■ Peripheral vasodilation ■ Coronary vasodilation ■ Negative chronotropy ■ Negative inotropy	■ Extreme bradycardia ■ AV node block and PR prolongation ■ Blood pressure reduction ■ Exacerbation of chronic and acute heart failure	■ Resting bradycardia ■ Prolonged PR interval (>220-240 ms) ■ Baseline low blood pressure ■ Acute decompensated heart failure ■ Ejection fraction < 40% ■ Usually, patients already on β-blockers
Calcium-channel blockers: amlodipine and felodipine	■ Peripheral vasodilation ■ Coronary vasodilation ■ No net negative chronotropic or inotropic effects	■ Blood pressure reduction ■ Peripheral edema	■ Baseline low blood pressure

AV, Atrioventricular.

treatment is associated with a 33% reduction in the risk of vascular events (nonfatal MI, nonfatal stroke, and vascular death). Over the course of a couple of years of treatment, aspirin would be expected to prevent about 10 to 15 vascular events for every 1000 people treated.

18. Should patients with chronic stable angina be on clopidogrel?
Clopidogrel is a reasonable alternative in the patient with stable CAD who is allergic to or cannot tolerate aspirin. However, the use of aspirin and clopidogrel in combination is no more effective than aspirin alone at reducing vascular events in patients with stable CAD.

19. Should patients with chronic stable angina be treated with an ACE inhibitor?
The addition of an ACE inhibitor to standard therapy does not reduce the risk of CV events In "low-risk" stable CAD patients (i.e., those with normal ejection fraction in whom CV risk factors are well controlled and revascularization has been performed). Conversely, in "high-risk" patients, ACE inhibitors reduce the incidence of MI, stroke, or CV death by approximately 20%. Thus, ACE inhibitors are started and continued indefinitely in all patients with a left ventricular ejection fraction (LVEF) of 0.40 or below, and in those with hypertension, diabetes, or chronic kidney disease, unless contraindicated.

20. What's the proper statin dose for the patients with chronic stable angina?
The dose of statin is gradually increased until the target serum LDL cholesterol concentration is achieved. The goal for patients with stable CAD or a CAD equivalent is less than 100 mg/dL, and for those at "very high risk" (i.e., established CAD and multiple risk factors), the LDL cholesterol goal is less than 70 mg/dL.

21. Which patients with chronic stable angina should be referred for stress testing?
The two purposes of stress testing are *diagnosis* of CAD and *prognosis* in patients with presumed or known CAD. Stress testing performed for diagnostic purposes is usually performed with the patient off antianginal therapy, whereas stress testing performed for prognostic purposes may sometimes be performed with the patient on antianginal agents.

An estimation of the pretest probability of CAD—based on an assessment of the patient's chest pain and his or her risk factors for atherosclerosis—is essential in determining if further testing is warranted. In general, diagnostic testing is appropriate for the patient with an intermediate pretest probability of CAD, but it is not recommended for those with a low (10% or less pretest probability) or high (90% or more pretest probability) risk.

For example, an abnormal exercise test in a 35-year-old woman with atypical chest pain and no risk factors for atherosclerosis (pretest probability of clinically significant CAD is less than 5%) is likely to be falsely positive, thereby prompting the use of unnecessary medications or invasive diagnostic testing; a negative test would simply support a low clinical suspicion of CAD. Similarly, testing of high-risk patients is unlikely to provide information that will alter the diagnosis of CAD. A positive exercise test will only confirm the high clinical suspicion of CAD; a negative result would only lower the estimate of likelihood of CAD into the moderate range and would not exclude the diagnosis.

The results of noninvasive diagnostic testing are most likely to influence subsequent decisions when the pretest probability of CAD is in the intermediate range. For example, a positive exercise test in a 55-year-old man with atypical chest pain and no risk factors for atherosclerosis (pretest probability of clinically significant CAD, approximately 50%) substantially increases the likelihood of clinically important CAD (posttest probability, 85%), whereas a negative exercise test dramatically reduces the likelihood (posttest probability, 15%).

The chronic stable angina guidelines advocate obtaining a stress test for prognostic reasons in many cases—if the stress test reveals low-risk findings, then the patient can be managed medically, whereas if the stress test reveals high-risk findings, the patient is usually referred for cardiac catheterization.

22. **Which patients with chronic stable angina should have a cardiac catheterization?**
    - High risk findings on stress testing
    - Symptoms not adequately controlled with antianginal medications
    - Depressed ejection fraction
    - Unstable symptoms develop

23. **Which patients with chronic stable angina should be referred for revascularization?**

    In most individuals, survival with optimal medical therapy is similar to that observed following revascularization. In the patient with stable angina and preserved ejection fraction receiving optimal medical therapy, percutaneous coronary intervention (PCI) does not reduce the incidence of subsequent MI or cardiac death. Although PCI-treated patients initially may experience a greater improvement in symptom control and quality of life, these salutary effects largely disappear within 24 months. Hence intensive medical therapy and lifestyle intervention are appropriate as initial therapy for most patients with chronic stable angina.

    Revascularization should be reserved for those with (1) symptoms that interfere with the patient's lifestyle despite optimal medical therapy or (2) coronary anatomic findings that indicate that revascularization would provide a survival benefit, including
    - Left main CAD
    - 3 vessel CAD and depressed ejection fraction (less than 50%)
    - Multivessel CAD with stenosis of the proximal left anterior descending (LAD) artery.

    The optimal method of revascularization—coronary artery bypass graft (CABG) or PCI—is selected based on the coronary angiographic findings, the likelihood of success (or complications) of each procedure, and the subject's preferences. Ideally, both an interventional cardiologist and cardiac surgeon should review the patient's data (including the angiogram) and reach agreement on which procedure(s) should be offered, after which the patient is presented with the advantages and disadvantages of each and allowed to choose between them. Among subjects with left main CAD (or in those with extensive 2- or 3-vessel CAD), either procedure could be considered, but the weight of published evidence supports the more durable benefit afforded by CABG (mortality reduction and lower incidence of repeat revascularization).

24. **Is there an easy way to remember how to manage the patient with chronic stable angina?**

    The "ABCDEs" of treatment for patients with chronic stable angina
    - A = Aspirin and antianginal therapy: ACE inhibitors in patients not considered "low risk"
    - B = β-blocker and blood pressure control
    - C = Cigarette smoking and cholesterol
    - D = Diet and diabetes
    - E = Education and exercise

BIBLIOGRAPHY, SUGGESTED READINGS, AND WEBSITES

1. 2012 ACCF/AHA/ACP/AATS/PCNA/SCAI/STS guideline for the diagnosis and management of patients with stable ischemic heart disease: executive summary: a report of the American College of Cardiology Foundation/American Heart Association Task Force on Practice Guidelines, and the American College of Physicians, American Association for Thoracic Surgery, Preventive Cardiovascular Nurses Association, Society for Cardiovascular Angiography and Interventions, and Society of Thoracic Surgeons. *Circulation.* 2012;126:3097–3137. Available at: http://circ.ahajournals.org/content/126/25/3097.full.pdf+html. Accessed Feb 9, 2013.

2. Bhatt DL, Fox KA, Hacke W, et al: Clopidogrel and aspirin versus aspirin alone for the prevention of atherothrombotic events, *N Engl J Med* 354:1706–1717, 2006.

3. Boden WE, O'Rourke RA, Teo KK, et al: Optimal medical therapy with or without PCI for stable coronary disease, *N Engl J Med* 356:1503–1516, 2007.

4. Braunwald E, Domanski MJ, Fowler SE, et al: Angiotensin-converting-enzyme inhibition in stable coronary artery disease, *N Engl J Med* 351:2058–2068, 2004.

5. Antithrombotic Trialists' Collaboration: Collaborative meta-analysis of randomised trials of antiplatelet therapy for prevention of death, myocardial infarction, and stroke in high risk patients, *BMJ* 324:71–86, 2002.

6. Fox KM: Efficacy of perindopril in reduction of cardiovascular events among patients with stable coronary artery disease: randomised, double-blind, placebo-controlled, multicentre trial (the EUROPA study), *Lancet* 362:782–788, 2003.

7. Gerstein HC, Miller ME, Genuth S, et al: Long-term effects of intensive glucose lowering on cardiovascular outcomes, *N Engl J Med* 364:818–828, 2011.

8. Hillis LD, Smith PK, Anderson JL, et al: 2011 ACCF/AHA Guideline for coronary artery bypass graft surgery: Executive Summary: A report of the American College of Cardiology Foundation/American Heart Association Task Force on Practice Guidelines, *J Am Coll Cardiol* 58:2584–2614, 2011.

9. Levine GN, Bates ER, Blankenship JC, et al: 2011 ACCF/AHA/SCAI Guideline for percutaneous intervention: Executive summary: A report of the American College of Cardiology Foundation/American Heart Association Task Force on Practice Guidelines, *J Am Coll Cardiol* 58:2550–2583, 2011.

10. Serruys PW, Morice MC, Kappetein AP, et al: Percutaneous coronary intervention versus coronary-artery bypass grafting for severe coronary artery disease, *N Engl J Med* 360:961–972, 2009.

11. Trikalinos TA, Alsheikh-Ali AA, Tatsioni A, Nallamothu BK, Kent DM: Percutaneous coronary interventions for non-acute coronary artery disease: a quantitative 20-year synopsis and a network meta-analysis, *Lancet* 373:911–918, 2009.

12. Weintraub WS, Spertus JA, Kolm P, et al: Effect of PCI on quality of life in patients with stable coronary disease, *N Engl J Med* 359:677–687, 2008.

NON–ST SEGMENT ELEVATION ACUTE CORONARY SYNDROME

Paul A. Schurmann, MD, and Glenn N. Levine, MD, FACC, FAHA

1. What is non–ST segment elevation acute coronary syndrome?

It is now recognized that unstable angina, non–Q wave myocardial infarction (MI), non–ST segment elevation MI, and ST segment elevation myocardial infarction (STEMI) are all part of a continuum of the pathophysiologic process in which a coronary plaque ruptures, thrombus formation occurs, and partial or complete, transient or more sustained vessel occlusion may occur (Fig. 17-1). This process is deemed acute coronary syndrome when it is clinically recognized and causes symptoms. Acute coronary syndromes can be subdivided for treatment purposes into non–ST segment elevation acute coronary syndrome (NSTE-ACS) and ST segment elevation acute coronary syndrome (STE-ACS).

The American College of Cardiology Foundation/American Heart Association (ACCF/AHA) guidelines have traditionally used the terms *unstable angina/non–ST elevation MI* (UA/NSTEMI) when referring to patients with NSTE-ACS, whereas the European Society of Cardiology (ESC) guidelines prefer the term *acute coronary syndrome without ST elevation.*

2. What is the current definition of a myocardial infarction?

According to the 2007 joint ESC/ACCF/AHA/World Heart Federation statement, the term *myocardial infarction* should be used "when there is evidence of myocardial necrosis in a clinical setting consistent with myocardial ischemia." For patients with acute coronary syndromes, this includes detection of the rise or fall of cardiac biomarkers (preferably troponin) with at least one value above the ninety-ninth percentile of the upper reference limit, and evidence of myocardial ischemia with at least one of the following:

- Symptoms of ischemia
- Electrocardiogram (ECG) changes indicative of new ischemia (new ST-T changes or new left bundle branch block)
- Development of pathologic Q waves in the ECG
- Imaging evidence of new loss of viable myocardium or new regional wall motion abnormalities

Note that using this definition, patients admitted with anginal chest pains and troponin elevations of as little as 0.04 to 0.08 ng/mL may now be diagnosed as having myocardial infarction, depending on locally established ninety-ninth percentile ranges of troponin values.

3. What other conditions besides epicardial coronary artery disease and acute coronary syndrome can cause elevations in troponin?

Although troponins have extremely high myocardial tissue specificity and sensitivity with new assay, numerous conditions besides epicardial coronary artery disease and acute coronary syndromes *may cause* elevations of troponins. Such conditions include noncoronary cardiac disease (myocarditis, acute congestive heart failure [CHF] exacerbation, cardiac contusion, apical ballooning syndrome), acute vascular pathology (hypertensive crisis, aortic dissection, pulmonary embolus), infiltrative diseases (amyloidosis, sarcoidosis), and systemic illnesses (anemia, chromic kidney disease [CKD], hypothyroidism, hypoxemia). Conditions that have been associated with elevation of troponin levels are given in Table 17-1.

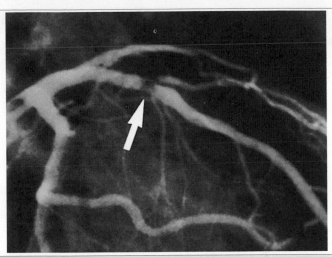

Figure 17-1. Plaque rupture in the proximal left anterior descending (LAD) coronary artery has led to thrombus formation *(arrow)* and partial occlusion of the vessel. (Reproduced with permission from Cannon CP, Braunwald E: Unstable angina and non–ST elevation myocardial infarction. In Libby P, Bonow R, Mann D, et al, editors: *Braunwald's heart disease: a textbook of cardiovascular medicine*, ed 8, Philadelphia, 2008, Saunders, p. 1179)

4. **What are the factors that make up the Thrombolysis in Myocardial Infarction (TIMI) Risk Score?**
   The seven factors that make up the TIMI Risk Score are shown in the list that follows. Each factor counts as 1 point. A total score of 0 to 2 is a low TIMI Risk Score and is associated with a 4.7% to 8.3% 2-week risk of adverse cardiac events; a total score of 3 to 5 is an intermediate TIMI Risk Score and is associated with a 13.2 to 26.2% 2-week risk of adverse cardiac events; and a total score of 6 to 7 is a high TIMI Risk Score and is associated with a 40.9% risk of adverse cardiac events.
   - Age greater than 65 years
   - Three or more risk factors for coronary artery disease (CAD)
   - Prior catheterization demonstrating CAD
   - ST segment deviation
   - Two or more anginal events within 24 hours
   - Acetylsalicylic acid (ASA) use within 7 days
   - Elevated cardiac markers

5. **What are the components of the Global Registry of Acute Coronary Events (GRACE) ACS Risk Model (at the time of admission)?**
   The components of the GRACE ACS Risk Model at the time of admission consist of:
   - Age
   - Heart rate (HR)
   - Systolic blood pressure (SBP)
   - Creatinine
   - Congestive heart failure Killip class
   - Cardiac arrest at admission (yes/no)
   - ST segment deviation (yes/no)
   - Elevated cardiac enzymes/markers

   Scores are calculated based on established criteria. Calculation algorithms are easily download-able to computers and handheld devices. A low-risk score is considered 108 or less and is associated with a less than 1% risk of in-hospital death. An intermediate score is 109 to 140 and is associated

TABLE 17–1. CONDITIONS OTHER THAN CORONARY ARTERY DISEASE ASSOCIATED WITH ELEVATION IN CARDIAC TROPONIN

System	Causes of Troponin Elevation
Cardiovascular	Acute aortic dissection
	Arrhythmia
	Medical ICU patients
	Hypotension
	Heart failure
	Apical ballooning syndrome
	Cardiac inflammation
	Endocarditis, myocarditis, pericarditis
	Hypertension
	Infiltrative disease
	Amyloidosis, sarcoidosis, hemochromatosis, scleroderma
	Left ventricular hypertrophy
Myocardial injury	Blunt chest trauma
	Cardiac surgeries
	Cardiac procedures
	Ablation, cardioversion, percutaneous intervention
	Chemotherapy
	Hypersensitivity drug reactions
	Envenomation
Respiratory	Acute PE
	ARDS
Infectious/Immune	Sepsis/SIRS
	Viral illness
	Thrombotic thrombocytopenic purpura
Gastrointestinal	Severe GI bleeding
Nervous system	Acute stroke
	Ischemic stroke
	Hemorrhagic stroke
	Head trauma
Renal	Chronic kidney disease
Endocrine	Diabetes
	Hypothyroidism
Musculoskeletal	Rhabdomyolysis
Integumentary	Extensive skin burns
Inherited	Neurofibromatosis
	Duchenne muscular dystrophy
	Klippel-Feil syndrome
Others	Endurance exercise
	Environmental exposure
	Carbon monoxide, hydrogen sulfide

Reproduced with permission from Januzzi JL Jr: Causes of Non-ACS Related Troponin Elevations. Available at http://www.cardiosource.org. Accessed February 16, 2013.
ARDS, Acute respiratory distress syndrome; *GI*, gastrointestinal; *ICU*, intensive care unit; *PE*, pulmonary embolism; *SIRS*, systemic inflammatory response syndrome.

with a 1% to 3% risk of in-hospital death. A high-risk score is greater than 140 and associated with a more than 3% risk of in-hospital death.

6. What other biomarkers and measured blood levels have been shown to correlate with increased risk of adverse cardiovascular outcome?

Multiple biomarkers can be measured in the blood, but it is important to understand what they represent. The most common are creatine kinase—MB (CK-MB) and troponin T and I levels, which are related to myocardial injury and are independent predictors of adverse cardiovascular outcomes.

Common inflammatory biomarkers like C-reactive protein (CRP), matrix metalloproteinase (MMP-9), myeloperoxidase (MPO), B-type natriuretic peptide (BNP), and ischemia modified albumin (IMA) have been shown to be independent predictors of adverse cardiovascular outcomes. How these findings should be used in clinical practice is subject to continued investigation and debate. Additional markers are expected to emerge over the next several years.

7. What are the differences between the oral antiplatelet agents?

The first thienopyridine was ticlopidine (Ticlid), which was used along with aspirin for the prevention of stent thrombosis. Ticlopidine was replaced in clinical practice by clopidogrel, which was a once-daily agent with similar efficacy to ticlopidine, but better tolerated.

More recently, the thienopyridine prasugrel and the triazolopyrimidine ticagrelor have been approved for use. These two agents have been studied in patients with ACS undergoing stent implantation. Like clopidogrel, both are P2Y$_{12}$ blockers. Both these newer agents are more potent than clopidogrel, leading to greater and more reliable platelet inhibition than clopidogrel. They also both have a shorter onset of action than clopidogrel. Like clopidogrel, prasugrel irreversibly inhibits the platelet. Although ticagrelor does not irreversibly inhibit the platelet, there nevertheless is effective platelet inhibition for days following discontinuation of ticagrelor. The characteristics of these 3 agents are summarized in Table 17-2.

8. What antiplatelet agents are recommended in the ACCF/AHA and ESC guidelines?

Both organizations recommend that aspirin should be administered as soon as possible and that in patients with true aspirin allergies or aspirin contraindications, clopidogrel should be administered as a substitute for aspirin.

The ACCF/AHA guidelines recommend administration of either clopidogrel, ticagrelor, or a glycoprotein (GP) IIb/IIIa inhibitor (in addition to aspirin) in patients who are to be treated with an early invasive

TABLE 17-2.	CHARACTERISTICS OF THE THREE ORAL P2Y$_{12}$ INHIBITOR ANTIPLATELET AGENTS USED IN THE TREATMENT OF PATIENTS WITH NSTE-ACS		
	Clopidogrel	**Prasugrel**	**Ticagrelor**
Class	Thienopyridine	Thienopyridine	Triazolopyrimidine
Reversibility	Irreversible	Irreversible	Reversible
Activation	Prodrug	Prodrug	Active drug
Onset of action	2-4 hr	30 min	30 min
Duration	3-10 days	5-10 days	3-4 days
Withdrawal before CABG	5 days	7 days	5 days

Reproduced with permission from Hamm CW, Bassand JP, Agewall S, et al: ESC Guidelines for the management of acute coronary syndromes in patients presenting without persistent ST-segment elevation: The Task Force for the management of acute coronary syndromes (ACS) in patients presenting without persistent ST-segment elevation of the European Society of Cardiology (ESC). *Eur Heart J* 32:2999-3054, 2011.
NSTE-ACS, Non—ST segment elevation acute coronary syndrome.

strategy. Administration of both an oral $P2Y_{12}$ inhibitor and an intravenous antiplatelet agent can be considered in certain circumstances in which a patient with high risk characteristics is to be treated with an early invasive strategy. Prasugrel can be considered as the $P2Y_{12}$ agent in patients who are undergoing PCI with coronary stent implantation. The ACCF/AHA guidelines recommend clopidogrel or ticagrelor (in addition to aspirin) in patients to be treated with an initial conservative strategy.

The ESC guidelines recommend that all patients receive a $P2Y_{12}$ inhibitor, with ticagrelor or prasugrel generally being preferred over clopidogrel. The additional use of GP IIb/IIIa inhibitors in high-risk patients is also recommended.

The antiplatelet recommendations of the ACCF/AHA and the ESC NSTE-ACS guidelines are summarized in Table 17-3.

TABLE 17-3. ACCF/AHA AND ESC GUIDELINES FOR ANTIPLATELET THERAPIES IN PATIENTS WITH NSTE-ACS

ACCF/AHA Guidelines

Class I

- Aspirin
- Clopidogrel if ASA allergic/intolerant
- Clopidogrel or ticagrelor in addition to ASA if initial conservative strategy
- Clopidogrel, ticagrelor, or GP IIb/IIIa (in addition to ASA) upstream if early invasive strategy
- Prasugrel (in addition to ASA) *at the time* of the percutaneous coronary intervention
- Clopidogrel, ticagrelor or prasugrel should be administered at least 12 months in patient who underwent percutaneous coronary intervention.

Class IIa

- It is reasonable to omit GP IIb/IIIa if early invasive strategy and patient treated with bivalirudin and with clopidogrel (>6 hr).
- For initial conservative strategy, if already on ASA and clopidogrel (or ticagrelor) and has recurrent ischemia, add GP IIb/IIIa inhibitors.

Class IIb

- Clopidogrel *and* GP IIb/IIIa (in addition to ASA) upstream if early invasive strategy

Class III—No benefit

- Abciximab should not be administered to patient in whom PCI is not planned.

Class III—Harm

- Prasugrel use in patient with prior history of stroke or TIA for whom PCI is planned

ESC Guidelines

Class I

- Aspirin should be given *to all patients* without contraindications.
- $P2Y_{12}$ inhibitor (in addition to ASA) *for all patients*, except if they are high risk for bleeding.
- Ticagrelor is recommended for all patients at mod-high ischemic events regardless of initial treatment strategy.
- Prasugrel is recommended for $P2Y_{12}$ inhibitor naive patient with known coronary anatomy and planned for PCI without contraindications.
- Clopidogrel is recommended for patients who cannot receive ticagrelor or prasugrel.
- In patients considered for invasive procedure/PCI, 600 mg loading dose of clopidogrel may be used.

Continued

TABLE 17-3.   ACCF/AHA AND ESC GUIDELINES FOR ANTIPLATELET THERAPIES IN PATIENTS WITH NSTE-ACS—CONT'D

- GP IIb/IIIa (in addition to dual oral antiplatelet agents) in high-risk patients (elevated troponin, visible thrombus) is recommended if the risk of bleeding is low.

Class IIa

- Eptifibatide and tirofiban added to aspirin should be considered prior to angiography in high-risk patients not preloaded with $P2Y_{12}$ inhibitors.

Class IIb

- Platelets function analysis or genotyping might be considered in selected cases where result may alter the management.

Class III

- NSAIDs (nonselective or COX-2 inhibitors) should not be administered during UA/NSTEMI, except aspirin.
- Routine GP IIb/IIIa inhibitors with ASA and/or $P2Y_{12}$ inhibitor is not recommended, particularly in those undergoing medical management without PCI.

Modified from Wright RS; Anderson JL, Adams CD, et al: 2011 ACCF/AHA Focused Update of the Guidelines for the Management of Patients With Unstable Angina/Non–ST-Elevation Myocardial Infarction (Updating the 2007 Guideline): a report of the American College of Cardiology Foundation/American Heart Association Task Force on Practice Guidelines. *Circulation* 123:2022-2060, 2011; Jneid H, Anderson JL, Wright RS, et al: 2012 ACCF/AHA Focused update of the guideline for the management of patients with unstable angina/non-ST-elevation myocardial infarction (updating the 2007 guideline and replacing the 2011 focused update). *J Am Coll Cardiol* 2012:645-81; and Hamm CW, Bassand JP, Agewall S, et al: ESC Guidelines for the management of acute coronary syndromes in patients presenting without persistent ST-segment elevation: The Task Force for the management of acute coronary syndromes (ACS) in patients presenting without persistent ST-segment elevation of the European Society of Cardiology (ESC). *Eur Heart J* 32:2999-3054, 2011.
ACCF, American College of Cardiology Foundation; *AHA*, American Heart Association; *ASA*, acetylsalicylic acid; *ESC*, European Society of Cardiology; *GP*, glycoprotein; *NSAID*, nonsteroidal antiinflammatory drug; *NSTE-ACS*, non–ST segment elevation acute coronary syndrome; *PCI*, percutaneous coronary intervention; *TIA*, transient ischemic attack; *UA/NSTEMI*, unstable angina/non–ST segment elevation myocardial infarction.

9. **What are the differences between the intravenous antiplatelet agents?**
Eptifibatide (Integrilin) and tirofiban (Aggrastat) are small-molecule GP IIb/IIIa inhibitors that are used both for "upfront" treatment of NSTE-ACS and during percutaneous coronary intervention (PCI). Abciximab (ReoPro) is an antibody fragment that is used predominantly at the time of PCI (although there is a very specific circumstance in which it can be considered in NSTE-ACS patients before PCI is performed). Eptifibatide and tirofiban lead to reversible platelet inhibition, whereas abciximab leads to irreversible platelet inhibition. All 3 agents lead to a high degree of platelet inhibition, are associated with a small but real increased risk of major bleeding, and are associated with a small (1% to 4%) incidence of thrombocytopenia. Thrombocytopenia can occur rapidly and be profound, and careful monitoring of platelet counts is warranted when these agents are begun. The characteristics of these 3 agents are summarized in Table 17-4.

10. **What anticoagulant agents are recommended by the ACCF/AHA and ESC guidelines?**
The ACCF/AHA guidelines give a Class I recommendation to unfractionated heparin (UFH), enoxaparin, fondaparinux, and bivalirudin.
   The ESC guidelines place a strong emphasis on the prevention of bleeding complications and preferentially recommend fondaparinux, with a single bolus of UFH (85 IU/kg or 60 IU/kg in the case of concomitant use of GP IIb/IIIa) at the time of the PCI. If fondaparinux is not available, enoxaparin

TABLE 17-4.   CHARACTERISTICS OF THE 3 INTRAVENOUS ANTIPLATELET AGENTS USED IN THE TREATMENT OF PATIENTS WITH NSTE-ACS

	Abciximab	Eptifibatide	Tirofiban
Class	GP IIb/IIIa	GP IIb/IIIa	GP IIb/IIIa
Reversibility	Irreversible	Reversible	Reversible
Activation	Active drug	Active drug	Active drug
Onset of action	10 min	15 min	30 min
Duration	2 days, low levels up to 10 days	6 hr	4-8 hr
Withdrawal before CABG	At least 12 hr	At least 2-4 hr	At least 2-4 hr

Modified with permission from Hamm CW, Bassand JP, Agewall S, et al: ESC Guidelines for the management of acute coronary syndromes in patients presenting without persistent ST-segment elevation: The Task Force for the management of acute coronary syndromes (ACS) in patients presenting without persistent ST-segment elevation of the European Society of Cardiology (ESC). *Eur Heart J* 32:2999-3054, 2011.
CABG, coronary artery bypass graft; *GP*, glycoprotein.

(1 mg/kg twice daily) is recommended. If fondaparinux or enoxaparin are not available, UFH with a target aPTT of 50-70 sec (or other low molecular weight heparin) is recommended.

Bivalirudin plus provisional GP IIb/IIIa inhibitors are recommended as an alternative to UFH plus GP IIb/IIIa inhibitors, particularly in patients with a high risk of bleeding who are subject to invasive strategy. Anticoagulant agents recommendations are summarized in Table 17-5.

11. **What is the recommended dosing of unfractionated heparin?**
The dosing recommendations vary slightly between ACCF/AHA and ESC, as well as with the American College of Chest Physicians (ACCP).
   - ACCF/AHA: 60 U/kg bolus (max. 4000 U), then initial infusion of 12 U/kg (max. initial infusion 1000 U/hr). Target anti-Xa is 0.3 to 0.7; target activated partial thromboplastin time (aPTT) is 1.5 to 2.5 times control (60 to 80 seconds per ACCP guidelines).
   - ESC: 60 to 70 U/kg bolus (max. 5000 U), then initial infusion of 12 to 15 U/kg (initial max. 1000 U/hr). Target aPTT is 50 to 75 seconds (1.5 to 2.5 times control).

12. **Which patients with NSTE-ACS should be treated with a strategy of early catheterization and revascularization?**
Studies performed in the 1980s comparing a strategy of early catheterization and revascularization with a strategy of initial medical therapy failed to show benefits of early catheterization and revascularization. More recent studies have demonstrated benefits of early catheterization and revascularization in appropriately selected patients with high-risk features.

An *early invasive* strategy is considered to be the performance of catheterization (and PCI if appropriate) within 2 to 48 hours of admission. Patients who should be treated with early invasive strategy are those without clear contraindications to catheterization, revascularization, and elevated risk for clinical events.

The ACCF/AHA criteria for elevated risk for clinical events (Fig. 17-2) include recurrent angina/ischemia, elevated troponin, new ST depression, CHF exacerbation, reduced left ventricular (LV) function, high-risk findings on noninvasive testing, hemodynamic instability, sustained ventricular tachycardia (VT), PCI within 6 months, prior coronary artery bypass graft (CABG), and high risk score (TIMI ≥ 6, GRACE > 140).

The ESC criteria of high-risk features (Fig. 17-3) include elevated troponin, dynamic ST or T-wave changes, diabetes mellitus (DM), reduced renal function (glomerular filtration rate [GFR] less than

TABLE 17–5. ACCF/AHA AND ESC GUIDELINES FOR ANTITHROMBIN THERAPIES IN PATIENTS WITH NSTE-ACS*

ACCF/AHA Guidelines

Class I

- UFH (early invasive or initial conservative strategies)
- Enoxaparin (early invasive or initial conservative strategies)
- Fondaparinux (early invasive or initial conservative strategies)
- Bivalirudin (early invasive strategy only)
- Fondaparinux preferred for conservative strategy in patients with increased risk of bleeding.
- For initial conservative treatment, enoxaparin or fondaparinux preferred over UFH.

ESC Guidelines

Class I

- Anticoagulation is recommended for all patients in addition to antiplatelet therapy.
- Anticoagulant should be selected according to risk of both ischemic and bleeding events.
- In conservative treatment, anticoagulation should be maintained up to hospital discharge.
- Fondaparinux (2.5 mg SC daily) is recommended as having the best efficacy–safety profile.
- If initial anticoagulant is fondaparinux, a single bolus of UFH 85 IU/kg or 60 IU/kg in the case of concomitant use of GP IIb/IIIa should be added at the time of PCI.
- Enoxaparin (1 mg/kg twice daily) is recommended when fondaparinux is not available.
- If fondaparinux or enoxaparin are not available, UFH with a target PTT of 1.5 to 2.5 times control is indicated.
- Bivalirudin plus provisional GP IIb/IIIa are recommended as an alternative to UFH plus GP IIb/IIIa particularly in patients with a high risk of bleeding planned for urgent or early invasive strategy.

Class III

- Crossover of heparins (UFH and LMWH) is not recommended.

Modified from Wright RS; Anderson JL, Adams CD, et al: 2011 ACCF/AHA Focused Update of the Guidelines for the Management of Patients With Unstable Angina/Non–ST-Elevation Myocardial Infarction (Updating the 2007 Guideline): a report of the American College of Cardiology Foundation/American Heart Association Task Force on Practice Guidelines. *Circulation*. 123:2022-2060, 2011; and Hamm CW, Bassand JP, Agewall S, et al: ESC Guidelines for the management of acute coronary syndromes in patients presenting without persistent ST-segment elevation: The Task Force for the management of acute coronary syndromes (ACS) in patients presenting without persistent ST-segment elevation of the European Society of Cardiology (ESC). *Eur Heart J* 32:2999-3054, 2011.
ACCF, American College of Cardiology Foundation; *AHA*, American Heart Association; *ESC*, European Society of Cardiology; *GP*, glycoprotein; *LMWH*, low-molecular-weight heparin; *NSTE-ACS*, non–ST segment elevation acute coronary syndrome; *PCI*, percutaneous coronary intervention; *PTT*, partial thromboplastin time; *SC*, subcutaneous; *UFH*, unfractionated heparin.

60 mL/min/1.73 m^2), ejection fraction (EF) less than 40%, early post-MI angina, PCI within the past 6 months, prior CABG, and intermediate to high GRACE risk score. Urgent invasive strategy (within 120 minutes after first medical contact) should be for very high-risk patients: refractory angina, recurrent angina despite intense anti-anginal treatment, with ST depression or deep negative T wave, hemodynamic instability (shock), and life-threatening arrhythmias (ventricular fibrillations or ventricular tachycardia).

Hemodynamically unstable patients should generally undergo immediate catheterization.

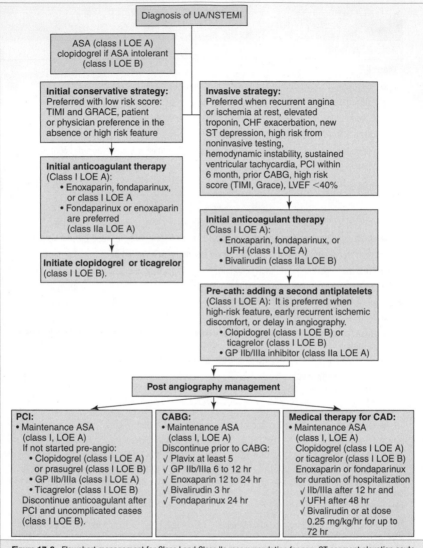

Figure 17-2. Flowchart management for Class I and Class IIa recommendation for non–ST segment elevation acute cardiac syndrome (NSTE-ACS) by the American College of Cardiology Foundation and the American Heart Association. *ASA*, acetylsalicylic acid; *CABG*, coronary artery bypass graft; *CAD*, coronary artery disease; *CHF*, congestive heart failure; *GP*, glycoprotein; *GRACE*, Global Registry of Acute Coronary Events; *LOE*, level of evidence; *LVEF*, left ventricular ejection fraction; *PCI*, percutaneous coronary intervention; *TIMI*, Thrombolysis in Myocardial Infarction Study Group; *UA/NSTEMI*, unstable angina/non–ST segment elevation myocardial infarction.

13. **Should platelet function testing be used routinely to determine platelet inhibitory response?**

    No. Currently the routine use of platelet function test in NSTE-ACS is not recommended by the ACCF/AHA or ESC. However, it may be considered in selected cases if the results of testing may alter management (Class IIb; level of evidence [LOE] B).

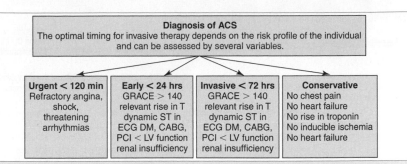

Figure 17-3. Flowchart management for non−ST segment elevation acute cardiac syndrome (NSTE-ACS) by the European Society of Cardiology (ESC). *ACS,* Acute cardiac syndrome; *CABG,* coronary artery bypass graft; *DM,* diabetes mellitus; *ECG,* electrocardiogram; *GRACE,* Global Registry of Acute Coronary Events; *PCI,* percutaneous coronary intervention.

14. **Should nonsteroidal antiinflammatory drugs (NSAIDs) or COX-2 inhibitors (other than aspirin) be continued in patients admitted for NSTE-ACS?**

    No. Recent data suggest potential adverse effects of these agents, and it is now recommended to stop such therapy in patients admitted for NSTE-ACS.

15. **Can nitrate therapy be administered to patients currently taking erectile dysfunction agents?**

    No. Concurrent use of nitrates and currently available erectile dysfunction (ED) agents may lead to profound hypotension because of increased levels of the vasodilator nitric oxide. Patients who have taken an ED agent should not be treated with nitrates for the following periods:

    - Sildenafil (Viagra): 24 hours
    - Tadalafil (Cialis): 48 hours
    - Vardenafil (Levitra): not established at the time of this writing, but common sense would dictate at least 24 hours and perhaps a little longer

16. **Can statin therapy be safely started in patients admitted with acute coronary syndromes?**

    Yes. Several trials, among them Myocardial Ischemia Reduction with Acute Cholesterol Lowering (MIRACL) and Pravastatin or Atorvastatin Evaluation and Infection Therapy—Thrombolysis in Myocardial Infarction (PROVE IT–TIMI 22) demonstrated a very low incidence of liver function test (LFT) elevation and rhabdomyolysis in appropriately selected patients. These patients presented acute coronary syndrome and were started on high-dose/high-intensity lipid therapy (e.g., atorvastatin 80 mg). Based on these and other studies, it is now recommended that statin therapy, when appropriate, be initiated during the hospital stay.

17. **What are the recommendations regarding drug discontinuation in patients who are to undergo CABG?**

    The following recommendations have been made regarding these medications commonly used in patients with NSTE-ACS who are to undergo CABG. When possible, for elective CABG:

    - Wait at least 5 days after the last dose of clopidogrel or ticagrelor before CABG.
    - Wait at least 7 days after the last dose of prasugrel before CABG.
    - Discontinue eptifibatide or tirofiban at least 2 to 4 hours before CABG; discontinue abciximab at least 12 hours before CABG.
    - Discontinue enoxaparin 12 to 24 hours before CABG and dose with UFH.
    - Discontinue fondaparinux 24 hours before CABG and dose with UFH.
    - Discontinue bivalirudin 3 hours before CABG and dose with UFH.

REFERENCES, SUGGESTED READINGS, AND WEBSITES

1. Cannon CP, Braunwald E: Unstable angina and non–ST-elevation myocardial infarction. In Bonow R, Mann D, Zipes P, editors: *Braunwald's heart disease: a textbook of cardiovascular medicine*, ed 9, Philadelphia, 2012, Saunders, pp. 1178-1209.

2. Center for Outcomes Research, University of Massachusetts Medical School. Global Registry of Acute Coronary Events (GRACE) Risk Calculator. Available at: http://www.outcomes-umassmed.org/grace/acs_risk/acs_risk_content.html. Accessed March 28, 2013

3. Hamm C, Bassand JP, Agewall S, et al: Task Force for management acute coronary syndromes in patient presenting without-ST-Segment Elevation of the European Society of Cardiology: ESC guidelines for the management of acute coronary syndromes of patients presenting without ST-segment elevation, *Eur Heart J* 32:2999–3054, 2011.

4. Thygesen K, Alpert JS, White HD: Universal definition of myocardial infarction, *Circulation* 116(22):2634–2653, 2007.

5. Wright RS, Anderson JL, Adams CD, et al: ACC/AHA 2011 guidelines for the management of patients with unstable angina/non–ST-elevation myocardial infarction, *Circulation* 123:2022–2060, 2011.

CHAPTER 18

ST SEGMENT ELEVATION MYOCARDIAL INFARCTION

Glenn N. Levine, MD, FACC, FAHA

1. **What are the electrocardiograph (ECG) criteria for the diagnosis of ST segment elevation myocardial infarction (STEMI)?**

   Criteria for the diagnosis of STEMI can derive from criteria established for the administration of thrombolytic therapy, which evolved in the late 1980s and 1990s. ECG criteria for suspected coronary artery occlusion include:

   - American College of Cardiology Foundation/American Heart Association (ACCF/AHA) criteria for STEMI consist of ST segment elevation greater than 0.1 mV (one small box) in at least two contiguous leads (e.g., leads III and aVF, or leads V2 and V3). The European Society of Cardiology (ESC) STEMI guidelines require 0.2 mV or greater ST elevation when analyzing leads V1 through V3 (but similarly, 0.1 mV elevation for other leads and/or territories). Figure 18.1 demonstrates the ECG finding of ST elevation in a patient with acute myocardial infarction.
   - New or presumably new left bundle branch block (LBBB)

2. **Is intracoronary thrombus common in STEMI?**

   Yes. The majority of STEMI is due to plaque rupture, fissure, or disruption, leading to superimposed thrombus formation and vessel occlusion. Angioscopy demonstrates coronary thrombus in more than 90% of patients with STEMI (as opposed to 35% to 75% of patients with non–ST segment elevation acute coronary syndrome [NSTE-ACS] and 1% of patients with stable angina).

3. **What is primary PCI?**

   Primary percutaneous coronary intervention (PCI) refers to the strategy of taking a patient who presents with STEMI directly to the cardiac catheterization laboratory to undergo mechanical revascularization using balloon angioplasty, coronary stents, aspiration thrombectomy, and other measures. Patients

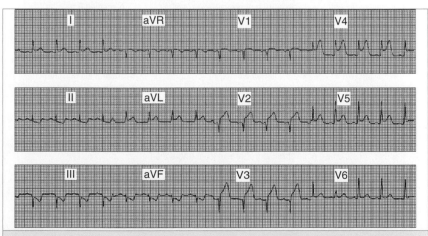

Figure 18-1. ST elevation in a patient with acute myocardial infarction (MI). There are 3 to 4 mm ST elevation in the anterior leads (V2 through V4), with lesser degrees of ST elevation in the lateral leads (I, aVL, V5, V6).

are not treated with thrombolytic therapy in the emergency room (or ambulance) but preferentially taken directly to the cardiac catheterization laboratory for primary PCI. Studies have demonstrated that primary PCI is superior to thrombolytic therapy when it can be performed in a timely manner by a skilled interventional cardiologist with a skilled and experienced catheterization laboratory team.

4. **What are considered to be contraindications to thrombolytic therapy?**
Several absolute contraindications to thrombolytic therapy and several relative contraindications (or cautions) must be considered in deciding whether to treat a patient with lytic agents. As would be expected, these are based on the risks and consequences of bleeding resulting from thrombolytic therapy. These contraindications and cautions are given in Box 18-1.

BOX 18-1. CONTRAINDICATIONS AND CAUTIONS OR RELATIVE CONTRAINDICATIONS FOR FIBRINOLYTIC THERAPY, AS GIVEN BY THE AMERICAN COLLEGE OF CARDIOLOGY/AMERICAN HEART ASSOCIATION (ACC/AHA) AND BY THE EUROPEAN SOCIETY OF CARDIOLOGY (ESC)

ACC/AHA

Absolute Contraindications:
- Any prior intracranial hemorrhage (ICH)
- Known structural cerebral vascular lesion (e.g., arteriovenous malformation)
- Known malignant intracranial neoplasm (primary or metastatic)
- Ischemic stroke within 3 months (except acute ischemic stroke within 4.5 hours)
- Suspected aortic dissection
- Active bleeding (excluding menses) or bleeding diathesis
- Significant closed-head or facial trauma within 3 months

Cautions/Relative Contraindications:
- History of chronic, severe, poorly controlled hypertension
- Severe uncontrolled hypertension of presentation (systolic blood pressure [SBP] > 180 mm Hg or diastolic blood pressure [DBP] > 110 mm Hg)
- Traumatic or prolonged (>10 minutes) cardiopulmonary resuscitation (CPR) or major surgery within 3 weeks
- Recent (within 2-4 weeks) internal bleeding
- Noncompressible vascular punctures
- Pregnancy
- Active peptic ulcer
- Current use of anticoagulants with high international normalized ratio (INR); the higher the INR, the higher the risk of bleeding
- For streptokinase or anistreplase: prior exposure (more than 5 days ago) or prior allergic reaction to these agents

ESC

Absolute Contraindications:
- Hemorrhagic stroke or stroke of unknown origin at any time
- Ischemic stroke in preceding 6 months
- Central nervous system (CNS) damage or neoplasms
- Recent major trauma/surgery/head injury (within preceding 3 weeks)
- Gastrointestinal bleeding within the last month
- Known bleeding disorder
- Aortic dissection

Relative Contraindications:
- Transient ischemic attack in preceding 6 months
- Oral anticoagulant therapy
- Pregnancy or within 1 week post-partum
- Non-compressible punctures
- Traumatic resuscitation
- Refractory hypertension (SBP > 180 mm Hg)
- Advanced liver disease
- Infective endocarditis
- Active peptic ulcer

Modified from Antman EM, Anbe DT, Armstrong PW, et al: ACC/AHA guidelines for the management of patients with ST-elevation myocardial infarction. *J Am Coll Cardiol* 44:E1-E211, 2004, and from Van de Werf F, Ardissino D, Betriu A, et al: Management of acute myocardial infarction in patients presenting with ST-segment elevation. The Task Force on the Management of Acute Myocardial Infarction of the European Society of Cardiology. *Eur Heart J* 24:28-66, 2003.

5. **What is door-to-balloon time?**

Door-to-balloon time is a phrase that denotes the time it takes from when a patient with STEMI sets foot in the emergency room until the time that a balloon is inflated in the occluded, culprit coronary artery. More recently, the concept of *medical contact-to-balloon time* has been emphasized, given that STEMI may first be diagnosed in the transporting ambulance in some cases. Because balloon angioplasty is no longer always the first intervention performed on an occluded artery, the term has further evolved to *medical contact-to-device time*. The generally accepted medical contact-to-device time goal is 90 minutes or less in cases in which the patient presents or is taken directly to a hospital that performs PCI. In cases in which the patient must be transferred from a hospital that does not perform PCI to a hospital that does perform PCI, the goal is a medical contact-to-device time of no more than 120 minutes.

6. **What is door-to-needle time?**

Door-to-needle time is a phrase that denotes the time it takes from when a patient with STEMI sets foot in the emergency room until the beginning of thrombolytic therapy administration. The generally accepted goal for door-to-needle time is 30 minutes or less.

7. **In patients treated with thrombolytic therapy, how long should antithrombin therapy be continued?**

Patients who are treated with unfractionated heparin (UFH) should be treated for 48 hours. Studies of low-molecular-weight heparins (EXTRACT, CREATE) and of direct thrombin inhibitors (OASIS-6) have suggested that patients treated with these agents should be treated throughout their hospitalizations, up to 8 days maximum. Guidelines for adjunctive antiplatelet and antithrombin therapy in patients treated with thrombolytic therapy are given in Table 18-1.

8. **Which patients with STEMI should undergo cardiac catheterization?**

Patients with STEMI who should undergo immediate coronary angiography include those who are candidates for primary PCI, those with severe heart failure or cardiogenic shock (if they are suitable candidates for revascularization), and many of those with moderate to large areas of myocardium at risk and evidence of failed fibrinolysis. Cardiac catheterization is reasonable in hemodynamically stable patients with evidence of successful fibrinolysis. Recommendations from the 2011 ACCF/AHA/ Society for Cardiovascular Angiography and Interventions (SCAI) Guidelines on PCI regarding coronary angiography in patients with STEMI are given in Table 18-2.

9. **Which patients with STEMI should undergo primary PCI?**

Primary PCI should be performed in patients with STEMI who present within 12 hours of symptom onset, in patients with severe heart failure or cardiogenic shock, and in those with contraindications to fibrinolytic therapy. PCI can also be considered in those who have clinical evidence for fibrinolytic failure or infarct artery reocclusion after fibrinolytic failure, as well as those treated with likely successful fibrinolytic failure. Recommendations from the 2011 ACCF/AHA/SCAI Guidelines on PCI regarding PCI in patients with STEMI are given in Table 18-3.

10. **What is facilitated PCI?**

Facilitated PCI refers to a strategy of planned PCI immediately or shortly after administration of an initial pharmacologic regimen intended to improve coronary artery patency before the PCI procedure. Such regimens have included full-dose or reduced-dose thrombolytic therapy, glycoprotein IIb/IIIa inhibitors, antithrombin agents, and combinations of agents. The concept is to restore at least some coronary blood flow as the cardiac catheterization laboratory is getting activated and the patient is being transported to the hospital's catheterization laboratory. Although this strategy is intuitively appealing, studies of such a strategy generally have not demonstrated any advantage of facilitated PCI over primary PCI and it is no longer generally recommended. The term itself is controversial, and there has been a movement to abolish this phrase.

11. **What is rescue PCI?**

Rescue PCI is the performance of PCI after thrombolytic therapy has *failed* in a patient. Studies of rescue PCI versus medical management generally have shown a modest benefit with rescue PCI

TABLE 18–1.	2013 ACCF/AHA GUIDELINES FOR ADJUNCTIVE ANTITHROMBOTIC THERAPY TO SUPPORT REPERFUSION WITH FIBRINOLYTIC THERAPY		
		COR	LOE
Antiplatelet therapy			
Aspirin			
■ 162- to 325-mg loading dose		I	A
■ 81- to 325-mg daily maintenance dose (indefinite)		I	A
■ 81 mg daily is the preferred maintenance dose		IIa	B
P2Y$_{12}$ receptor inhibitors			
■ Clopidogrel:		I	A
○ Age ≤75 y: 300-mg loading dose			
Followed by 75 mg daily for at least 14 d and up to 1 y in absence of bleeding		I	A (14 d) C (up to 1 y)
○ Age >75 y: no loading dose, give 75 mg		I	A
Followed by 75 mg daily for at least 14 d and up to 1 y in absence of bleeding		I	A (14 d) C (up to 1 y)
Anticoagulant therapy			
■ UFH:		I	C
○ Weight-based IV bolus and infusion adjusted to obtain aPTT of 1.5 to 2.0 times control for 48 h or until revascularization. IV bolus of 60 U/kg (maximum 4000 U) followed by an infusion of 12 U/kg/h (maximum 1000 U) initially, adjusted to maintain aPTT at 1.5 to 2.0 times control (approximately 50 to 70 s) for 48 h or until revascularization			
■ Enoxaparin:		I	A
○ If age <75 y: 30-mg IV bolus, followed in 15 min by 1 mg/kg subcutaneously every 12 h (maximum 100 mg for the first 2 doses)			
○ If age ≥75 y: no bolus, 0.75 mg/kg subcutaneously every 12 h (maximum 75 mg for the first 2 doses)			
○ Regardless of ages, if CrCl < 30 mL/min: 1 mg/kg subcutaneously every 24 h			
○ Duration: For the index hospitalization, up to 8 d or until revascularization			
■ Fondaparinux:		I	B
○ Initial dose 2.5 mg IV, then 2.5 mg subcutaneously daily starting the following day, for the index hospitalization up to 8 d or until revascularization			
○ Contraindicated if CrCl < 30 mL/min			

Reproduced with permission from O'Gara P, Kushner FG, Ascheim D, et al. 2013 ACCF/AHA Guideline for the Management of ST-Elevation Myocardial Infarction. *J Am Coll Cardiol* 2013;61(4):e78-e140.
ACC, American College of Cardiology; *AHA,* American Heart Association; *aPPT,* activated partial thromboplastin time; *COR,* Class of Recommendation; *CrCl,* creatinine clearance; *IV,* intravenous; *LOE,* Level of Evidence; *N/A,* not available; *STEMI,* ST segment elevation myocardial infarction; *UFH,* unfractionated heparin.

TABLE 18-2. RECOMMENDATIONS FROM THE 2011 ACCF/AHA/SCAI GUIDELINES ON PCI REGARDING CORONARY ANGIOGRAPHY IN PATIENTS WITH STEMI

Indications	COR	LOE
Immediate Coronary Angiography		
Candidate for primary PCI	I	A
Severe heart failure or cardiogenic shock (if suitable revascularization candidate)	I	B
Moderate to large area of myocardium at risk and evidence of failed fibrinolysis	IIa	B
Coronary Angiography 3 to 24 Hours after Fibrinolysis		
Hemodynamically stable patients with evidence for successful fibrinolysis	IIa	A
Coronary Angiography before Hospital Discharge		
Stable patients	IIb	C
Coronary Angiography at Any Time		
Patients in whom the risks of revascularization are likely to outweigh the benefits or the patient or designee does not want invasive care	III: No benefit	C

Modified from Levine GN, Bates ER, Blankenship JC, et al. 2011 ACCF/AHA/SCAI Guideline for Percutaneous Coronary Intervention. A report of the American College of Cardiology Foundation/American Heart Association Task Force on Practice Guidelines and the Society for Cardiovascular Angiography and Interventions. *J Am Coll Cardiol* 58:e44-e122, 2011.
ACCF, American College of Cardiology Foundation; *AHA*, American Heart Association; *COR*, class of recommendation; *LOE*, level of evidence; *PCI*, percutaneous coronary intervention; *SCAI*, Society for Cardiovascular Angiography and Interventions; *STEMI*, ST segment elevation myocardial infarction.

in appropriately selected patients. The problem with rescue PCI is that clinical and electrocardiographic criteria for predicting which patients have actually failed thrombolytic therapy (have not had successful lysis of coronary thrombosis and restoration of coronary perfusion) are imprecise. Thus, some patients with continued occluded arteries may not be referred for rescue PCI and some patients with successful reperfusion will be referred for unnecessary cardiac catheterization. As with the term *facilitated PCI*, some have advocated for elimination of the term *rescue PCI*.

12. **Which patients should not be treated with beta-adrenergic blocking agent (β-blocker) therapy?**
β-Blockers have been a mainstay of STEMI therapy for decades. However, in the Clopidogrel and Metoprolol in Myocardial Infarction Trial/Second Chinese Cardiac (COMMIT/CCS-2) study, the potential benefits of β-blocker therapy were offset by an increased incidence of cardiogenic shock and shock-related death with β-blocker therapy. Therefore, in patients with signs of heart failure, evidence of a low-output state, or increased risk for cardiogenic shock, β-blocker therapy should not be initiated. Risk factors for cardiogenic shock include age older than 70 years, systolic blood pressure less than 120 mm Hg, sinus tachycardia greater than 110 beats/min, and heart rate less than 60 beats/min. Other contraindications to initiating β-blocker therapy include PR interval more than 0.24 seconds, second- or third-degree heart block, active asthma, or severe reactive airway disease.

13. **Which patients should be treated with nitrate therapy?**
Sublingual (SL) nitroglycerin (0.4 mg) every 5 minutes, up to three doses, should be administered for ongoing ischemic discomfort. Intravenous nitroglycerin is indicated for relief of ongoing ischemic discomfort that responds to nitrate therapy, for control of hypertension, and

TABLE 18-3. RECOMMENDATIONS FROM THE 2011 ACCF/AHA/SCAI GUIDELINES ON PCI REGARDING PCI IN PATIENTS WITH STEMI

Indications	COR	LOE
Primary PCI		
STEMI symptoms within 12 hours	I	A
Severe heart failure or cardiogenic shock	I	B
Contraindications to fibrinolytic therapy with ischemic symptoms <12 hours	I	B
Asymptomatic patient presenting between 12 and 24 hours after symptoms onset and higher risk	IIB	C
Noninfarct artery PCI at the time of primary PCI in patients without hemodynamic compromise	III: Harm	B
Delayed or elective PCI in patients with STEMI (i.e., nonprimary PCI)		
Clinical evidence for fibrinolytic failure or infarct artery reocclusion	IIA	B
Patient infarct artery 3 to 24 hours after fibrinolytic therapy	IIA	B
Ischemia on noninvasive testing	IIA	B
Hemodynamically significant stenosis in a patient infarct artery >24 hours after STEMI	11B	B
Totally occluded infarct artery >24 hours after STEMI in a hemodynamically stable asymptomatic patient without evidence of severe ischemia	III: No benefit	B

Modified from Levine GN, Bates ER, Blankenship JC, et al. 2011 ACCF/AHA/SCAI Guideline for Percutaneous Coronary Intervention. A report of the American College of Cardiology Foundation/American Heart Association Task Force on Practice Guidelines and the Society for Cardiovascular Angiography and Interventions. *J Am Coll Cardiol* 58:e44-e122, 2011.
ACCF, American College of Cardiology Foundation; *AHA*, American Heart Association; *COR*, class of recommendation; *LOE*, level of evidence; *PCI*, percutaneous coronary intervention; *SCAI*, Society for Cardiovascular Angiography and Interventions; *STEMI*, ST segment elevation myocardial infarction.

for management of pulmonary edema. Nitrates should not be administered to patients who have received a phosphodiesterase inhibitor for erectile dysfunction within 24 to 48 hours (depending on the specific agent). Nitrates should also not be administered to those with suspected right ventricular (RV) infarction, systolic blood pressure less than 90 mm Hg (or 30 mm Hg or more below baseline), severe bradycardia (less than 50 beats/min), or tachycardia (more than 100 beats/min) (Box 18-1).

14. **Should patients with STEMI be continued on nonselective nonsteroidal antiinflammatory drugs (NSAIDs) (other than aspirin) or COX-2 inhibitors?**
    No. Use of these agents has been associated with increased risk of reinfarction, hypertension, heart failure, myocardial rupture, and death. Therefore, such agents should be discontinued at the time of admission.

15. **What are the main mechanical complications of myocardial infarction?**
    - **Free wall rupture:** Acute free wall rupture is almost always fatal. In some cases of *subacute free wall rupture,* only a small quantity of blood initially reaches the pericardial cavity and

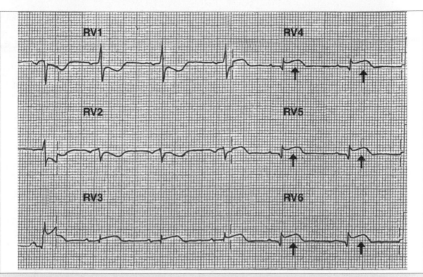

Figure 18-2. Right-sided leads demonstrating ST segment elevation *(arrows)* in leads RV4 through RV6, highly suggestive of right ventricular infarction.

begins to cause signs of pericardial tamponade. Emergent echocardiography and immediate surgery are indicated.

- **Ventricular septal rupture:** A ventricular septal defect (VSD) caused by myocardial infarction and septal rupture occurred in 1% to 2% of all patients with infarction in older series, though the incidence in the fibrinolytic age is 0.2% to 0.3%. Patients may complain of a chest pain somewhat different than their MI pain and will usually develop cardiogenic shock. A new systolic murmur may be audible, often along the left sternal border. Mortality without surgery is 54% in the first week and up to 92% within the first year.
- **Papillary muscle rupture:** Papillary muscle rupture leads to acute and severe mitral regurgitation. It occurs in approximately 1% of STEMI patients. Because of the abrupt elevation in left atrial pressure, there may not be an audible murmur of mitral regurgitation. Pulmonary edema and cardiogenic shock usually develop. Treatment is urgent or emergent mitral valve replacement (or in rare cases, mitral valve repair).

16. What is the triad of findings suggestive of RV infarction?

The triad of findings suggestive of RV infarction is hypotension, distended neck veins, and clear lungs. Clinical RV infarction occurs in approximately 30% of inferior MI patients. Because the infarcted right ventricle is dependent on preload, administration of nitroglycerin (or morphine), which leads to venous pooling and decreased blood return to the right ventricle, may lead to profound hypotension. When such hypotension occurs, patients should be placed in reverse Trendelenburg position (legs above chest and head) and treated with extremely aggressive administration of several liters of fluid through large-bore intravenous needles. Those who do not respond to such therapy may require treatment with agents such as dopamine.

In patients with inferior MI, a *right-sided* ECG should be obtained. The precordial leads are placed over the right side of the chest in a mirror-image pattern to normal. The finding of 1 mm or greater ST elevation in leads RV4 through RV6 is highly suggestive of RV infarction (Fig. 18-2), although the absence of this often-transient finding should not be used to dismiss a diagnosis of RV infarction made on clinical grounds.

17. **Besides plaque rupture and thrombotic occlusion, what are other causes of STEMI?**

Although plaque rupture with subsequent thrombus formation is the most common etiology of STEMI, other causes to consider include:

- Coronary vasospasm, such as what can occur with cocaine use
- Coronary artery embolism, such as in a patient with atrial fibrillation, left ventricular thrombus, endocarditis, or cardiac or valvular tumor
- Spontaneous coronary artery dissection
- Ascending thoracic aortic dissection with compromise of the right coronary artery ostium
- Tako-tsubo cardiomyopathy (stress cardiomyopathy, "broken heart syndrome")

BIBLIOGRAPHY, SUGGESTED READINGS, AND WEBSITES

1. Antman EM: ST-elevation myocardial infarction: management. In Libby P, Bonow R, Mann D, editors: *Braunwald's heart disease: a textbook of cardiovascular medicine*, ed 8, Philadelphia, 2008, Saunders.

2. Antman EM, Anbe DT, Armstrong PW, et al: ACC/AHA guidelines for the management of patients with ST-elevation myocardial infarction: a report of the American College of Cardiology/American Heart Association Task Force on Practice Guidelines (Committee to Revise the 1999 Guidelines for the Management of Patients with Acute Myocardial Infarction), *J Am Coll Cardiol* 44:E1–E211, 2004.

3. Antman EM, Hand M, Armstrong PW, et al: focused update of the ACC/AHA 2004 guidelines for the management of patients with ST-elevation myocardial infarction: a report of the American College of Cardiology/American Heart Association Task Force on Practice Guidelines, *J Am Coll Cardiol* 51:210–247, 2007. 2008.

4. Zafari AM: Myocardial infarction. Available at: http://emedicine.medscape.com/article/155919-overview. Accessed March 28, 2013.

5. CM Gibson, JP Carrozza, RJ Laham, Primary PCI versus Fibrinolysis (Thrombolysis) in Acute ST Elevation (Q Wave) Myocardial Infarction: Clinical Trials. Available at: http://www.uptodate.com/contents/primary-percutaneous-coronary-intervention-versus-fibrinolysis-in-acute-st-elevation-myocardial-infarction-clinical-trials. Accessed March 28, 2013.

6. GS Reeder, HL Kennedy, RS Rosenson, Overview of the Management of Acute ST Elevation (Q Wave) Myocardial Infarction. Available at: http://www.uptodate.com/contents/overview-of-the-acute-management-of-st-elevation-myocardial-infarction. Accessed March 28, 2013.

7. Van de Werf F, Ardissino D, Betriu A, et al: Management of acute myocardial infarction in patients presenting with ST-segment elevation. The Task Force on the Management of Acute Myocardial Infarction of the European Society of Cardiology, *Eur Heart J* 24:28–66, 2003.

CHAPTER 19

CARDIOGENIC SHOCK

Hani Jneid, MD, and Mahboob Alam, MD

1. **Define cardiogenic shock.**
   Cardiogenic shock is a state of end-organ hypoperfusion due to cardiac failure and the inability of the cardiovascular system to provide adequate blood flow to the extremities and vital organs. In general, patients with cardiogenic shock manifest persistent hypotension (systolic blood pressure less than 80 to 90 mm Hg or a mean arterial pressure 30 mm Hg below baseline) with severe reduction in cardiac index (less than 1.8 L/min/m^2) in the presence of adequate or elevated filling pressure (left ventricular end-diastolic pressure more than 18 mm Hg or right ventricular end-diastolic pressure more than 10 to 15 mm Hg).

2. **What are the various types of shock?**
   Blood flow is determined by three entities: blood volume, vascular resistance, and pump function. There are three main types of shock: (1) hypovolemic, (2) vasogenic or distributive, and (3) cardiogenic. Examples of causes of *hypovolemic shock* include gastrointestinal bleeding, severe hemorrhage, and severe diabetic ketoacidosis (as a result of volume depletion). Examples of *vasogenic shock* include septic shock, anaphylactic shock, neurogenic shock, and shock from pharmacologic causes. There are many causes of *cardiogenic shock,* although acute myocardial infarction (MI) is the most common. Cardiogenic shock can be separated into *true cardiac causes*, such as MI, and *extracardiac causes*, such as obstruction to inflow (tension pneumothorax, cardiac tamponade) or outflow (pulmonary embolus).

3. **Describe the clinical signs observed in cardiogenic shock and other types of shock?**
   The medical history and clinical examination help in making the diagnosis of cardiogenic shock. Feeling the extremities and examining the jugular veins provide vital clues: warm skin is suggestive of a vasogenic cause; cool, clammy skin reflects enhanced reflex sympathoadrenal discharge leading to cutaneous vasoconstriction, suggesting hypovolemia or cardiogenic shock. Distended jugular veins, rales, and an S3 gallop suggest a cardiogenic cause rather than hypovolemia. Figure 19-1 presents an algorithm for the evaluation and treatment of cardiogenic shock.

   It is important to note that the clinical examination and chest radiograph may not be reliable predictors of the pulmonary capillary wedge pressure (PCWP). Neither clinically reflect an elevated PCWP in up to 30% of cardiogenic shock patients. In addition, both cardiac tamponade and massive pulmonary embolism can present as cardiogenic shock without associated pulmonary congestion. Right-sided heart catheterization with intracardiac pressure and cardiac pressure measurements is important to confirm the diagnosis of cardiogenic shock.

4. **Do all patients with cardiogenic shock have an increased heart rate?**
   No. Patients with cardiogenic shock related to third-degree heart block or drug overdose (such as β-blockers and calcium channel antagonists overdose) can present with bradycardia and require temporary transvenous pacemaker implantation.

5. **What are the determinants of central venous pressure (CVP)?**
   The normal CVP is 5 to 12 cm H$_2$O. Intravascular volume, intrathoracic pressure, right ventricular function, and venous tone all affect the CVP. To reduce variability caused by intrathoracic pressure, CVP should be measured at the end of expiration.

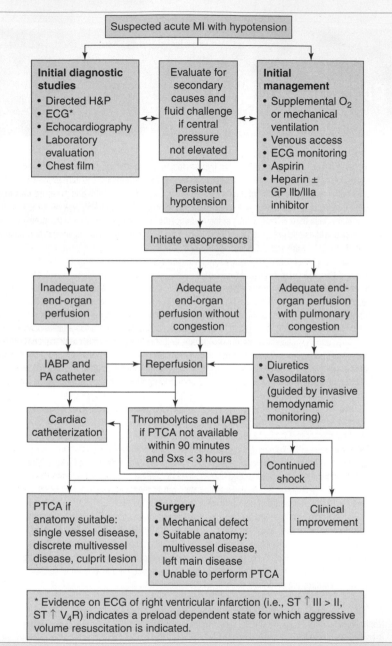

Figure 19-1. Evaluation and treatment algorithm for cardiogenic shock. (Modified from Hollenberg SM, Kavinsky CJ, Parillo JE: Cardiogenic shock. *Ann Intern Med* 131:47-59, 1999.) *ECG,* Electrocardiogram; *GP,* glycoprotein; *H&P,* history and physical examination; *IABP,* intraaortic balloon pump; *MI,* myocardial infarction; *PA,* pulmonary artery; *PTCA,* percutaneous transluminal coronary angioplasty; *Sxs,* symptoms.

6. **What is the significance of a loud holosystolic murmur in a patient with shock after acute myocardial infarction?**
New loud holosystolic murmurs with MI indicate either papillary muscle rupture or an acute ventricular septal defect (VSD). These may be indistinguishable, but acute VSD usually occurs with an anteroseptal MI and has an associated palpable thrill. Papillary rupture often does not have a thrill and is usually seen in inferior MI. These often cause shock on the basis of reduced forward blood flow and can be differentiated by echocardiography or pulmonary artery catheterization. Both require emergent cardiothoracic surgery for early repair. Note that in some patients, particularly those who develop acute mitral regurgitation, the murmur may be soft or inaudible (as a result of a small pressure gradient between the left ventricle and left atrium [or right ventricle]).

7. **How can one differentiate cardiogenic from septic shock?**
In classic septic shock, the systemic vascular resistance (SVR) and the PCWP are reduced and the cardiac output is increased. These are usually opposite to the findings in cardiogenic shock. However, a significant decrease in cardiac output may occur in advanced and late stages of sepsis (*cold* septic shock, which carries a very high mortality rate). Many patients with cardiogenic shock may have normal SVR (i.e., relatively low), even while on vasopressor therapy. Patients with cardiogenic shock may also become *dry* (normal or low PCWP) with overzealous diuresis. Conversely, septic shock patients may become *wet* (high PCWP) with overzealous volume replacement. It is therefore ill advised to depend solely on the aforementioned hemodynamic criteria to differentiate cardiogenic shock from septic shock.

8. **What is the most common cause of cardiogenic shock?**
Acute MI remains the leading cause of cardiogenic shock in the United States. In fact, despite the decline in its incidence with progressive use of timely primary percutaneous coronary intervention (PCI), cardiogenic shock still occurs in 5% to 8% of hospitalized patients with ST segment elevation myocardial infarction (STEMI). Unlike what is commonly believed, cardiogenic shock may also occur in up to 2% to 3% of patients with non–ST segment elevation myocardial infarction (NSTEMI). Overall, 40,000 to 50,000 cases of cardiogenic shock occur annually in the United States.

9. **Describe the pathophysiology of cardiogenic shock among patients with acute myocardial infarction?**
Left ventricular (LV) pump failure is the primary insult in most forms of cardiogenic shock. The degree of myocardial dysfunction that initiates cardiogenic shock is often, but not always, severe. Hypoperfusion causes release of catecholamines, which increase contractility and peripheral blood flow, but this comes at the expense of increased myocardial oxygen demand and its proarrhythmic and cardiotoxic effects. The decrease in cardiac output also triggers the release of vasopressin and angiotensin II, which lead to improvement in coronary and peripheral perfusion at the cost of increased afterload. Neurohormonal activation also promotes salt and water retention, which may improve perfusion but exacerbates pulmonary edema.
The reflex mechanism of increased SVR is in some cases not fully effective, and many patients have normal SVR even while on vasopressor therapy. Systemic inflammation, including expression of inducible nitric oxide synthase and generation of excess nitric oxide, is believed to contribute to the pathogenesis and inappropriate vasodilatation in some cases of cardiogenic shock.

10. **Describe other mechanisms that cause or contribute to cardiogenic shock after myocardial infarction.**
It is critical to exclude mechanical complications after MI, which may cause or exacerbate cardiogenic shock in some patients. These mechanical complications include ventricular septal rupture, ventricular free wall rupture, and papillary muscle rupture. Two-dimensional (2-D) echocardiography is the preferred diagnostic modality and should be promptly performed when mechanical complications are suspected. Among STEMI patients with suspected mechanical complications in whom a 2-D echocardiogram is not available, diagnostic pulmonary artery catheterization should be performed

(class I recommendation by the 2004 American College of Cardiology/American Heart Association [ACC/AHA] guidelines). The detection of mechanical complications before coronary angiography may help in dictating the revascularization strategy (surgical revascularization with mechanical repair of the complication rather than primary PCI of the infarct vessel without mechanical repair of the complication).

Additional contributing factors to shock after MI include hemorrhage, infection, and bowel ischemia (the latter may be related to embolization after large anterior MI or persistent hypotension, or may be a complication of prolonged intraaortic balloon pump placement).

11. **Can right ventricular (RV) dysfunction result in cardiogenic shock?**
RV dysfunction may cause or contribute to cardiogenic shock. Predominant RV shock represents 5% of all cardiogenic shock cases complicating MI. RV failure may limit LV filling via a decrease in the RV output, ventricular interdependence, or both. Treatment of patients with RV dysfunction and shock has traditionally focused on ensuring adequate right-sided filling pressures to maintain cardiac output and adequate left ventricular preload. However, caution should be undertaken not to overfill the RV and compromise LV filling (via ventricular interdependence).

Shock caused by isolated RV dysfunction carries nearly as high a mortality as LV shock and benefits equally from revascularization.

12. **List the other major causes of cardiogenic shock.**
Cardiovascular causes of cardiogenic shock are given in Table 19-1.

13. **What is the mainstay therapy for patients with cardiogenic shock complicating myocardial infarction?**
Acute reperfusion and prompt revascularization for cardiogenic shock improves survival substantially and is considered the mainstay therapy for cardiogenic shock after acute MI. The Should We Emergently Revascularize Occluded Coronaries for Cardiogenic Shock (SHOCK) study was a landmark trial conducted in the 1990s enrolling patients with acute MI complicated by cardiogenic shock and randomizing patients to emergency revascularization or initial medical stabilization. Six-month mortality was lower in the early revascularization group than in the medical stabilization group (50% versus 63%, P = 0.03). At

---

TABLE 19-1.   CARDIOVASCULAR CAUSES OF CARDIOGENIC SHOCK

- Acute myocardial infarction with severe left ventricular dysfunction
- Acute myocardial infarction with mechanical complication (ruptured papillary muscle, ventricular septal defect, free wall rupture)
- Aortic dissection (+/− acute aortic regurgitation)
- Endocarditis leading to mitral and/or aortic regurgitation
- Cardiac tamponade
- Massive pulmonary embolism
- Chronic congestive cardiomyopathy
- Tako-tsubo cardiomyopathy
- Acute myopericarditis
- Brady- or tachyarrhythmias
- Critical mitral or aortic stenosis
- Hypertrophic cardiomyopathy
- Toxins or drugs (negative inotropes, negative chronotropes, vasodilators)
- Traumatic cardiogenic shock (cardiac penetration with subsequent tamponade, myocardial contusion, or tension pneumothorax)
- Left atrial myxoma

1 year, survival was 47% for patients in the early revascularization group compared with 34% in the initial medical stabilization group (P < 0.03). The benefits of early revascularization persisted at long-term follow-up, and the strategy of early revascularization was associated with 67% relative improvement in 6-year survival compared with initial medical stabilization. Currently, the ACC/AHA guidelines recommend early revascularization in cardiogenic shock for those aged 75 years or younger.

14. **Which is the best revascularization strategy in patients with cardiogenic shock complicating myocardial infarction?**
   Among patients assigned to revascularization in the SHOCK trial, PCI accounted for 64% of initial revascularization attempts and coronary artery bypass grafting (CABG) for 36%. Although those treated with CABG had more diabetes and worse coronary disease, survival rates were similar with both revascularization strategies. Therefore, emergency CABG is an important treatment strategy in patients with cardiogenic shock and should be considered a complementary revascularization option to PCI in patients with extensive coronary disease.
   The ACC/AHA guidelines recommend CABG in cardiogenic shock patients with multivessel coronary artery disease. However, staged multivessel PCI may be performed if surgery is not an option. A single-stage procedure may be considered if the patient remains in shock after PCI of the infarct-related artery and if the other vessel has a critical flow-limiting lesion and supplies a large myocardium at risk.

15. **Does the timing of revascularization matter in the treatment of cardiogenic shock?**
   It is essential that revascularization and reperfusion are conducted promptly. Among patients with STEMI and cardiogenic shock, primary PCI should be done within a door-to-balloon time of less than 90 minutes. Although fibrinolytic therapy is less effective, it is indicated when timely PCI is unlikely to occur and when MI and cardiogenic shock onset are within 3 hours. Unlike what is commonly believed, prompt CABG is feasible. In the SHOCK trial, patients underwent CABG at a median time of 2.7 hours after randomization. It is also important to emphasize that approximately three-fourths of patients with cardiogenic shock after MI develop shock after hospital admission. Therefore, prompt revascularization and early reperfusion after acute MI may serve as a strategy to prevent the occurrence of cardiogenic shock.

16. **Describe the common medical therapies for cardiogenic shock.**
   Antiplatelet and antithrombotic therapies with aspirin and heparin should be administered to all patients with MI. Negative inotropes and vasodilators (including nitroglycerin) should be avoided. Optimal oxygenation and a low threshold to institute mechanical ventilation should be considered. Antiarrhythmic therapies (intravenous amiodarone) should be instituted when needed.
   Pharmacologic support with inotropic and vasopressor agents may be needed for short-term hemodynamic improvement. Although inotropic agents have a central role in cardiogenic shock treatment because the initiating event involves contractile failure, these agents increase myocardial adenosine triphosphate (ATP) consumption and hence their short-term hemodynamic benefits occur at the cost of increased oxygen demand. Higher vasopressor doses have also been associated with poorer survival. Therefore, these agents should be used in the lowest possible doses and for the shortest time possible. The ACC/AHA guidelines recommend norepinephrine for more severe hypotension because of its high potency. Often, dobutamine is needed as an additional inotropic agent.

17. **What is the mainstay mechanical therapy for cardiogenic shock?**
   Intraaortic balloon pump counterpulsation (IABP) has long been the mainstay of mechanical therapy for cardiogenic shock. IABP support should be instituted promptly, even before transfer for revascularization. IABP improves coronary and peripheral perfusion via diastolic balloon inflation (perfusion augmentation) and augments LV performance via systolic balloon deflation (afterload reduction). Thus, accurate timing of IABP inflation and deflation is important for the optimal hemodynamic support of the failing heart. IABP was performed in 86% of patients in the SHOCK trial. The overall and major

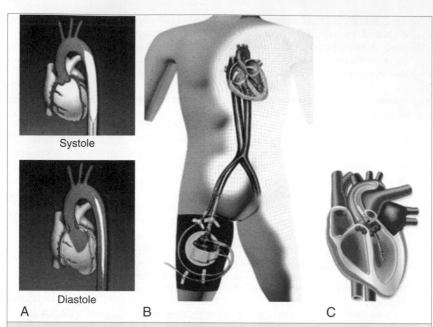

Systole

Diastole

A   B   C

Figure 19-2. Percutaneous left ventricular support devices. **A,** Intraaortic balloon counterpulsation device inflating in systole and deflating during diastole. **B,** The TandemHeart inflow cannula enters the left atrium transseptally; its outflow cannula is inserted into the arterial circulation. **C,** The Impella 2.5 L/min device enters the ventricle in a retroaortic manner.

complication rates were 7% and 3%, respectively, and were more evident among women and in patients with small body size and peripheral arterial disease.

18. **What is the role of total circulatory support in cardiogenic shock?**
    Temporary mechanical circulatory support with LV assist devices (LVADs) interrupts the vicious cycles of ischemia, hypotension, and myocardial dysfunction and allows the recovery of stunned and hibernating myocardium and reversal of neurohormonal derangements. LVAD support involves circulation of oxygenated blood through a device that drains blood from the left side of the heart and returns blood to the systemic arteries with pulsatile or continuous flow. These devices are advocated as a bridge to surgical revascularization, although they have been used as destination therapy for patients with end-stage cardiomyopathy and no alternative therapeutic options. Device-related complications and irreversible organ failure remain their major limitations. Surgically implanted LVADs remove blood through a cannula placed at the LV apex and return blood to the ascending aorta.

    Percutaneous LVADs are currently available and can be placed in the cardiac catheterization laboratory. The TandemHeart (CardiacAssist, Inc., Pittsburgh) removes blood from the left atrium using a cannula placed through the femoral vein and into the left atrium via transseptal puncture. Blood is then returned to a systemic artery, usually the femoral, with retrograde perfusion of the abdominal and thoracic aorta. Another percutaneous device, the Impella (Abiomed, Danvers, Mass.), is a novel intravascular microaxial blood pump, which can be introduced via the femoral artery and placed across the aortic valve into the left ventricle to unload the left ventricle and provide a short-term mechanical support for the failing heart (Fig. 19-2). Extracorporeal life support (ECLS) involves extracorporeal circulation of blood through a membrane oxygenator, which relieves both the right side and left side of the heart and the lungs of part of their workload.

19. **What are the mortality and morbidity rates of cardiogenic shock?**

In the modern era, the mortality rate of cardiogenic shock is approximately 50%. In the SHOCK trial, the 3- and 6-year survival rates among patients in the early revascularization group were 41% and 33%, respectively, with persistence of treatment benefits for up to 6 years. Importantly, 83% of 1-year survivors in the SHOCK trial were in New York Heart Association (NYHA) classes I or II and many of them enjoyed an acceptable quality of life at 6-year follow-up. Therefore, cardiogenic shock should be regarded as a very serious but treatable (and possibly preventable) condition that, when treated aggressively and in a timely manner, carries a reasonable chance for full recovery.

BIBLIOGRAPHY, SUGGESTED READINGS, AND WEBSITES

1. Anderson JL, Adams CD, Antman EM, et al: ACC/AHA 2007 guidelines for the management of patients with unstable angina/non–ST-elevation myocardial infarction, *J Am Coll Cardiol* 50:e1–e157, 2007.

2. Hochman JS, Sleeper LA, Webb JG, et al: Early revascularization in acute myocardial infarction complicated by cardiogenic shock. SHOCK Investigators. Should we emergently revascularize occluded coronaries for cardiogenic shock, *N Engl J Med* 341:625–634, 1999.

3. Hochman JS, Sleeper LA, Webb JG, et al: Early revascularization and long-term survival in cardiogenic shock complicating acute myocardial infarction, *JAMA* 295:2511–2515, 2006.

4. Jneid H, Anderson JL, Wright RS, et al: 2012 ACCF/AHA focused update of the guideline for the management of patients with unstable angina/non-ST-elevation myocardial infarction (updating the 2007 guideline and replacing the 2011 focused update): a report of the American College of Cardiology Foundation/American Heart Association Task Force on Practice Guidelines. *J Am Coll Cardiol* 60(7):648–681, 2012.

5. Levine GN, Bates ER, Blankenship JC, et al: 2011 ACCF/AHA/SCAI Guideline for Percutaneous Coronary Intervention: a report of the American College of Cardiology Foundation/American Heart Association Task Force on Practice Guidelines and the Society for Cardiovascular Angiography and Interventions, *Circulation* 124:e574–e651, 2011.

6. O'Gara PT, Kushner FG, Ascheim DD, et al: American College of Cardiology Foundation/American Heart Association Task Force on Practice Guidelines: 2013 ACCF/AHA guideline for the management of ST-elevation myocardial infarction: a report of the American College of Cardiology Foundation/American Heart Association Task Force on Practice Guidelines, *Circulation* 127(4):e362–e425, 2013.

CHAPTER 20

PERCUTANEOUS CORONARY INTERVENTION

Ahmad Munir, MD, Theodore L. Schreiber, MD, and Cindy L. Grines, MD

1. **What does the term percutaneous coronary intervention mean?**

   Percutaneous coronary intervention (PCI) is a common term used to describe both percutaneous transluminal coronary angioplasty (PTCA), which implies the use of balloon angioplasty but not stenting, and coronary stent placement. The first successful balloon angioplasty procedure in humans was performed by Dr. Andreas Gruentzig in 1977. Since then, there has been tremendous development in the field of interventional cardiology. The development of coronary stents was a major boost to interventional cardiology, addressing many of the complications and limitations associated with balloon angioplasty. Eighty percent of the PCIs performed currently involve stent placement. PCI has become one of the most commonly performed medical procedures in the United States, with more than about 600,000 procedures performed annually. PCI is performed for coronary revascularization in patients with stable coronary disease, as well as those with acute coronary syndromes (ACS) in the appropriate clinical settings.

2. **Which patients with chronic stable angina benefit from PCI?**

   The goals of treatment in patients with coronary artery disease are to:
   - Relieve symptoms.
   - Prevent adverse outcomes such as cardiovascular death, myocardial infarction (MI), left ventricular (LV) dysfunctions, and arrhythmias.
   - Prevent or slow the progression of disease and symptoms.

   Multiple clinical trials of PCI plus medical therapy or medical therapy alone involving patients with chronic stable angina over the last two decades have consistently shown improvement in angina, exercise duration, and quality of life with PCI. However, they have not demonstrated any difference in death and MI between treatment with PCI plus medical therapy compared to medical therapy alone. In contrast, the use of PCI in patients with ACS has been shown to decrease recurrent ischemia, nonfatal MI, and death.

   In general, patients with chronic stable angina in whom PCI should be considered are those with symptom-limiting angina, one or more significant coronary arteries stenoses, a high likelihood of technical success, and a low risk of complications.

   In patients with 3-vessel coronary artery disease (CAD), particularly if they have complex and/or extensive CAD (reflected in a high SYNTAX score or diabetes), bypass surgery is generally preferred over multivessel PCI. Unprotected left main PCI can be considered in those with a stenosis that has a high likelihood of procedural success and long-term durability, especially in cases in which the patient is at high risk for surgery (reflected by a high Society of Thoracic Surgeons [STS] risk score).

3. **Which patients with unstable angina/non–ST elevation myocardial infarction (UA/NSTEMI) should undergo a strategy of early cardiac catheterization and revascularization?**

   Two major strategies, conservative (medical therapy without an initial strategy of catheterization and revascularization) and early invasive, are employed in treating patients with UA/NSTEMI. The early invasive approach involves performing diagnostic angiography with intent to perform PCI along with administering the usual antiischemic, antiplatelet, and anticoagulant medications. Evidence from clinical trials suggests that an early invasive approach with UA/NSTEMI leads to a reduction in adverse cardiovascular outcomes, such as death and nonfatal MI, especially in high-risk patients.

Several risk-assessment tools are available that assign a score based upon the patient's clinical characteristics (e.g., TIMI and GRACE scores). Patients who present with UA/NSTEMI should be risk stratified to identify those who would benefit most from an early invasive approach. Patients with the following clinical characteristics indicative of high risk should be taken for early coronary angiography with intent to perform revascularization:

- Recurrent angina or ischemia at rest or with low-level activities
- Elevated cardiac biomarkers (troponin T or I)
- New or presumably new ST segment deviation
- Congestive heart failure [CHF], new or worsening mitral regurgitation, or hypotension
- Reduced LV function (ejection fraction less than 40%)
- Hemodynamic instability
- Sustained ventricular tachycardia
- High-risk findings from noninvasive testing
- PCI within the last six months or prior coronary artery bypass graft (CABG)
- High risk score as per risk-assessment tools (e.g., TIMI, GRACE)

Initially stabilized patients without the above risk factors (low-risk patients) may be treated with an initial conservative (or selective invasive) strategy. An early invasive approach should not be undertaken in patients with extensive comorbidities, organ failure, or advanced cancer, in which the risk of revascularization is greater than the benefit, or in patients who do not consent to the procedure.

4. **What are the contraindications to PCI and the predictors of adverse outcomes?**
   The only absolute contraindication to PCI is lack of any vascular access or active severe bleeding, which precludes the use of anticoagulation and antiplatelet agents. Relative contraindications include the following:

   - Bleeding diathesis or other conditions that predispose to bleeding during antiplatelet therapy
   - Severe renal insufficiency unless the patient is on hemodialysis, or severe electrolyte abnormalities
   - Sepsis
   - Poor patient compliance with medications
   - A terminal condition that indicates short life expectancy such as advanced or metastatic malignancy
   - Other indications for open heart surgery
   - Failure of previous PCI or not amenable to PCI based upon previous angiograms
   - Patients with severe cognitive dysfunction or advanced physical limitations

   Patients generally should not undergo PCI if the following conditions are present:

   - There is only a very small area of myocardium at risk.
   - There is no objective evidence of ischemia (unless patient has clear anginal symptoms and has not had a stress test).
   - There is a low likelihood of technical success.
   - The patient has left-main or multivessel CAD with high SYNTAX score and is a candidate for CABG.
   - There is insignificant stenosis (less than 50% luminal narrowing).
   - The patient has end-stage cirrhosis with portal hypertension resulting in encephalopathy or visceral bleeding.

   Clinical predictors of poor outcomes include older age, an unstable condition (ACS, acute MI, decompensated CHF, cardiogenic shock), LV dysfunction, multivessel coronary disease, diabetes mellitus, renal insufficiency, small body size, and peripheral artery disease.

   Angiographic predictors of poor outcomes include the presence of thrombus, degenerated bypass graft, unprotected left main disease, long lesions (more than 20 mm), excessive tortuosity of proximal segment, extremely angulated lesions (more than 90 degrees), a bifurcation lesion with involvement of major side branches, or chronic total occlusion.

5. **What are the major complications related to PCI?**

   The incidence of major complications has constantly decreased over the last two decades as a result of the use of activated clotting time to measure degree of anticoagulation, better antithrombotic and antiplatelet agents, advanced device technology, more skilled operators, and superior PCI strategies. These factors have particularly lowered the incidence of MI and the need for emergent CABG. Major complications of PCI include the following:

   Death: The overall in-hospital mortality rate is 1.27% ranging from 0.65% in elective PCI to 4.81% in ST elevation myocardial infarction (STEMI) (based on the National Cardiac Data Registry [NCDR] CathPCI database of patients undergoing PCI between 2004 and 2007).

   MI: The incidence of PCI-related MI is 0.4% to 4.9%; the incidence varies depending on the acuity of symptoms, lesion morphology, definition of MI, and frequency of measurement of biomarkers.

   Stroke: The incidence of PCI-related stroke is 0.22%. In-hospital mortality in patients with PCI-related stroke is 25% to 30% (based on a contemporary analysis from the NCDR).

   Emergency CABG: The need to perform emergency CABG in the stent era is extremely low (between 0.1% and 0.4%).

   Vascular complications: The incidence of vascular complications ranges from 2% to 6%. These include access-site hematoma, retroperitoneal hematoma, pseudoaneurysm, arteriovenous fistula, and arterial dissection. In randomized trials, closure devices were only beneficial in reducing time to hemostasis but did not reduce the incidence of vascular complications.

   Radial artery access complications: There is significant reduction of vascular complications with the use of radial arterial access as compared to femoral artery access. Complications include loss of the radial pulse in fewer than 5% of cases, compartment syndrome, pseudoaneurysm in fewer than 0.01% of cases, sterile abscess, and radial artery spasm.

   Other complications associated with PCI: Other complications include transient ischemic attack (TIA), renal insufficiency, and anaphylactoid reactions to contrast agents.

6. **When should cardiac biomarkers be assessed in patients undergoing PCI?**

   The American College of Cardiology/American Heart Association (ACC/AHA) guidelines recommend measuring the myocardium-associated isozyme of creatine kinase (CK-MB), or troponin I or T in all patients who have signs or symptoms suggestive of MI during or after PCI, and in those who undergo complicated procedures. Currently, there are no compelling data to support routinely measuring cardiac biomarkers for all PCI procedures.

7. **What is abrupt vessel closure?**

   Abrupt vessel closure is when the artery becomes completely occluded within hours of the PCI procedure. This can be due to stent thrombosis, dissection flap, vessel spasm, or side-branch occlusion. The incidence has decreased to less than 1% in the modern era of stents and antiplatelet therapies.

8. **What is stent thrombosis?**

   Stent thrombosis is when there is complete occlusion of the artery due to thrombus formation in the stent. This may occur in the first 24 hours after stent deployment (acute stent thrombosis); in the first month after implantation (subacute stent thrombosis); between 1 and 12 months after implantation (late stent thrombosis); or even more than 1 year after implantation, most notably after drug-eluting stent (DES) implantation (very late stent thrombosis). Most instances of stent thrombosis occur in the first thirty days after implantation, at a rate of less than 1% per year. Beyond 30 days, the incidence is 0.2% to 0.6% per year depending on patient characteristics and type of stent used. Stent thrombosis is a potentially catastrophic event and often presents as STEMI, requiring emergency revascularization. Stent thrombosis carries a mortality rate of 20% to 45%. The primary factors contributing to stent thrombosis are inadequate stent deployment, incomplete stent apposition, residual stenosis, unrecognized dissection impairing blood flow, and noncompliance with dual antiplatelet therapy (DAPT). Noncompliance to DAPT is the most common cause of stent thrombosis. Resistance to aspirin and clopidogrel, and hypercoagulable states, such as those associated with malignancy, are additional, less common causes of stent thrombosis.

9. **What do the terms slow-flow and no-reflow mean?**

   Slow-flow is the term applied when contrast agent injection of the coronary artery reveals delayed clearing of the contrast down the coronary artery; *no-reflow* is the more extreme form, when the contrast does not appear to flow down the coronary artery at all. These entities are caused by vasospasm, distal embolization, and microvascular plugging resulting in impaired epicardial blood flow, quantified as abnormal TIMI frame rates and myocardial blush scores. It occurs more commonly in the setting of atherectomy, thrombus, or degenerated saphenous vein graft (SVG) PCI. Another form of no-reflow is seen when reperfusion in the infarct-related artery is suboptimal. The etiology includes myocardial edema and endothelial injury, in addition to vasospasm and embolization.

10. **Are bleeding complications related to PCI clinically important?**

    A bleeding complication is an independent predictor of early and late mortality in patients undergoing elective or urgent PCI. The potential for bleeding complications is always present, due to the routine use of potent antithrombin and antiplatelet agents during PCI. Bleeding can adversely affect a patient, not only due to ensuing severe anemia, but also due to the potential of ischemic events when anticoagulation is reversed. Additionally, accumulating data suggest a possible direct link between blood transfusion and poor outcomes. Proinflammatory and prothrombotic effects of red blood cell transfusion have been demonstrated. Use of a restrictive transfusion policy has been associated with improved outcomes.

    Factors contributing towards the risk of bleeding include advanced age, low body mass index, renal insufficiency, anemia at baseline, difficult vascular access, site and condition of access vessel, sheath size, and degree of anticoagulation and platelet inhibition. Measures to reduce the bleeding complications include using weight-based anticoagulation regimens, frequent assessment of anticoagulation status to prevent over-anticoagulation, use of bivalirudin, and adjustment of the dosing of certain medications when chronic kidney disease is present. Use of the radial access may also decrease bleeding complications.

11. **What are the important complications that can occur at the access site?**

    Potential complications of vascular access include retroperitoneal bleeding, pseudoaneurysm, arteriovenous fistula, arterial dissection, thrombosis, distal artery embolization, groin hematoma, infection and/or abscess, and femoral neuropathy. Risk factors for access-site complications include older age, female gender, morbid obesity or low body weight, hypertension, low platelet count, peripheral artery disease, larger sheath size, prolonged sheath time, intraaortic balloon pump use, concomitant venous sheath, over-anticoagulation, thrombolytic therapy use, and repeat intervention. Patients with a femoral puncture site above the most inferior border of the inferior epigastric artery are at an increased risk for retroperitoneal bleeding. Conversely, development of pseudoaneurysm and arteriovenous fistula are associated with a puncture site at or below the level of the femoral bifurcation.

    Arteriotomy closure devices (vascular closure devices) have emerged as an alternative to mechanical compression for achieving rapid vascular hemostasis. These devices are categorized based on the principle mechanism of hemostasis, which includes biodegradable plug, suture, or staples. Although arteriotomy closure devices offer advantages over mechanical compression (shorter time to hemostasis and patient ambulation, high rate of patient satisfaction, and greater cost effectiveness), no prospective randomized study has been able to show a clear-cut reduction in vascular complications with these devices.

12. **What are some treatment options for various vascular complications?**

    Pseudoaneurysm: For small pseudoaneurysms, observation is recommended. For larger pseudoaneurysms, ultrasound-guided compression or percutaneous thrombin injection under ultrasound guidance is the treatment of choice. For pseudoaneurysms with a large neck, simultaneous balloon inflation to occlude the entry site can be helpful. In cases of thrombin failure, surgical repair should be considered. Endovascular repair with stent-graft implantation can also be used in the treatment of pseudoaneurysms.

Arteriovenous fistula: For small arteriovenous fistulae, observation is recommended; most close spontaneously or remain stable. For a large fistula or when significant shunting is present, options include ultrasound-guided compression, covered stent, or surgical repair.

Dissection: If there is no effect on blood flow, a conservative approach is indicated. In the presence of flow impairment (distal limb ischemia), angioplasty, stenting, and surgical repair are the treatment options.

Retroperitoneal bleeding: This should always be suspected with unexplained hypotension, marked decrease in hematocrit, flank/abdominal or back pain, and high arterial sticks. Treatment includes intravascular volume replacement, reversal of anticoagulation, blood transfusion, and, occasionally, vasopressor agents and monitoring in the intensive care unit with serial hemoglobin and hematocrit checks. Endovascular management with covered stents, prolonged balloon inflation, or surgical repair are options, but are rarely necessary.

13. What is contrast nephropathy?

Contrast nephropathy is a worsening in renal function, as assessed by creatinine levels, due to administration of intravascular iodinated contrast agent, such as is used during cardiac catheterization and PCI. Contrast nephropathy usually first manifests clinically 48 hours after contrast administration, and peaks approximately 5 days after contrast administration. Contrast-induced nephropathy (CIN) has been associated with increased mortality and morbidity. Several predisposing factors for CIN have been identified, including chronic renal insufficiency (the risk of CIN is directly proportional to the severity of preexisting renal insufficiency), diabetes, CHF, intravascular volume depletion, multiple myeloma, and the use of a large volume of contrast. The most widely accepted measure to prevent CIN consists of assuring adequate hydration with isotonic saline (such as 1.0 to 1.5 mL/kg/hr for 3 to 12 hours before and continuing for 6 to 24 hours after the procedure). In patients with creatinine clearance of less than 60 mL/min, contrast volume should be kept to a minimum and adequate intravenous hydration initiated. Diuretics, nonsteroidal antiinflammatory agents, and other nephrotoxic drugs should be held before PCI.

Both a recent meta-analysis and a recent large randomized trial assessing the efficacy of *N*-acetylcysteine for CIN found no benefit with *N*-acetylcysteine administration. Based upon these data, the 2011 ACC/AHA guidelines on PCI do not recommend the use of *N*-acetylcysteine for prevention of CIN, giving it a "class III–no benefit" indication. Studies of administration of bicarbonate or hemofiltration (ultrafiltration) have produced conflicting results.

14. What is restenosis?

Restenosis is the process by which the treated stenosis in a coronary artery recurs over time. Restenosis usually clinically manifests itself over the 1 to 6 month period after PCI. Patients with restenosis present most commonly with exertional angina and less frequently with unstable angina or MI. The process of restenosis is driven by the following mechanisms:

- Neointimal hyperplasia caused by smooth muscle cell migration and proliferation and extracellular matrix production
- Platelet deposition and thrombus formation
- Vessel elastic recoil after balloon inflation and vessel negative remodeling over time

Restenosis occurs more commonly in patients with diabetes, renal insufficiency, ostial, bifurcation or SVG locations, small vessels (less than 2.5 mm diameter), and long lesions (longer than 40 mm).

Angiographic restenosis rates after balloon PTCA range from 32% to 42%, based upon randomized controlled trials, and approximately half of these patients with restenosis require clinically driven repeat target lesion revascularization within the first year.

Coronary stents prevent vessel elastic recoil and negative remodeling, and significantly reduce both angiographic and clinical restenosis rates. The main factor leading to restenosis in coronary arteries treated with bare metal stents (BMS) is neointimal hyperplasia as a result of smooth muscle cell proliferation and extracellular matrix production. Angiographic restenosis rates with BMS range from 16% to 32% with a target lesion revascularization rate of 12% and target-vessel revascularization rate of 14% at 1 year. Similar to PTCA, restenosis after BMS typically occurs within the first 6 months.

Drug-eluting stents (DES) are coated with a polymer that contains antirestenotic (antiproliferative) medication that is slowly released over a period of weeks. Restenosis after DES ranges from 5% to 10%, depending on the type of DES, stent size, length, lesion morphology, and presence of diabetes. Compared with BMS, DES significantly reduce the rates of target lesion revascularization (approximately 6.2% versus 16.6%), without any effect on all-cause mortality.

Options to treat restenosis include aggressive medical therapy, repeat PCI and CABG. Patient factors such as compliance with DAPT, the type of intervention (PTCA, BMS, or DES) initially performed, chances of recurrence of restenosis, and appropriateness of CABG should be considered when addressing restenotic lesions. For restenosis after PTCA, stent placement is recommended; for restenosis after BMS, repeat stenting with DES is the preferred treatment. For DES restenosis, there is a lack of robust clinical data for the most appropriate therapy. In current interventional practice, focal DES restenosis is treated mostly by PTCA. For diffuse DES restenosis, repeat DES placement, and CABG can be considered, taking into account patient and angiographic characteristics.

15. **What are the recommendations regarding antiplatelet therapy after PCI?**
Patients undergoing PCI should receive dual antiplatelet therapy with aspirin and a $P2Y_{12}$ inhibitor. The duration of antiplatelet therapy depends upon the type (PTCA, BMS or DES) and setting (elective vs. ACS) of intervention performed.
Recommendations for aspirin:
- Patients who are already on aspirin should continue with 81 to 325 mg of aspirin. Those who are not on aspirin should receive 325 mg of non–enteric-coated aspirin preferably 24 hours prior to PCI, after which it should be continued indefinitely at a dose of 81 mg daily.
Recommendations for $P2Y_{12}$ receptor inhibitors:
- A loading dose of a $P2Y_{12}$ inhibitor should be given prior to PCI with stent placement. The loading doses for the three recommended drugs are clopidogrel 600 mg, prasugrel 60 mg, and ticagrelor 180 mg.
- Following a loading dose of a $P2Y_{12}$ inhibitor, a maintenance dose is continued. The recommendations for dose and duration are as follows:
  ○ For patients undergoing stent BMS or DES implantation in the setting of ACS, clopidogrel 75 mg daily or prasugrel 10 mg daily or ticagrelor 90 mg twice daily should be continued for at least 12 months.
  ○ For patients undergoing elective DES implantation, the duration of $P2Y_{12}$ inhibitor therapy should be at least 12 months. Prasugrel and ticagrelor are more effective at reducing stent thrombosis in patients with ACS or STEMI.
  ○ In patients undergoing elective BMS implantation, the duration of $P2Y_{12}$ inhibitor therapy should be a minimum of one month, and preferably up to 12 months. In patients who are at high risk of bleeding, a minimum duration of 2 weeks is recommended.
Prior to PCI, the ability of the patient to comply with DAPT should be assessed and therapy tailored accordingly.

16. **What steps should be taken to prevent premature discontinuation of dual antiplatelet therapy?**
Although stent thrombosis most commonly occurs in the first month after stent implantation, numerous cases of late stent thrombosis (1 month to 1 year) or even very late stent thrombosis (after 1 year) have been reported, particularly in patients who have been treated with DES.

Premature discontinuation of antiplatelet therapy markedly increases the risk of stent thrombosis, and with this, MI or death. Factors contributing to premature cessation of $P2Y_{12}$ therapy include drug cost, inadequate patient and health care provider understanding about the importance of continuing therapy, and requests to discontinue therapy before noncardiac procedures.

To eliminate premature discontinuation of $P2Y_{12}$ therapy, the following recommendations should be followed:
- Patients should be clearly educated about the rationale for not stopping antiplatelet therapy and the potential consequences of stopping such therapy. Each should be instructed to call

their cardiologist if bleeding develops or if another physician advises them to stop antiplatelet therapy.

- Health care providers who perform invasive or surgical procedures and are concerned about periprocedural bleeding must be made aware of the potentially catastrophic risks of premature discontinuation of $P2Y_{12}$ therapy. The professionals who perform these procedures should contact the patient's cardiologist to discuss optimal patient management strategy.
- Any elective procedure for which there is significant risk of perioperative bleeding should be deferred until patients have completed an appropriate course of $P2Y_{12}$ therapy (12 months after DES implantation if they are not at high risk of bleeding, and a minimum of 1 month for BMS implantation).
- For patients treated with DES who are to undergo procedures that mandate discontinuation of $P2Y_{12}$ therapy, aspirin should be continued if at all possible, and thienopyridine restarted as soon as possible after the procedure.

17. What should be the management of a patient with a DES who requires urgent noncardiac surgery?

If at all possible, elective surgery should be avoided until the patient has received a minimum of 1 year of dual antiplatelet therapy after DES. Aspirin should not be discontinued in the perioperative period unless a significant bleeding situation arises (and continuation of $P2Y_{12}$ therapy is also preferred). Use of heparin or short-acting GP IIb/IIIa inhibitors is not routinely recommended in patients being withdrawn from $P2Y_{12}$ therapy, because of lack of evidence and concern for rebound platelet hyperactivity, especially in absence of aspirin, with or without clopidogrel treatment.

Surgery should be performed in an institution with 24-hour catheterization laboratory availability, in case of stent thrombosis; emergency PCI is strongly preferred over thrombolysis in cases of stent thrombosis, and thrombolytic therapy is contraindicated in patients with recent surgery.

BIBLIOGRAPHY, SUGGESTED READINGS, AND WEBSITES

1. Investigators ACT: Acetylcysteine for prevention of renal outcomes in patients undergoing coronary and peripheral vascular angiography. main results from the randomized Acetylcysteine for Contrast-Induced Nephropathy Trial (ACT), *Circulation* 124:1250–1259, 2011.

2. Anderson JL, Adams CD, Antman EM, et al: ACCF/AHA Focused Update Incorporated Into the ACC/AHA 2007 Guidelines for the Management of Patients With Unstable Angina/Non–ST-Elevation Myocardial Infarction A Report of the American College of Cardiology Foundation/American Heart Association Task Force on Practice Guidelines, *Circulation* 123:e426–e579, 2011. 2011.

3. Bavry AA, Kumbhani DJ, Rassi AN, Bhatt DL, Askari AT: Benefit of early invasive therapy in acute coronary syndromes a meta-analysis of contemporary randomized clinical trials, *J Am Coll Cardiol* 48:1319–1325, 2006.

4. Boden WE, O'Rourke RA, Teo KK, et al: Optimal medical therapy with or without PCI for stable coronary disease, *N Engl J Med* 356:1503–1516, 2007.

5. Gonzales DA, Norsworthy KJ, Kern SJ, et al: A meta-analysis of N-acetylcysteine in contrast-induced nephrotoxicity: unsupervised clustering to resolve heterogeneity, *BMC Med* 5:32, 2007.

6. Grines CL, Bonow RO, Casey DE, et al: Prevention of premature discontinuation of dual antiplatelet therapy in patients with coronary artery stents, *J Am Coll Cardiol* 49:734–739, 2007.

7. Keeley EC, Boura JA, Grines CL: Comparison of primary and facilitated percutaneous coronary interventions for ST-elevation myocardial infarction: quantitative review of randomised trials, *Lancet* 367:579–588, 2006.

8. Levine GN, Bates ER, Blankenship JC, et al: ACCF/AHA/SCAI Guideline for Percutaneous Coronary Intervention. A report of the American College of Cardiology Foundation/American Heart Association Task Force on Practice Guidelines and the Society for Cardiovascular Angiography and Interventions, *J Am Coll Cardiol* 58:e44–e122, 2011.

9. Levine GN, Kern MJ, Berger PB, et al: For the American Heart Association Diagnostic and Interventional Cardiac Catheterization Committee: management of patients undergoing percutaneous coronary revascularization, *Ann Intern Med* 139:123–136, 2003.

10. Patel MR, Dehmer GJ, Hirshfeld JW, Smith PK, Spertus JA: ACCF/SCAI/STS/AATS/AHA/ASNC/HFSA/SCCT 2012 Appropriate use criteria for coronary revascularization focused update: a report of the American College of Cardiology Foundation Appropriate Use Criteria Task Force, Society for Cardiovascular Angiography and Interventions, Society of Thoracic Surgeons, American Association for Thoracic Surgery, American Heart Association, American Society of Nuclear Cardiology, and the Society of Cardiovascular Computed Tomography, *J Am Coll Cardiol* 59:857–881, 2012.

11. Shaw LJ, Berman DS, Maron DJ, et al: Optimal Medical Therapy With or Without Percutaneous Coronary Intervention to Reduce Ischemic Burden Results From the Clinical Outcomes Utilizing Revascularization and Aggressive Drug Evaluation (COURAGE) Trial Nuclear Substudy, *Circulation* 117:1283–1291, 2008.

12. Serruys PW, Morice MC, Kappetein AP, et al: Percutaneous Coronary Intervention versus Coronary-Artery Bypass Grafting for Severe Coronary Artery Disease, *N Engl J Med* 360:961–972, 2009.

13. Stergiopoulos K, Brown DL: Initial coronary stent implantation with medical therapy vs medical therapy alone for stable coronary artery disease: meta-analysis of randomized controlled trials, *Arch Intern Med* 172:312–319, 2012.

CHAPTER 21

CORONARY ARTERY BYPASS SURGERY

Lorraine D. Cornwell, MD, Ourania Preventza, MD, and Faisal Bakaeen, MD

1. **What are the indications for coronary artery bypass grafting (CABG)?**
   According to the latest published guidelines from the American College of Cardiology Foundation/ American Heart Association (ACCF/AHA), class I indications for CABG include significant left main stenosis and three-vessel coronary artery disease (CAD). Class I indications also include two-vessel disease involving the proximal left anterior descending (LAD) artery. CABG should be considered as a reasonable treatment strategy (class IIa) in patients with proximal LAD artery disease, and in 2-vessel disease without proximal LAD artery disease but with extensive ischemia.

   After myocardial infarction (MI), primary surgical revascularization should be considered in patients not suitable for percutaneous coronary intervention (PCI), patients who have failed PCI, or patients with ongoing ischemia or symptoms. After a transmural infarct, mechanical complications such as a postinfarction ventricular septal defect (VSD), acute mitral regurgitation (MR) as a result of papillary rupture, and free-wall pseudoaneurysm should be considered as indications for primary surgical intervention.

2. **How does CABG compare with medical management for CAD?**
   Three early prospective randomized trials comparing CABG with medical therapy were conducted in the late 1970s and were reported in the early 1980s. The Veterans Affairs (VA) cooperative trial, European Coronary Surgery Study (ECSS), and Coronary Artery Surgery Study (CASS) showed long-term superiority of surgery over medical therapy in patients with left main (LM) artery CAD, significant CAD involving the LAD artery, and multivessel disease.

3. **How does CABG compare with stents?**
   The Arterial Revascularization Therapies Study (ARTS) was the largest trial comparing CABG with bare metal stents in patients (1) with ejection fraction (EF) greater than 30% and (2) where there was consensus between surgeon and cardiologist that the disease was suitable for both therapies. The study showed improved event-free survival in the CABG group at 1, 2, and 5 years.

4. **What about with drug-eluting stents (DES)?**
   Drug-eluting stents have reduced the problem of restenosis, but data directly comparing DES with CABG is limited and still relatively short-term. In a registry study from the New York state cardiovascular database, CABG resulted in improved survival at 3 years compared with DES for patients with double- and triple-vessel disease. ARTS II randomized patients to DES or CABG, and showed that the primary composite outcomes at one year were similar. The international SYNTAX trial, involving 85 centers and 1800 patients with multivessel or left main CAD, recently published 3-year follow-up data in 2011. This showed worse outcomes in the PCI group as compared to the CABG group at 3 years, with increased composite major adverse cardiac and cerebrovascular events (MACCE: death, stroke, MI, or repeat revascularization). Although there was no significant difference in all-cause mortality and stroke at 3 years, MI and repeat revascularization were both increased in the PCI group. The study concluded that patients with more complex disease (three-vessel CAD with intermediate-high SYNTAX scores and LM artery CAD with high SYNTAX scores) have an increased risk of MACCE with PCI, and CABG is the preferred treatment option.

5. **What is the SYNTAX score?**

The SYNTAX score derives from a scoring system developed by the SYNTAX trial investigators to quantify the extent and complexity of CAD based on findings at cardiac catheterization. Scores are divided into tertiles: low (0-22), intermediate (23-32), and high (≥33), with higher scores representing more extensive and complex CAD. The SYNTAX score was found to correlate with PCI risk and outcome, but not with CABG risk and outcome. Patients with higher SYNTAX scores generally benefited from a revascularization strategy of CABG in preference to PCI. This is reflected in current guidelines, which state that it is reasonable to choose CABG over PCI as a revascularization strategy in patients with complex three-vessel disease and high SYNTAX scores (class IIa recommendation).

6. **Which patients benefit most from CABG?**

The decision for surgery is made based on the comprehensive evaluation of the patient. Anatomic considerations that favor recommendation for CABG include presence of significant LM or proximal LAD coronary artery disease, multivessel CAD, and presence of lesions not amenable to stenting. The presence of diabetes also favors surgical revascularization over stenting in operable patients. Depressed ejection fraction has been recognized as an additional indication for CABG.

Although the coronary anatomy may be suitable for bypass, each patient's comorbidities should be considered in the overall risk-benefit analysis. Preoperative renal insufficiency, peripheral vascular disease, recent MI, or recent stroke, as well as emergency operation and cardiogenic shock, have been identified as factors that increase mortality.

7. **What is the cardiopulmonary bypass (CPB) pump, and how is it used?**

The "pump" involves temporarily placing a patient on a machine to supply circulation and oxygenation during an operation, so that the heart can be stopped to facilitate the procedure. The bypass circuit consists of the tubing, a collection chamber, oxygenator, heater-cooler machines to control temperature, and the pump. An aortic cannula is placed in the distal ascending aorta, and this is connected to tubing that will be used to bring artificially oxygenated blood from the pump back to the patient's arterial bloodstream. A venous cannula is placed in the right atrium, and advanced down into the inferior vena cava, to collect venous blood and return it towards the pump. Once the venous blood is oxygenated, it is pumped back into the arterial line to the patient's aorta. A perfusionist runs the pump under the direction of the surgeon.

8. **Why is heparin required for CPB?**

The CPB circuit is thrombogenic, and systemic anticoagulation is required to prevent clotting and embolization. The standard anticoagulant is heparin (300 U\kg), which is administered to produce a target activated clotting time (ACT) of greater than 480 seconds. In patients with previously documented heparin-induced thrombocytopenia, direct thrombin inhibitors have been used for anticoagulation. Heparin is used in off-pump CABG at partial dose. After termination of CPB and decannulation, heparin-related anticoagulation is reversed with protamine.

9. **How is the heart stopped while on CPB?**

The heart is stopped by placing a completely occluding cross-clamp across the ascending aorta, below the aortic cannula, eliminating arterial blood flow to the coronary arteries. Cardioplegia solution is then used to induce arrest of the heart, and can be given antegrade and/or retrograde. Components of cardioplegia solution are varied in different institutions but include potassium to achieve diastolic arrest. Cardioplegia solution administered into the aortic root, via a small cannula below the cross-clamp, is delivered in an antegrade fashion to the myocardium via the coronary ostia. Retrograde cardioplegia is also used frequently, by infusing cardioplegia solution into the coronary sinus with backward filling of the cardiac veins to reach the myocardium, and is especially important in situations where antegrade may not be as effective, such as with severe CAD and aortic valve insufficiency. Most commonly, cold cardioplegia at 4° C is administered intermittently in 15- to 20-minute intervals. Blood can be mixed to the crystalloid component of cardioplegia in a 4:1 mix to provide oxygenated blood to the myocardium and to buffer the pH of the tissue (Fig. 21-1).

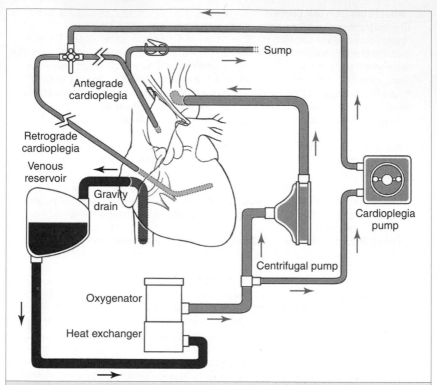

Figure 21-1. Schematic of total cardiopulmonary bypass circuit. All returning venous blood is siphoned into a venous reservoir and is oxygenated and temperature regulated before being pumped back through a centrifugal pump into arterial circulation. The common site for inflow into the patient is the ascending aorta, but alternate sites include the femoral arteries or the right axillary artery in special circumstances (see later). A parallel circuit derives oxygenated blood that is mixed with cold (4° C) cardioplegic solution in the ratio of 4:1 and administered in an antegrade or retrograde fashion to accomplish cardiac arrest. Antegrade cardioplegia is administered into the aortic root and retrograde through the coronary sinus. During the administration of retrograde cardioplegia, the efflux of blood from the coronary ostium is siphoned off via the sump drain. The sump drain, a return parallel circuit connected to the venous reservoir (not shown), also helps to keep the heart decompressed during the arrest phase. (From Townsend CM Jr, Beauchamp RD, Evers BM, Mattox KL: *Sabiston Textbook of Surgery,* ed 19, Philadelphia, 2012, Saunders.)

10. **How is the myocardium protected during cardiac arrest during bypass surgery?**
   Myocardial ischemia occurs when the aortic cross-clamp is applied, at which time the coronary arteries no longer perfuse the myocardium. Strategies to protect the myocardium during this time include cooling the heart, unloading the ventricle, and arresting the heart. Systemic cooling of the heart and the body is accomplished with the cardiopulmonary bypass machine. Direct cooling of the heart is also accomplished with cold cardioplegic solution and topical ice solution. Unloading the ventricles is accomplished by the CPB machine, which empties the heart. The greatest decrease in oxygen demand (by as much as 80%) occurs with the diastolic arrest of the heart using cardioplegia solution, which eliminates the electrical and mechanical work of the myocardium.

11. **What are the benefits of using the internal mammary artery for bypass?**
   Use of the internal mammary artery (IMA) was first described by Kolessov in 1967, but its impact on survival wasn't noted until the mid-1980s. Left IMA (LIMA) anastomosed to the LAD artery has an approximately 90% patency at 10 years and offers an advantage in both survival and freedom from

reoperation. The current guidelines for CABG include a class I recommendation for use of the LIMA to bypass the LAD artery when bypass of the LAD artery is indicated (Fig. 21-2).

12. **What about other arterial conduits?**
The right IMA (RIMA), radial artery, gastroepiploic artery, and inferior epigastric arteries have also been used as bypass conduits, and some surgeons have favored all-arterial strategies for bypass grafting, with hopes to improve long-term patency over saphenous vein grafts (SVG). However, these other arterial grafts have not duplicated the success of the LIMA to the LAD artery. The radial artery has been recently evaluated in several randomized trials using follow-up angiography, and results are mixed, with some showing a small incremental benefit in patency over SVG at 1 year. A recent VA cooperative study randomized 733 patients to radial artery versus saphenous vein graft, and showed equivalent graft patency at one year (89% in each group). Because the important question is long-term patency, 5 year patency rates will be the subject of ongoing investigations.

13. **What is the long-term patency of the saphenous vein?**
The saphenous vein is readily available and relatively easy to procure, provides multiple graft segments, and is the most common bypass graft used other than the LIMA. The major limitation of the SVG is its long-term patency. Early attrition of up to 15% can occur by 1 year, with 10-year patency

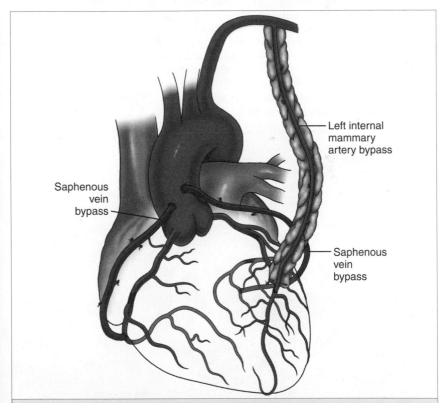

Figure 21-2. Typical configuration for a three-vessel coronary artery bypass. The left internal mammary artery is anastomosed to the left anterior descending artery. Aortocoronary bypasses are created using the reversed saphenous vein to the distal right coronary artery and an obtuse marginal branch of the circumflex coronary artery. The circumflex coronary artery is usually avoided as a target for bypass because it is located well into the atrioventricular groove and difficult to visualize. (From Townsend CM Jr, Beauchamp RD, Evers BM, Mattox KL: *Sabiston Textbook of Surgery*, ed 19, Philadelphia, 2012, Saunders.)

traditionally cited at 60%. Early patency has been shown to be improved by use of aspirin postoperatively. SVG can be harvested using a single long leg incision, multiple short incisions with intervening skin islands, or endoscopic techniques. Early patency has largely been found to be equivalent both clinically and angiographically between open and endoscopic techniques.

14. **What is off-pump CABG, and what are the differences between on-pump and off-pump CABG?**

Off-pump bypass is CABG surgery performed without use of the CPB machine. The heart remains beating throughout the procedure, and stabilizers and coronary occlusion and shunts are used to perform the bypass graft to native coronary artery anastomoses (Fig. 21-3). Because off-pump surgery avoids CPB, it should lessen the side effects of the extracorporeal circulation, such as activation of inflammatory mediators, coagulopathy, and risk of embolic events. Surgeons have debated the merits of off-pump verses on-pump bypass for many years, and the goal of demonstrating differences between the two techniques in hard endpoints, such as mortality, stroke, and renal failure, has been elusive. In fact, the literature largely shows equivalency in these major early outcomes. In some studies, slightly shorter lengths of hospital stay and lower transfusion rates have been noted with off-pump surgery.

Surgeons that prefer on-pump bypass surgery argue that the use of CPB allows maintenance of hemodynamic stability and aids in complete revascularization. The motionless and bloodless field allows precise and exact anastomoses. Off-pump revascularization on a beating heart is technically more demanding, especially with small or diffusely diseased targets, and the technical difficulty may result in decreased long-term patency of the grafts.

The technique of off-pump revascularization can be particularly useful in selected cases, such as in patients with a heavily calcified aorta (often called a "porcelain aorta"). In experienced centers, patency rates of the bypass grafts performed on-pump versus off-pump should not differ greatly. Most centers use off-pump selectively. In the United States, currently approximately 80% of CABG operations are performed on-pump using CPB, whereas 20% are performed off-pump.

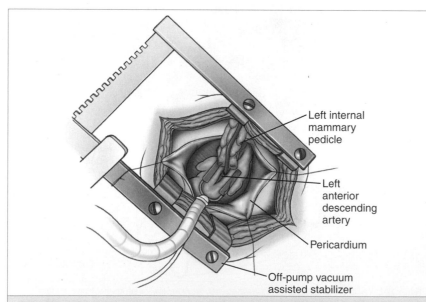

Left internal mammary pedicle

Left anterior descending artery

Pericardium

Off-pump vacuum assisted stabilizer

Figure 21-3. Left thoracotomy approach for performing off-pump left internal mammary to left anterior descending bypass. This is commonly used in the minimally invasive direct coronary artery bypass (MIDCAB) approach. Multiarticulating stabilizers are essential for this technique. (From Townsend CM Jr, Beauchamp RD, Evers BM, Mattox KL: *Sabiston Textbook of Surgery,* ed 19, Philadelphia, 2012, Saunders.)

15. **What are minimally invasive, robotic, and hybrid CABG procedures, and what are their current roles in coronary revascularization?**

   Minimally invasive CABG involves the use of smaller incisions, sometimes with videoscopic guidance, and is often referred to by the acronym "MICS," for minimally invasive cardiac surgery. The most common minimally invasive bypass surgery is known as the "MID-CAB," which consists of a single vessel LIMA to LAD artery, done through a small left anterior thoracotomy, using off-pump technique. The rationale for such minimally invasive operations is that avoiding a full sternotomy should help avoid some serious potential complications of CABG, such as mediastinitis, and allow for quicker recovery, because patients could theoretically return to full activity and lifting sooner, without the risk for sternal dehiscence. However, mini-thoracotomy, which usually employs rib spreading, can sometimes be more painful for the patient than a median sternotomy, and the benefits of such techniques are not well established. Some surgeons have also pursued multivessel off-pump "MICS" CABG through mini-thoracotomy, but such efforts are technically very demanding and may have substantial risk without proven benefit.

   There has been a good deal of fanfare about robotic cardiothoracic surgery over the past decade. Robotic CABG consists of robotically controlled endoscopic instruments and a three-dimensional camera set up through ports placed in the patient's chest, controlled remotely by a surgeon sitting at a console in the same operating room. For CABG, the robotic instruments are often used mainly to mobilize the internal mammary artery, but can also be used to perform the anastomoses; however, this is technically very challenging and has no proven benefit over hand-sewn anastomoses. High cost and cumbersome setup, in addition to technical difficulties and lack of evidence for overwhelming benefit, have limited the applicability of robotics to coronary surgery.

   Some centers have popularized performing "hybrid" procedures, where a patient will receive a single-vessel CABG with LIMA to LAD artery, most commonly using a mini-thoracotomy, and other non-LAD artery coronary lesions will be treated with coronary stents, either at the same or staggered settings. One rationale for this strategy is to attempt to capitalize on the high long-term patency and mortality benefit demonstrated with the LIMA to LAD artery graft, while avoiding the downside of sternotomy. In the current CABG guidelines, hybrid CABG has a class IIa indication if there are limitations to traditional CABG, such as heavily calcified aorta, poor target vessels, lack of suitable conduit, or unfavorable LAD artery for PCI. Otherwise, indications for hybrid CABG are deemed class IIb, or a "may be reasonable alternative," in an attempt to improve the overall risk-benefit ratio. These techniques are used in a minority of CABG procedures performed in the US.

16. **What complications can occur following CABG?**

   Operative mortality is currently less than 2% overall, and less than 1% in low-risk patients. Sentinel complications include stroke, MI, renal failure, respiratory failure, and mediastinitis (see the following question). The incidence of each is approximately 1% to 5% and varies with age and preoperative comorbidities of the patient.

   Atrial fibrillation is the most common complication after cardiothoracic surgery, with an incidence of 20% to 40%. The incidence of atrial fibrillation increases with age, duration of CPB, presence of chronic obstructive pulmonary disease (COPD), and preexisting heart failure, among other risk factors. The peak incidence of postoperative atrial fibrillation is between 2 to 4 days after surgery, is usually self-limited, and usually resolves over time as the inflammatory state of the heart improves. Use of beta-adrenergic blocking agents (β-blockers) postoperatively is routine and is useful to decrease the risk of atrial fibrillation. Goals of therapy are rate control and conversion to normal sinus rhythm, if possible. Anticoagulation may be advisable if timely conversion cannot be accomplished, or if the arrhythmia recurs intermittently.

17. **Who is at risk for mediastinitis?**

   Mediastinitis is a deep surgical-site infection following sternotomy. The infection involves the sternal bone and underlying heart and mediastinum. The organism most commonly recovered is *Staphylococcus,* but gram-negative organisms can also be found. The incidence of mediastinitis has been reported in the past to be 1% to 4%, but a recent Society of Thoracic Surgeons (STS) database study has shown an incidence less than 1%. The incidence of mediastinitis increases with the presence of diabetes, morbid obesity, COPD, and when bilateral mammary harvesting is performed. Perioperative prophylactic antibiotics, proper skin preparation and clipping, and active control of hyperglycemia in the postoperative setting are important measures believed to decrease the incidence of mediastinitis.

18. **What causes strokes during coronary bypass?**

Incidence of stroke (type I neurologic deficit) in the perioperative period after cardiac surgery is 1% to 6% and varies with age. The risk of stroke is dependent on the atherosclerotic burden in the cerebrovascular circulation and in the aorta. Atherosclerotic plaques in the ascending aorta can be the source of atheroemboli during aortic cannulation, cross-clamping, or manipulation of the ascending aorta. Microemboli may also be due to fat and to air that can arise during extracorporeal circulation. Regional hypoperfusion can occur in the brain as a result of intracranial and extracranial vascular lesions when there are significant fluctuations in the blood pressure during on-pump or off-pump surgery.

19. **What is a type II neurologic deficit?**

A type II neurologic deficit is a neurocognitive change after CABG, and its true incidence remains controversial. Changes in intellectual abilities, memory, and mood are often based on subjective assessment and often difficult to quantitatively evaluate. Reported incidence ranges widely from 2% to 50%. Studies have shown decreases in neurocognitive functioning after CABG, but in small series, similar declines over time have been noted in on-pump, off-pump, PCI, and CAD "control patients" not undergoing intervention.

20. **How should clopidogrel be managed preoperatively?**

Preoperative clopidogrel use increases blood transfusion during cardiac surgery and increases the risk of reoperation after surgery for mediastinal bleeding. The current recommendation is to avoid clopidogrel for 5 days before CABG, unless the need for urgent or emergent revascularization for ongoing ischemia exceeds the risk of bleeding.

21. **What factors are important in the follow-up of CABG patients?**

Secondary prevention and control of atherosclerotic risk factors are important in maintaining the long-term clinical success of the operation. Use of statins, β-blockers, and aspirin is advised in all post-CABG patients who do not have strong contraindications to those medications. Angiotensin-converting enzyme (ACE) inhibitors are also recommended in patients with low left ventricular ejection fraction (less than 40%). In addition, control of hypertension and diabetes, and smoking cessation are also essential aspects of secondary prevention.

22. **What is the incidence of recurrent disease requiring redo-CABG?**

Reoperation may be required because of progression of native coronary disease or failure of previous grafts. The incidence of reoperation in studies has been reported to be approximately 10% by 10 years, although aggressive secondary prevention and advances in the use of PCI for the treatment of native and graft disease may decrease the need for reoperation. Redo CABG is technically more challenging. Scarring of the mediastinum increases the risk of complications, including damage to the LIMA graft. Lack of suitable bypass conduits is also a concern in patients undergoing redo bypass surgery.

BIBLIOGRAPHY, SUGGESTED READINGS, AND WEBSITES

1. Collins P, Webb CM, Chong CF, et al: Radial artery versus saphenous vein patency (RSVP) randomized trial: five-year angiographic follow-up, *Circulation* 117:2859–2864, 2008.
2. Goldman S, Sethi GK, Holman W, et al: Radial artery grafts vs saphenous vein grafts in coronary artery bypass surgery. A randomized trial, *JAMA* 305:167–174, 2011.

3. Goldman S, Zadin K, Moritz T, et al: Long-term patency of saphenous vein and left internal mammary artery grafts after coronary artery bypass surgery: results from a Department of Veterans Affairs cooperative study, *J Am Coll Cardiol* 44:2149–2156, 2004.

4. Hannan EL, Wu C, Walford G, et al: Drug-eluting stents vs. coronary artery bypass grafting in multivessel coronary disease, *N Engl J Med* 358:331–334, 2008.

5. Hillis LD, Smith PK, Anderson JL, et al: 2011 ACCF/AHA guideline for coronary artery bypass graft surgery: executive summary: A report of the American College of Cardiology Foundation/ American Heart Association Task Force on Practice Guidelines, *J Thorac Cardiovasc Surg* 143:4–34, 2012.

6. Kappetein AP, Feldman TE, Mack MJ, et al: Comparison of coronary bypass surgery with drug-eluting stenting for the treatment of left main and/or three-vessel disease: 3-year follow-up of the SYNTAX trial, *Eur Heart J* 32:2125–2134, 2011.

7. Lamy A, Devereaux PJ, Prabhakaran D, et al: Off-pump or on-pump coronary-artery bypass grafting at 30 days. (CORONARY investigators), *N Engl J Med* 366:1489–1497, 2012.

8. McKhann GM, Grega MA, Borowicz LM Jr, et al: Is there cognitive decline 1 year after CABG? Comparison with surgical and nonsurgical controls, *Neurology* 65:991–999, 2005.

9. Sellke FW, DiMaio JM, Caplan LR, et al: Comparing on-pump and off-pump coronary artery bypass grafting: numerous studies but few conclusions: a scientific statement from the American Heart Association Council on Cardiovascular Surgery and Anesthesia in collaboration with the Interdisciplinary Working Group on Quality of Care Outcomes Research, *Circulation* 111:2858–2864, 2005.

10. Shroyer AL, Grover FL, Hattler B, et al: Veterans Affairs randomized on/off bypass (ROOBY) study group. On-pump versus off-pump coronary artery bypass surgery, *N Eng J Med* 361:1827–1837, 2009.

11. Smith SC Jr, Allen J, Blair SN, et al: AHA\ACC Guidelines for secondary prevention for patients with coronary and other atherosclerotic vascular disease: 2006 update, *Circulation* 113:2363–2372, 2006.

CHAPTER 22

ACUTE DECOMPENSATED HEART FAILURE

G. Michael Felker, MD, MHS, FACC

1. **What is acute decompensated heart failure? Isn't it just a worsening of chronic heart failure?**

   Acute decompensated heart failure (ADHF) is a clinical syndrome of worsening signs or symptoms of heart failure requiring hospitalization or other unscheduled medical care. For many years, ADHF was viewed as simply an exacerbation of chronic heart failure as a result of volume overload, with few implications beyond a short-term need to intensify diuretic therapy (a similar paradigm to exacerbations of chronic asthma). Recent decades have seen an explosion of research into the epidemiology, pathophysiology, outcomes, and treatment of ADHF. Multiple lines of evidence now support the concept that ADHF is a unique clinical syndrome with its own epidemiology and underlying mechanisms and a need for specific therapies. ADHF is not just a worsening of chronic heart failure, any more than an acute myocardial infarction (MI) is just a worsening of chronic angina.

   Outcomes data from a variety of studies now support the concept that hospitalization for ADHF can often signal a dramatic change in the natural history of the heart failure syndrome. Rates of rehospitalization or death are as high as 50% within 6 months of the initial ADHF event, which is a much higher event rate than is seen with acute MI.

2. **Are there clinically important subcategories of ADHF?**

   There is great interest in developing a framework for understanding ADHF that would assist in stratifying patients, guiding therapy, and developing new treatments, similar to the basic framework developed for acute coronary syndromes (i.e., ST segment elevation myocardial infarction [STEMI], non–ST segment elevation myocardial infarction [NSTEMI], and unstable angina). Although this area is rapidly evolving, a few general clinical *phenotypes* of ADHF have emerged.

   - **Hypertensive acute heart failure:** Data from large registries such as ADHERE and OPTIMIZE have shown that a substantial portion of ADHF patients are hypertensive on initial presentation to the emergency department. Such patients often have relatively little volume overload, preserved or only mildly reduced ventricular function, and are more likely to be older and female. Symptoms often develop quickly (minutes to hours), and many such patients have little or no history of chronic heart failure. Hypertensive urgency with acute pulmonary edema represents an extreme form of this phenotype.
   - **Decompensated heart failure:** This describes patients with a background of significant chronic heart failure, who develop symptoms of volume overload and congestion over a period of days to weeks. These patients typically have significant left ventricular dysfunction and chronic heart failure at baseline. Although specific triggers are poorly understood, episodes are often triggered by noncompliance with diet or medical therapy.
   - **Cardiogenic shock/advanced heart failure:** Although patients with advanced forms of heart failure are often seen in tertiary care centers, they are relatively uncommon in the broader population (probably fewer than 10% of ADHF hospitalizations). These patients may present with so called *low-output* symptoms (e.g., confusion, fatigue, abdominal pain, or anorexia) that may make diagnosis challenging. Hypotension (systolic blood pressure [SBP] less than 90 mm Hg) and significant end-organ dysfunction (especially renal dysfunction) are common features. Many of these patients have concomitant evidence of significant right ventricular dysfunction, with ascites or generalized anasarca.

3. **What is the role of biomarkers like B-type natriuretic peptides (BNPs) in the diagnosis of ADHF?**

   Although the clinical symptoms (dyspnea, paroxysmal nocturnal dyspnea [PND], orthopnea, fatigue) and signs (elevated jugular venous pressure, pulmonary rales, edema) of ADHF are well known, the diagnosis can often be challenging in patients presenting to acute care settings. This is especially true in the elderly and patients with significant comorbid conditions such as chronic obstructive pulmonary disease (COPD). The development of natriuretic peptides as a diagnostic tool has been a major advance in ADHF diagnosis. The clinically available natriuretic peptides for ADHF diagnosis include BNP and its biologically inert amino-terminal fragment, N-terminal prohormone of B-type natriuretic peptide (NT-proBNP). Despite some subtle differences between these two biomarkers, they provide similar diagnostic information when used in patients presenting to the emergency department with unexplained dyspnea, although the range of values is significantly different (in general, NT-proBNP levels are approximately 5 to 10 times greater than BNP levels in the same patient). The landmark Breathing Not Properly Study measured BNP levels in 1586 patients presenting to the emergency department with unexplained dyspnea. In this study, treating physicians were blinded to BNP values and a panel of cardiologists adjudicated whether hospitalizations were due to ADHF or other causes (based on all clinical data other than the BNP values). As shown in Figure 22-1, a cutoff of 100 pg/mL of BNP had a positive predictive value of 79% and a negative predictive value of 89% for the diagnosis of ADHF. The area under the receiver operating characteristic (ROC) curve was 0.91, suggesting a very high degree of accuracy for establishing the diagnosis of ADHF. Subsequent studies have demonstrated similar findings for NT-proBNP, although optimal diagnostic cutoffs are different (450 pg/mL for patients younger than 50 years and 900 pg/mL for patients older than 50 years). The use of natriuretic peptide has now become the standard of care in the diagnosis of patients with dyspnea presenting to acute care settings, and has a class I indication ("should be done") in clinical practice guidelines.

4. **What features suggest patients who are particularly high risk?**

   Analysis of large datasets from both clinical trials and registries of ADHF patients have identified a few features that consistently suggest a high risk of short-term morbidity and mortality in patients hospitalized with ADHF (Box 22-1). Across studies, the most consistent of these are blood urea nitrogen (BUN), serum creatinine, SBP, and hyponatremia. Interestingly, BUN has consistently proved to be

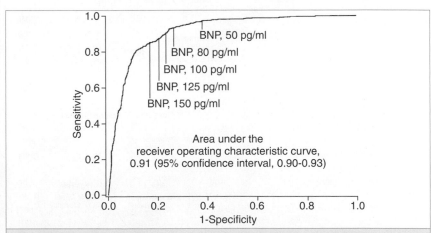

Figure 22-1. Receiver operating characteristic curve for use of B-type natriuretic peptide *(BNP)* in making diagnosis of acute decompensated heart failure in patients with acute unexplained dyspnea. (Adapted from Maisel AS, Krishnaswamy P, Nowak RM, et al: Rapid measurement of B-type natriuretic peptide in the emergency diagnosis of heart failure. *N Engl J Med* 347:161-167, 2002.)

a stronger predictor of outcomes than creatinine (Fig. 22-2). One potential explanation of this finding is that BUN may integrate both renal function and hemodynamic information. Unlike the situation in many other cardiovascular conditions, *higher* blood pressure has consistently been associated with *lower* risk. Hyponatremia appears to be associated with lower output and greater neurohormonal activation, and risk appears to be increased with even mild forms of hyponatremia. A variety of biomarkers also appear to have strong prognostic implications in ADHF, in particular the natriuretic peptides (BNP or NT-proBNP) and troponin.

Box 22-1 HIGH-RISK FEATURES IN PATIENTS HOSPITALIZED WITH ACUTE DECOMPENSATED HEART FAILURE

- Lower systolic blood pressure
- Elevated blood urea nitrogen (BUN)
- Hyponatremia
- History of prior heart failure hospitalization
- Elevated BNP or NT-proBNP
- Elevated troponin T or I

BNP, B-Type natriuretic peptide; *NT-proBNP*, N-terminal prohormone of B-type natriuretic peptide.

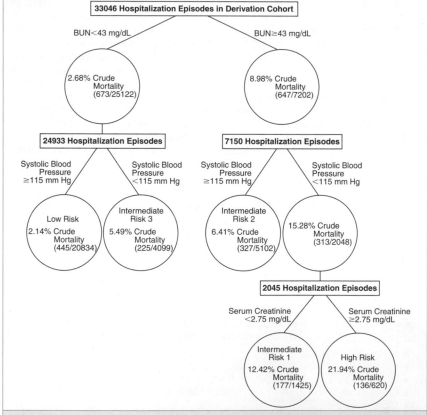

Figure 22-2. Predictors of in-hospital mortality in the ADHERE database. (Reprinted with permission from Fonarow GC, Adams KF Jr, Abraham WT, et al: Risk stratification for in-hospital mortality in acutely decompensated heart failure: classification and regression tree analysis. *JAMA* 293:572-580, 2005.) *BUN*, Blood urea nitrogen.

5. **What are the goals of therapy in ADHF?**

Specific therapies for ADHF should be assessed in the context of the overall goals of therapy. A summary of suggested goals of therapy based on current guidelines from the Heart Failure Society of America (HFSA) and European Society of Cardiology (ESC) are shown in Box 22-2.

6. **How should we give diuretics in ADHF?**

Because most episodes of ADHF are associated with some degree of congestion or volume overload, intravenous (IV) loop diuretics remain a cornerstone of ADHF therapy. Because many symptoms in ADHF (in particular dyspnea) appear to be closely related to elevated ventricular filling pressures, reduction of filing pressures in order to improve acute symptoms is a major goal of therapy. Recently, however, observational data from a variety of sources have led to questions about the appropriate use of diuretics in patients with ADHF. Studies of patients with both chronic heart failure and ADHF have shown that higher diuretic use is associated with a higher incidence of adverse events (especially worsening renal function) and mortality. Interpreting this type of data is highly problematic because of the issue of confounding by indication (i.e., patients who need higher diuretic doses are typically sicker, and thus it is impossible to determine if higher doses of diuretics are simply a marker of greater disease severity or whether they directly contribute to worsening outcomes). Controversy also exists regarding whether continuous infusion (as opposed to intermittent bolus administration) may be a safer and more efficacious way of administering IV diuretics in ADHF. These questions have been recently addressed by a National Institutes of Health (NIH)–sponsored randomized clinical trial (the Diuretic Optimization Strategies Evaluation [DOSE]).

Using a 2×2 factorial design, DOSE randomized 308 patients to either high ($2.5 \times$ chronic oral dose given IV) or low ($1 \times$ chronic oral dose given IV) dosages of diuretics, and also to either continuous infusion or every-12-hour IV bolus. With regard to route of administration, there was no significant difference in either efficacy or safety when diuretics were given as intermittent boluses or as continuous infusion. With regard to dosing, there was a general trend towards greater decongestion and improved symptoms with higher-dose diuretics (although the study did not meet its nominal primary efficacy endpoint of patient global assessment with a P value $= 0.06$). This suggestion of improved efficacy did appear to come at a cost of more episodes of renal dysfunction in the higher-dose arm, but these changes were transient and did not appear to have any impact on postdischarge clinical outcomes. Taken as a whole, the results from DOSE appear to generally support an aggressive approach to decongestion of volume overloaded patients with ADHF, although renal function, electrolytes, and volume status need to be carefully monitored.

7. **What about using vasodilators such as nesiritide?**

Nesiritide, a recombinant form of human BNP, is a vasodilator with similar hemodynamic effects to other parenteral vasodilators, such as nitroglycerin and sodium nitroprusside. Nesiritide was approved for ADHF therapy based on its ability to speed the resolution of symptoms in patients with ADHF in the Vasodilation in the Management of Acute Congestive Heart Failure (VMAC) study. Subsequently, several retrospective meta-analyses have suggested the possibility that nesiritide therapy could be associated with adverse effects on renal function or even increased mortality. This led to

---

Box 22-2 TREATMENT GOALS FOR ACUTE DECOMPENSATED HEART FAILURE HOSPITALIZATION

- Improve symptoms of congestion.
- Optimize volume status.
- Identify and address triggers for decompensation.
- Optimize chronic oral therapy.
- Minimize side effects.
- Identify patients who might benefit from revascularization.
- Educate patients concerning medications and disease management.

substantial controversy about the appropriate role of nesiritide in ADHF management. The ASCEND-HF study was a large international randomized controlled trial designed to assess the impact of nesiritide on symptoms, renal function, and 30-day clinical outcomes. ASCEND-HF randomized 7141 patients with ADHF within 24 hours of initial IV treatment for heart failure. This study showed statistically significant (but clinically very modest) improvements in dyspnea with nesiritide at both 6 and 24 hours from randomization. There was no significant difference in either death or the composite of death or heart failure hospitalization at 30 days. Overall, the ASCEND-HF results do not support the routine use of nesiritide in patients with ADHF.

8. **What is the role of inotropes like dobutamine or milrinone in patients with ADHF?**

   Inotropic drugs, which increase cardiac contractility, are theoretically appealing as a therapy for ADHF. Despite this theoretical appeal, however, available data clearly demonstrate that such agents are not indicated for the vast majority of ADHF patients. In the OPTIME-CHF study, a large randomized trial of IV milrinone therapy in ADHF, randomization to milrinone did not shorten length of stay or improve other clinical outcomes, and it was associated with significantly higher rates of arrhythmias and hypotension than was the placebo. These data suggest that the routine use of inotropes is not indicated in ADHF management. Importantly, OPTIME-CHF specifically excluded patients with shock or other apparent indications for inotropes. As noted earlier, the vast majority of ADHF patients do not have evidence of end-organ hypoperfusion or shock. In the subset of patients with cardiogenic shock or severe end-organ dysfunction, inotropic therapy may still be indicated as a method of achieving short-term stabilization until more definitive long-term therapy (such are revascularization, cardiac transplantation, or mechanical cardiac support) can be employed.

9. **What is the role for invasive hemodynamic monitoring in patients with ADHF?**

   The routine use of invasive hemodynamic monitoring (such as with pulmonary artery catheters) is not indicated in patients with ADHF. This recommendation is based primarily on the results of the ESCAPE study, which demonstrated no advantage in terms of days alive and free from hospitalization when patients hospitalized with advanced heart failure were randomized to pulmonary artery catheter-guided therapy versus usual care. Invasive hemodynamic monitoring may be indicated to guide therapy in selected patients who are refractory to initial therapy, particularly those with hypotension or worsening renal function.

10. **What is cardiorenal syndrome in ADHF?**

    Worsening renal function during hospitalization for ADHF represents a major clinical challenge. Often termed *cardiorenal syndrome* (CRS), this clinical syndrome is characterized by persistent volume overload accompanied by worsening of renal function. Development of CRS, as defined by an increase in serum creatinine of 0.3 mg/dL or more from admission, occurs in as many as one-third of patients hospitalized with ADHF. Development of CRS is associated with higher mortality and increased length of stay in patients with ADHF. Although the underlying mechanisms of CRS remain ill defined, data suggest that higher diuretic doses, preexisting renal disease, and diabetes mellitus are associated with an increased risk. The optimal therapeutic strategy for patients with ADHF and CRS remains unknown. A variety of clinical approaches (hemodynamically guided therapy, inotropes, temporarily holding diuretics, etc.) have all been used with varying results, and there are no large outcomes studies to guide management of these challenging patients. Ultrafiltration therapy, which results in the removal of both free water and sodium, is currently being studied as an approach to CRS in an NIH-sponsored, randomized clinical trial that has recently completed enrollment.

11. **How should we determine when to discharge patients?**

    The decision of when to discharge a patient with ADHF from the hospital is often based on clinical judgment rather than objective criteria. Criteria that should be met before consideration of hospital discharge have been published in the HFSA guidelines (Box 22-3). Most patients should have follow-up scheduled within 7 to 10 days of discharge, and high-risk patients should be considered for earlier

---

Box 22-3 CRITERIA FOR HOSPITAL DISCHARGE IN ACUTE DECOMPENSATED HEART FAILURE

- Exacerbating factors addressed
- Near optimal volume status achieved
- Transitioned from intravenous to oral therapy (consider 24 hours of stability on oral therapy for high-risk patients)
- Education of patient and family
- Near optimal chronic heart failure therapy achieved
- Follow-up appointment scheduled in 7 to 10 days (earlier if high risk)

---

follow-up (by phone or in person) or referral to a comprehensive disease management program. Early adjustment of diuretics may be required as patients make the transition from the hospital environment (with IV diuretics and controlled low-sodium diet) to home.

BIBLIOGRAPHY, SUGGESTED READINGS, AND WEBSITES

1. Adams KF, Lindenfeld J, Arnold JM, et al: HFSA 2006 comprehensive heart failure practice guideline, *J Card Fail* 12:1–119, 2006.

2. Cotter G, Felker GM, Adams KF, et al: The pathophysiology of acute heart failure–is it all about fluid accumulation? *Am Heart J* 155(1):9–18, 2008.

3. ESCAPE Investigators, ESCAPE Study Coordinators: Evaluation Study of Congestive Heart Failure and Pulmonary Artery Catheterization Effectiveness: the ESCAPE trial, *JAMA* 294:1625–1633, 2005.

4. Felker GM, Lee KL, Bull DA, et al: Diuretic strategies in patients with acute decompensated heart failure, *N Engl J Med* 364:797–805, 2011.

5. Fonarow GC, Adams KF Jr, Abraham WT, et al: Risk stratification for in-hospital mortality in acutely decompensated heart failure: classification and regression tree analysis, *JAMA* 293:572–580, 2005.

6. Forman DE, Butler J, Wang Y, et al: Incidence, predictors at admission, and impact of worsening renal function among patients hospitalized with heart failure, *J Am Coll Cardiol* 43:61–67, 2004.

7. Gheorghiade M, Zannad F, Sopko G, et al: Acute heart failure syndromes: current state and framework for future research, *Circulation* 112:3958–3968, 2005.

8. Hasselblad V, Stough WG, Shah MR, et al: Relation between dose of loop diuretics and outcomes in a heart failure population: results of the ESCAPE trial, *Eur J Heart Fail* 9:1064–1069, 2007.

9. Maisel AS, Krishnaswamy P, Nowak RM, et al: Rapid measurement of B-type natriuretic peptide in the emergency diagnosis of heart failure, *N Engl J Med* 347:161–167, 2002.

10. Nieminen MS, Bohm M, Cowie MR, et al: Executive summary of the guidelines on the diagnosis and treatment of acute heart failure: the Task Force on Acute Heart Failure of the European Society of Cardiology, *Eur Heart J* 26:384–416, 2005.

11. O'Connor CM, Starling RC, Hernandez AF, et al: Effect of nesiritide in patients with acute decompensated heart failure, *N Engl J Med* 365:32–43, 2011.

12. Sackner-Bernstein D, Kowalski M, Fox M, et al: Short-term risk of death after treatment with nesiritide for decompensated heart failure: a pooled analysis of randomized controlled trials, *JAMA* 293:1900–1905, 2005.

CHAPTER 23

HEART FAILURE EVALUATION AND LONG-TERM MANAGEMENT

Arunima Misra, MD, FACC, Kumudha Ramasubbu, MD, FACC, Shawn T. Ragbir, MD, Glenn N. Levine, MD, FACC, FAHA, and Biykem Bozkurt, MD, PhD, FACC, FAHA

This chapter deals specifically with the evaluation and long-term management of patients with heart failure caused by depressed ejection fraction. The management of patients with heart failure with preserved ejection fraction *(diastolic dysfunction)* is discussed in Chapter 24. The management of patients with acute decompensated heart failure is discussed in Chapter 22. Specific discussions of the evaluation and management of myocarditis, dilated cardiomyopathy, hypertrophic cardiomyopathy, and restrictive/infiltrative cardiomyopathy, as well as consideration with cardiac transplantation, are discussed in other dedicated chapters in this section of the book. The roles of pacemakers and implantable cardioverter-defibrillators in patients with heart failure are discussed in this chapter, as well as in the chapters on pacemakers (Chapter 37) and implantable cardioverter-defibrillators (Chapter 38).

1. **What are the most common causes of heart failure?**
   Ischemic heart disease, hypertension, and valvular heart disease are the most common causes of heart failure. Less common causes include diabetes; microvascular disease; genetic cardiomyopathies and muscular dystrophies; autoimmune and collage vascular diseases such as systemic lupus, dermatomyositis, or scleroderma; toxic cardiomyopathies, including alcohol or illicit drugs such as cocaine; chemotherapy induced cardiomyopathies (e.g., Adriamycin); myocarditis and viral cardiomyopathy; postpartum cardiomyopathy; tachycardia-mediated heart failure; hypothyroidism- or hyperthyroidism-related cardiomyopathies; infiltrative disorders such as sarcoidosis, hemochromatosis, and amyloidosis; high-output states (thyrotoxicosis, beriberi, systemic arteriovenous shunting, chronic anemia); and stress-induced (Tako-tsubo) cardiomyopathy.

2. **What elements should the initial assessment of the patient with heart failure include?**
   Initial assessment of the patient with heart failure should include:
   - Evaluation of heart failure symptoms and functional capacity (dyspnea on exertion, orthopnea, paroxysmal nocturnal dyspnea [PND], fatigue, and lower extremity edema)
   - Evaluation for the presence of diabetes; hypertension; smoking; prior cardiac disease; family history of cardiac disease; history of heart murmur, congenital heart disease, or rheumatic fever; sleep disturbances (obstructive sleep apnea [OSA]); thyroid disease history; exposure to infectious agents; exposure to cardiotoxins; mediastinal irradiation; and past or current use of alcohol and illicit drugs
   - Physical examination, including heart rate and rhythm; blood pressure and orthostatic blood pressure changes; measurements of weight, height, and body mass index; overall volume status; jugular venous distension; carotid upstroke and presence or absence of bruits; lung examination for rales or effusions; cardiac examination for systolic or diastolic murmurs; displaced point of maximal impulse (PMI); presence of left ventricular heave; intensity of S2; presence of S3 or S4; liver size; presence of ascites; presence of renal bruits; presence of abdominal aortic aneurysm; peripheral edema; peripheral pulses; and checking whether the extremities are cold and clammy
   - Laboratory tests, including complete blood cell count (CBC), creatinine and blood urea nitrogen (BUN), serum electrolytes, natriuretic peptide (BNP or NT-proBNP), fasting blood glucose, lipid

profile, liver function tests, thyroid-stimulating hormone (TSH), and urine analysis; and screening for hemochromatosis and human immunodeficiency virus (HIV), pheochromocytoma, amyloidosis, or rheumatologic diseases reasonable in selected patients, particularly if there is clinical suspicion for testing

- Twelve-lead electrocardiogram (ECG), assessing for rhythm, conduction abnormalities, QRS voltage and duration, QT duration, chamber enlargement, presence of ST/T changes, and Q waves
- Chest radiograph
- Transthoracic echocardiogram to asses for left ventricular (LV) and right ventricular (RV) function: wall motion; chamber sizes; filling pressures; morphology of the valves; presence of ventricular hypertrophy; and diastolic parameters
- Consideration of ischemia workup; depending on patient's age, history, symptoms, and ECG, this may be no workup, stress testing, or cardiac catheterization.
- Endomyocardial biopsy is not part of routine workup but can be considered in highly specific circumstances (see later).
- Consider cardiac MRI if infiltrative causes, such as cardiac sarcoidosis or amyloidosis, are suspected.

3. How are heart failure symptoms classified?

Symptoms are most commonly classified using the New York Heart Association (NYHA) classification system:

- **Class I:** No limitation; ordinary physical activity does not cause excess fatigue, shortness of breath, or palpitations.
- **Class II:** Slight limitation of physical activity; ordinary physical activity results in fatigue, shortness of breath, palpitations, or angina.
- **Class III:** Marked limitation of physical activity; ordinary activity will lead to symptoms.
- **Class IV:** Inability to carry on any physical activity without discomfort; symptoms of congestive heart failure (CHF) are present even at rest; increased discomfort is experienced with any physical activity.

4. What is the stage system for classifying heart failure?

In 2001, the American College of Cardiology/American Heart Association (ACC/AHA) introduced a system to categorize the stages of heart failure. This system is somewhat different in focus than the previous NYHA classification system and was intended, in part, to emphasize the prevention of the development of symptomatic heart failure. In addition, the 2009 update on the 2005 Heart Failure Guidelines suggest appropriate therapy for each stage (Figure 23-1).

- **Stage A:** Patient is at high risk for developing heart failure but is without structural heart disease or symptoms of heart failure. Includes patients with hypertension, coronary artery disease (CAD), obesity, diabetes, history of drug or alcohol abuse, history of rheumatic fever, family history of cardiomyopathy, or treatment with cardiotoxins
- **Stage B:** Patient with structural heart disease but is without signs or symptoms of heart failure. Includes patients with previous myocardial infarction (MI), LV remodeling (including left ventricular hypertrophy [LVH] or low ejection fraction), or asymptomatic valvular disease
- **Stage C:** Patient with structural heart disease and with prior or current symptoms of heart failure
- **Stage D:** Patient with refractory heart failure requiring specialized interventions

5. Which patients with heart failure should be considered for endomyocardial biopsy (EMB)?

In 2007, the ACC/AHA/European College of Cardiology (ACC/AHA/ECC) issued a scientific statement on the role of EMB. Most patients who are seen for heart failure should not be referred for EMB. Biopsy results are often nonspecific or unrevealing, and in most cases there is no specific therapy based on biopsy results that have been shown to improve prognosis. However, in certain clinical scenarios, EMB

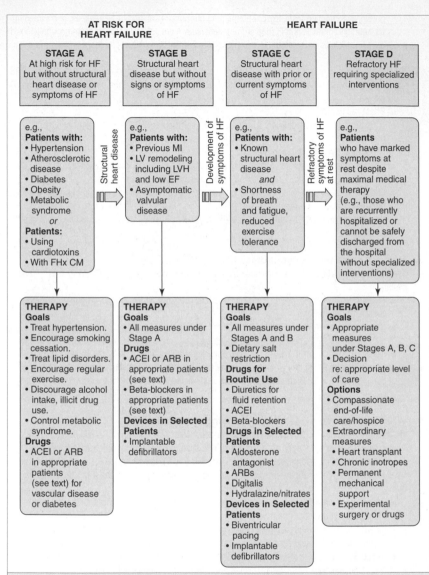

Figure 23-1. American College of Cardiology/American Heart Association Stages in the Development of Heart Failure/Recommended Therapy by Stage. (From Jessup M, Abraham WT, Casey DE, et al: ACC/AHA 2009 focused update: ACCF/AHA guidelines for the diagnosis and management of heart failure in adults : a report of the American College of Cardiology Foundation/American Heart Association Task Force on Practice Guidelines: Developed in collaboration with the International Society for Heart and Lung Transplantation, *Circulation* 119:1977-2016, 2009; originally published online March 26, 2009.) *ACEI,* Angiotensin-converting enzyme inhibitor; *ARB,* angiotensin II receptor blocker; *EF,* ejection fraction; *FHx CM,* family history of cardiomyopathy; *HF,* heart failure; *LV,* left ventricle; *LVH,* left ventricular hypertrophy; *MI,* myocardial infarction.

should be performed (class I recommendation) or can be considered and is considered reasonable (class IIa recommendation). As given in that document, these scenarios include the following:

- New-onset heart failure of less than 2 weeks duration associated with a normal-sized or dilated left ventricle and hemodynamic compromise (class I; level of evidence B)
- New-onset heart failure of 2 weeks to 3 months duration associated with a dilated left ventricle and new ventricular arrhythmias, second- or third-degree heart block, or failure to respond to usual care within 1 to 2 weeks (class I; level of evidence B)
- Heart failure of more than 3 months duration associated with a dilated left ventricle and new ventricular arrhythmias, second- or third-degree heart block, or failure to respond to usual care within 1 to 2 weeks (class IIa; level of evidence C)
- Heart failure associated with a dilated cardiomyopathy of any duration associated with suspected allergic reaction or eosinophilia (class IIa; level of evidence C)
- Heart failure associated with suspected anthracycline cardiomyopathy (class Ia; level of evidence C)
- Heart failure with unexplained restrictive cardiomyopathy (class IIa; level of evidence C)

6. **What are the general treatments for patients with heart failure?**
- Diuretics are indicated for volume overload. Starting doses of furosemide are often 20 to 40 mg once or twice a day, but higher doses will be required in patients with significant renal dysfunction. The dose should be uptitrated to a maximum of up to 600 mg daily in divided doses. Failure of therapy is often the result of inadequate diuretic dosing. Torsemide is more expensive than furosemide but has superior absorption and longer duration of action. Bumetanide is approximately 40 times more potent milligram-for-milligram than furosemide and can also be used in patients who are unresponsive or poorly responsive to furosemide. Synergistic diuretics that act on the distal portion of the tubule (thiazides such as metolazone, or potassium-sparing agents) are often added in those who fail to respond to high-dose loop diuretics alone. In addition, a new recommendation from 2009 Focused Update states that for hospitalized heart failure patients, if diuresis is inadequate to relieve congestion, higher doses of loop diuretics should be used, addition of second diuretic should be made or continuous infusion of a loop diuretic should be considered.
- Inhibition of the renin-angiotensin-aldosterone system should be initiated. Angiotensin-converting enzyme (ACE) inhibitors are first-line agents in those with depressed ejection fraction because they have been convincingly shown to improve symptoms, decrease hospitalizations, and reduce mortality. Angiotensin II receptor blockers (ARBs) are used in those who are ACE-inhibitor intolerant because of persistent cough. ARBs may also be considered *in addition* to ACE inhibitors in select patients (this latter decision is best left to a heart failure specialist). The aldosterone antagonists spironolactone or eplerenone can be considered as additional therapy in carefully selected patients with preserved renal function already on standard heart failure therapies.
- Hydralazine and isosorbide are used in patients who are unable to tolerate both ACE inhibitors and ARBs because of renal failure. Hydralazine and isosorbide should be considered *in addition* to an ACE inhibitor or ARB in African Americans, and can be considered as an add-on therapy in others. They may be considered in patients who are ACE inhibitor and ARB intolerant.
- The beta-adrenergic blocking agents (β-blockers) metoprolol succinate (Toprol XL), carvedilol (Coreg), and bisoprolol have been shown to decrease mortality in appropriately selected patients. These agents should be initiated in euvolemic patients on stable background heart failure therapy, including ACE inhibitors or ARBs.
- Implantable cardioverter-defibrillators (ICDs) are considered for primary prevention in patients whose ejection fractions remain less than 30% to 35% despite optimal medical therapy, and who have a good-quality life expectancy of at least 1 year.
- Biventricular pacing for resynchronization therapy should be considered. According to the 2009 American College of Cardiology Foundation/AHA (ACCF/AHA) guidelines, biventricular pacing for cardiac resynchronization therapy (CRT) should be considered for patients in sinus rhythm with NYHA class III-IV symptoms, left ventricular ejection fraction (LVEF) less than 35%, and QRS greater than 120 ms. Consultation with an electrophysiologist is recommended.

The elements of long-term management of patients with CHF resulting from depressed LV systolic function are summarized in Table 23-1.

TABLE 23-1.   ELEMENTS OF THE LONG-TERM MANAGEMENT OF PATIENTS WITH CONGESTIVE HEART FAILURE DUE TO LEFT VENTRICULAR SYSTOLIC DYSFUNCTION

Treatment/Intervention	Recommendation (Level of Evidence)
Diuretics for fluid retention	Class I (LOE: C)
Salt restriction	Class I (LOE: C)
ACE inhibitors (ACEIs)	Class I (LOE: A)
Angiotensin II receptor blockers (ARB) in ACEI-intolerant patients	Class I (LOE: A)
ARB in persistently symptomatic patients with reduced LVEF already being treated with conventional therapy	Class IIb (LOE: C)
Hydralazine + Isosorbide in patients ACEI and ARB intolerant	Class IIb (LOE: C)
Hydralazine + Isosorbide in patients already on ACEI and β-blocker with persistent symptoms	Class IIa (LOE: A)
β-Blockers	Class I (LOE: A)
Digoxin in patients with heart failure symptoms. Generally used in those with continued symptoms and/or hospitalizations despite good therapy with diuretics and ACEIs	Class IIa (LOE: B)
Aldosterone antagonists in patients with moderate-severe symptoms who can carefully be monitored for renal function and potassium level and with baseline creatinine < 2-2.5 mg/dL and potassium < 5.0 mEq/L	Class I (LOE: B)
Exercise training in ambulatory patients	Class I (LOE: B)
ICD for "secondary prevention" (history of cardiac arrest, ventricular fibrillation, or hemodynamically destabilizing ventricular tachycardia)	Class I (LOE: A)
ICD for "primary prevention" for LVEF < 30%-35% and symptomatic heart failure (see text)	Class I-IIa (LOE: A-B)
Cardiac resynchronization therapy for patients in sinus rhythm with class III-IV symptoms despite medical therapy, LVEF < 35%, and QRS > 120 ms (see text)	Class I (LOE: A)

Modified from Hunt SA, Abraham WT, Chin MH, et al: ACC/AHA 2005 guideline update for the diagnosis and management of chronic heart failure in the adult: a report of the American College of Cardiology/American Heart Association Task Force on Practice Guidelines (Writing Committee to Update the 2001 Guidelines for the Evaluation and Management of Heart Failure). *J Am Coll Cardiol* 46:e1-e82, 2005.
ACE, Angiotensin-converting enzyme; *ICD*, implantable cardioverter-defibrillator; *LVEF*, left ventricular ejection fraction.

7. How do ACE inhibitors and ARBs work?

ACE inhibitors inhibit ACE, thus blocking the conversion of angiotensin I to angiotensin II. ACE is predominantly found in the pulmonary and to a lesser extent in the renal endothelium. By decreasing the production of angiotensin II, ACE inhibitors attenuate sympathetic tone, decrease arterial vasoconstriction, and attenuate myocardial hypertrophy. Because angiotensin II stimulates aldosterone production, circulating levels of aldosterone are reduced. This results in decreased in sodium chloride absorption, decreased potassium excretion in the distal tubules, and decreased water retention. Through a decrease in antidiuretic hormone (ADH) production, ACE inhibitors also decrease water absorption in the collecting ducts.

ARBs selectively block the binding of angiotensin II to the AT_1 receptor, thereby blocking the effect of angiotensin II on end organs. This results in attenuation of sympathetic tone, decrease in arterial vasoconstriction, and attenuation of myocardial hypertrophy. Because angiotensin II stimulates aldosterone production, circulating levels of aldosterone are reduced. This results in a decrease in sodium chloride absorption, potassium excretion in the distal tubules, and water retention.

8. **What approach should be taken if a patient treated with an ACE inhibitor develops a cough?**
Nonproductive cough related to ACE inhibitors occurs in 5% to 10% of white patients of European descent and in up to 50% of Chinese patients. The cough is believed related to kinin potentiation. The cough usually develops within the first months of therapy and disappears within 1 to 2 weeks of discontinuation of therapy. ACC/AHA guidelines suggest one should first make sure the cough is related to treatment and not to another condition. The guidelines state that the demonstration that the cough disappears after drug withdrawal and recurs after rechallenge with another ACE inhibitor strongly suggests that ACE inhibition is the cause of the cough. They emphasize that patients should be *rechallenged,* because many will not redevelop a cough, suggesting the initial development of cough was coincidental and may have been related to heart failure. Patients who do have ACE inhibitor–related cough and cannot tolerate symptoms should be treated with an ARB.

9. **What is the efficacy of ARBs compared with ACE inhibitors in patients with chronic heart failure?**
Trials comparing the efficacy of ARBs with ACE inhibitors in chronic heart failure revealed that treatment with ARB was equivalent to ACE inhibition (trials using valsartan and candesartan); however, a trend toward improved outcomes was noted with ACE inhibitors in a trial using the ARB losartan.
In view of the vast experience with the ACE inhibitors as compared with ARBs, ACE inhibitors continue to be the recommended agents of choice for patients with heart failure and depressed LV systolic function. That said, ARBs—specifically, candesartan and valsartan—confer significant benefit on mortality and morbidity in patients with heart failure who are intolerant of ACE inhibitors, and therefore offer a good alternative strategy in these patients. Candesartan and valsartan are the recommended ARBs for patients with heart failure who are intolerant of ACE inhibitors.

10. **When should ARBs be added to ACE inhibitors in patients with chronic heart failure?**
Theoretically, the more complete angiotensin II inhibition using a combination of ACE inhibitors and ARBs in patients with heart failure may translate into improved clinical outcomes.
Two large clinical trials in patients with heart failure, the Val-HeFT and the CHARM-Added trial, evaluated the impact on morbidity and mortality of adding ARBs to ACE inhibitors. Both trials suggest that adding an ARB to an ACE inhibitor leads to a reduction in heart failure hospitalizations, although combination therapy had no impact on mortality. Thus, the current Heart Failure Society of America guidelines recommend the addition of ARBs to ACE inhibitors in patients who meet the following conditions:
- Continue to have symptoms of heart failure despite receiving target doses of ACE inhibitors and β-blockers
- Are taking ACE inhibitors but are unable to tolerate β-blockers and have persistent symptoms, if there are no contraindications

11. **How do aldosterone antagonists work?**
Aldosterone receptor blockers block the mineralocorticoid receptor in the distal renal tubules, thereby decreasing sodium chloride absorption, potassium excretion, and water retention. In addition, they block the direct deleterious effects of aldosterone on the myocardium and may thus decrease myocardial fibrosis and its consequences.

12. **List the indications and recommended dosing of aldosterone antagonists in heart failure.**
Current indications include the following:
- Chronic NYHA class III-IV heart failure and left ventricular ejection fraction 35% or less; already receiving standard therapy for heart failure, including ACE inhibitors, β-blockers, and diuretics

(based on the RALES trial with spironolactone [Aldactone]). The recent EMPHASIS trial with eplerenone demonstrated improvement in survival and heart failure hospitalizations in patients with mild (NYHA class II) heart failure symptoms and systolic heart failure suggesting a wider class of patients (NYHA class II-IV) may benefit from aldosterone antagonism.

■ Post-MI LV dysfunction (ejection fraction less than 40%) and heart failure; already receiving standard therapy, including ACE inhibitors and β-blockers (EPHESUS study of eplerenone)

Dosing is as follows:

■ **Spironolactone:** 12.5 mg daily, increased to 25 mg daily
■ **Eplerenone:** 25 mg daily, increased to 50 mg daily

The initial and target doses for aldosterone antagonists and other drugs used to treat patients depressed systolic ejection fraction and/or CHF are listed in Table 23-2.

13. **Can all patients with heart failure safely be started on an aldosterone antagonist?**

No. Aldosterone antagonists should not be started in men with creatinine more than 2.5 mg/dL or women with creatinine more than 2 mg/dL, patients with potassium more than 5 mEq/L, those in whom monitoring for hyperkalemia and renal function is not anticipated to be feasible, and those not already on other diuretics.

14. **Describe common adverse effects of ACE inhibitors, ARBs, and aldosterone antagonists.**

Common adverse effects include the following:

■ **ACE inhibitors:** hypotension, worsening renal function, hyperkalemia, cough, angioedema
■ **ARBs:** hypotension, worsening renal function, hyperkalemia
■ **Aldosterone antagonists:** hyperkalemia; renal dysfunction may be aggravated, may cause hypotension and hyponatremia

ARBs are as likely as ACE inhibitors to produce hypotension, worsening renal function, and hyperkalemia. Otherwise, ARBs are better tolerated than ACE inhibitors. The incidence of cough is much lower in ARBs (approximately 1%) compared with ACE inhibitors (approximately 10%). The incidence of angioedema with ACE inhibitors is rare (less than 1%; more common in African Americans) and even more rare with ARBs. However, because there have been case reports of patients developing angioedema on ARBs, the guidelines advise that ARBs may be considered in patients who have had angioedema while taking an ACE inhibitor, albeit with extreme caution. Practically, if a patient develops angioedema while taking an ACE inhibitor, an ARB is generally not initiated.

Gynecomastia and other antiandrogenic effects can occur with spironolactone and are not generally seen with eplerenone.

15. **What are the indications and dosing of nitrates/hydralazine in patients with chronic heart failure?**

The vasodilator combination of isosorbide dinitrate (Isordil) and hydralazine (I/H) has been shown to produce modest benefit in patients with heart failure, compared with placebo. The combination has, however, been shown to be less effective than ACE inhibitors. The recent A-Heft trial, which was limited to African-American patients with class III-IV heart failure, showed that the addition of I/H to standard therapy with ACE inhibitor or a β-blocker conferred significant morbidity and mortality benefit.

Taking all the evidence together, the I/H combination is indicated in the following patients:

■ Those who cannot take an ACE inhibitor or ARB because of renal insufficiency or hyperkalemia
■ Those who are hypertensive and/or symptomatic despite taking ACE inhibitor, ARB, and β-blockers
■ The combination of hydralazine and nitrates is recommended to improve outcomes for patients self-described as African Americans with moderate-severe symptoms on optimal medical therapy with ACE inhibitors, β-blockers, and diuretics.

TABLE 23-2.   INITIAL AND TARGET DOSES FOR COMMONLY USED DRUGS FOR PATIENTS WITH DEPRESSED SYSTOLIC EJECTION FRACTION AND/OR CONGESTIVE HEART FAILURE

Drug	Initial Daily Doses	Target/Maximum Doses
ACE Inhibitors		
Captopril	6.25 mg tid	50 mg tid
Enalapril	2.5 mg bid	10-20 mg bid
Lisinopril	2.5-5 mg qd	20-40 mg qd
Perindopril	2 mg qd	8-16 mg qd
Ramipril	1.25-2.5 mg qd	10 mg qd
Trandolapril	1 mg qd	4 mg qd
Angiotensin Receptor Blockers (ARBs)		
Candesartan	4-8 mg qd	32 mg qd
Valsartan	20-40 mg bid	160 mg bid
Losartan	25-50 mg	50-100 mg
Aldosterone Antagonists		
Spironolactone	12.5-25 mg qd	25 mg qd
Eplerenone	25 mg qd	50 mg qd
β-Blockers		
Bisoprolol	1.25 mg qd	10 mg qd
Carvedilol*	3.125 mg bid	25 mg bid (50 mg bid if >85 kg)
Metoprolol succinate	12.5-25 mg qd	200 mg qd
Loop Diuretics		
Bumetanide	0.5-1.0 mg qd-bid	Max daily dose 10 mg
Furosemide	20-40 mg qd-bid	Max daily dose 600 mg
Torsemide	10-20 mg qd	Max daily dose 200 mg
Thiazide Diuretics		
Chlorothiazide	250-500 mg qd-bid	Max daily dose 1000 mg
Chlorthalidone	12.5-25 mg qd	Max daily dose 100 mg
Hydrochlorothiazide	25 mg qd-bid	Max daily dose 200 mg
Metolazone	2.5 mg qd	Max daily dose 20 mg
Potassium-Sparing Diuretics		
Amiloride	5 mg qd	Max daily dose 20 mg
Eplerenone	25 mg qd	50 mg qd
Spironolactone	12.5-25 mg qd	Max daily dose 50 mg
Triamterene	50-75 mg bid	Max daily dose 200 mg

Modified from Hunt SA, Abraham WT, Chin MH, et al: ACC/AHA 2005 guideline update for the diagnosis and management of chronic heart failure in the adult: a report of the American College of Cardiology/American Heart Association Task Force on Practice Guidelines (Writing Committee to Update the 2001 Guidelines for the Evaluation and Management of Heart Failure). *J Am Coll Cardiol* 46:e1-e82, 2005.
ACE, Angiotensin-converting enzyme; *bid*, twice a day; *qd*, one a day; *tid* three times a day.
*Extended-release carvedilol now available, although this preparation not specifically tested in heart failure.

Dosages are as follows:

- Hydralazine: start at 37.5 mg three times a day and increase to a goal of 75 mg three times a day.
- Isosorbide dinitrate: start at 20 mg three times a day and increase to a goal of 40 mg three times a day.

16. How should patients be treated with β-blockers?

Certain β-blockers have been convincingly shown to decrease mortality in patients with depressed ejection fraction and symptoms of heart failure, and thus it is a class I indication to treat such patients with β-blockers, with an attempt to reach target doses. The β-blockers shown to decrease mortality, their starting doses, and their target doses are given in Table 2. Recommendations from the Heart Failure Society of America and other organizations include the following:

- Patients should not be initiated on β-blocker therapy during decompensated or hemodynamically unstable state heart failure.
- β-Blocker therapy should only be initiated when patients are euvolemic and hemodynamically stable, are usually on a good maintenance dose of diuretics (if indicated), and receiving ACE inhibitors or ARBs.
- β-Blockers should be initiated at low doses, uptitrated gradually (in at least 2-week intervals), and titrated to target doses shown to be effective in clinical trials (see Table 23-2). Practitioners should aim to achieve target doses in 8 to 12 weeks from initiation of therapy and to maintain patients at maximal tolerated doses.
- If patient symptoms worsen during initiation or dose titration, the dose of diuretics or other concomitant vasoactive medications should be adjusted, and titration to target dose should be continued after the patient's symptoms return to baseline.
- If uptitration continues to be difficult, the titration interval can be prolonged, the target dose may have to be reduced, or the patient should be referred to a heart failure specialist.
- If an acute exacerbation of chronic heart failure occurs, therapy should be maintained if possible; the dose can be reduced if necessary, but abrupt discontinuation should be avoided. If the dose is reduced (or discontinued), the β-blocker (and prior dose) should be gradually reinstated before discharge, if possible.

17. What is the mechanism of action of digoxin?

Digoxin is a cardiac glycoside and is an inhibitor of the Na^+,K^+-ATPase pump in the sarcolemmal membrane of the myocyte and other cells. This inhibition causes intracellular accumulation of Na^+, which makes the Na^+-Ca^{2+} pump extrude less Ca^{2+}, causing Ca^{2+} to accumulate inside the cell. This effect results in increased force of contraction. Cardiac glycosides also have effects in the central nervous system, enhancing parasympathetic and reducing sympathetic outputs to the heart, through carotid sinus baroreceptor reflex sensitization. This is the mechanism that underlies the reduction in sinus node activity and slowing in atrioventricular (AV) conduction, which makes digoxin the only agent with a positive inotropic-bradycardic effect and is the basis for its use in the control of some supraventricular arrhythmias.

18. Is there scientific evidence for the use of digoxin?

The Digitalis Investigation Group (DIG) trial was a multicenter, randomized, double-blinded, placebo-controlled study of 6801 symptomatic patients with heart failure and ejection fraction less than 45%, who were in sinus rhythm. Mean follow-up was 37 months. Patients already receiving digoxin were allowed into the trial and randomized to digoxin or placebo without a washout period. About 95% of patients in both groups received ACE inhibitors; β-blockers were not in use for heart failure at the time. The primary outcome was total mortality. Digoxin did not improve total mortality (34.8% versus 35.1% in the placebo group, $P = 0.80$) or deaths from cardiovascular causes (29.9% versus 29.5%, $P = 0.78$). Hospitalizations as a result of worsening heart failure (a secondary endpoint) were significantly reduced by digoxin (26.8% versus 34.7% in the placebo group, risk ratio 0.72, $P < 0.001$). Hospitalizations for suspected digoxin toxicity were higher in the digoxin group (2% versus 0.9%, $P < 0.001$). In an ancillary, parallel trial in patients with ejection fraction greater than 45% and sinus rhythm, the findings were consistent with the results of the main trial. Whether these results hold with contemporary heart failure treatment that includes β-blockers, aldosterone-receptor blockers, and resynchronization therapy is not known.

19. **What are some of the relevant drug interactions of digoxin?**
    - Quinidine, verapamil, amiodarone, propafenone, and quinine (used for muscle cramps) may double digoxin levels, and the dose of digoxin should be halved when used in combination with any of these drugs.
    - Tetracycline, erythromycin, and omeprazole can increase digoxin absorption, whereas cholestyramine and kaolin-pectin can decrease it.
    - Thyroxine and albuterol increase the volume of distribution, resulting in decreased digoxin levels.
    - Cyclosporine and paroxetine and other selective serotonin reuptake inhibitors (SSRIs) can increase serum digoxin levels.

20. **What are the clinical manifestations of digoxin toxicity?**
    Digoxin has a narrow safety margin (the difference in plasma drug concentrations between therapeutic and toxic levels is small). Patients with digoxin toxicity may manifest nausea, vomiting, anorexia, diarrhea, fatigue, generalized malaise, visual disturbances (green or yellow halos around lights and objects), and arrhythmias. In the presence of hypokalemia, digoxin toxicity may occur within the therapeutic level. Digoxin dose should be reduced in elderly patients, in patients with renal insufficiency (glomerular filtration rate [GFR] less than 60 mL/min), and when combined with certain drugs. To guide dosing during chronic therapy, digoxin levels should be measured 6 to 8 hours after a dose.

21. **What are the electrocardiographic findings of digoxin toxicity?**
    Digoxin toxicity can result in a variety of ventricular and supraventricular arrhythmias and AV conduction abnormalities, including:
    - Sinus bradycardia
    - Sinus arrest
    - First- and second-degree AV block
    - AV junctional escape
    - Paroxysmal atrial tachycardia with AV block (common)
    - Bidirectional ventricular tachycardia (rare but typical)
    - Premature ventricular beats
    - Bigeminy
    - Regularized atrial fibrillation or atrial fibrillation with slow ventricular response (common)
    These arrhythmias result from the electrophysiologic effects of digoxin: Increased intracellular Ca^{2+} levels predispose to Ca^{2+}-induced delayed afterdepolarizations and, hence, increased automaticity (especially in the junction, Purkinje system, and ventricles); excessive vagal effects predispose to sinus bradycardia and/or arrest, and AV block. Bradyarrhythmias and blocks are more common when the patient is also taking amiodarone.

22. **How is digoxin toxicity treated?**
    It depends on the clinical severity. Digoxin withdrawal is sufficient with only suggestive symptoms. Activated charcoal may enhance the gastrointestinal (GI) clearance of digoxin if given within 6 hours of ingestion. Drugs that increase plasma digoxin levels (see Question 19) should be discontinued (except amiodarone, because of its long half-life). Correction of hypokalemia is vital (intravenous [IV] replacement through a large vein is preferred with life-threatening arrhythmias), but judgment is needed in the presence of high degrees of AV block. Symptomatic AV block may respond to atropine or to phenytoin (100 mg IV every 5 minutes up to 1000 mg until response or side effects); if no response, use digoxin immune Fab (ovine) (Digibind). The use of temporary transvenous pacing should be avoided. Patients with severe bradycardia should be given Digibind, even if they respond to atropine. Lidocaine and phenytoin may be used to treat ventricular arrhythmias, but for potentially life-threatening bradyarrhythmias or tachyarrhythmias, Digibind should be used. IV magnesium may

be given 2 grams over 5 minutes and has been shown to help with digoxin toxicity related arrhythmias. Dialysis has no role because of the high tissue-binding of digoxin.

23. **What are the indications for Digibind?**

The indications for Digibind include life-threatening bradyarrhythmias and tachyarrhythmias; hemodynamic instability caused by digoxin, potassium level of more than 5 mEq/L in the setting of acute ingestion, regardless of symptoms or ECG findings; and digoxin level of more than 10 ng/mL or the ingestion of more than 10 mg of digoxin, regardless of symptoms or ECG findings. Digibind is an antibody that binds to digoxin in the plasma and interstitial space, creating a concentration gradient for the exit of intracellular digoxin. As poisoning of the Na^+,K^+-ATPase is relieved, K^+ is pumped intracellularly with the potential of causing hypokalemia; potassium levels should be monitored when Digibind is used. The half-life of the digoxin-Digibind complex is 15 to 20 hours if renal function is normal. Serum digoxin concentration rises significantly after Digibind use (as tissue digoxin is released into the bloodstream, bound to the antibody) and should not be measured.

24. **What three classes of drugs exacerbate the syndrome of CHF and should be avoided in most CHF patients?**

a. Antiarrhythmic agents. They can exert cardiodepressant and proarrhythmic effects. Only amiodarone and dofetilide have been shown not to adversely affect survival.

b. Calcium channel blockers. The nondihydropyridines can lead to worsening heart failure and have been associated with an increased risk of cardiovascular events. Only the dihydropyridines or vasoselective calcium channel blockers have been shown not to adversely affect survival.

c. NSAIDs. According to the ACC/AHA guidelines, nonsteroidal antiinflammatory drugs (NSAIDs) can cause sodium retention and peripheral vasoconstriction and can attenuate the efficacy and enhance the toxicity of diuretics and ACE inhibitors. The European Society of Cardiology also cautions against the use of NSAIDs.

25. **Is dietary restriction of sodium recommended in patients with symptomatic heart failure?**

Yes. In general, patients should restrict themselves to 2 to 3 g sodium daily, and less than 2 g daily in moderate to severe cases of heart failure.

26. **Is fluid restriction recommended in all patients with heart failure?**

Not necessarily. Expert opinion differs, although some believe fluid restriction generally is not necessary unless the patient (a) is hyponatremic (sodium less than 130 mEq/L) or (b) fluid retention is difficult to control despite high doses of diuretics and sodium restriction. In such cases, patients are generally restricted to less than 2 L/day.

27. **Should patients with CHF be told to use salt substitutes instead of salt?**

In some cases, the answer is no. Many salt substitutes contain potassium chloride in place of sodium chloride. This could lead to potential hyperkalemia in patients on potassium-sparing diuretics, ACE inhibitors or ARBs, or aldosterone antagonists, and those with chronic kidney disease (or those with the potential to develop acute renal failure). Patients who are permitted to use salt substitutes need to be cautioned about potassium issues.

28. **What are the current criteria for consideration of CRT with biventricular pacing?**

Patients who should be considered for referral of CRT (class I indication) with or without ICD are those who meet the following criteria:

- Presence of sinus rhythm
- Class III or ambulatory class IV symptoms despite good medical therapy
- LVEF less than or equal to 35%
- QRS more than 120 ms (especially if left bundle branch block morphology present)

29. Which patients with heart failure should be considered for an ICD?

In the 2008 ACC/AHA/Heart Rhythm Society (ACC/AHA/HRS) guidelines on device-based therapy, the writing group stated that they believed guidelines for ICD implantation should reflect the ICD trials that were conducted. Thus, there are many very specific indications for ICD placement, based on symptom class, ischemic or nonischemic causes of heart failure, and ejection fraction. Because ejection fraction may improve significantly after MI (as a result of myocardial salvage and myocardial stunning) and with optimal medical therapy (including ACE inhibitors/ARBs and β-blockers), patients being considered for ICD implantation for primary prevention should be optimally treated and have their ejection fraction reassessed on optimal medical therapy. ICD should only be considered in patients with a reasonable expectation of survival with an acceptable functional status for at least 1 year. Class I recommendations for ICD include the following:

- Secondary prevention (cardiac arrest survivors of ventricular tachycardia/ventricular fibrillation [VT/VF], hemodynamically unstable sustained VT)
- Structural heart disease and sustained VT, whether hemodynamically stable or unstable
- Syncope of undetermined origin with hemodynamically significant sustained VT or VF induced at electrophysiologic study
- LVEF less than or equal to 35% at least 40 days after MI and NYHA functional class II-III
- LVEF less than 30% at least 40 days after MI and NYHA functional class I
- LVEF less than or equal to 35% despite medical therapy in patients with nonischemic cardiomyopathy and NYHA functional class II-III
- Nonsustained VT caused by prior MI, LVEF less than 40%, and inducible VF or sustained VT at electrophysiologic study

The 2005 European Society of Cardiology guidelines for the diagnosis and treatment of CHF distill their recommendations into three concise points:

- ICD therapy is recommended to improve survival in patients who have survived cardiac arrest or who have sustained VT, which is either poorly tolerated or associated with reduced systolic LV function (class I; level of evidence A).
- ICD implantation is reasonable in selected patients with LVEF less than 30% to 35%, not within 40 days of an MI, on optimal background therapy including ACE inhibitor, ARB, β-blocker, and an aldosterone antagonist, where appropriate, to reduce likelihood of sudden death (class I; level of evidence A).
- ICD implantation in combination with biventricular pacing can be considered in patients who remain symptomatic with severe heart failure, NYHA class III-IV, with LVEF 35% or less and QRS 120 ms or more to improve mortality or morbidity (class IIa; level of evidence B).

BIBLIOGRAPHY, SUGGESTED READINGS, AND WEBSITES

1. Arnold JMO: Heart Failure (HF). 2012. Available at http://www.merckmanuals.com/professional/cardiovascular_disorders/heart_failure/heart_failure_hf.html. Accessed March 19, 2013.

2. Cooper LT, Baughman KL, Feldman AM, et al: The role of endomyocardial biopsy in the management of cardiovascular disease: a scientific statement from the American Heart Association, the American College of Cardiology, and the European Society of Cardiology. Endorsed by the Heart Failure Society of America and the Heart Failure Association of the European Society of Cardiology, *J Am Coll Cardiol* 50:1914–1931, 2007.

3. Epstein AE, DiMarco JP, Ellenbogen KA, et al: ACC/AHA/HRS 2008 guidelines for device-based therapy of cardiac rhythm abnormalities: a report of the American College of Cardiology/American Heart Association Task Force on Practice Guidelines (Writing Committee to Revise the ACC/AHA/NASPE 2002 Guideline Update for Implantation of Cardiac Pacemakers and Antiarrhythmia Devices) developed in collaboration with the American Association for Thoracic Surgery and Society of Thoracic Surgeons, *J Am Coll Cardiol* 51:e1–e62, 2008.

4. Heart Failure Society of America: The HFSA *website*. Available at http://www.hfsa.org. Accessed March 19, 2013.

5. Heart Failure Society of America: Heart failure in patients with left ventricular systolic dysfunction, *J Card Fail* 12:e38–e57, 2006.

6. Hunt SA, Abraham WT, Chin MH, et al: ACC/AHA 2005 guideline update for the diagnosis and management of chronic heart failure in the adult: a report of the American College of Cardiology/American Heart Association Task Force on Practice Guidelines (Writing Committee to Update the 2001 Guidelines for the Evaluation and Management of Heart Failure), *J Am Coll Cardiol* 46:e1–e82, 2005.

7. Jessup M, Abraham WT, Casey DE, et al: Focused Update: ACCF/AHA Guidelines for the Diagnosis and Management of Heart Failure in Adults, *Circulation* 119:1977–2016, 2009.

8. Mann DL: Management of heart failure patients with reduced ejection fraction. In Libby P, Bonow R, Mann D, editors: *Braunwald's heart disease: a textbook of cardiovascular medicine*, ed 8, Philadelphia, 2008, Saunders.

9. Swedberg K, Cleland J, Dargie H, et al: Guidelines for the diagnosis and treatment of chronic heart failure: executive summary (update 2005): the Task Force for the Diagnosis and Treatment of Chronic Heart Failure of the European Society of Cardiology, *Eur Heart J* 26:1115–1140, 2005.

10. Dumitru, I: Heart Failure. Available at http://www.emedicine.com. Accessed March 19, 2013.

CHAPTER 24

HEART FAILURE WITH PRESERVED EJECTION FRACTION

Sameer Ather, MD, PhD, and Anita Deswal, MD, MPH

1. What is diastolic dysfunction?

Diastolic dysfunction occurs when there is an abnormality in the mechanical function of the myocardium during the diastolic phase of the cardiac cycle. This mechanical abnormality can occur with or without systolic dysfunction, as well as with or without the clinical syndrome of heart failure. Diastolic dysfunction may include abnormalities in left ventricular (LV) stiffness and relaxation that impair filling and/or result in elevated LV filling pressure to achieve adequate LV preload (end-diastolic volume) at rest or during physiologic stress.

2. What is diastolic heart failure?

Whereas diastolic dysfunction describes abnormalities in mechanical function, diastolic heart failure is a clinical syndrome characterized by the signs and symptoms of heart failure, a preserved LV ejection fraction (LVEF ≥ 45% to 50%), and evidence of diastolic dysfunction. Earlier studies of patients with heart failure with preserved LVEF uniformly referred to this condition as *diastolic heart failure,* based on the premise that diastolic dysfunction was the sole mechanism for this syndrome. However, more recent studies suggest that a number of other abnormalities, both cardiac and noncardiac, may play an important role in the pathophysiology of heart failure with normal or near-normal LVEF. Therefore, the term *heart failure with preserved ejection fraction* (HFpEF) is more commonly used to refer to this clinical syndrome.

3. What is the prevalence of HFpEF?

Approximately 5 million Americans currently have a diagnosis of heart failure, and more than half a million new cases of heart failure are diagnosed annually. Epidemiologic studies of various heart failure cohorts have documented a prevalence of HFpEF ranging from 40% to 71% (average approximately 50%). In addition, the prevalence of this condition is increasing as the population ages.

4. What is the morbidity and mortality associated with HFpEF compared with heart failure with reduced ejection fraction?

Compared with age-matched controls without heart failure, patients with HFpEF have a significantly higher mortality. However, studies examining the risk of death in patients with HFpEF compared with patients with heart failure and reduced ejection fraction (LVEF < 40% to 50%), commonly known as systolic heart failure, show a somewhat lower or similar mortality in patients with HFpEF. Once hospitalized for heart failure, mortality in patients with HFpEF may be as high as 22% to 29% at 1 year and approximately 65% at 5 years. Although survival has significantly improved over time for patients with systolic heart failure, there has been no similar improvement in survival for HFpEF patients. In contrast to mortality, both the groups have similar morbidity as reflected by hospital admissions. Although the total or all-cause admissions are similar between the 2 groups, patients with HFpEF have higher non–heart failure related admissions that are driven by the higher prevalence of non-cardiac comorbidities in this population.

5. Which patients are at the highest risk for developing HFpEF?

Patients with HFpEF are generally elderly and are predominantly women (60% to 70%). Reasons for the female predominance in HFpEF are not entirely clear but may be related to the fact that women have a greater tendency for the left ventricle to hypertrophy in response to load, and lesser predisposition for the ventricle to dilate. Hypertension is the most common cardiac condition associated with HFpEF. Hypertensive heart disease results in LV hypertrophy with resultant impairment in relaxation and increase in LV stiffness. Acute myocardial ischemia results in diastolic dysfunction, although its role in chronic diastolic dysfunction and chronic HFpEF remains uncertain. Valvular heart diseases, including regurgitant and stenotic aortic and mitral valve disease, can also result in the development of HFpEF. Other recognized risk factors associated with HFpEF include obesity, diabetes mellitus, and renal insufficiency. Onset of atrial fibrillation with rapid ventricular rate may precipitate decompensation of HFpEF, and the presence of diastolic dysfunction in general is also a risk factor for the development of this arrhythmia.

6. What are proposed pathophysiologic mechanisms of HFpEF?

Diastolic dysfunction has been thought to be the major mechanism contributing to HFpEF, with abnormalities in active LV relaxation and in LV passive diastolic stiffness. LV relaxation is an active, energy-dependent process that may begin during the ejection phase of systole and continue throughout diastole. Animal studies and various models have shown that impaired LV relaxation can contribute to elevated mean LV diastolic filling pressures in HFpEF when the heart rate is increased (as during exercise or uncontrolled atrial fibrillation). On the other hand, LV stiffness consists of the passive viscoelastic properties that contribute to returning the ventricular myocardium to its resting force and length. These viscoelastic properties are dependent on both intracellular and extracellular structures. The greater the stiffness of the LV myocardium, for any given change in LV volume during diastolic filling, the higher the corresponding filling pressures. In other words, when comparing a left ventricle with normal diastolic function with that of a left ventricle with diastolic dysfunction, for any given left ventricle volume during diastole, LV pressure will be higher in the ventricle with diastolic dysfunction compared with normal. The net result of these processes is that LV diastolic pressures and left atrial pressures become elevated at rest and/or during exercise, with resultant elevation of pulmonary capillary wedge pressure and pulmonary vascular congestion.

Clinically, this manifests as dyspnea at rest or with exertion, paroxysmal nocturnal dyspnea, and orthopnea. Furthermore, these stiffer hearts have an inability to increase end-diastolic volume and stroke volume via the Frank-Starling mechanism despite significantly elevated LV filling pressure. The resultant decrease in augmentation of cardiac output, which normally occurs with exercise, results in reduced exercise tolerance and fatigue.

In addition to diastolic dysfunction, a number of additional factors are now thought to contribute to the development of HFpEF. For example, increased arterial vascular stiffness along with LV systolic stiffness may increase systolic blood pressure sensitivity to circulating intravascular volume and may predispose to rapid-onset pulmonary edema. On the other hand, vascular-ventricular stiffening also predisposes to the hypotensive effects of preload or afterload reduction, thus potentially limiting the efficacy of vasodilators or diuretics in HFpEF. Neurohormonal activation may result in increased venous vascular tone, which in turn may result in a shift of the blood volume to the central circulation. Concomitant renal dysfunction may contribute to sodium and water retention and may precipitate symptoms of volume overload and heart failure in patients with the above substrate. Concurrent atrial dysfunction may result in further elevation in left atrial pressures and pulmonary vascular congestion.

In the elderly, chronotropic incompetence with exercise is more commonly seen and may contribute to limitation in exercise cardiac output with resultant exertional fatigue. Pulmonary hypertension is common in HFpEF. The pulmonary hypertension may be related to both pulmonary venous as well as reactive pulmonary arterial hypertension in both HFpEF and systolic heart failure. As the right ventricle is very sensitive to afterload, resting and exercise-induced pulmonary hypertension may contribute to progressive right ventricular dysfunction.

7. What factors may precipitate decompensated HFpEF?

In patients with underlying diastolic dysfunction and other abnormalities detailed in Question 6, acute decompensation of heart failure may often be contributed to by uncontrolled hypertension, atrial fibrillation or flutter (especially with rapid ventricular rates), myocardial ischemia, hyperthyroidism, medication noncompliance (especially diuretics and antihypertensives), dietary indiscretion (e.g., high-sodium foods), anemia, and infection.

8. How is the diagnosis of HFpEF made?

The clinical diagnosis of HFpEF depends on the presence of signs and symptoms of heart failure and documentation of normal or near-normal LVEF (greater than 45% to 50%) by echocardiography, radionuclide ventriculography, or contrast ventriculography.

9. What common tests are useful in the diagnosis of HFpEF, and what do they often reveal?

- Chest radiographs may demonstrate cardiomegaly (as a result of hypertrophy), pulmonary venous congestion, pulmonary edema, or pleural effusions.
- The electrocardiogram (ECG) may demonstrate hypertrophy, ischemia, or arrhythmia.
- Echocardiography can be used to assess ventricular function; atrial and ventricular size; hypertrophy; diastolic function and filling pressures (see Question 11); wall motion abnormalities; and pericardial, valvular, or myocardial (hypertrophic or infiltrative) disease. By definition, the LVEF is normal or near normal. Echocardiography often demonstrates LV hypertrophy, enlarged left atrium, diastolic dysfunction, and pulmonary hypertension. Left ventricular volumes are usually normal or even small in HFpEF. Valvular heart disease, such as significant aortic or mitral stenosis and/or regurgitation, can lead to a presentation of HFpEF but needs to be differentiated, as management often requires surgical intervention for the valvular pathology.
- Stress testing and coronary angiography can identify contributory coronary artery disease.
- Routine laboratory analysis can help identify renal failure or anemia as factors associated with decompensation, electrolyte abnormalities such as hyponatremia seen with heart failure, and transaminase or bilirubin elevation resulting from hepatic congestion. In addition, thyroid function tests can rule out hyperthyroidism (a consideration particularly in patients who develop atrial fibrillation). Studies have shown that B-type natriuretic peptide (BNP) and N-terminal prohormone of B-type natriuretic peptide (NT-proBNP) levels are elevated in HFpEF patients compared with persons without heart failure. However, BNP and NT-proBNP levels in HFpEF patients are usually lower compared with systolic heart failure patients. Of note, increased BNP levels may identify patients with elevation of the LV diastolic pressure, but may not be clinically useful in individual patients to predict preserved versus reduced LVEF. Also, it should be kept in mind that BNP levels increase with age and are higher in women, both of which are common features of HFpEF. Levels of BNP are also higher with worsening renal insufficiency. On the other hand, obesity is associated with lower levels of BNP, making the diagnosis of HFpEF more difficult in this group of patients.

10. What is the clinical approach to further evaluate patients with HFpEF?

A diagnostic algorithm, based on the 2006 Heart Failure Society of America Heart Failure Practice Guidelines, provides a systematic approach for the clinical workup and classification of HFpEF (Fig. 24-1). This framework addresses the common clinical conditions presenting as HFpEF, including hypertensive heart disease, hypertrophic cardiomyopathy, ischemic heart failure, valvular heart disease, infiltrative (restrictive) cardiomyopathy, pericardial constriction, high-cardiac-output state, and right ventricular dysfunction.

11. What tests are available to evaluate diastolic function?

Cardiac catheterization with a high-fidelity pressure manometer allows for precise intracardiac pressure measurements. This information can be used to estimate the rate of LV relaxation by calculation of indices such as peak instantaneous LV pressure decline (-dP/dt max) and the time constant of LV relaxation, tau. Estimation of LV myocardial stiffness requires simultaneous assessment of LV volume and pressure to evaluate the end-diastolic pressure-volume relationship. However, these measurements are invasive and cannot be made on a routine basis. Therefore, noninvasive markers of diastolic dysfunction are more commonly used in clinical practice.

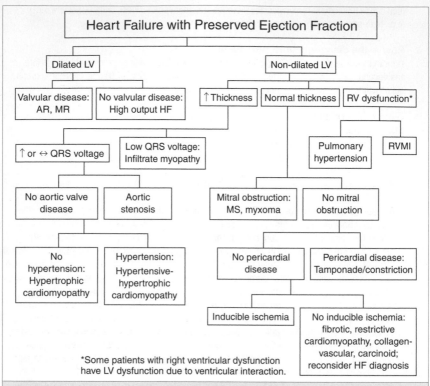

Figure 24-1. Diagnostic considerations in patients with heart failure with preserved ejection fraction. (From Adams, KF, Lindenfeld J, Arnold JMO, et al: Executive summary: HFSA 2006 Comprehensive heart failure practice guideline. *J Cardiac Failure* 12:10-38, 2006.) *AR,* Aortic regurgitation; *HF,* heart failure; *LV,* left ventricle; *MR,* mitral regurgitation; *MS,* mitral stenosis; *RV,* right ventricle; *RVMI,* right ventricular myocardial infarction.

Echocardiography with Doppler examination offers a noninvasive method of evaluating diastolic function. In addition to the Doppler criteria for diastolic dysfunction, enlargement of the left atrium on two-dimensional (2-D) echocardiography suggests the presence of significant diastolic dysfunction (in the absence of significant mitral valvular disease). The degree of left atrial (LA) enlargement estimated either by LA diameter or more accurately by LA volume is a marker of the severity and duration of diastolic dysfunction. Importantly, left atrial function index, which is a function of LA emptying, portends a poor prognosis in HFpEF patients that is independent of the severity of diastolic dysfunction and LA volumes.

Doppler measurements of mitral and pulmonary venous flow, as well as Doppler tissue imaging (DTI), allow for determination of ventricular and atrial filling patterns and estimation of LV diastolic filling pressures. The normal transmitral filling pattern consists of early rapid filling (E wave) and atrial contraction (A wave). The contribution of each of these stages of diastole is expressed as the E/A ratio. Mitral annular tissue Doppler velocities (which measure tissue velocities rather than the conventional Doppler, which measures blood flow velocities) are relatively independent of preload conditions. As such, the early diastolic filling annular tissue velocity (E') is a marker of LV relaxation and correlates well with hemodynamic catheter-derived values of tau. The ratio of the transmitral early filling velocity to the annular DTI early filling velocity (E/E') has been shown to accurately estimate mean LA pressure. Using these various echocardiographic parameters, the severity of diastolic dysfunction and of elevated LV diastolic pressures can be assessed. These issues are also discussed in Chapter 5 on echocardiography.

Nuclear imaging is another, less commonly used, noninvasive modality for evaluating diastolic dysfunction. Certain diastolic parameters, such as peak filling rate and time to peak rate, can be calculated using this modality.

12. How do you treat acutely decompensated HFpEF?

The cornerstones of treatment of acute decompensated HFpEF are blood pressure control, volume management, and treatment of exacerbating factors.

Systemic blood pressure control is of paramount importance because blood pressure directly affects LV diastolic pressure and thus LA pressures. The goal of blood pressure control should be a systolic blood pressure less than 140/90 and possibly even less than 130/80 mm Hg.

Volume management in the inpatient setting often requires use of intravenous diuretics. Loop diuretics (e.g., furosemide) are the primary diuretics of choice but may be combined with thiazide-like diuretics (e.g., metolazone) for additional effect. Although treatment of pulmonary vascular congestion with diuresis is a primary goal of therapy, rapid or aggressive diuresis in patients who have a combination of severe LV hypertrophy and small LV volume may result in development of hypotension and renal insufficiency. While a patient is undergoing diuresis, it is imperative to monitor electrolytes (particularly potassium, sodium, and magnesium), renal function (serum blood urea nitrogen [BUN] and creatinine), clinical response (daily weights, meticulous fluid balance, blood pressure), and perform physical examinations (jugular venous distension, lung examination, and peripheral edema) in order to appropriately adjust diuretic doses.

Apart from diuretics, nitrates may also provide symptomatic benefit by reducing preload, leading to a reduction in ventricular filling pressures and pulmonary congestion. In acute decompensated heart failure, they can be used intravenously and may improve symptoms by reducing filling pressures, as well as by controlling systemic hypertension. Theoretically, by releasing nitric oxide, nitrates may improve the diastolic distensibility of the ventricle. Again, as with diuretics, caution is required when nitrates are used in patients without hypertension or with severe diastolic dysfunction, and patients should be closely monitored for a significant reduction in blood pressure and/or cardiac output as a result of preload reduction.

Patients with significant volume overload and resistance to diuretics may benefit from ultrafiltration. Lastly, patients with advanced renal failure and volume overload who are refractory to diuretics may require urgent dialysis.

Evaluation and treatment of exacerbating factors form a crucial part of the treatment of acutely decompensated HFpEF. Uncontrolled atrial arrhythmias such as atrial fibrillation or atrial flutter can be detrimental in HFpEF. The combination of the loss of atrial contraction to LV diastolic filling and shortened diastolic filling time with tachycardia can cause marked elevation of mean LA pressure and result in pulmonary edema. Rate control alone with β-blockers, nondihydropyridine calcium channel blockers (verapamil or diltiazem), or digoxin, with a target heart rate less than 70 to 90 beats/min at rest, may improve symptoms. When ventricular rates remain uncontrolled or there is inadequate response to treatment of heart failure, direct-current cardioversion with restoration of sinus rhythm may be beneficial. In addition to the previously described measures, management of other factors, such as myocardial ischemia, anemia, medical noncompliance, and infections, is important in the treatment of the patient with HFpEF.

13. How do you treat patients with chronic HFpEF?

Nonpharmacologic therapy for HFpEF is the same as therapy for heart failure with reduced ejection fraction, including daily home monitoring of weight, compliance with medical treatment, dietary sodium restriction (2-3 g sodium daily), and close medical follow-up. Similar to heart failure with reduced ejection fraction, structured exercise training improves exercise capacity and leads to atrial reverse remodeling and improvement in LV diastolic function in HFpEF patients.

Large clinical trials have not shown consistent improvement in morbidity or mortality with ACE inhibitors and/or angiotensin receptor blockers (ARBs), or with digoxin. Large trials evaluating β-blockers specifically in HFpEF are not available. A large trial examining the efficacy of spironolactone, an aldosterone receptor blocker, in patients with HFpEF is ongoing. Current therapeutic

---

Box 24-1 TREATMENT RECOMMENDATIONS FOR PATIENTS WITH CHRONIC HEART FAILURE WITH PRESERVED EJECTION FRACTION (HFpEF)

- Control of systolic and diastolic hypertension as per published hypertension guidelines
- Control of ventricular rate in atrial fibrillation
- Diuretics to control pulmonary congestion and peripheral edema
- Consider revascularization in patients with significant coronary artery disease and symptoms and/or demonstrable ischemia, where ischemia may be regarded as a contributor to abnormal cardiac function
- Restoration and maintenance of sinus rhythm in certain patients with atrial fibrillation may be useful to control symptoms
- β-blockers can be considered for HFpEF with:
  - Prior myocardial infarction
  - Hypertension
  - Atrial fibrillation
- ACE inhibitors or ARBs can be considered for HFpEF with:
  - Hypertension
  - Diabetes
  - Atherosclerotic vascular disease
- Calcium channel blockers can be considered for HFpEF with:
  - Atrial fibrillation requiring control of ventricular rate in patients for whom blockers have proven inadequate: consider diltiazem or verapamil
  - Symptom-limiting angina
  - Hypertension: consider amlodipine
- Digitalis may be considered for rate control in atrial fibrillation if not responsive to other agents listed above.

ACE, Angiotensin-converting enzyme; *ARB*, angiotensin II receptor blocker.

---

recommendations for HFpEF are aimed at symptom management and treatment of concomitant comorbidities, as outlined in Box 24-1.

HFpEF patients usually have several non–heart failure related comorbidities. These comorbidities lead to non–heart failure related admissions that are even higher than in heart failure with reduced LVEF. Overall, the comorbidities in the HFpEF population require aggressive management as they have significant impact on overall outcomes in this population. The most common among these is hypertension, and its aggressive management is strongly recommended, especially as hypertension can lead to HFpEF. Small trials have demonstrated improvement in outcomes in HFpEF patients with the treatment of anemia and sleep disordered breathing. Overall, in contrast to heart failure with reduced EF, there is a paucity of evidence-based treatment options for patients with HFpEF.

BIBLIOGRAPHY, SUGGESTED READINGS, AND WEBSITES

1. Ahmed A, Rich MW, Fleg JL, et al: Effects of digoxin on morbidity and mortality in diastolic heart failure: the ancillary digitalis investigation group trial, *Circulation* 114:397–403, 2006.

2. Ather S, Chan W, Bozkurt B, et al: Impact of non-cardiac comorbidities on morbidity and mortality in a predominantly male population with heart failure and preserved versus reduced ejection fraction, *J Am Coll Cardiol* 59:998–1006, 2012.

3. Borlaug BA, Paulus WJ: Heart failure with preserved ejection fraction: pathophysiology, diagnosis, and treatment, *Eur Heart J* 32:670–679, 2011.

4. Cleland JGF, Tenderar M, Adamus J, et al: The Perindopril in Elderly People with Chronic Heart Failure (PEP-CHF) study, *Eur Heart J* 27:2338–2345, 2006.

5. Deswal A: Treatment of heart failure with a positive ejection fraction. In Mann DL, editor: *Heart failure: a companion to Braunwald's Heart Disease*, St Louis, 2011, Saunders.

6. Hogg K, Swedberg K, McMurray J: Heart failure with preserved left ventricular systolic function; epidemiology, clinical characteristics, and prognosis, *J Am Coll Cardiol* 43:317–327, 2004.

7. Lindenfeld J, Albert NM, Boehmer JP, et al: HFSA 2010 comprehensive heart failure practice guideline, *J Card Fail* 16:e126–e133, 2010.

8. Massie BM, Carson PE, McMurray JJ, et al: Irbesartan in patients with heart failure and preserved ejection fraction, *N Engl J Med* 359:2456–2467, 2008.

9. Paulus WJ, Tschöpe C, Sanderson JE, et al: How to diagnose diastolic heart failure: a consensus statement on the diagnosis of heart failure with normal left ventricular ejection fraction by the Heart Failure and Echocardiography Associations of the European Society of Cardiology, *Eur Heart J* 28:2539–2550, 2007.

10. Yusuf S, Pfeffer MA, Swedberg K, et al: Effects of candesartan in patients with chronic heart failure and preserved left-ventricular ejection fraction: the CHARM-Preserved Trial, *Lancet* 362:777–781, 2003.

11. Zile MR, Baicu CF: 2011 Alterations in ventricular function: diastolic heart failure. In Mann DL, editor: *Heart failure: a companion to Braunwald's Heart Disease*, St Louis, 2011, Saunders.

CHAPTER 25

MYOCARDITIS

Chantal El Amm, MD, and Leslie T. Cooper Jr., MD

1. **What is myocarditis?**

   Myocarditis is an inflammatory disease of the heart muscle that can cause acute heart failure, heart block, sudden death, and chronic dilated cardiomyopathy.

   Myocarditis can be classified by cause, histology, immunohistology clinicopathologic, and clinical criteria. The clinicopathologic classification consists of the following four categories:
   - Fulminant myocarditis
   - Acute myocarditis
   - Chronic active myocarditis
   - Chronic persistent myocarditis

   Most myocarditis in developed countries results from a viral infection and the immune reaction to viral injury.

2. **What is the pathogenesis of myocarditis?**

   Most of the information about the pathogenesis of myocarditis derives from animal models rather than human studies. From these experiments, the progression from acute viral injury to chronic dilated cardiomyopathy can be simplified into a three-phase process:
   - Phase 1, sometimes called *acute viral*, occurs after viral entry and proliferation in the myocardium and results in direct tissue injury even before an inflammatory reaction.
   - Phase 2, called *subacute immune*, is characterized by activation of the innate and acquired immune response. The innate immune response leads to upregulation of a variety of inflammatory mediators like interferons, tumor necrosis factor, and nitric oxide, which ultimately result in an influx of tissue-specific T and B cells (acquired immune response) into the heart. If the inflammatory response persists, a chronic myopathic phase (phase 3) with fibrosis and remodeling with dilation of the ventricles may develop in susceptible individuals.
   - In phase 3, immune activation may persist and contribute to progressive cardiomyopathy.

   In any phase, inflammation and fibrosis may lead to ventricular arrhythmias or heart block.

3. **What is the clinical presentation of myocarditis?**

   The clinical presentation of myocarditis in adults is highly variable. Patients may report a viral prodrome of fever, rash, myalgias, arthralgias, fatigue, and respiratory or gastrointestinal symptoms in the days to weeks before cardiac symptoms, which range from mild dyspnea to chest pain and cardiogenic shock. Chest pain in myocarditis can mimic typical angina and be associated with electrocardiographic (ECG) changes, including ST segment elevation. There may be a rise in biomarkers of cardiac injury (e.g., troponins). The pattern of troponin elevation is typically longer than is seen following an acute coronary thrombosis. If the pericardium is involved, patients can present with symptoms typical of pericarditis. Cardiac rhythm disturbances are not uncommon and may include new-onset atrial or ventricular arrhythmias or high-grade atrioventricular (AV) block with syncope.

   In contrast to adults with myocarditis, children often have a more fulminant presentation and may require advanced circulatory support for ventricular failure in early stages of their disease. Despite a severe presentation, recovery after a period of hemodynamic support is not uncommon.

4. **What is the incidence of myocarditis and who does it affect?**
The population-based incidence of myocarditis is not known because of the variable clinical presentation and lack of a specific, noninvasive diagnostic test. In referral cohorts of patients with otherwise unexplained acute to subacute heart failure, the incidence of biopsy-proven myocarditis is 9% to 10% using histologic criteria, and up to 40% using newer immunostain-based diagnostic standards. Recently, inflammation (using newer immunostains) has been observed in up to 40% of biopsies from patients with chronic, severe dilated cardiomyopathy.
The mean age of adults diagnosed with myocarditis ranges from 20 to 51 years in most series. Most studies report a slight predominance of men, which may be partly mediated by testosterone. Testosterone increases post-viral inflammation in animal models of myocarditis. Myocarditis should be considered in select patients who develop cardiac symptoms and who also have risk factors for human immunodeficiency virus (HIV) infection, Chagas disease, and rheumatic fever.

5. **What are the causative agents of myocarditis?**
Myocarditis can be triggered by many infectious pathogens, including viruses, bacteria, *Chlamydia*, rickettsia, fungi, and protozoans, as well as systemic toxic and hypersensitivity reactions (Table 25-1).
Viral infection is the most commonly reported cause of myocarditis in Western Europe and North America. Currently, the most commonly identified viruses in reports from Germany and the United States are parvovirus B19 and human herpesvirus 6 (HHV-6). Enteroviruses, in particular coxsackievirus B (CVB), were the most commonly identified viruses from the 1950s until the 1990s. CVB still causes regional clusters of myocarditis, although the overall reported rate of CVB infection had declined.
Cytomegalovirus (CMV) can cause myocarditis in patients posttransplant and early infection posttransplant correlates with coronary allograft vasculopathy.

TABLE 25-1. CAUSES OF MYOCARDITIS

Viruses	Bacteria	Cardiotoxins	Hypersensitivity
Adenovirus*	*Chlamydia*	Ethanol*	Cephalosporins
Coxsackievirus B*	Cholera	Anthracycline drugs*	Clozapine
Cytomegalovirus*	*Mycoplasma*	Arsenic	Diuretics
Epstein-Barr virus	*Neisseria*	Carbon monoxide	Insect bites
Hepatitis C virus	*Salmonella*	Catecholamines	Lithium
Herpes simplex virus	*Staphylococcus*	Cocaine*	Snake bites
HIV*	*Streptococcus*	Heavy metals	Sulfonamides
Influenza virus	Tetanus	Copper	Tetanus toxoid
Mumps	Tuberculosis	Mercury	Tetracycline
Parvovirus B19		Lead	
Poliovirus	**Spirochetal**		**Systemic Disorders**
Rabies	Leptospirosis	**Protozoa**	Hypereosinophilia
Rubella	Lyme disease	Chagas disease	Kawasaki disease
Varicella zoster virus	Relapsing fever	Leishmaniasis	Sarcoidosis
Yellow fever	Syphilis	Malaria	Wegener granulomatosis

From Elamm C, Fairweather D, Cooper LT: Pathogenesis and diagnosis of myocarditis, *Heart* 98:835-840, 2012.
HIV, Human immunodeficiency virus.
*Frequent cause of myocarditis.

In the developing world, rheumatic carditis and, to a lesser degree, *Trypanosoma cruzi*, still contribute substantially to the global burden of disease. Scorpion bites have been reported to have a high rate of myocarditis in India.

Hypersensitivity myocarditis is an autoimmune reaction that is often drug-related and should be suspected when there is a temporal association between the onset of heart failure and the start of a new medication. Numerous medications, including the antipsychotic clozapine (Clozaril), anticonvulsants, and antibiotics have been implicated.

6. **What are some of the clinical presentations of nonviral infectious myocarditis?**
   - Bacteria: Bacterial myocarditis is far less common than viral-induced myocarditis. *Corynebacterium diphtheriae* can cause myocarditis associated with bradycardia in people not previously immunized. *Clostridium* organisms and bacteremia from any source may result in endocarditis and adjacent myocarditis. Other bacterial pathogens to consider include meningococci, streptococci, and *Listeria* organisms.
   - Spirochetes: The tick-borne spirochete *Borrelia burgdorferi* causes Lyme disease. The initial infection is often marked by a rash followed in weeks or months by involvement of other organ systems, including the heart and nervous system, and joints. Heart block or symptomatic ventricular arrhythmias in the setting of cardiomyopathy should raise suspicion for Lyme disease, particularly in endemic areas such as parts of New England or the upper Mississippi River valley. Full recovery is typical, although carditis sometimes persists. Co-infection with *Ehrlichia* organisms has been reported.
   - Protozoa: Infection with the protozoa *Trypanosoma cruzi* causes Chagas disease, which is encountered in Central and South America. It may be transmitted by direct inoculation by reduviid insects, through blood transfusions, or, rarely, oral inoculation. Chagas disease can present as acute myocarditis, but more commonly presents as a chronic cardiomyopathy characterized by segmental wall motion abnormalities, apical aneurysms, and ECG changes, including right bundle branch block (RBBB), left anterior fascicular block (LAFB), and AV block.

7. **What is giant cell myocarditis?**
   Giant cell myocarditis (GCM) is a fulminant, rapidly progressive disease that is usually fatal and that affects young, otherwise healthy individuals. It is considered to be primarily autoimmune in nature because of its association with a variety of autoimmune disorders and with thymoma. GCM presents most commonly with a few days to weeks of new heart failure symptoms, often associated with ventricular arrhythmias or, sometimes, heart block. Unlike lymphocytic myocarditis, patients do not usually improve with guideline-based treatment. The diagnosis requires an endomyocardial biopsy.

   The initial treatment may include mechanical circulatory support and sometimes transplantation. Immunosuppression that includes cyclosporine may prolong transplant-free survival.

8. **What are the ECG findings in myocarditis?**
   The ECG has a low sensitivity for diagnosing myocarditis. Nonspecific ECG changes in myocarditis include sinus tachycardia, ST and T wave abnormalities, and ST segment elevation mimicking an acute myocardial infarction. There may also occasionally be atrial or ventricular conduction delays, or supraventricular and ventricular arrhythmias. The presence of a widened QRS or Q waves are associated with higher rates of cardiac death or heart transplantation.

9. **What are the echocardiographic findings in myocarditis?**
   There are no specific echocardiographic features of myocarditis. Echocardiography is used mainly to exclude other causes of heart failure, such as valvular, congenital, or pericardial disease. Impaired right ventricular (RV) function is an independent predictor of death or the need for cardiac transplantation. Patients with fulminant myocarditis tend to present with near normal cardiac chamber dimensions and thickened walls compared with patients with a longer duration of symptoms who have greater left ventricular (LV) dilation and normal wall thickness. Patients who meet the clinicopathologic criteria for fulminant myocarditis have a greater rate of full recovery if they survive their initial illness. Therefore, echocardiography has a value in classifying patients with acute myocarditis and may provide prognostic information.

10. **Are cardiac biomarkers useful?**

Troponin I was found to be elevated in only 34% of subjects with acute myocarditis in the US Myocarditis Treatment trial cohort who were enrolled an average of 1 month after symptom onset. In a study of more acutely ill patients seen in a hospital setting, creatine kinase MB isozyme (CK-MB) levels greater than 29.5 ng/mL predicted in-hospital mortality with a sensitivity of 83% and a specificity of 73%. B-type natriuretic peptide (BNP) or N-terminal prohormone of BNP (NT-proBNP) are probably useful confirmatory tests for the diagnosis of heart failure in cases of suspected myocarditis.

11. **Are inflammatory markers and viral serology useful?**

Nonspecific serum markers of inflammation, including erythrocyte sedimentation rate (ESR), C-reactive protein (CRP), and leukocyte count, are often elevated in myocarditis patients, but normal values do not exclude an acute myocardial inflammatory process. The diagnostic value of viral serology is limited by the fact that most viral infections believed to be involved in the pathogenesis of myocarditis are highly prevalent in the general population. Antibody levels also vary over the time course of the disease. For example, IgM antibodies against parvovirus B19 are only detectable for a short period after acute infection. In a recent study, there was a poor correlation between myocardial viral genome polymerase chain reaction (PCR) results and viral serology. Therefore, routine viral serology for the diagnosis of a specific pathogen in suspected acute myocarditis is not recommended.

12. **What is the gold standard to diagnose myocarditis?**

Endomyocardial biopsy (EMB) remains the gold standard for diagnosing myocarditis. According to the Dallas criteria, acute myocarditis is defined as histologic evidence of inflammatory cell infiltrates associated with myocyte necrosis. However, sampling error caused by patchy involvement of the myocardium, high interobserver variability, and lack of correlation with clinical outcomes limit the utility of these criteria. Although approximately 6 biopsy samples are routinely obtained (using a Stanford Caves bioptome), a post mortem analysis of histologically proven myocarditis cases found that more than 17 samples are needed to diagnose myocarditis with an 80% sensitivity.

Figure 25-1 presents histologic examples of myocarditis.

13. **Should an endomyocardial biopsy be performed on every patient with suspected myocarditis?**

Because of the limitations mentioned above, as well as cost and risk of the procedure, EMB should be used selectively in those patients in whom the likely incremental information gained will meaningfully impact prognosis or treatment. The 2007 American Heart Association/American College of Cardiology/European Society of Cardiology (AHA/ACC/ESC) Scientific Statement limited the class I indications to only two clinical scenarios:

- EMB should be performed in that subset of adults who present with recent-onset severe heart failure requiring inotropic or mechanical circulatory support within two weeks of a viral illness, because they frequently can be bridged to recovery if they have lymphocytic myocarditis.
- Patients who present with fulminant or acute dilated cardiomyopathy with sustained or symptomatic ventricular tachycardia or high-degree heart block, or who fail to respond to standard heart failure treatment should be biopsied for possible giant cell myocarditis. The sensitivity of biopsy in this setting is reported to range between 80% and 85%.

14. **Is there a role for cardiac magnetic resonance imaging (CMR) in myocarditis?**

CMR is useful to distinguish ischemic from nonischemic cardiomyopathy in the setting of acute dilated cardiomyopathy. Criteria suggested by an expert panel recommended that both T1- and T2-weighted imaging be used when myocarditis is suspected. CMR in acute myocarditis may demonstrate regional rather than global involvement. CMR may have a diagnostic synergy when combined with EMB, and may also be useful in guiding EMB to suspected areas of myocardial involvement.

15. **What is the treatment of lymphocytic myocarditis?**

The mainstay of treatment for myocarditis presenting as recent-onset dilated cardiomyopathy is supportive therapy for LV dysfunction. Most patients with acute myocarditis presenting with dilated

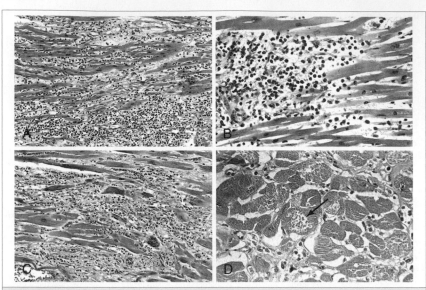

Figure 25-1. Myocarditis. **A,** Lymphocytic myocarditis, associated with myocyte injury. **B,** Hypersensitivity myocarditis, characterized by interstitial inflammatory infiltrate composed largely of eosinophils and mononuclear inflammatory cells, predominantly localized to perivascular and expanded interstitial spaces. **C,** Giant cell myocarditis, with mononuclear inflammatory infiltrate containing lymphocytes and macrophages, extensive loss of muscle and multinucleated giant cells. **D,** The myocarditis of Chagas disease. A myofiber distended with trypanosomes *(arrow)* is present along with inflammation and necrosis of individual myofibers. (From Kumar V, Abbas AK, Fausto N, Aster J: *Robbins and Cotran Pathologic basis of disease, professional edition*, ed 8, Philadelphia, 2009, Saunders.

cardiomyopathy respond well to standard heart failure therapy, including diuretics and angiotensin-converting enzyme (ACE) inhibitors or angiotensin receptor antagonists, as well as treatment with β-blockers once clinically stabilized.

Therapy for nonsustained arrhythmias is also supportive, as arrhythmias usually resolve after the acute phase of the disease. However, patients with symptomatic or sustained ventricular tachycardia that persists after the acute inflammatory phase of myocarditis usually require an implantable cardioverter-defibrillator (ICD).

Digoxin and nonsteroidal antiinflammatory drugs (NSAIDs) should be avoided, as they have been associated with increased mortality in animal models. Sustained aerobic exercise during acute viral myocarditis leads to increased mortality in animals. Therefore, strictly limiting aerobic physical activity until myocarditis is resolved is recommended.

16. **Is there a role for antiviral and immunosuppressive therapy?**
    In the setting of acute lymphocytic myocarditis, there is no established role for immunosuppressive or antiviral therapy. In patients with acute GCM, however, transplant-free survival is probably improved with cyclosporine and corticosteroids treatment. The role of antiviral and immunosuppressive treatments in select groups of patients with chronic dilated cardiomyopathy and evidence of either viral infection or myocarditis is an area of current research.

17. **When does the patient with myocarditis need mechanical circulatory support and when should patients be considered for cardiac transplantation?**
    Mechanical circulatory support may be effective in patients presenting with cardiogenic shock despite optimal medical intervention. Extracorporeal membrane oxygenation support may be beneficial for adult and pediatric patients with fulminant myocarditis and profound shock, as short-term recovery

can occur within days. For patients with cardiogenic shock due to acute myocarditis who deteriorate despite optimal medical management, recovery is more likely to be prolonged, and implantation of a ventricular assist device as a bridge to transplantation or recovery may be a more effective alternative. For those patients who are refractory to medical therapy and mechanical circulatory support, cardiac transplantation should be considered. The overall rate of survival after cardiac transplantation for myocarditis in adults is similar to that for other causes of cardiac failure.

18. **What is the prognosis of myocarditis?**
Prognosis is overall very good for adult patients with acute lymphocytic myocarditis who have mild symptoms and preserved LV ejection fraction (LVEF). Predictors of death or need for cardiac transplantation from various case series include presentation with syncope, RV systolic dysfunction, lower LVEF, elevated pulmonary artery pressure, advanced New York Heart Association (NYHA) class, and widened QRS and Q waves on presenting ECG.

CHAPTER 26

DILATED CARDIOMYOPATHY

Arunima Misra, MD, FACC, Shawn T. Ragbir, MD, and Biykem Bozkurt, MD, FACC

1. **What is the definition of dilated cardiomyopathy?**

   Dilated cardiomyopathy (DCM) refers to a spectrum of heterogeneous myocardial disorders characterized by ventricular dilation and depressed myocardial contractility in the absence of abnormal loading conditions (e.g., hypertension or valvular heart disease) or ischemic heart disease sufficient to cause global systolic impairment. Thus, DCM can be envisioned as the final common pathway for myriad cardiac disorders that either damage the heart muscle or, alternatively, disrupt the ability of the myocardium to generate force and subsequently cause chamber dilation.

   In practice and clinical trials, DCM is used interchangeably with *nonischemic cardiomyopathy* (NICM), although the latter includes systolic heart failure (heart failure) related to hypertension or valvular disease.

2. **How prevalent is DCM?**

   The incidence of DCM is 5 to 8 per 100,000 persons, whereas the prevalence is 36 per 100,000. DCM accounts for 10,000 deaths annually and represents approximately 30% to 40% of heart failure cases (as defined by NICM). African Americans are three times more likely to develop DCM than whites, and more likely to die from DCM compared with age-matched whites.

3. **How does DCM present?**

   The presenting features of DCM are typical of heart failure and include symptoms of left ventricular (LV) failure, including progressive exertional dyspnea, fatigue, weakness, diminished exercise capacity, orthopnea, paroxysmal nocturnal dyspnea, and nocturnal cough. Abdominal distension, right upper quadrant abdominal pain, early satiety, postprandial fullness, and nausea are seen with the development of right-sided heart failure. In advanced heart failure, cardiac cachexia may develop. Approximately 4% to 13% of the patients with DCM will present with asymptomatic LV dysfunction and LV dilation.

4. **What kind of diagnostic studies should be carried out for DCM?**

   The diagnostic evaluation is similar to those with ischemic heart failure and should include routine assessment of serum electrolytes, liver function tests, complete blood cell count, cardiac enzymes, serum natriuretic peptide levels (B-type natriuretic peptide [BNP] or N-terminal prohormone of BNP [NT-proBNP]), chest radiograph, electrocardiogram, and assessment of LV function by echocardiography or radionuclide imaging.

   Echocardiography typically shows four-chamber dilation, wall thinning, global hypokinesis, and left ventricular ejection fraction (LVEF) less than 35% to 40%. LV apical thrombi can be identified in up to 40% of patients with DCM. Tricuspid and mitral regurgitation may be present as a result of annular dilation and altered LV geometry. Doppler mitral inflow patterns may reveal elevated filling pressures.

   Multigated radionuclide angiocardiography (MUGA) may be used to assess LV systolic function in those with poor echocardiographic windows. Compared with echo assessment of LVEF, MUGA may have less interobserver and intertest variability. Thallium-201 myocardial scintigraphy is not a reliable technique for differentiating patients with ischemic cardiomyopathy (ICM) from those with DCM, as patients with DCM may have both reversible and fixed perfusion abnormalities related to the presence of myocardial fibrosis, although a completely normal scan (without reversible or fixed defects) would favor the diagnosis of NICM.

Cardiac catheterization may be performed if symptoms suggestive of ischemia are present or if coronary artery disease is strongly suspected. Catheterization in DCM generally shows normal coronary arteries or mild, nonobstructive, isolated atherosclerotic lesions that are insufficient to explain the extent of cardiomyopathy.

Endomyocardial biopsy may be performed if and only if a specific diagnosis is suspected in which specific therapy may be efficacious upon establishment of diagnosis (see Chapter 23 on endomyocardial biopsy).

5. **What is the natural history of DCM?**
The natural history of DCM depends on the underlying cause. Generally, symptomatic patients have a 25% mortality at 1 year and 50% mortality at 5 years. The prognosis in those with asymptomatic LV dysfunction is less clear. Pump failure accounts for approximately 70% of deaths, whereas sudden cardiac death accounts for approximately 30%.

Approximately 25% of symptomatic DCM patients will improve spontaneously. Idiopathic DCM has a lower total mortality compared with ischemic cardiomyopathy, although the risk of sudden death may be higher.

6. **What are the prognostic features of DCM?**
Many of the prognostic features are similar to those in ischemic cardiomyopathy, including age, LVEF, New York Heart Association (NYHA) class, lack of heart rate variability, elevated levels of neurohormones, and elevated markers of myocardial cell death. However, certain causes of DCM carry a more favorable prognosis and are potentially reversible—for example, cardiomyopathy associated with alcohol, peripartum, trastuzumab, or tachycardia. Other causes, such as anthracyclines or human immunodeficiency virus (HIV), have a worse prognosis.

7. **What are the common causes of DCM?**
The term nonischemic cardiomyopathy may include cardiomyopathies commonly caused by hypertension or valvular heart disease, which are not conventionally accepted under the definition of DCM. Causes for DCM include genetic causes (familial cardiomyopathies), toxins (alcohol, cocaine, chemotherapy such as anthracycline), infection (such as Coxsackie virus, HIV, *Trypanosoma cruzi*), inflammatory disorders (such as collagen vascular disease, hypersensitivity myocarditis), nutritional causes (such as thiamine deficiency), pregnancy, endocrine causes (such as diabetes, hyperthyroidism), tachycardia, and stress-induced (tako-tsubo) cardiomyopathy.

8. **What are the features of alcohol-induced cardiomyopathy?**
Alcohol-induced cardiomyopathy is said to occur when cardiomyopathy is noted in a heavy drinker in the absence of other causes (i.e., by exclusion). Alcoholic patients consuming more than 90 g of alcohol a day (approximately 7 to 8 standard drinks per day) for more than 5 years are at risk for this entity. Symptoms may develop with continued drinking. Approximately 20% of subjects with excessive drinking may demonstrate clinical heart failure. The typical patient is a man 30 to 55 years old who has been a heavy alcohol consumer for 10 years. Women may be more susceptible to the cardiodepressive effects of alcohol. Death rates are higher in African Americans (compared with whites). Abstinence may partially or completely reverse the cardiomyopathy. Overall prognosis remains poor, with a mortality of 40% to 50% at 3 to 6 years without abstinence.

9. **What are the features of cocaine-induced cardiomyopathy?**
Approximately 4% to 18% of cocaine users have depressed LV function. Cardiac catheterization reveals normal or mildly diseased coronary arteries, insufficient to explain the extent of myocardial dysfunction. Abstinence may lead to reversal.

10. **What are the features of chemotherapy-induced cardiomyopathy?**
Anthracyclines and trastuzumab are among the more prominent chemotherapeutic agents associated with cardiomyopathy. Three major types of anthracycline cardiotoxicity are distinguished: acute,

chronic, and late onset, which differ considerably in clinical picture and prognosis. Cardiac failure is rare with acute toxicity. Chronic cardiotoxicity is observed in 0.4% to 23%, several weeks or months after chemotherapy. Such anthracycline-induced cardiomyopathy carries a 27% to 61% mortality rate despite aggressive medical treatment. Late cardiotoxicity occurs years after chemotherapy, at 5% at 10 years, and presents as heart failure, arrhythmia, or conduction abnormalities. The primary risk factor for cardiomyopathy is cumulative dose administered. Toxicity is rare (less than 3%) with cumulative doses below 400 mg/m^2. Other risk factors include extremes of age and coexisting cardiac disease. Elevated cardiac troponin and BNP after chemotherapy may allow identification of patients who may develop cardiac toxicity. Anthracyclines should *not* be administered to patients with a baseline LVEF of 30% or less. LV function should be assessed repeatedly before each subsequent dose (or if the initial ejection fraction [EF] is more than 50%, after a cumulative dose of 350 to 500 mg/m^2), and treatment stopped if EF declines by 10% or more, or to a value less than 30% (or less than 50% if EF was normal at baseline). Reversibility has been documented anecdotally. The most effective protection is dexrazoxane (an iron chelator), with a two- to threefold decrease in the risk of cardiomyopathy.

Trastuzumab is a monoclonal antibody that selectively binds human epidermal growth factor receptor 2 (HER2), which is expressed in 25% of cases of breast cancer. In earlier trials in advanced breast cancer, trastuzumab was associated with the development of heart failure in up to 27% of patients. The majority of these patients, however, had received significant cumulative doses of anthracyclines or had preexisting cardiac disease. Risk factors for development of trastuzumab-associated heart failure include increasing age, lower LVEF, and higher anthracycline dose. Trastuzumab-associated heart failure responds better to standard therapy than does anthracycline-induced heart failure, with complete recovery usually seen within 6 months of discontinuing trastuzumab.

11. What are the features of HIV-related cardiomyopathy?

HIV-related cardiomyopathy accounts for up to 4% of DCM. The incidence is higher among patients with a CD4 count less than 400 cells/mm^3. HIV-related cardiomyopathy is discussed in detail in Chapter 46 on cardiac manifestations of HIV and acquired immunodeficiency syndrome (AIDS).

12. What are the associations between collagen vascular disease and DCMs?

In systemic lupus erythematosus (SLE), global LV dysfunction has been reported in 5% of patients, segmental LV wall motion abnormalities in 4% of patients, and right ventricular enlargement in 4% of patients, but DCM is rare. In rheumatoid arthritis, symptomatic cardiac disease, including myocarditis, develops in 8% of patients. Progressive systemic sclerosis can rarely lead to heart failure through myocardial fibrosis, arrhythmia, or intermittent vascular spasm. Dermatomyositis may be associated with cardiomyopathy in some patients. For further discussion, see Chapter 47 on cardiac manifestations of connective tissue disorders and vasculitides.

13. What is peripartum cardiomyopathy?

Peripartum cardiomyopathy (PPCM) is the development of symptomatic heart failure in the last trimester of pregnancy or within 6 months of parturition. Other causes of DCM must be excluded in such patients before making the PPCM diagnosis. PPCM occurs in 1 per 2289 to 4000 live births. Risk factors may include older age, multiparity, African American ancestry, multiple gestation, toxemia, chronic hypertension, and use of tocolytics. In recent case series, up to 50% of PPCM developed with the first two pregnancies. Fifty percent of women recover baseline cardiac function within 6 months. Even though the prognosis in subsequent pregnancies is better if cardiac function recovers, 21% of these patients will develop heart failure symptoms. The prognosis in subsequent pregnancies is poorer if cardiac function remains abnormal—37% deliver prematurely and 19% die.

14. What are the features of tachycardia-induced cardiomyopathy?

Sustained elevated ventricular rates have been shown to cause changes in LV geometry and dilation. This entity should be considered in patients with no other explanation for LV dysfunction and a concomitant tachyarrhythmia. Hyperthyroid-induced sinus tachycardia or atrial fibrillation should be excluded in such patients. Treatment involves restoration of normal sinus rhythm or control of ventricular rate, with which there is typically resolution as quickly as 4 to 6 weeks.

15. **What are the features of nutritional causes of DCM?**

Thiamine deficiency causes cardiovascular beriberi, in which the circulation is hyperkinetic and DCM results. Treatment for beriberi should consist of administration of thiamine, along with standard heart failure therapy. DCM may occur with chronic alcoholism and with anorexia nervosa.

16. **What are the features of cardiomyopathy caused by iron overload?**

Iron-overload cardiomyopathy occurs as a result of increased cardiac iron deposition, commonly in disorders such as hereditary hemochromatosis and β-thalassemia major. Extracardiac manifestations typically precede symptomatic heart failure. Initially, the hemodynamic profile represents a restrictive pattern. As cardiomyopathy advances, DCM ensues. The diagnosis of iron overload is suggested by elevated serum ferritin and a ratio of iron to total iron-binding capacity greater than 50%. The most definitive test for calculation of iron stores is measurement of iron concentration by liver biopsy.

The mainstays of therapy are phlebotomy (in hereditary hemochromatosis) and chelation therapy (in secondary iron overload related to blood transfusions, prophylactically after transfusion of 20 to 30 units of red blood cells [RBCs] or when serum ferritin is more than 2500 ng/mL). Early diagnosis and treatment before tissue damage has occurred is essential, because life span seems to be normal in treated patients but markedly shortened in those who are not.

17. **What are the pharmacologic treatments to be used in DCM?**

Similar to therapy for chronic stable heart failure, standard medical therapy with β-blockers and angiotensin-converting enzyme (ACE) inhibitors (or angiotensin-receptor blockers) is indicated per current guidelines from the American College of Cardiology/American Heart Association (ACC/AHA). Intake of salt should be restricted. Depending on the circumstances, spironolactone, or a combination of isosorbide dinitrate and hydralazine, may be added in *symptomatic* heart failure, and in some patients digoxin may be considered. Use of spironolactone should entail judicious adjustment of potassium supplements and close laboratory follow-up. Diuretics should be used to manage volume overload symptoms.

Antiarrhythmic therapy is reserved for individualized treatment of symptomatic arrhythmias, especially for suppression of ventricular arrhythmias after an implantable cardioverter-defibrillator (ICD). Recent data suggest that use of such agents for maintaining sinus rhythm in heart failure patients with atrial fibrillation may not be better than rate control.

18. **What are the device treatments to be used in DCM?**

Defibrillators are indicated for secondary prevention in survivors of ventricular fibrillation (VF) or hemodynamically significant ventricular tachycardia (VT); in patients with structural heart disease or unexplained syncope with hemodynamically significant VF or VT on electrophysiologic study; and in patients with NICM who have an LVEF 35% or lower.

Recent trials of cardiac resynchronization therapy (with or without concomitant defibrillator) have shown a 50% decrease in all-cause mortality versus placebo among subjects with NICM or DCM. In addition to the mortality benefit, resynchronization improves quality of life. Thus, resynchronization therapy, with or without defibrillator, should be offered to patients who have an LVEF 35% or less, a QRS duration 0.12 seconds or more, and sinus rhythm who continue to be categorized as NYHA functional class III or IV despite optimal recommended medical therapy. Recent studies in patients with mild heart failure symptoms (NYHA class II) also demonstrated survival benefit, especially in patients with left bundle branch block (LBBB) and QRS greater than 150 ms. According to the 2009 heart failure guidelines, symptomatic patients with atrial fibrillation may also be considered for resynchronization therapy, a class IIa indication.

19. **Should DCM patients be anticoagulated?**

Patients with DCM have multiple risk factors that predispose to thromboembolic events—with the incidence ranging from 0.8 to 2.5 per 100 patient-years. Pooled data from small, randomized, controlled clinical trials and current guidelines do not support routine anticoagulation in heart failure with sinus rhythm. The results of the Warfarin versus Aspirin in Reduced Cardiac Ejection Fraction (WARCEF) trial showed that in a large randomized comparison of aspirin versus warfarin in patients with heart failure and reduced ejection fraction (not in atrial fibrillation) there was no overall difference in the combined primary outcome of death, ischemic stroke, or intracranial hemorrhage between treatment groups. Available data do support the use of anticoagulants in the presence of atrial fibrillation, previous stroke or other thromboembolic events, or visible protruding or mobile thrombus on echocardiography.

20. What is the role of exercise therapy?

Exercise training should be considered in stable patients. Training has been shown to decrease symptoms, improve exercise tolerance, and improve quality of life beyond that provided by pharmacologic treatment. Long-term outcomes, however, are not entirely known, although small studies have shown reduction in mortality or readmission for heart failure. The Heart Failure and a Controlled Trial Investigating Outcomes of Exercise Training (HF-ACTION) trial failed to demonstrate a reduction in all-cause mortality or all-cause hospitalization in patients randomized to a structured exercise program when compared to "usual care," although secondary analysis did suggest some benefit.

BIBLIOGRAPHY, SUGGESTED READINGS, AND WEBSITES

1. Arnold JMO: *Heart Failure*. Available at: http://www.merckmanuals.com/professional/cardiovascular_disorders/heart_failure/heart_failure_hf.html; Last full review/revision January 2010; last modified April 2012. Accessed March 19, 2013.

2. Cooper LT, Baughman KL, Feldman AM, et al: The role of endomyocardial biopsy in the management of cardiovascular disease: a scientific statement from the American Heart Association, the American College of Cardiology, and the European Society of Cardiology. Endorsed by the Heart Failure Society of America and the Heart Failure Association of the European Society of Cardiology, *J Am Coll Cardiol* 50:1914–1931, 2007.

3. Desai AS, Fang JC, Maisel WH, Baughman KL: Implantable defibrillators for the prevention of mortality in patients with nonischemic cardiomyopathy: a meta-analysis of randomized controlled trials, *JAMA* 292:2874–2879, 2004.

4. Dries D, Exner D, Gersh B, et al: Racial differences in the outcome of left ventricular dysfunction, *N Engl J Med* 340:609–616, 1999.

5. Epstein AE, DiMarco JP, Ellenbogen KA, et al: ACC/AHA/HRS 2008 Guidelines for Device-Based Therapy of Cardiac Rhythm Abnormalities: a report of the American College of Cardiology/American Heart Association Task Force on Practice Guidelines (Writing Committee to Revise the ACC/AHA/NASPE 2002 Guideline Update for Implantation of Cardiac Pacemakers and Antiarrhythmia Devices) developed in collaboration with the American Association for Thoracic Surgery and Society of Thoracic Surgeons, *J Am Coll Cardiol* 51(21):e1–e62, 2008.

6. Heart Failure Society of America: Heart failure in patients with left ventricular systolic dysfunction, *J Card Fail* 12:e38–e57, 2006.

7. Heart Failure Society of America: *HFSA website*. Available at: http://www.hfsa.org. Accessed March 19, 2013.

8. Homma S, Thompson JLP: *Results of the Warfarin versus Aspirin in Reduced Cardiac Ejection Fraction (WARCEF) trial. International Stroke Conference 2012*. New Orleans, February 3, 2012, Abstract LB. 12–4372.

9. Hunt SA: American College of Cardiology; American Heart Association Task Force on Practice Guidelines (Writing Committee to Update the 2001 Guidelines for the Evaluation and Management of Heart Failure): ACC/AHA 2005 guideline update for the diagnosis and management of chronic heart failure in the adult, *J Am Coll Cardiol* 46:1–82, 2005.

10. Koniaris L, Goldhaber S: Anticoagulation in dilated cardiomyopathy, *J Am Coll Cardiol* 31:745–748, 1998.

11. Mann DL: Management of heart failure patients with reduced ejection fraction. In Libby P, Bonow R, Mann D, editors: *Braunwald's heart disease: a textbook of cardiovascular medicine*, ed 8, Philadelphia, 2008, Saunders.

12. Piano M: Alcoholic cardiomyopathy: incidence, clinical characteristics, and pathophysiology, *Chest* 121:1638–1650, 2002.

13. Richardson P, McKenna W, Bristow M, et al: Report of the 1995 World Health Organization/International Society and Federation of Cardiology Task Force on the Definition and Classification of Cardiomyopathies, *Circulation* 93:841–842, 1996.

14. Saxon L, De Marco T: Arrhythmias associated with dilated cardiomyopathy, *Card Electrophysiol Rev* 6:18–25, 2002.

15. Sliwa K, Fett J, Elkayam U: Peripartum cardiomyopathy, *Lancet* 368:687–693, 2006.

16. Swedberg K, Cleland J, Dargie H, et al: Guidelines for the diagnosis and treatment of chronic heart failure: executive summary (update 2005): The Task Force for the Diagnosis and Treatment of Chronic Heart Failure of the European Society of Cardiology, *Eur Heart J* 26:1115–1140, 2005.

17. Wigner M, Morgan JP: *Causes of dilated cardiomyopathy*. In Basow, DS, editor: UpToDate, Waltham, MA, 2013, UpToDate. Available at: http://www.uptodate.com/contents/causes-of-dilated-cardiomyopathy. Accessed March 26, 2013.

18. Dumitru, I: *Heart Failure*. Available at: http://www.emedicine.com. Accessed March 19, 2013.

CHAPTER 27

HYPERTROPHIC CARDIOMYOPATHY

Luke Cunningham, MD, and Kumudha Ramasubbu, MD, FACC

1. **What is hypertrophic cardiomyopathy?**

   Hypertrophic cardiomyopathy (HCM) is a primary disorder of the cardiac muscle characterized by inappropriate myocardial hypertrophy of a nondilated left ventricle (LV) in the absence of a cardiovascular or systemic disease (i.e., aortic stenosis or systemic hypertension). Historically, HCM has been known by a confusing array of names, such as idiopathic hypertrophic subaortic stenosis (IHSS), muscular subaortic stenosis, and hypertrophic obstructive cardiomyopathy (HOCM). Currently, *hypertrophic cardiomyopathy* is the preferred term.

2. **What is the prevalence of HCM?**

   The reported prevalence of HCM from epidemiologic studies is about 1:500 in the general population (0.2%). HCM affects men and women equally and occurs in many races and countries.

3. **What are the genetic mutations that cause HCM, and how are they transmitted?**

   Thus far, more than 400 mutations in 11 genes have been identified that can cause HCM. These genes encode for cardiac sarcomere proteins that serve contractile, structural, and regulatory functions. They are cardiac troponin T, cardiac troponin I, myosin regulatory light chain, myosin essential light chain, cardiac myosin-binding protein C, α- and β-cardiac myosin heavy chain, cardiac α actin, α tropomyosin, titin, and muscle LIM protein (MLP). Mutations in cardiac myosin-binding protein C and β-cardiac myosin heavy chain are the most common and account for 82% of all mutations. HCM is inherited as an autosomal dominant trait; therefore, patients with HCM have a 50% chance of transmitting the disease to each of their offspring.

4. **Who should be screened for HCM?**

   Patients with known HCM mutations, but without evidence of disease, and first-degree relatives of patients with HCM should be screened. Screening is performed primarily with history, physical examination, 12-lead electrocardiogram (ECG), and two-dimensional echocardiography. Traditionally, screening was performed on a 12- to 18-month basis, usually beginning by age 12 until age 18 to 21. However, it is now recognized that development of the HCM phenotype uncommonly can occur later in adulthood. Therefore, the current recommendation is to extend clinical surveillance into adulthood at about 5-year intervals or to undergo genetic testing (Table 27-1).

5. **Who should undergo genetic testing?**

   Genetic testing, which is not commercially available, has become recognized as an important aspect in the evaluation of HCM. It is strongly recommended that patients diagnosed with HCM be evaluated by a genetics specialist. In an index patient, genetic testing is also recommended in order to identify the risk in first-degree family members of developing HCM. First-degree relatives of patients with HCM should undergo the previously discussed clinical screening, with or without genetic testing based on genetic counseling. However, genetic testing is not helpful in first-degree family members of an HCM patient without identifiable pathologic mutation.

6. **What are the histologic characteristics of HCM?**

   The histology of HCM is characterized by hypertrophy of cardiac myocytes and myocardial fiber disarray. The abnormal myocytes contain bizarrely shaped nuclei and are arranged in disorganized

---

TABLE 27-1. CLINICAL SCREENING STRATEGIES FOR DETECTION OF HYPERTROPHIC CARDIOMYOPATHY IN FAMILIES*

<12 years old

Optional unless:
   Malignant family history of premature HCM death or other adverse complications
   Competitive athlete in an intense training program
   Onset of symptoms
   Other clinical suspicion of early LV hypertrophy

12 to 18-21 years old

Every 12-18 months

>18-21 years old

Probably approximately every 5 years or more frequent intervals with a family history of late-onset hypertrophic cardiomyopathy and/or malignant clinical course

From Maron BJ, Seidman JG, Seidman CE: Proposal for contemporary screening strategies in families with hypertrophic cardiomyopathy. *J Am Coll Cardiol* 44:2125-2132, 2004.
*In the absence of laboratory-based genetic testing.

---

patterns. The volume of the interstitial collagen matrix is greatly increased, and the arrangement of the matrix components is also disorganized. Myocardial disarray is seen in substantial portions of hypertrophied and nonhypertrophied LV myocardium. Almost all HCM patients have some degree of disarray, and in the majority, at least 5% of the myocardium is involved.

7. **What are the common types of HCM?**
   The distribution and severity of LV hypertrophy in patients with HCM can vary greatly. Even first-degree relatives, with the same genetic mutation, usually show different patterns of hypertrophy. Various patterns of LV hypertrophy have been reported. The most common site of hypertrophy is the anterior interventricular septum (Fig. 27-1), which is seen in more than 80% of HCM patients and is known as *asymmetrical septal hypertrophy* (ASH). *Concentric LV hypertrophy*, with maximal thickening at the level of the papillary muscles, is seen in 8% to 10% of patients with HCM. A variant with primary involvement of the apex *(apical HCM)* is common in Japan and rare in the U.S. (less than 2%) and is characterized by spadelike deformity of the LV.

8. **What are the most common symptoms in patients with HCM?**
   Most patients with HCM have no or only minor symptoms and often are diagnosed during family screening. The most common symptoms are as follows:
   - Dyspnea
     - Present in more than 90% of symptomatic patients
     - Caused mainly by LV diastolic dysfunction with impaired filling caused by abnormal relaxation and increased chamber stiffness
     - Also caused by dynamic LV outflow tract (LVOT) obstruction (see Fig. 27-1) leading to elevated intraventricular pressures.
   - Angina pectoris
     - May occur in both obstructive and nonobstructive HCM
     - Caused by a mismatch of supply and demand in myocardial perfusion
     - Several mechanisms have been proposed, including increased muscle mass and wall stress, decreased coronary perfusion pressure secondary to LV outflow obstruction, elevated diastolic filling pressures, systolic compression of large intramural coronary arteries, inadequate capillary density, impaired vasodilatory reserve, and abnormally narrowed small intramural coronary arteries

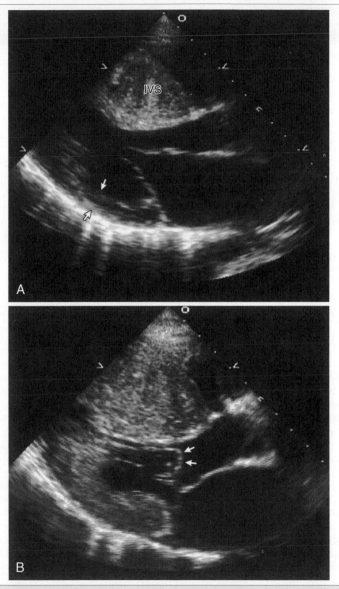

Figure 27-1. A, Echocardiogram of a patient with hypertrophic cardiomyopathy, demonstrating a markedly thickened interventricular septum compared with the normal wall thickness of the posterior wall *(arrows)*. **B,** During systole, there is systolic anterior motion (SAM) and buckling of the anterior mitral leaflet *(arrows)*, obstructing the left ventricular outflow tract.

- Syncope and presyncope
  - Caused by inadequate cardiac output with exertion (as a result of LVOT obstruction) or as a result of cardiac arrhythmia
  - Identifies patients at risk for sudden death

TABLE 27-2. CLINICAL PARAMETERS USED TO DISTINGUISH HYPERTROPHIC CARDIOMYOPATHY FROM ATHLETE'S HEART

Parameters	HCM	Athlete's Heart
LV wall thickness	>16 mm	<16 mm
Pattern of hypertrophy	Asymmetric, symmetric or apical	Symmetric
LV end-diastolic dimension	<45 mm	>55 mm
Left atrium size	Enlarged	Normal
LV diastolic filling pattern	Impaired relaxation	Normal
Response to deconditioning	None	LV wall thickness decreases
ECG findings	Very high QRS voltage; Q waves; deep negative T waves	Criteria for LVH but without unusual features
Family history of HCM	Present	Absent
Sarcomeric protein mutation	Present	Absent

Modified from Elliott PM, McKenna WJ: *Diagnosis and evaluation of hypertrophic cardiomyopathy.* Available at: www.UpToDate.com. Accessed February 2008.
HCM, Hypertrophic cardiomyopathy; *LV,* left ventricular; *LVH,* left ventricular hypertrophy.

9. **How is HCM differentiated from athlete's heart?**
   Long-term athletic training can lead to cardiac hypertrophy, known as *athlete's heart.* This clinically benign physiologic condition must be differentiated from HCM, because HCM is the most common cause of sudden death in competitive athletes. Clinical parameters that support the diagnosis of HCM instead of athlete's heart are asymmetric hypertrophy greater than 16 mm, LV end-diastolic dimension less than 45 mm, enlarged left atrium, impaired LV relaxation on Doppler mitral valve inflow parameters and tissue Doppler echocardiography, absent response to deconditioning (e.g., hypertrophy does not regress with absence of exercise), family history of HCM, and sarcomeric protein mutation identified by genetic testing. These parameters are summarized in Table 27-2.

10. **Describe the classic murmur of obstructive HCM and bedside maneuvers that differentiate it from other cardiac abnormalities**
    The classic murmur of obstructive HCM is a harsh crescendo–decrescendo systolic murmur and is heard best between the left sternal border and apex. It often radiates to the axilla and base but not into the neck vessels. A variety of provocative maneuvers can augment or suppress the murmur to help differentiate it from other systolic murmurs.
    Maneuvers that increase intracardiac blood volume or decrease contractility typically lead to a decrease in murmur intensity, and maneuvers that decrease intracardiac blood volume or increase contractility lead to an increase in murmur intensity (Table 27-3).

11. **How does the carotid pulse in obstructive HCM differ from that in valvular aortic stenosis?**
    In patients with obstructive HCM, the carotid pulse has an initial brisk rise, followed by midsystolic decline as a result of LVOT obstruction, then a second rise *(pulsus bisferiens).* In contrast, as a result of the fixed obstruction in aortic stenosis, the carotid upstroke is diminished in amplitude and delayed *(pulsus parvus and tardus).*

12. **What noninvasive studies are helpful in making the diagnosis of HCM?**
    The ECG is abnormal in the majority of patients with HCM; however, no changes are pathognomonic for HCM. The common abnormalities are ST-segment and T-wave changes, voltage criteria for left

TABLE 27-3.   EFFECT OF BEDSIDE MANEUVERS ON SYSTOLIC MURMURS

Maneuver	HCM	AS	MR	VSD
Valsalva	↑	↓	↓	↓
Handgrip	↓	↓	↑	↑
Squatting	↓	↑	↑	↑
Amyl nitrite	↑	↑	↓	↓
Leg raise	↓	↑	↑	↑

AS, Aortic stenosis; *HCM*, hypertrophic cardiomyopathy; *MR*, mitral regurgitation; *VSD*, ventricular septal defect.

ventricular hypertrophy (LVH), prominent Q waves in the inferior (II, III, aVF) or precordial (V2 to V6) leads, left axis deviation, and left atrial enlargement. Apical HCM, seen predominantly in Japanese patients, is characterized by giant negative T waves in the precordial leads.

Echocardiography is the primary and preferred diagnostic modality for HCM. The cardinal feature is LVH with diastolic wall thickness 15 mm or greater. Other findings include a septal-to-posterior wall ratio 1.3 or more (seen in patients with ASH), small LV cavity, reduced septal motion and thickening, normal or increased motion of the posterior wall, systolic anterior motion of the mitral leaflets, mitral regurgitation (mid- to late systolic), partial midsystolic closure of aortic valve with coarse fluttering of the leaflets in late systole, and diastolic dysfunction. In the setting of dynamic LVOT obstruction, a resting LVOT gradient may or may not be detected. A significant gradient is defined as a resting gradient more than 30 mm Hg and a provocable gradient more than 50 mm Hg. The LVOT Doppler signal in HCM is typically late peaking and is referred to as *dagger shaped*.

Magnetic resonance imaging (MRI) is becoming a valuable tool to complement echocardiographic findings. It offers high-resolution images, three-dimensional imaging, and tissue characterization. MRI is especially useful to detect LVH in areas that may be difficult to assess by echocardiography, or if the technical quality of echocardiographic images is inadequate.

13. **What is systolic anterior motion and what causes it?**
Systolic anterior motion (SAM) is the abnormal anterior displacement of the anterior mitral leaflet toward the septum during midsystole. Several mechanisms have been proposed for SAM:
- The anterior mitral leaflet is drawn toward the septum by a Venturi effect produced by the lower pressure in the LVOT that occurs as blood is ejected at a high velocity.
- The anterior mitral leaflet is pulled against the septum by contraction of abnormally inserted and oriented papillary muscles.

This typically results in eccentric mitral regurgitation directed posteriorly. Because SAM worsens during the course of systole, the mitral regurgitation also becomes more prominent during mid- to late systole.

14. **Describe the mechanism of LVOT obstruction in HCM**
LVOT obstruction in HCM is produced by SAM of the anterior mitral leaflet and midsystolic contact with the hypertrophic ventricular septum. The magnitude of the subaortic gradient is directly related to the duration of contact between the mitral leaflet and the septum. The subaortic gradient is often dynamic and responds to provocative maneuvers in the same manner as the systolic murmur (see Question 9 and Table 27-3).

15. **What are the characteristic hemodynamic findings during cardiac catheterization in obstructive HCM?**
Cardiac catheterization is not required for the diagnosis of HCM, and the diagnosis is usually made using noninvasive tests. Cardiac catheterization is generally reserved for assessment of coronary

artery disease and evaluation before surgical procedures, such as myectomy. The typical findings during cardiac catheterization are subaortic or midventricular outflow gradient on catheter pullback, spike-and-dome pattern of aortic pressure tracing, elevated left atrial and LV end-diastolic pressures, elevated pulmonary capillary wedge pressure, increased V wave on wedge tracing (as a result of mitral regurgitation), and elevated pulmonary arterial pressure.

16. What is the Brockenbrough-Braunwald sign?
Normally, following a premature ventricular contraction (PVC), with the subsequent sinus beat there is increased contractility and stroke volume, leading to an increase in the systolic blood pressure and thus an increase in the pulse pressure (the difference between systolic and diastolic pressure). However, in patients with HCM, the increased contractility after a PVC results in increased LVOT obstruction, leading to a decrease in stroke volume and systolic pressure, and thus a decrease in pulse pressure. This phenomenon is known as the Brockenbrough-Braunwald sign.

17. What are the risk factors for sudden cardiac death in patients with HCM?
Sudden cardiac death (SCD) is the most devastating consequence of HCM and is often the initial clinical manifestation in asymptomatic individuals. The most common cause of SCD in HCM patients is ventricular tachyarrhythmias. Seven major risk factors for SCD have been identified:
- prior cardiac arrest or sustained ventricular tachycardia (VT)
- family history of SCD
- unexplained syncope
- hypotensive blood pressure response to exercise
- nonsustained VT on ambulatory (Holter) monitoring
- identification of a high-risk mutant gene
- massive LVH with wall thickness 30 mm or greater

18. What medications should generally be avoided in patients with obstructive HCM?
Medications that decrease preload and afterload and increase contractility will worsen LVOT obstruction and therefore should be avoided.
- **Preload reducing** agents are diuretics and nitroglycerin. Diuretics may be used cautiously in patients with persistent heart failure symptoms and volume overload.
- **Afterload reducing** agents include dihydropyridine calcium channel blockers (CCB), nitroglycerin, angiotensin-converting enzyme (ACE) inhibitors, and angiotensin II receptor blockers.
- **Increased contractility** is produced by medications such as digoxin, dobutamine, and phosphodiesterase inhibitors (milrinone).

19. What are the pharmacologic therapies for patients with HCM?
Pharmacologic therapy is primarily used to alleviate symptoms of heart failure, angina, and syncope in HCM patients. Routine pharmacologic therapy is not recommended in asymptomatic patients.
- **Beta-adrenergic blocking agents (β-blockers)** are generally considered first-line therapy for HCM. The beneficial effects of β-blockers are mediated by their negative chronotropic property, which increases ventricular diastolic filling time, and by the negative inotropic property.
- **Nondihydropyridine calcium channel blockers** are an alternative to β-blockers in the treatment of HCM. Verapamil has been the most widely used CCB and improves symptoms by increasing LV relaxation and diastolic filling and by decreasing LV contractility. However, because of its vasodilatory effect, verapamil should be avoided in patients with marked outflow obstruction. Diltiazem has been used less often but may improve LV diastolic function. Dihydropyridine CCBs should be avoided in patients with HCM because of their predominantly vasodilatory properties, which can result in worsening of the LVOT obstruction.
- **Disopyramide** is a class IA antiarrhythmic drug with potent negative inotropic effect that is used when β-blockers and CCBs have failed to improve symptoms. Disopyramide is used in combination with a β-blocker because it may accelerate AV nodal conduction.

20. **What nonpharmacologic treatments are available to patients with HCM?**
   - **Septal myectomy** surgery has been the gold standard for more than 45 years for patients with severe symptoms that are refractory to medical therapy. Septal myectomy, known as the Morrow procedure, uses a transaortic approach to resect a small amount of muscle from the proximal septum. It is associated with persistent and long-lasting improvement in symptoms, exercise capacity, and possibly survival.
   - **Alcohol septal ablation (ASA)** has gained tremendous popularity in recent years as a new treatment modality for HCM. The procedure is performed by injecting 1 to 3 mL of 96% to 98% ethanol into a septal perforator branch of the left anterior descending coronary artery to create a limited myocardial infarction in the proximal septum. This scarring leads to progressive thinning and hypokinesis of the septum, increases LVOT diameter, improves mitral valve function, and ultimately reduces LVOT obstruction. The procedure-related mortality rate is 1% to 2%, which is similar to that of surgery. ASA is generally reserved for patients in whom surgery is contraindicated or is considered high risk, and is not indicated in children. It has also been noted that those with a septal wall thickness greater than 30 mm are likely to receive little benefit.
   - **Dual-chamber pacing** was promoted to be an alternative to myectomy to improve symptoms and reduce LVOT obstruction in the early 1990s. However, subsequent randomized studies have shown that subjectively perceived symptomatic improvement was not accompanied by objective evidence of improved exercise capacity and may be due to a placebo effect. Dual-chamber pacing has a limited role in the contemporary management of HCM, mainly in the subgroup of elderly patients who are not candidates for myectomy or ASA.

21. **What are the indications for an implantable cardioverter-defibrillator (ICD) in HCM?**
   An ICD is the preferred therapy for prevention of SCD in HCM patients. The recommended indications are as follows:
   - ICD can be used for secondary prevention in survivors of cardiac arrest or sustained VT.
   - ICD is indicated for high-risk patients, defined as having two or more of the major risk factors for SCD (see Question 17).
   - In patients with one major risk factor, care needs to be individualized. The decision to implant an ICD should take into account the age of the patient, strength of the risk factor, the level of risk acceptable to the patient and family, and the potential complications.
   - ICD can be used in patients with end-stage HCM, characterized by LV systolic dysfunction, LV wall thinning, and chamber dilation.

22. **What is the natural history of HCM?**
   The clinical course of patients with HCM is variable. Clinical manifestation can present at any age, from birth to age 90 or older. Many patients remain asymptomatic or mildly symptomatic for many years and achieve normal life expectancy. Others develop progressive symptoms of heart failure with exertional dyspnea and functional limitation despite medical therapy. Increase in LVH is predominately seen in adolescents and young adults. In older adults, LV wall thickness generally remains stable. Approximately 10% to 15% of patients will progress to end-stage HCM as described earlier. Atrial fibrillation occurs in 10% to 20% of HCM patients and may lead to clinical deterioration. The annual mortality rate in patients with HCM is about 1% in adults and 2% in children.

BIBLIOGRAPHY, SUGGESTED READINGS, AND WEBSITES

1. Arnold JMO: *Hypertrophic cardiomyopathy.* Available at http://www.merckmanuals.com/professional/cardiovascular_disorders/cardiomyopathies/hypertrophic_cardiomyopathy.html. Accessed May 1, 2012.

2. Elliot PM, McKenna WJ: *Diagnosis and Evaluation of Hypertrophic Cardiomyopathy.* Available at: www.UpToDate.com. Accessed February 2008.

3. Fatkin D, Seidman JG, Seidman CE: Hypertrophic cardiomyopathy. In Willerson JT, Cohn JN, Wellens HJJ, Holmes DR, editors: *Cardiovascular medicine*, ed 3, New York, 2007, Springer, pp 1261–1284.

4. Gersh BJ, Maron BJ, Bonow RO, et al: ACCF/AHA Guideline for the Diagnosis and Treatment of Hypertrophic Cardiomyopathy: A Report of the American College of Cardiology Foundation/American Heart Association Task Force on Practice Guidelines, *Circulation* 124:e783–e831, 2011.

5. Kimmelstiel CD, Maron BJ: Role of percutaneous septal ablation in hypertrophic obstructive cardiomyopathy, *Circulation* 109:452–456, 2004.

6. Maron BJ: Hypertrophic cardiomyopathy: a systematic review, *JAMA* 287:1308–1320, 2002.

7. Maron BJ: Hypertrophic cardiomyopathy. In Libby P, Bonow RO, Mann DL, Zipes DP, editors: *Braunwald's Heart Disease: A Textbook of Cardiovascular Medicine*, ed 8, Philadelphia, 2007, Saunders.

8. Maron BJ, Dearani JA, Ommen SR, et al: The case for surgery in obstructive hypertrophic cardiomyopathy, *J Am Coll Cardiol* 44:2044–2053, 2004.

9. Maron BJ, Pelliccia A: The heart of trained athletes: cardiac remodeling and the risks of sports, including sudden death, *Circulation* 114:1633–1644, 2006.

10. Maron BJ, Seidman JG, Seidman CE: Proposal for contemporary screening strategies in families with hypertrophic cardiomyopathy, *J Am Coll Cardiol* 44:2125–2132, 2004.

11. NHLBI Program for Genomic Applications, Harvard Medical School. Genomics of Cardiovascular Development, Adaptation, and Remodeling: *Sarcomere Protein Gene Mutation Database*. Available at: http://genepath.med.harvard.edu/~seidman/cg3. Accessed May 1, 2012.

12. Ommen SR, Maron BJ, Olivotto I, et al: Long-term effects of surgical septal myectomy on survival in patients with obstructive hypertrophic cardiomyopathy, *J Am Coll Cardiol* 46:470–476, 2005.

13. Richard P, Charron P, Carrier L, et al: Hypertrophic cardiomyopathy: distribution of disease genes, spectrum of mutations, and implications for a molecular diagnosis strategy, *Circulation* 107:2227–2232, 2003.

14. Sherrid MV, Barac I, McKenna WJ, et al: Multicenter study of the efficacy and safety of disopyramide in obstructive hypertrophic cardiomyopathy, *J Am Coll Cardiol* 45:1251–1258, 2005.

15. Shah SN: *Hypertrophic cardiomyopathy*. Available at: http://www.emedicine.com. Accessed May 1, 2012.

CHAPTER 28

RESTRICTIVE CARDIOMYOPATHY

Ravi S. Hira, MD, and Glenn N. Levine, MD, FACC, FAHA

1. **What is the basic physiologic problem in restrictive cardiomyopathy?**

   The basic physiologic problem in restrictive cardiomyopathy is increased *stiffness* of the ventricular walls, causing impaired diastolic filling of the ventricles that leads to a precipitous rise in pressure within the ventricles with small increases in volume. Systolic function is usually preserved (at least in the early stages of disease, although it may become severely impaired in the later stages of amyloidosis). The condition can affect either or both of the ventricles and they may not be uniformly affected.

2. **What are the main causes of restrictive cardiomyopathy?**

   Approximately half the cases of restrictive cardiomyopathy have an identifiable cause. The most common identifiable cause is myocardial infiltration from amyloidosis. Other infiltrative diseases include sarcoidosis, Gaucher disease, and Hurler disease. Storage diseases include hemochromatosis, glycogen storage disease, and Fabry disease. Endomyocardial involvement from endomyocardial fibrosis, radiation, and anthracycline treatment can also lead to restrictive cardiomyopathy. Although restrictive cardiomyopathy is a rather uncommon cause of heart failure in North America and Europe, it is a common cause of heart failure and death in tropical regions, including parts of Africa, Central and South America, India, and other parts of Asia (where the incidence of endomyocardial fibrosis is relatively high). Causes of restrictive cardiomyopathy are summarized in Table 28-1.

   Secondary restrictive physiology develops in the advanced stages of dilated, hypertensive, and ischemic heart disease. While both are associated with elevated left ventricular (LV) filling pressures, one should be sure to distinguish "restrictive cardiomyopathy" from "restrictive physiology" (as may be reported on an echocardiogram report).

3. **What are the usual echocardiographic findings in restrictive cardiomyopathy?**

   Echocardiography usually demonstrates normal or near-normal systolic function, ventricles of normal or decreased volumes, normal or only minimally increased ventricular wall thickness, impaired ventricular relaxation and filling *(diastolic dysfunction),* and biatrial enlargement. As discussed in Question 4, these findings may be different in later stages of amyloidosis and certain other conditions (Fig. 28-1, *A*). On Doppler echocardiography, one observes accentuated early diastolic filling of the ventricles (prominent E wave), shortened deceleration time, and diminished atrial filling (diminutive A wave) resulting in a high E-to-A wave ratio on the mitral inflow velocities (see Fig. 28-1, *B*).

4. **How does amyloidosis affect the heart?**

   As with other organs, in amyloidosis there may be protein deposition in myocardial tissue. The term *amyloidosis* was reportedly coined by Virchow and means "starchlike." The affected myocardium is found to be firm, rubbery, and noncompliant. This protein deposition leads to *restrictive physiology,* as well as to eventual systolic heart dysfunction and possible conduction abnormalities. Patients are often extremely fluid sensitive, and management is complicated by having to walk a fine line between volume overload and inadequate preload. Patients with amyloidosis often manifest orthostatic hypotension and may develop additional conduction-related disorders. The prognosis is generally extremely poor.

TABLE 28-1. CLASSIFICATION OF TYPES OF RESTRICTIVE CARDIOMYOPATHY ACCORDING TO CAUSE
Infiltrative
Amyloidosis
Sarcoidosis
Gaucher disease
Hurler disease
Fatty infiltration
Storage Disease
Hemochromatosis
Fabry disease
Glycogen storage disease
Endomyocardial
Endomyocardial fibrosis
Radiation
Hypereosinophilic syndrome (Löffler disease)
Carcinoid syndrome
Myocardial Noninfiltrative
Idiopathic cardiomyopathy
Familial cardiomyopathy
Hypertrophic cardiomyopathy
Scleroderma
Modified from Kushwaha S, Fallon, JT, Fuster V: Restrictive cardiomyopathy, *N Engl J Med* 336:267-276, 1997.

5. **How is cardiac amyloidosis diagnosed?**

   If the patient is not otherwise known to have amyloidosis, cardiac amyloidosis may be suggested by symptoms and signs of heart failure, an echocardiogram that demonstrates impaired filling and often thickened ventricular walls, a "sparkling" pattern on echocardiography (Fig. 28-2), and low voltage on the electrocardiogram (in spite of the thickened ventricular walls). Radionuclide imaging showing increased diffuse uptake of technetium-99m (^{99m}Tc) pyrophosphate and indium-111 (^{111}In) antimyosin in cardiac amyloidosis can also be used to make the diagnosis. The diagnosis is usually confirmed, if necessary, by biopsy.

6. **What are the main cardiac manifestations of sarcoidosis?**

   Sarcoidosis can lead to noncaseating granulomas infiltrating the myocardium, leading to fibrosis and scar formation. Infiltration may be patchy throughout the myocardium. Myocardial radionuclide imaging with thallium demonstrates patchy abnormal uptake in the affected segments. Myocardial infiltration can lead to congestive heart failure, heart block and syncope (as a result of infiltration of the conduction system), and ventricular arrhythmias (including syncope and sudden death). Pulmonary involvement may lead to pulmonary hypertension and its associated effects on right-sided heart function.

7. **Is endomyocardial biopsy useful in cases of suspected restrictive cardiomyopathy?**

   Endomyocardial biopsy is considered *reasonable* in the setting of heart failure associated with unexplained restrictive cardiomyopathy (it is a class IIa, level-of-evidence C, recommendation in the scientific statement on endomyocardial biopsy by the American College of Cardiology/American Heart Association/European Society of Cardiology [ACC/AHA/ESC]). Endomyocardial biopsy may reveal specific disorders, such as amyloidosis or hemochromatosis, or myocardial fibrosis and myocyte

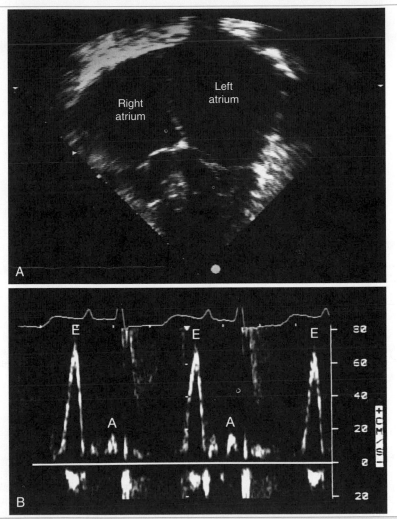

Figure 28-1. Echocardiogram of a patient with familial restrictive cardiomyopathy. **A,** Apical 4-chamber view with dilated atria and normal ventricles. **B,** Mitral inflow pattern showing augmented early filling E waves *(E)* with shortened deceleration time and attenuated A waves *(A)* with minimal respiratory variation in velocity. (Modified from Schwartz ML, Colan SD: Familial restrictive cardiomyopathy with skeletal abnormalities. *Am J Cardiol* 92:636-639, 2003.)

hypertrophy consistent with idiopathic restrictive cardiomyopathy. Endomyocardial biopsy should not be performed if computed tomography (CT) or magnetic resonance imaging (MRI) suggests the patient instead has pericardial constriction or if other less invasive tests and studies can identify a specific cause of the restrictive cardiomyopathy.

8. **Is cardiac CT or cardiac MRI useful in cases of possible restrictive cardiomyopathy?**
Both cardiac CT and cardiac MRI can be useful in cases of restrictive cardiomyopathy. Both imaging modalities can demonstrate a thickened pericardium, which may suggest constrictive pericarditis as

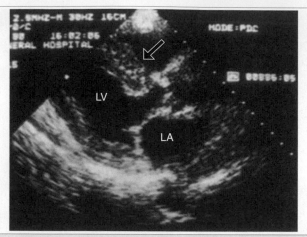

Figure 28-2. Echocardiogram demonstrating the *sparkling* pattern that can be seen in patients with cardiac amyloidosis. This sparkling pattern is best seen in this picture in the thickened ventricular septum *(arrow)*. (Modified from Levine RA: Echocardiographic assessment of the cardiomyopathies. In Weyman AE: *Principles and practice of echocardiography*, ed 2, Philadelphia, 1994, Lea & Febiger, p 810.) *LA*, Left atrium; *LV*, left ventricle.

the actual cause of the patient's ailment. Cardiac MRI, with the use of delayed hyperenhancement in many cases, may demonstrate findings suggestive of sarcoidosis, eosinophilic endomyocardial disease, amyloidosis, and other causes of restrictive cardiomyopathy. Cardiac MRI can also be used to make the diagnosis of cardiac hemochromatosis. In some cases, MRI may also be used to guide endomyocardial biopsy and to assess the likelihood of obtaining diagnostic biopsy samples.

9. **What are hypereosinophilic syndrome (HES) and Löffler disease?**
   HES and Löffler (sometimes spelled "Loeffler") disease are similar (and possibly the same) diseases characterized by persistent marked eosinophilia, absence of a primary cause of eosinophilia (e.g., parasitic or allergic disease), and eosinophil-mediated end-organ damage. The most common cardiac manifestation of HES is endomyocardial fibrosis, which was first described in the 1930s by Löffler. Secondary thrombosis may contribute to ventricular cavity obliteration, and thus these conditions are sometimes referred to as "restrictive obliterative cardiomyopathies" (Fig. 28-3). The reader should be aware that there is a confusing and variable use of the terms *HES, Löffler disease, Löffler endomyocardial fibrosis,* and *endomyocardial fibrosis* throughout the literature, with some authorities believing the syndromes are related and others treating them as distinct entities.

10. **What is Gaucher disease?**
    Gaucher disease is a disease in which there is deficiency of the enzyme β-glucocerebrosidase, resulting in the accumulation of cerebroside in the heart and other organs.

11. **How does Hurler syndrome affect the heart?**
    Hurler syndrome leads to the deposition of mucopolysaccharides in the myocardium, cardiac valves, and coronary arteries.

12. **What are the clinical features of restrictive cardiomyopathy?**
    Reduced LV filling leads to reduced stroke volume resulting in low cardiac output symptoms such as fatigue and lethargy. Increased filling pressures cause pulmonary and systemic congestion and symptomatic dyspnea. On physical exam, the pulse may reflect low stroke volume with low amplitude and tachycardia. Jugular venous pulse is often elevated with prominent y descent

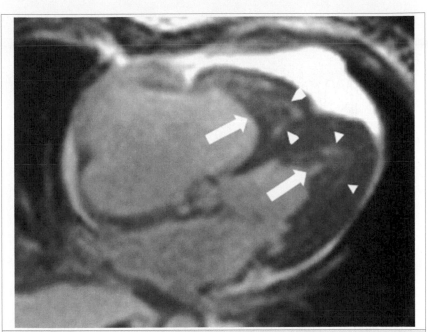

Figure 28-3. Cardiac magnetic resonance imaging demonstrating endomyocardial fibrosis and intracardiac thrombus, partially obliterating the left and right ventricles. The *long arrows* point to ventricular thrombus; the *arrow heads* demonstrate areas of endomyocardial fibrosis. (Modified with permission from Salanitri GC: Endomyocardial fibrosis and intracardiac thrombus occurring in idiopathic hypereosinophilic syndrome. *AJR Am J Roentgenol* 184:1432-1433, 2005.)

consistent with rapid early ventricular filling. Inspiratory rise in venous pressure (the Kussmaul sign) may be seen. On heart exam, S3 gallop may be heard due to abrupt cessation of rapid ventricular filling.

13. **What drugs can cause restrictive cardiomyopathy?**
    Certain drugs such as serotonin, methysergide, ergotamine, busulfan, and mercurial agents cause fibrous endocarditis, which leads to restrictive cardiomyopathy.

14. **What is the prognosis of idiopathic restrictive cardiomyopathy?**
    In a series of 94 symptomatic patients, 5-year survival was 64% (vs. 85% in age- and gender-matched controls). Adverse risk factors were male gender, age greater than 70 years, New York Heart Association (NYHA) class, and left atrial diameter greater than 6 cm.

15. **What are the treatment options for idiopathic restrictive cardiomyopathy?**
    Symptomatic treatment includes loop diuretics to treat systemic and pulmonary venous congestion. Caution should be exercised, because patients are frequently extremely sensitive to alterations in LV volume. Heart-rate lowering agents such as calcium channel blockers and beta-adrenergic blocking agents (β-blockers) may improve diastolic function by increasing diastolic filling time. Angiotensin converting enzyme (ACE) inhibitors and angiotensin receptor blockers (ARBs) counteract compensatory neurohormonal changes of heart failure as well. Digoxin increases intracellular calcium, thus worsening diastolic function, and may increase the risks of arrhythmias, and should be used with caution. The development of atrial fibrillation leads to the loss of "atrial kick" and exacerbates ventricular filling perturbations. Maintenance of sinus rhythm, if possible, is thus desirable. As stroke

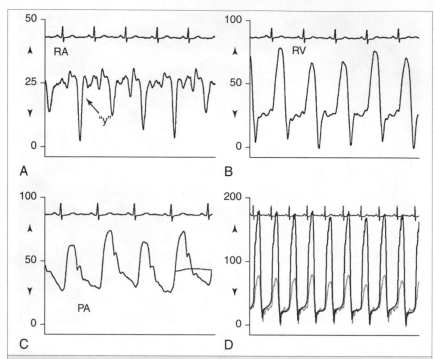

Figure 28-4. Hemodynamics obtained from right heart catheterization in a patient with restrictive cardiomyopathy. Note **A,** prominent *y* descent on the RA waveform; **B,** "square-root" sign in diastole on the RV waveform; **C,** PA systolic pressure above 50 mm Hg; and **D,** systolic concordance and lack of ventricular interdependence. (Modified from Ragosta M: Pericardial disease and restrictive cardiomyopathy. In Ragosta M, editor: *Textbook of clinical hemodynamics*, Philadelphia, 2008, Saunders, p. 144.) *PA,* Pulmonary artery; *RA,* right atrium; *RV,* right ventricle.

volume tends to be fixed, bradyarrhythmias will lead to further decreases in cardiac output, and pacing of patients with bradycardia is often indicated. In patients with intractable heart failure, cardiac transplantation should be considered.

16. **What are the hemodynamic findings on cardiac catheterization?**
It may be difficult to distinguish restrictive cardiomyopathy from constrictive pericarditis in the catheterization laboratory. The diastolic "dip-and-plateau" or "square-root sign" and prominent y descent in right atrial (RA) pressure are seen in both conditions. Features more consistent with restriction include difference in ventricular diastolic pressure greater than 5 mm Hg, pulmonary artery (PA) systolic pressure greater than 50 mm Hg, ratio of right ventricular (RV) diastolic to systolic pressure of less than 1:3, and lack of ventricular interdependence with inspiration (Fig. 28-4).

17. **What is diabetic cardiomyopathy?**
Diabetic cardiomyopathy is defined as ventricular dysfunction which occurs in diabetic patients independent of a recognized cause, such as coronary artery disease (CAD) or hypertension. Diabetics have higher LV mass, wall thickness, arterial stiffness, and increased diastolic dysfunction. Common findings on biopsy include interstitial fibrosis, myocyte hypertrophy, increase in contractile protein glycosylation and deposition of advanced glycation end products (AGEs), and collagen, all leading to ventricular wall stiffness.

BIBLIOGRAPHY, SUGGESTED READINGS, AND WEBSITES

1. Ammash NM, Tajik AJ: *Idiopathic Restrictive Cardiomyopathy*. In Basow DS, editor: UpToDate, Waltham, MA, 2013, UpToDate. Available at: http://www.uptodate.com/contents/idiopathic-restrictive-cardiomyopathy. Accessed February 8, 2013.

2. Arnold JMO: *Restrictive Cardiomyopathy*. Available at: http://www.merckmanuals.com/professional/cardiovascular_disorders/cardiomyopathies/restrictive_cardiomyopathy.html. Accessed February 8, 2013.

3. Cooper LT: *Definition and Classification of the Cardiomyopathies*. In Basow DS, editor: UpToDate, Waltham, MA, 2013, UpToDate. Available at: http://www.uptodate.com/contents/definition-and-classification-of-the-cardiomyopathies. Accessed February 8, 2013.

4. Cooper LT, Baughman K, Feldman AM, et al: AHA/ACC/ESC joint scientific statement: the role of endomyocardial biopsy in the management of cardiovascular disease, *Circulation* 116:2216–2233, 2007.

5. Hare JM: The dilated, restrictive, and infiltrative cardiomyopathies. In Libby P, Bonow RO, Mann DL, Zipes DP, editors: *Braunwald's Heart Disease: A Textbook of Cardiovascular Medicine*, ed 9, Philadelphia, 2012, Saunders, pp. 1571-1578.

6. Kushwaha SS, Fallon JT, Fuster V: Restrictive cardiomyopathy, *N Engl J Med* 335:267–276, 1997.

7. Murarka S, Movahed MR: Diabetic cardiomyopathy, *J Card Fail* 16:971–979, 2010.

8. Ragosta M: Pericardial disease and restrictive cardiomyopathy. In Ragosta M, editor: *Textbook of clinical hemodynamics*, Philadelphia, 2008, Saunders. pp. 136-146.

9. Viccellio AW: *Restrictive cardiomyopathy*. Available at: http://www.emedicine.com. Accessed February 8, 2013.

CHAPTER 29

CARDIAC TRANSPLANTATION

Kumudha Ramasubbu, MD, FACC

1. **How many heart transplantations are performed in the U.S. each year? What are the most frequent causes of heart disease requiring cardiac transplantation?**
   Dr. Christiaan Barnard performed the first human allograft transplantation in 1967. Approximately 2000 to 2200 hearts are currently transplanted each year, most commonly for nonischemic cardiomyopathy (46%) and coronary artery disease (40%), as well as for congenital heart disease, valvular heart disease, and other indications, including retransplantation.

2. **List common indications for heart transplantation.**
   - Severe heart failure (New York Heart Association [NYHA] class III or IV) with poor short-term prognosis despite maximal medical therapy, requiring continuous inotropic therapy, requiring mechanical support (e.g., balloon pump, left ventricular assist device [LVAD], extracorporeal membrane oxygenation [ECMO])
   - Restrictive or hypertrophic cardiomyopathy with NYHA class III or IV symptoms
   - Refractory angina despite medical therapy, not amenable to revascularization, with poor short-term prognosis
   - Recurrent or refractory ventricular arrhythmias, despite medical and/or device therapy
   - Complex congenital heart disease with progressive ventricular failure not amenable to surgical or percutaneous repair
   - Unresectable low-grade tumors confined to the myocardium, without evidence of metastasis

3. **What baseline evaluations are obtained in the pretransplantation workup?**
   Pretransplantation evaluation serves the purpose of assessing a patient's severity of heart failure, mortality benefit from surgery, comorbidities, and potential contraindications to surgery. Factors important in transplantation evaluation are given in Box 29-1.

4. **What are contraindications to heart transplantation?**
   Contraindications include any noncardiac conditions that may decrease a patient's survival, and increase risk of rejection or infection, and are listed in Box 29-2.

5. **Define allotransplantation versus xenotransplantation, and orthotopic versus heterotopic transplantation.**
   Allotransplantation involves transplantation of cells, tissue, or organs between *same* species *Xenotransplantation* involves transplantation of cells, tissue, or organs between *different* species. During *orthotopic heart transplantation*, the donor heart is transplanted *in place of* the recipient's heart. There are two anastomotic approaches used (Fig. 29-1).
   - **Biatrial approach:** The donor atrial cuff is anastomosed to the recipient left atrium, right atrium, followed by aortic and pulmonary artery anastomosis.
   - **Bicaval approach:** The donor left atrial cuff is anastomosed to the recipient left atrium, followed by inferior vena cava, superior vena cava, aortic, and pulmonary artery anastomosis. This approach may be associated with improved atrial function, lower incidence of atrial arrhythmias, sinus node dysfunction, and tricuspid insufficiency.
   During *heterotopic heart transplantation*, the recipient's heart is *left in the mediastinum*, and the donor heart is attached "parallel" to the recipient heart (see Fig. 29-1).

Box 29-1 FACTORS IMPORTANT IN THE EVALUATION OF PATIENTS FOR CARDIAC TRANSPLANTATION

Immunocompatibility
- ABO and human leukocyte antigen (HLA) typing
- Panel-reactive antibody (PRA) or flow-PRA

Infection
- Screen for hepatitis B & C, human immunodeficiency virus (HIV), syphilis, tuberculosis (tuberculin purified protein derivative [PPD] skin test).
- Check titers for immunoglobulin (Ig) G for herpes simplex virus (HSV), cytomegalovirus (CMV), toxoplasma, Epstein-Barr virus (EBV), and varicella.

Organ function
- Basic metabolic panel
- Complete blood count
- Liver function tests
- Prothrombin time and international normalized ratio (PT-INR)
- Urinalysis
- Glomerular filtration rate, urine proteins
- Pulmonary function test with arterial blood gas
- Posterior-anterior and lateral chest radiograph
- Abdominal ultrasound
- Carotid Doppler
- Ankle-brachial index (ABI)
- Dual energy x-ray absorptiometry (DEXA)
- Dental exam
- Ophthalmologic exam if patient has diabetes mellitus (DM)

Heart Failure (HF) Severity
- Cardiopulmonary exercise test with respiratory exchange ratio
- Echocardiogram (echo)
- Right heart catheter with vasodilator challenge (if indicated)
- Electrocardiogram (ECG)

Vaccination History
- Influenza
- Pneumococcal
- Hepatitis B

Preventive and Age-Appropriate Screening
- Colonoscopy
- Mammography
- Gynecologic examination and Pap test
- Prostate evaluation

Psychosocial Evaluation

6. **Define ischemic time of the donor heart. Why is it important?**
   The *cold ischemic time* is the time interval between removal of the donor heart and the implantation in the recipient. During this interval, ischemic injury can occur to the heart due to lack of perfusion. Myocardial preservation is achieved with hypothermia and placement of the heart in a solution mimicking intracellular milieu to prevent cellular edema and/or acidosis, and maintain ATP supply for membrane function. A prolonged ischemic time can lead to irreversible damage to the harvested

---

Box 29-2 ABSOLUTE AND RELATIVE CONTRAINDICATIONS TO HEART TRANSPLANTATION

Absolute Contraindications

- Systemic illness limiting survival despite heart transplantation (e.g., malignancy, HIV/AIDS with CD4 count <200 cells/mm^3, systemic lupus erythematosus)
- Systemic illness with high probability of recurrence in the transplanted heart (e.g., amyloidosis)
- Fixed pulmonary hypertension (pulmonary vascular resistance >5 Wood units, transpulmonary gradient >15 mm Hg) unresponsive to pulmonary vasodilators
- Presence of any noncardiac conditions that would limit life expectancy
  - ○ Irreversible hepatic disease
  - ○ Irreversible renal failure
  - ○ Severe symptomatic cerebrovascular disease
  - ○ Severe symptomatic peripheral vascular disease irremediable to surgical or percutaneous intervention
  - ○ Severe pulmonary dysfunction (FVC and FEV$_1$ <40% of predicted)

Relative Contraindications

- Age >65 years (program dependent)
- Diabetes mellitus with end organ damage
- Morbid obesity (body mass index cutoff is program dependent, typically >35)
- Psychosocial impairment (tobacco/alcohol/polysubstance abuse, psychiatric instability, noncompliance, poor social support)

AIDS, acquired immunodeficiency syndrome; *FEV$_1$*, forced expiratory volume in 1 s; *FVC*, forced vital capacity; *HIV*, human immunodeficiency virus.

---

organ. A cold ischemic time of more than 5 hours is associated with a higher incidence of cardiac allograft dysfunction and decreased transplant recipient survival.

7. **What is the estimated graft survival at 1 year, 3 years, 5 years, and 10 years posttransplantation? What are the common causes of death?**
   Based on the 2007 U.S. Organ Procurement and Transplantation Network (OPTN) and Scientific Registry of Transplant Recipients (SRTR) report, graft survival approximates 88% at 1 year, 73% at 5 years, and 50% at 10 years posttransplantation.
   The major causes of death posttransplantation are as follows:
   - **Less than 30 days:** graft failure, multiorgan failure, infection
   - **Less than 1 year:** infection, graft failure, acute allograft rejection
   - **More than 5 years:** allograft vasculopathy, late graft failure, malignancies, infection

8. **What is cardiac allograft vasculopathy (CAV)? Describe its pathophysiology, incidence, risk factors, and outcome.**
   Also known as transplant vasculopathy or transplant coronary artery disease (CAD), CAV is the progressive narrowing of the coronary arteries of the transplanted heart. Angiographic incidence of CAV is approximately 30% at 5 years and 50% at 10 years. CAV is associated with a significantly increased risk of death. After the first year posttransplantation, CAV is the second most common cause of death (after malignancy). In CAV, there is diffuse, concentric proliferation of the intimal smooth muscle cells and it typically involves the entire length of the coronary artery. In contrast, conventional atherosclerosis results from fibrofatty plaque resulting in concentric or eccentric focal lesions. The etiology of CAV remains unclear, but both immunologic (cellular and/or humoral rejection, human leukocyte antigen [HLA] mismatch) and nonimmunologic (cytomegalovirus [CMV] infection, hypercholesterolemia, older age and/or male donors,

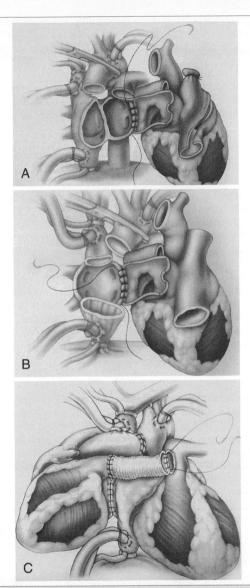

Figure 29-1. Anastomotic approaches used in cardiac transplantation. **A,** Biatrial approach. The donor atrial cuff is anastomosed to the recipient left atrium, right atrium, followed by aortic and pulmonary artery anastomosis. **B,** Bicaval approach. The donor left atrial cuff is anastomosed to the recipient left atrium, followed by inferior vena cava, superior vena cava, aortic, and pulmonary artery anastomosis. This approach may be associated with improved atrial function, lower incidence of atrial arrhythmias, sinus node dysfunction, and tricuspid insufficiency. **C,** Heterotopic transplantation. The donor-recipient left atrial cuff is anastomosed, followed by superior vena cava, aortic, and pulmonary artery anastomosis via Dacron graft. This procedure is considered in donor-recipient body-size mismatch, when the recipient pulmonary artery systolic pressure is greater than 60 mm Hg, or when there is suboptimal donor heart systolic function. (From Kirklin JK, Young JB, McGiffin DC: *Heart transplantation*, Philadelphia, 2002, Churchill Livingstone.)

younger recipients, history of CAD, diabetes mellitus [DM], and insulin resistance) factors have been implicated

Note that cardiac transplant recipients can also develop conventional atherosclerosis through two main mechanisms:

- *Progression* of preexisting donor CAD, and
- *De novo* development as a result of transplantation-related hypertension, DM, or dyslipidemia.

9. List infections that are encountered early and late after cardiac transplantation.

Early (<1 month):
- Donor-transmitted pathogens
- Nosocomial infections related to surgery or invasive procedures (mediastinitis, wound/line/ urinary tract infections, ventilator-associated pneumonia)
- Early virus reactivation (typically herpes simplex virus, human herpesvirus 6)

Intermediate (1-6 months):
- Opportunistic infections
  - ○ Bacterial (*Mycobacteria, Listeria,* and *Nocardia* organisms)
  - ○ Viral (CMV, Epstein-Barr virus [EBV], varicella zoster virus [VZV], adenovirus, papovavirus)
  - ○ Fungal (*Aspergillus, Pneumocystis,* and *Cryptococcus* organisms)
  - ○ Protozoal (*Strongyloides* and *Toxoplasma* organisms)

Late (>6 months):
- Most patients have stable graft function by this time, therefore the immunosuppressive regimen is reduced, and the risk for opportunistic infection decreases. Typically encountered infections include common viral and bacterial respiratory pathogens, however, some patients may develop chronic or recurrent opportunistic infections (i.e., CMV-related superinfection, EBV-associated lymphoproliferative disease).

10. What type of malignancies are encountered posttransplantation? List incidence, time course, and prognosis.

Malignancy risk in cardiac transplant recipients approaches 1% to 4% per year and is 10 to 100 times higher than that in age-matched controls. Malignancy is the major cause of late death in heart transplant recipients and is thought to be a result of chronic immunosuppression. The most common malignancy encountered is skin cancer (29% at 15 years). Squamous cell carcinoma is more prevalent in transplantation patients compared to basal cell cancer, which is more prevalent in the general population. Non-skin malignancies are seen in 18% of cardiac transplant recipients at 15 years (prostate, lung, bladder, renal, breast, and colon cancer).

Posttransplantation lymphoproliferative disorder (PTLD) is diagnosed in 6% of cardiac transplant recipients at 15 years. PTLD can be associated with primary or reactivated EBV infection, which leads to abnormal proliferation of lymphoid cells and can involve gastrointestinal, pulmonary, and central nervous systems; PTLD usually presents as non-Hodgkin's lymphoma (predominately B cell type). Risk of PTLD varies with allograft type, immunosuppression, EBV immunity prior to transplantation, and previous CMV infection.

11. Describe potential arrhythmias encountered posttransplantation.

The donor heart is disconnected from sympathetic and parasympathetic innervation. Therefore, the resting heart rate is higher than normal (90-110 bpm) and atropine has no effect on the denervated heart. Early posttransplantation arrhythmias can be a result of surgical trauma to the sinoatrial (SA) or atrioventricular (AV) nodes, prolonged ischemic time, surgical suture lines, and rejection. Late-occurring arrhythmias may suggest rejection or the presence of transplant vasculopathy. Potential arrhythmias encountered posttransplantation include the following:

- **Sinus node dysfunction** occurs in up to 50% of cardiac transplant recipients. Sinus node dysfunction early after transplantation does not appear to affect mortality, but has been associated with increased morbidity. Treatment of sinus bradycardia includes temporary pacing, intravenous (isoproterenol or dobutamine) or oral (theophylline or terbutaline) therapy in the immediate postoperative period. However, severe persistent bradycardia may require permanent pace-maker placement (up to 15% of patients).

- **AV nodal block** is rarely encountered; its occurrence may indicate the presence of transplant vasculopathy and has been associated with increased mortality.
- **Atrial arrhythmias:** Transient atrial arrhythmias, especially *premature atrial contractions (PACs)* are common in the early postoperative period; their clinical significance remains unclear, but frequent occurrences should prompt evaluation for rejection. *Atrial fibrillation* or *flutter* can occur in up to 25% of cardiac transplant recipients; late occurrence warrants evaluation for rejection. Treatment includes rate control with beta-adrenergic blocking agents (β-blockers), calcium channel blockers, cardioversion, overdrive pacing, and treatment for rejection. Atrial flutter can be treated with radiofrequency ablation.
- **Ventricular arrhythmias:** *Premature ventricular contractions (PVCs)* are not uncommon early after cardiac transplantation, and their clinical significance is unknown. However, nonsustained ventricular tachycardia (>3 consecutive PVCs) has been associated with rejection and transplant vasculopathy. *Sustained ventricular tachycardia* or *ventricular fibrillation* are associated with poor prognosis and indicate severe transplant vasculopathy or high-grade rejection. Treatment includes correcting electrolyte abnormalities, intravenous amiodarone or lidocaine, defibrillation, and prompt evaluation for rejection and transplant vasculopathy.

12. **What are the clinical signs and symptoms associated with acute cardiac transplant rejection (allograft rejection)?**
Around 40% to 70% of cardiac transplant recipients experience rejection within the first year posttransplantation. Most episodes occur in the first 6 months, with a decrease in frequency after 12 months. Acute allograft rejection is the leading cause of death in the first year after transplantation; this emphasizes the importance of early diagnosis and treatment. The majority of patients are asymptomatic early in the course of rejection; therefore, routine biopsies are necessary to assist in the diagnosis of rejection.

The clinical presentation of rejection can be variable. Patients may present with nonspecific constitutional symptoms such as fever, malaise, fatigue, myalgias, joint pain, and flu-like symptoms. Signs and symptoms of LV and RV dysfunction including severe fatigue, loss of energy, listlessness, weight gain, sudden onset of dyspnea, syncope/presyncope, orthopnea/paroxysmal nocturnal dyspnea, and/or abdominal bloating/nausea/vomiting. Physical exam can reveal elevated jugular venous pulse, peripheral edema, hepatomegaly, S3 or S4 gallop, and lower than usual blood pressure. Signs of cardiac irritation may include sinus tachycardia, bradycardia, arrhythmias, pericardial friction rub, or new pericardial effusion by echo.

13. **List the different types of acute allograft rejection.**
Allograft rejection occurs as a result of recipient immune response to donor heart antigens.
- **Hyperacute rejection** occurs within minutes to hours of transplantation due to *preformed* recipient antibodies against donor ABO, HLA, and endothelial cell antigens. Hyperacute rejection often results in loss of the graft.
- **Cellular rejection** is a T lymphocyte predominant, mononuclear inflammatory response directed against the allograft.
- **Noncellular or humoral/antibody-mediated rejection** is the result of de novo antibodies formed by the donor against recipient HLA antigens expressed on the vascular endothelium of the graft. Complement-mediated cytokine release leads to microvascular damage to the donor heart.

14. **Describe the grading and immunohistologic findings of acute cellular rejection (ACR) and acute antibody-mediated rejection (AMR).**
The Standardized Biopsy Grading system for ACR and AMR was established in 1990 (later revised in 2004) by the International Society for Heart and Lung Transplantation (ISHLT):
- The rejection grades and corresponding histologic findings for ACR are presented in Table 29-1.
- The rejection grades and corresponding histologic findings for AMR are presented in Table 29-2.

TABLE 29-1. ACUTE CELLULAR REJECTION (ACR)	
Rejection Grade	**Histologic Findings**
Grade 0R	No rejection
Grade 1R, mild	Interstitial and/or perivascular infiltrate with ≤1 focus of myocyte damage
Grade 2R, moderate	≥2 Foci of infiltrate with associated myocyte damage
Grade 3R, severe	Diffuse infiltrate with multifocal myocyte damage, ± edema, hemorrhage, or vasculitis

TABLE 29-2. ACUTE ANTIBODY-MEDIATED REJECTION (AMR)	
Rejection Grade	**Histologic Findings**
AMR 0	Negative for acute AMR No histologic or immunopathologic features of AMR
AMR 1	Positive for AMR Histologic* features of AMR Positive immunofluorescence/immunoperoxidase[†] staining (+CD68, C4d)

*Histologic features of AMR: myocardial capillary injury with endothelial swelling and accumulation of perivascular macrophage.
[†]Immunohistochemistry shows deposition of immunoglobulin (IgG, M, A), complement (C3d, C4d, C1q), and CD68 staining for macrophage in capillaries (using CD31 or CD34 vascular markers).

15. **How is allograft rejection diagnosed?**
    - **Echocardiogram** may reveal increased ventricular wall thickness due to edema, alterations in diastolic function (decreased early diastolic filling velocity [Ea], pseudonormal and/or restrictive filling pattern, shortened isovolumic relaxation time), decreased systolic function, and pericardial effusion.
    - **Endomyocardial biopsy (EMB)** remains the gold standard for the diagnosis of allograft rejection. *ACR* is characterized by lymphocytic infiltration and myocyte damage. *AMR* is supported by findings of myocardial capillary injury with intravascular macrophages; immunologic staining will identify antibody and complement deposits within capillaries.
    - **Rejection is a clinical event.** Even if biopsies do not support rejection, treatment can still be initiated on the basis of symptoms.

16. **How is an EMB performed and what are potential complications?**
    During the first year posttransplantation, scheduled surveillance biopsies are performed. After the first year, the need for a biopsy is dictated by clinical suspicion for rejection. A sheath is placed into the right internal jugular vein or femoral vein, and a flexible bioptome is introduced via the sheath and advanced into the right ventricle by fluoroscopic guidance. Three to four samples are obtained, preferably from the interventricular septum.
    Potential complications of biopsies include:
    - Tricuspid valve or subvalvular damage, and chordal rupture can occur, resulting in flail leaflets and severe regurgitation
    - Right ventricular wall perforation resulting in cardiac tamponade

- Transient heart block and ventricular arrhythmia
- Complications associated with venous access that include hematomas, nerve paresis, pneumothorax, thrombosis, and thromboembolism

17. What is induction therapy? Describe its role in cardiac transplantation.

Induction therapy involves use of cytolytic antilymphocyte antibodies to suppress donor immune response, which is most vigorous shortly after transplantation. Induction agents have not consistently been shown to decrease rates of rejection and have been associated with increased risk of infection and malignancy. However, induction therapy is beneficial in certain situations.

- Steroid-refractory, recurrent rejection
- Inability to use calcineurin inhibitors in setting of profound renal insufficiency in the immediate postoperative period. Antilymphocyte antibodies can provide immunosuppression for at least 10 to 14 days, until recovery of renal function (Table 29-3).

18. What is the incidence of ACR? Describe predisposing factors and treatment.

Approximately 40% of cardiac transplant recipients have ACR (grade >1R) in the first year after transplantation. Rejection frequency declines after the first year posttransplantation. Risk factors for ACR include early posttransplantation period; female donor; young, African American, or female recipients; and HLA mismatches. Treatment generally consists of high-dose corticosteroids, antithymocyte globulin (ATG), or muromonab-CD3 (OKT3) (Table 29-4).

19. Describe predisposing risk factors and treatment for AMR?

AMR has a worse prognosis than ACR, with higher rates of mortality, graft loss, and incidence of transplant vasculopathy. Predisposing factors for AMR include prior cardiac transplantation, transfusion, pregnancy (exposure to husband's HLA through the fetus), ventricular assist device placement (which can result in prominent B cell activation and production of anti-HLA antibodies), CMV infection, and prior muromonab-CD3 therapy. AMR treatment has not been standardized. Therapies currently include high dose corticosteroids, plasmapheresis, intravenous immunoglobulins, rituximab, antilymphocyte antibodies (ATG or muromonab-CD3), intravenous heparin, target of rapamycin (TOR) inhibitors, cyclophosphamide, and photopheresis. Active CMV infection has been associated with AMR. Thus, patients with AMR should be evaluated for de novo or reactivation of CMV infection, and treated if infection is present.

20. Describe typical maintenance immunosuppression therapy.

The goal of maintenance immunosuppression is to suppress the recipient immune system from rejecting the transplanted heart. This "triple therapy" regimen consists of:

- Calcineurin inhibitors: cyclosporine or tacrolimus
- Antimetabolites or cell cycle modulators: mycophenolate mofetil (MMF) or azathioprine
- Corticosteroids

Approximately 60% of cardiac transplant recipients will not require long-term steroid use. Steroid withdrawal may be attempted after 1 year posttransplantation in patients without episodes of rejection. Newer agents include the TOR inhibitors (sirolimus, everolimus). Currently, the TOR inhibitors are not used as part of the standard maintenance therapy but are added in patients with accelerated transplant vasculopathy, worsening renal function on calcineurin inhibitors, and frequent rejections on standard triple maintenance therapy. Note that mycophenolate mofetil (MMF) or azathioprine are stopped when sirolimus or everolimus are added, to avoid excessive immunosuppression (Table 29-5).

21. What are common medical conditions encountered in posttransplantation patients?

- **Hypertension:** attributed to sympathetic stimulation, neurohormonal activation, renal vasoconstriction by calcineurin inhibitors and mineralocorticoid effect of steroids)

TABLE 29-3. INDUCTION AGENTS

Agent	Mechanism of Action	Adverse Effects	Therapeutic Target	Indications for Use
Polyclonal Antibodies*				
Antithymocyte globulin (ATG)	Inhibits T cell activation and B cell proliferation. Depletes T cells and B cells.	Serum sickness, infection (especially CMV), rash, thrombocytopenia, leukopenia, anaphylaxis	T cell to <10% of pretreatment level	a) Induction therapy b) Rejection grade >2R + symptoms/ hemodynamic compromise c) Steroid-refractory or recurrent rejection
Monoclonal Antibodies†				
Muromonab-CD3 (OKT3)	Inhibits T cell activation and B cell proliferation. Depletes T cells.	Cytokine release results in flu-like symptoms. Shock or anaphylaxis rarely occurs. Antimurine Ab production, increased infection, and PTLD risks	Target CD3+ cells to <10 cells/mL & <5% of total lymphocytes	a) Induction therapy b) Rejection grade >2R + symptoms/ hemodynamic compromise c) Steroid-refractory or recurrent rejection
Daclizumab (IL-2 receptor blocker)	Inhibits T and B cell proliferation.	Severe, acute hypersensitivity reaction		Induction therapy
Basiliximab (IL-2 receptor blocker)	Inhibits T and B cell proliferation.	Severe, acute hypersensitivity reaction		Induction therapy (shorter half-life of 7 d)

Ab, antibody; *CMV*, cytomegalovirus; *IL*, interleukin; *PTLD*, posttransplantation lymphoproliferative disorder.
*Derived from animals immunized with human thymocytes, cultured B cells.
†Genetically engineered from animal cells, typically mice.

- **Renal impairment:** as a result of low cardiac output pretransplantation, ischemic injury during transplantation, and calcineurin-related renal arteriolar vasoconstriction and tubulointerstitial fibrosis)
- **Dyslipidemia:** as a result of weight gain, corticosteroid, and cyclosporine use
- **Diabetes:** as a result of corticosteroid use, weight gain
- **Osteoporosis:** due to corticosteroid use
- **Gout:** hyperuricemia from decreased uric acid clearance with cyclosporine use

22. **Describe adverse effects encountered with calcineurin inhibitor use and potential drug interactions that may lead to calcineurin toxicity.**
    - **Hypertension:** greater than 70% by 1 year and 95% by 5 years after transplantation

TABLE 29-4. ACUTE CELLULAR REJECTION THERAPIES

Rejection Grade	Therapy
1R	No treatment
1R + sx/hemodynamic compromise	IV steroids followed by oral taper, repeat biopsy in 1 week
2R	High dose oral or IV steroids
2R + sx/hemodynamic compromise	IV steroids followed by taper, repeat biopsy in 1 week ATG or muromonab-CD3 if persistent rejection despite 2 courses of steroid therapy
3R	ATG or muromonab-CD3, repeat biopsy after course and again in 1 week
Recalcitrant rejection	Photopheresis, total lymphoid radiation

ATG, Antithymocyte globulin; *sx*, symptoms.

TABLE 29-5. MAINTENANCE IMMUNOSUPPRESSION

Agent	Mechanism of Action	Adverse Effects	Therapeutic Target (ng/mL)	Indications for Use
Calcineurin Inhibitors				
Cyclosporine	Inhibits IL-2 production, B cell proliferation.	Nephrotoxicity, HTN, dyslipidemia, hepatotoxicity, hirsutism, gingival hyperplasia, hyperuricemia, neurotoxicity, hyperkalemia, acidosis. Potential nephrotoxicity with aminoglycoside, amphotericin, NSAID, trimethoprim-sulfamethoxazole, sirolimus use. Metabolized by hepatic cytochrome P-450; therefore, monitor for potential drug interactions.	0-6 mo: 250-350 6-12 mo: 200-250 >12 mo: 100-200	Maintenance immunosuppression
Tacrolimus	Inhibits IL-2 production, B cell proliferation.	Nephrotoxicity, headache, tremor, glucose intolerance, hyperkalemia	0-6 mo: 12-15 6-12 mo: 8-12 >12 mo: 5-10	a) Alternative to cyclosporine as maintenance immunosuppression b) "Rescue" agent with recurrent rejection on cyclosporine

continued

TABLE 29-5. MAINTENANCE IMMUNOSUPPRESSION—cont'd

Agent	Mechanism of Action	Adverse Effects	Therapeutic Target (ng/mL)	Indications for Use
Antimetabolites				
MMF	Inhibits purine synthesis, B cell, and smooth muscle proliferation.	Gastrointestinal complaints (nausea, vomiting, diarrhea), and rarely leukopenia. Should be administered on an empty stomach (antacids decrease enteric absorption).	Blood levels not routinely monitored (2-5).	Maintenance immunosuppression
Azathioprine	Inhibits purine synthesis, B cell proliferation.	Bone marrow suppression, hepatotoxicity, pancreatitis, alopecia, cutaneous malignancies with chronic use. Allopurinol interferes with azathioprine metabolism; thus, potentiates myelosuppression.	Blood levels not monitored.	Maintenance immunosuppression
Other				
Corticosteroids	Inhibits T cell activation, B and T cell proliferation.	DM, impaired wound healing, HTN, peptic ulcer, obesity, avascular necrosis, osteoporosis, cataract, and psychosis	Blood levels not monitored.	Maintenance therapy and pulse therapy for acute rejection
Inhibitors of Target of Rapamycin (TOR)*				
Sirolimus (rapamycin) and everolimus	Inhibits G1-S of cell cycle progression, B and T cell, smooth muscle proliferation.	Thrombocytopenia, dyslipidemia, anemia, RI, and impaired wound healing	5-20	a) Can be used with lower dose of calcineurin inhibitor in calcineurin-related RI b) Alternative to antimetabolites in accelerated transplant vasculopathy c) Everolimus has been approved for use in Europe, but not in the US.

DM, diabetes mellitus; *HTN*, hypertension; *IL*, interleukin; *MMF*, mycophenolate mofetil; *mo*, month; *NSAID*, nonsteroidal antiinflammatory drug; *RI*, renal insufficiency.
*Not part of routine maintenance therapy. TOR inhibitors are added in certain situations (see text).

- **Renal dysfunction:** greater than 25% by 1 year and 5% progress to end-stage renal disease within 7 years after transplantation
- **Rhabdomyolysis** when used concurrently with HMG-CoA reductase inhibitors (statins), because calcineurin inhibitors inhibit metabolism of certain statins (lovastatin, simvastatin, cerivastatin, and atorvastatin). Fluvastatin, pravastatin, and rosuvastatin are less likely to be involved in this type of interaction.
- **Calcineurin toxicity** is characterized by neurologic symptoms (headaches, tremor, confusion, agitation, delirium, expressive aphasia, and seizures), nephrotoxicity, and hypertension. The enzyme CYP3A4 metabolizes calcineurin inhibitors, and inhibitors of CYP3A4 can lead to increased drug levels and adverse effects. CYP3A4 inhibitors include:
  - Azole antifungal agents (ketoconazole, itraconazole)
  - Macrolide antibiotics (erythromycin, clarithromycin)
  - Grapefruit juice
  - Nondihydropyridine calcium antagonists (diltiazem, verapamil)
  - Dihydropyridine calcium channel blockers (nicardipine, nifedipine); amlodipine has minimal effect on CYP3A4.

23. **How do patients with transplant vasculopathy clinically present? What invasive and noninvasive tests are used to assist in the diagnosis of transplant vasculopathy?**
Because transplanted hearts are denervated, cardiac transplant recipients typically do not present with angina when they develop transplant vasculopathy. Clinical manifestations include silent myocardial infarctions, symptoms of heart failure, syncope, sudden cardiac death, and arrhythmias.
   - **Coronary angiography:** Most centers have adopted surveillance angiographies for early diagnosis of CAV. However, CAV is often diffuse and concentric in its distribution and may be underestimated by angiography. To improve detection and sensitivity, intravascular ultrasound, and/or quantitative coronary angiography are used as adjunctive modalities.
   - **Noninvasive stress testing:** Dobutamine stress echo or myocardial perfusion imaging can be used to diagnose CAV, but have a lower sensitivity when compared to angiography. To avoid contrast-induced nephropathy, noninvasive stress testing is used in patients with renal insufficiency.

24. **Describe strategies to prevent and treat cardiac allograft vasculopathy.**
Although no effective preventive strategy for CAV has been identified, several factors have been associated with a lower incidence of CAV.
   - Lipid-lowering therapy (pravastatin has fewer drug interactions and is better tolerated than other statins)
   - TOR inhibitors (may decrease CAV incidence)
   - Blood pressure control (diltiazem may also limit intimal thickening)
Treatment of cardiac allograft vasculopathy may include the following:
   - Percutaneous and surgical revascularization have limited role in the setting of diffuse vasculopathy.
   - Retransplantation is the only definitive therapy.
   - Immunosuppression regimen adjustment and trial of TOR inhibitor may be attempted.

25. **When should mechanical circulatory support device (MCSD) implantation be considered?**
A limited number of donor hearts and an increasing number of patients with NYHA class IV symptoms have created a demand for alternative treatments for end-stage heart failure. One strategy is the implantation of an MCSD or left ventricular assist device (LVAD).
   Indications for LVAD implantation include:
   - An attempt to extend life in a deteriorating transplantation candidate who is listed for a donor heart (bridge-to-transplant)

- In patients with multiorgan failure, an LVAD may help determine transplantation eligibility. If pulmonary hypertension or renal insufficiency improves after LVAD, a heart transplantation would be more likely of benefit (bridge-to-decision).
- Support for patients whose surgery is complicated by cardiogenic shock
- Permanent support for patients who are not transplantation candidates (destination therapy)

26. What is gene expression profiling (GEP) and how is it used in the diagnosis of rejection?

GEP evaluates the transcription of genes involved in acute rejection and myocardial injury. GEP is performed on peripheral blood analysis. The AlloMap score (XDx, Inc., Brisbane, Calif.) uses GEP to grade the risk of presence of rejection. The AlloMap score has been shown to have a high negative predictive value for lower scores, but the positive predictive value for high scores is low. Thus, the use of AlloMap is recommended only in select patients: to rule out the presence of ACR of grade 2R or greater in low-risk patients, between 6 months and 5 years after cardiac transplantation.

BIBLIOGRAPHY, SUGGESTED READINGS, AND WEBSITES

1. Department of Transplantation Immunology, University of Heidelberg: Collaborative Transplant Study website. Available at: www.ctstransplant.org. Accessed May 1, 2012.

2. Eisen HJ: Immunosuppression on the horizon, *Heart Fail Clin* 3:43–49, 2007.

3. The International Society for Heart and Lung Transplantation: ISHLT website. Available at: www.ishlt.org. Accessed May 1, 2012.

4. Jessup M, Banner N, Brozena S, et al: Optimal pharmacologic and non-pharmacologic management of cardiac transplant candidates: approaches to be considered prior to transplant evaluation: International Society for Heart and Lung Transplantation guidelines for the care of cardiac transplant candidates—2006, *J Heart Lung Transplant* 25:1003–1023, 2006.

5. The Journal of Heat and Lung Transplantation: JHLT website. Available at: www.jhltonline.org. Accessed May 1, 2012.

6. Kirklin JK, Young JB, McGiffin DC: *Heart transplantation*, Philadelphia, 2002, Churchill Livingstone.

7. Kobashigawa JA: Contemporary concepts in noncellular rejection, *Heart Fail Clin* 3:11–15, 2007.

8. OPTN/SRTR: 2009 U.S. Organ Procurement and Transplantation Network (OPTN) and the Scientific Registry of Transplant Recipients (SRTR) Annual Report: Transplant Data 1999-2008. Available at: http://optn.transplant.hrsa.gov/ar2009/default.htm. Accessed May 1, 2012.

9. Sipahi I, Starling RC: Cardiac allograft vasculopathy: an update, *Heart Fail Clin* 3:87–95, 2007.

10. Steinman TI, Becker BN, Frost AE, et al: Guidelines for the referral and management of patients eligible for solid organ transplantation, *Transplantation* 71:1189–1204, 2001.

11. Stewart S, Winters GL, Fishbein MC, et al: Revision of the 1990 working formulation for the standardization of nomenclature in the diagnosis of heart rejection, *J Heart Lung Transplant* 24:1710–1720, 2005.

12. Stehlik J, Edwards LB, Kucheryavaya AY, et al: The Registry of the International Society of Heart and Lung Transplantation: Twenty-eighth official adult heart transplant report—2011, *J Heart Lung Transplant* 30:1078–1094, 2011.

13. United Network for Organ Sharing: UNOS website. Available at: www.unos.org. Accessed May 1, 2012.

AORTIC VALVE DISEASE

Blase A. Carabello, MD, FACC

1. What is the most common cause of aortic stenosis (AS) in developed countries today, and what is the current thinking about its pathogenesis?

Although rheumatic fever was once the most common cause of AS, today calcific disease of either bicuspid or tricuspid AS is the leading cause. Once considered a degenerative disease, it is now clear that calcific AS is an inflammatory process with many similarities to atherosclerosis. A normal aortic valve, and AS as a result of congenital bicuspid aortic valve, rheumatic AS, and calcific AS, are shown in Figure 30-1.

2. What is the pathophysiology of AS, and what effect does it have on the left ventricle (LV)?

AS exerts a pressure overload on the LV. Normally, pressure in the LV and aorta are similar during systole, as the normal aortic valve permits free flow of blood from LV to aorta. However, in AS, the stenotic valve forces the LV to generate higher pressure to drive blood through the stenosis, causing a pressure difference (gradient) from LV to aorta. The LV compensates for this pressure overload by

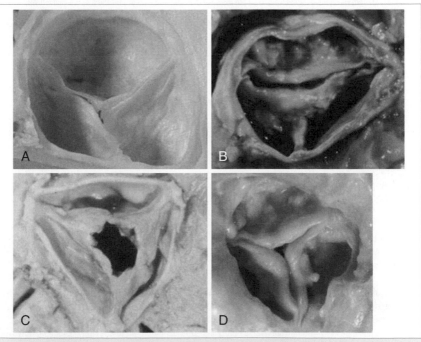

Figure 30-1. Normal and stenotic aortic valves. **A,** Normal aortic valve. **B,** Congenital bicuspid aortic stenosis. A false raphe is present at 6 o'clock. **C,** Rheumatic aortic stenosis. The commissures are fused with a fixed central orifice. **D,** Calcific degenerative aortic stenosis. (From Libby P, Bonow RO, Mann DL, Zipes DP: *Braunwald's heart disease: a textbook of cardiovascular medicine,* ed 8, Philadelphia, 2008, Saunders.)

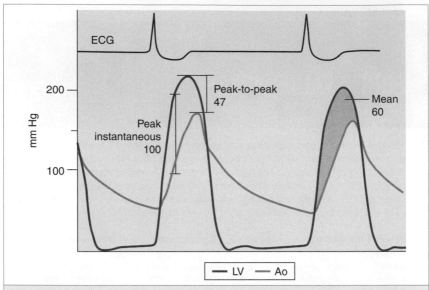

Figure 30-2. Various methods of describing an aortic transvalvular gradient. The figure shows representative pressure tracings measured during cardiac catheterization in a patient with aortic stenosis. One pressure transducer is placed in the left ventricle and a second pressure transducer is positioned in the ascending aorta. The peak-to-peak gradient (47 mm Hg) is the difference between the maximal pressure in the aorta *(Ao)* and the maximal left ventricle *(LV)* pressure. The peak instantaneous gradient (100 mm Hg) is the maximal pressure difference between the Ao and LV when the pressures are measured in the same moment (usually during early systole). The mean gradient *(shaded area)* is the integral of the pressure difference between the LV and Ao during systole (60 mm Hg). (From Bashore TM: *Invasive cardiology: principles and techniques*, Philadelphia, 1990, BC Decker, p. 258.) *ECG,* Electrocardiogram.

increasing its mass (left ventricular hypertrophy [LVH]). The ways in which the transvalvular gradient are measured and quantified are shown in Figure 30-2.

3. How is left ventricular hypertrophy compensatory?
The Law of Laplace states that systolic wall stress (σ) is equal to:

$$(pressure\ (p) \times radius\ (r))/2 \times thickness\ (h),\ or\ \sigma = p \times r/2h$$

As the pressure term in the numerator increases, it is offset by an increase in thickness in the denominator, thus normalizing afterload. Because afterload is a key determinant of ejection, LVH helps to maintain ejection fraction and cardiac output.

4. Are there downsides to LVH?
Yes. Although LVH is initially compensatory, as it progresses it takes on pathologic characteristics, leading to increased morbidity and mortality.

5. What are the classic symptoms of AS, and why are they important?
The classic symptoms of AS are angina and syncope and those of heart failure (dyspnea, orthopnea, paroxysmal nocturnal dyspnea, edema, etc.). Their importance is graphically displayed in Figure 30-3. In the absence of symptoms, survival is nearly the same as that of an unaffected population. However, at the onset of symptoms there is a dramatic demarcation such that mortality increases to 2% per month, so that three-quarters of all AS patients are dead within 3 years of symptom onset unless proper therapy is instituted. It should be noted that when the data for this figure were compiled, the etiology of AS was usually rheumatic or congenital heart disease and the average age of the

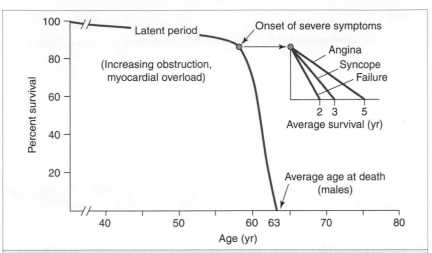

Figure 30-3. The natural history of medically treated aortic stenosis. Once symptoms develop in a patient with aortic stenosis, the average survival with medical treatment (e.g., no curative surgery) is only 2 to 5 years. (From Townsend CM Jr, Beauchamp RD, Evers BM, Mattox KL: *Sabiston textbook of surgery: the biological basis of modern surgical practice*, ed 18, Philadelphia, 2008, Saunders.)

patients was 48 years. Since then the etiology of AS has changed (as noted above) and with it the age at symptom onset has increased by about 15 years.

6. **What are findings of AS on physical examination?**
AS is usually recognized by the presence of a harsh systolic ejection murmur that radiates to the neck. In mild disease, the murmur peaks in intensity early in systole, peaking progressively later as severity of disease increases. The carotid upstrokes become delayed in timing and reduced in volume because the stenotic valve steals energy from the flow of blood as it passes the valve. The apical beat is forceful. Palpation of this strong apical beat with one examining hand while the other hand palpates the weakened delayed carotid upstroke is dynamic proof of the obstruction that exists between the LV and the systemic circulation. Because the severely stenotic aortic valve barely opens, there is little valve movement upon closing. Thus, the A2 component of S2 is lost, rendering a soft single second sound. An S4 is usually present in patients in sinus rhythm, reflecting impaired filling of the thickened, noncompliant LV.

7. **How is echocardiography used to assess the patient with AS?**
Currently, echocardiography is the central tool in diagnosing the presence and severity of AS. In severe AS, the aortic valve is calcified and has limited mobility. The amount of LVH and the presence or absence of LV dysfunction can be established. Because

$$flow = area \times velocity$$

as the valve area decreases, velocity of flow must increase for flow to remain constant (Fig. 30-4). This increase in blood velocity at the valve orifice is detected by Doppler ultrasound. The severity of AS is assessed using the factors given in Table 30-1. In general, if a patient has the symptoms of AS and assessment indicates severe disease, then the symptoms are attributed to AS. However, it must be emphasized that the benchmarks listed here are only guidelines to severity, and some patients exhibit exceptions to them.

8. **What other tests are useful in assessing AS?**
As noted earlier, the presence or absence of symptoms is a key determinant of outcome, yet in some patients an accurate history may be difficult to obtain. In such cases, more objective evidence of cardiac

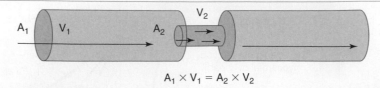

Figure 30-4. Determination of aortic valve area using the continuity equation. For blood flow ($A_1 \times V_1$) to remain constant when it reaches a stenosis (A_2), velocity must increase to V_2. Determination of the increased velocity V_2 by Doppler ultrasound permits calculation of both the aortic valve gradient and solution of the equation for A_2. (From Townsend CM Jr, Beauchamp RD, Evers BM, Mattox KL: *Sabiston textbook of surgery: the biological basis of modern surgical practice,* ed 18, Philadelphia, 2008, Saunders.) *A,* Area; *V,* velocity.

TABLE 30-1. ECHOCARDIOGRAPHIC CRITERIA FOR THE DEGREE OF AORTIC STENOSIS			
	Mild	**Moderate**	**Severe**
Peak jet velocity (m/s)	<3.0	3.0-4.0	>4.0
Mean gradient (mm Hg)	<25	25-40	>40
Aortic valve area (cm^2)	>1.5	1.0-1.5	<1.0
Valve area index (cm^2/m^2)			<0.6
Outflow track velocity-to-aortic valve velocity			<0.25

Modified from Bonow RO, Carabello BA, Chatterjee K, et al: ACC/AHA 2006 guidelines for the management of patients with valvular heart disease. *J Amer Coll Cardiol* 48:e1-e148, 2006.

compromise, such as exercise intolerance, may be helpful. Although exercise stress testing should *never* be performed in symptomatic AS patients, stress testing may be very helpful in establishing more objective evidence of symptomatic status when the history is unclear. As many as one-third of AS patients may become symptomatic for the first time during stress testing. This phenomenon probably indicates a previous denial of symptoms or a lifestyle altered to avoid symptoms. Such stress testing, if undertaken, should only be done with careful physician supervision.

Natriuretic peptides may also be useful in assessing the effects of AS on the heart. B-type natriuretic peptide (BNP) is released from the myocardium when sarcomere stretch increases to provide preload reserve. As such, increasing BNP indicates cardiac decompensation. Increasing BNP in AS patients is considered an ominous finding, although there is no agreement about what BNP level indicates the need for aortic valve replacement (AVR).

In some cases, the severity of AS is still uncertain following echocardiography. Cardiac catheterization to obtain invasive hemodynamics, including the transvalvular pressure gradient and cardiac output, is then used to derive the valve area (see Chapter 14).

9. **What is the therapy for AS?**
Because AS has many similarities to atherosclerosis, many have hypothesized that effective treatments for coronary disease might be able to retard the progression of AS. Although observational studies of the use of statins in AS have suggested those drugs might be effective, prospective trials have been, as yet, inconclusive.

No effective medical therapy is effective in the chronic treatment of this disease. The mainstay of therapy for this mechanical problem is mechanical relief of the obstruction, in the form of AVR. In most patients, AVR is performed surgically. However, for selected patients at prohibitive or high risk for surgical AVR, transcatheter placement of the aortic valve ("TAVI" or "TAVR") is now approved from the femoral and transapical approaches in the US (see Chapter 32, Prosthetic Heart Valves). It is almost certain that this field will evolve to have broader indications as devices become safer and easier to employ.

10. **What are the class I indications for aortic valve replacement?**
    According to the American College of Cardiology/American Heart Association (ACC/AHA) guidelines, AVR is indicated in the following situations:
    - Symptomatic patients with severe AS
    - Severe AS with LV systolic dysfunction (LV ejection fraction [LVEF] less than 50%)
    - Severe AS in patients undergoing coronary artery bypass grafting, other heart valve surgery, or thoracic aortic surgery (if AS is instead moderate, then AVR in these situations is considered a class IIa indication—*reasonable*)

11. **What is the outcome after AVR?**
    Survival of patients after AVR is dramatically improved compared with those who received only medical therapy.

12. **What are the causes of aortic regurgitation?**
    Abnormalities of either the aortic root or of the aortic valve leaflets can cause aortic regurgitation (AR). Common root abnormalities that cause AR include Marfan syndrome, annuloaortic ectasia, and aortic dissection. Leaflet abnormality causes include infective endocarditis, rheumatic heart disease, collagen vascular diseases, and previous use of anorectic drugs.

13. **What is the pathophysiology of aortic regurgitation?**
    The incompetent aortic valve allows ejected blood to return to the LV during diastole. This regurgitant volume is lost from the effective cardiac output. In turn, the LV must pump extra blood to make up for this loss; thus, AR constitutes an LV volume overload. Compensation comes from an increase in LV volume (eccentric hypertrophy). The larger LV can pump more blood to compensate for that lost to AR. Because all the stroke volume is pumped into the aorta during systole (while some leaks back into the LV during diastole), pulse pressure, which is dependent on stoke volume, widens as systolic pressure increases and diastolic pressure decreases. Thus, AR imparts not only a volume overload on the LV but also a pressure overload. Because of this second load, LV thickness in AR patients is slightly greater than normal. Increased wall thickness and the increased diastolic LV volume lead to increased LV diastolic filling pressure.

14. **What are the symptoms of aortic regurgitation?**
    Dyspnea and fatigue are the main symptoms of AR. Occasionally patients experience angina because reduced diastolic aortic pressure reduces coronary filling pressure, impairing coronary blood flow. Reduced diastolic systemic pressure may also cause syncope or presyncope.

15. **What are the findings of AR on physical examination?**
    Chronic AR produces myriad physical findings because of the large stroke volume pumped by the LV. The pulse pressure is wide. The dynamic LV apical beat is displaced downward and to the left and is often visible to an observer who is several feet away from the patient. A diastolic blowing murmur is present and is heard best along the left sternal border, with the patient sitting upward and leaning forward. A second murmur (Austin Flint) thought to be due to vibration of the mitral valve, caused by the impinging AR, is a low-pitched diastolic rumble heard toward the LV apex.
    The widened pulse pressure and high total stroke volume cause several physical signs of AR.
    - The head may bob with each heartbeat (de Musset sign).
    - Auscultation of the femoral artery may produce a sound similar to a pistol shot (pistol shot pulse).
    - If the bell of the stethoscope is compressed over the femoral artery, a to-and-fro bruit (Duroziez sign) may be heard.
    - Compression of the nailbed may demonstrate systolic plethora and diastolic blanching of the nail bed (Quincke pulse).

16. **How is the diagnosis of AR confirmed?**
    Although a chest radiograph is helpful in evaluating heart size and pulmonary congestion, echocardiography remains the mainstay of diagnosis. Cardiac size and function are evaluated using

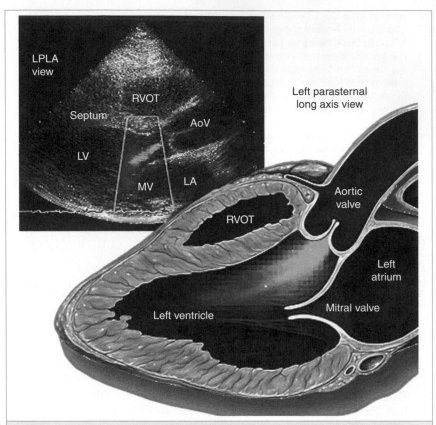

Figure 30-5. Aortic regurgitation. Left parasternal long-axis view of the heart, demonstrating aortic regurgitation seen on Doppler echocardiogram, along with the corresponding anatomic illustration. In actuality, the regurgitant jet is displayed in color, reflecting the direction of blood flow. (From Yale School of Medicine: Yale atlas of echocardiography. Available at: http://www.yale.edu/imaging/echo_atlas/entities/aortic_regurgitation.html. Accessed August 30, 2008.) *AoV*, Aortic valve; *LA*, left atrium; *LPLA*, left parasternal long axis; *LV*, left ventricle; *MV*, mitral valve; *RVOT*, right ventricular outflow tract.

this technique. Often the anatomic abnormality responsible for the patient's AR can be established. As shown in Figure 30-5, Doppler interrogation of the valve reveals the jet of blood leaking across the valve in diastole. Table 30-2 displays current criteria for establishing the severity of AR. Cardiac magnetic resonance imaging may also be useful in quantitating the magnitude of volume overload and in assessing left ventricular volume and mass.

17. **How is AR managed?**

Patients with severe AR should been seen at least once a year or more often to evaluate symptomatic status and to perform repeat echocardiograms to assess LV size and function.

AVR is indicated (ACC/AHA and European Society of Cardiology [ESC] class I recommendations) for the following patients:

- Symptomatic patients with severe AR, irrespective of LV systolic function
- Asymptomatic patients with chronic severe AR and LV systolic dysfunction (LVEF 50% or less)
- Patients with chronic severe AR who are undergoing coronary artery bypass grafting (CABG), other heart valve surgery, or thoracic aortic surgery

TABLE 30-2. CARDIAC CATHETERIZATION AND ECHOCARDIOGRAPHIC CRITERIA FOR THE DEGREE OF AORTIC REGURGITATION

	Mild	Moderate	Severe
Angiographic grade	1+	2+	3-4+
Color Doppler central jet width	<25% LVOT		>65% LVOT
Doppler vena contracta width	<0.3 cm	0.3-0.6 cm	>0.6 cm
Regurgitant volume (mL/beat)	<30 mL	30-59 mL	≥60 mL
Regurgitant fraction	<30%	30%-49%	≥50%
Regurgitant orifice area	<0.10 cm^2	0.10-0.29 cm^2	≥0.30 cm^2
LV size			Increased
Pressure half-time			<250 ms

Modified from Bonow RO, Carabello BA, Chatterjee K, et al: ACC/AHA 2006 guidelines for the management of patients with valvular heart disease. *J Amer Coll Cardiol* 48:e1-e148, 2006.
LV, Left ventricle; *LVOT,* left ventricular outflow tract.

AVR is considered reasonable (ACC/AHA and ESC class IIa recommendation) for asymptomatic patients with severe AR and with normal LV systolic function (LVEF more than 50%) but with severe LV dilation (end-diastolic dimension greater than 70-75 mm or end-systolic dimension greater than 50-55 mm).

As with AS, there is no proven medical therapy for AR, although vasodilator therapy can be considered in patients with severe AR who are not surgical candidates.

18. Is the presentation of acute AR different from that of chronic AR?
Yes, dramatically. In acute AR, there has been no time for LV dilation so that the increased forward stroke volume and widened pulse pressure that drive the dynamic examination of a patient with chronic AR are absent. Thus, the examination of a patient with severe acute AR may be misleadingly bland, belying a potentially fatal condition. Acute AR occurs most commonly in the patient with infective endocarditis. When such patients develop evidence of heart failure, AR should be suspected, even if there is only a faint murmur or no murmur at all.

BIBLIOGRAPHY, SUGGESTED READINGS, AND WEBSITES

1. Bekeredjian R, Grayburn PA: Valvular heart disease: aortic regurgitation, *Circulation* 112:125–134, 2005.
2. Bonow RO, Carabello BA, Chatterjee K, et al: ACC/AHA 2006 guidelines for the management of patients with valvular heart disease, *J Am Coll Cardiol* 48:e1–e148, 2006.
3. Carabello BA: Clinical practice. Aortic stenosis, *N Engl J Med* 346:677–682, 2002.
4. Carabello BA: Evaluation and management of patients with aortic stenosis, *Circulation* 105:1746–1750, 2002.
5. Enriquez-Sarano M, Tajik AJ: Clinical practice. Aortic regurgitation, *N Engl J Med* 351:1539–1546, 2004.
6. Gaasch WH: Course and management of chronic aortic regurgitation in adults. In Basow, DS, editor: UpToDate, Waltham, MA, 2013, UpToDate. Available at: http://www.uptodate.com/contents/course-and-management-of-chronic-aortic-regurgitation-in-adults. Accessed March 26, 2013.
7. Wang SS: Aortic regurgitation. Available at: http://www.emedicine.com. Accessed March 26, 2013.
8. Leon MB, Smith CR, Mack M, et al: Transcatheter aortic-valve implantation for aortic stenosis in patients who cannot undergo surgery, *N Engl J Med* 363:1597–1607, 2010.
9. Otto CM: Pathophysiology and clinical features of aortic stenosis in adults. In Basow, DS, editor: UpToDate, Waltham, MA, 2013, UpToDate. Available at: http://www.uptodate.com/contents/clinical-features-and-evaluation-of-aortic-stenosis-in-adults. Accessed March 26, 2013.
10. Vahanian A, Baumgartner H, Bax J, et al: Guidelines on the management of valvular heart disease: the Task Force on the Management of Valvular Heart Disease of the European Society of Cardiology, *Eur Heart J* 28:230–268, 2007.

CHAPTER 31

MITRAL STENOSIS, MITRAL REGURGITATION, AND MITRAL VALVE PROLAPSE

Blase A. Carabello, MD, FACC

1. **What is the usual cause of mitral stenosis (MS)?**

   Most cases of MS stem from previous episodes of rheumatic fever. Most cases of rheumatic heart disease are seen in patients who emigrate from areas of the world where rheumatic fever is still common, including the Middle East, Asia, and South Africa. Although the rate of rheumatic fever is similar in men and women, MS is three times more common in women than in men. However, as the population ages, mitral annular calcification is increasing as an etiology for MS.

2. **What is the pathophysiology of MS?**

   MS inhibits the normal free flow of blood from left atrium (LA) to left ventricle (LV) in diastole. Normally, diastolic LA and LV pressures equalize shortly after mitral valve opening. In MS, the stenotic valve impedes LA emptying, inducing a diastolic gradient between LA and LV (Fig. 31-1). Elevated LA pressure is referred to the lungs, where it causes pulmonary congestion. Simultaneously, impaired LA emptying reduces LV filling, limiting cardiac output. Thus, the combination of increased LA pressure and decreased cardiac output produce the syndrome of heart failure. Because increased LA pressure increases pulmonary pressure, the right ventricle (RV) becomes pressure overloaded, eventually leading to RV failure.

3. **What are the typical symptoms of MS?**

   Patients with mild disease are likely to be asymptomatic. As MS worsens, dyspnea appears, as does orthopnea and paroxysmal nocturnal dyspnea. If RV failure ensues, it may be accompanied by edema and ascites. During exercise, sudden increases in LA pressure and pulmonary venous pressure may cause rupture of anastomoses between pulmonary and systemic veins, leading to hemoptysis.

4. **What are the signs of MS at physical examination?**

   The gradient across the mitral valve holds the valve open throughout diastole, so that when it closes, S1 may be quite loud. The murmur of MS is a soft diastolic rumble heard near the apex. The murmur is often preceded by an opening snap, caused by sudden opening of the stiffened mitral valve from higher than normal atrial pressure. If pulmonary hypertension has developed, P2 is increased in intensity. If RV failure has occurred, elevated neck veins, ascites, and edema are likely to be present.

5. **How is the diagnosis of MS made?**

   The chest radiograph used to be at the forefront of diagnosis and still can be helpful today. It demonstrates an enlarged LA, seen as a double shadow along the right-sided heart border. Thickened lymphatics from high pulmonary venous pressure are seen as Kerley lines. The pulmonary artery (PA) is usually enlarged.

   Today, however, the echocardiogram is key to the diagnosis because it images the mitral valve so well. The valve is thickened and there is impaired opening of the mitral leaflets (Fig. 31-2). The LA is almost always enlarged. Valve area can be determined from direct visualization and planimetry of the mitral orifice, from Doppler assessment of the transvalvular gradient, and from measuring the delay in LA emptying. Pulmonary pressure, LV function, and RV function are also evaluated. In general, the main criteria for severe MS follow below. The severity of MS is estimated using the criteria given in Table 31-1.
   - Mean gradient more than 10 mm Hg
   - Valve area less than 1.0 cm^2
   - PA systolic pressure greater than 50 mm Hg

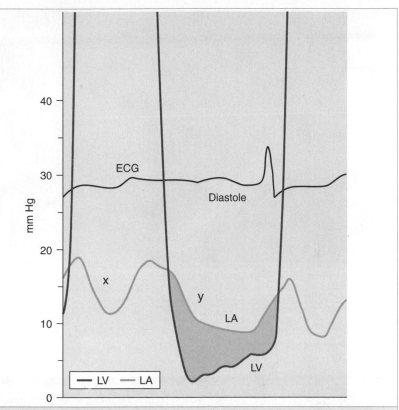

Figure 31-1. Pressure gradient in a patient with mitral stenosis. The pressure in the left atrium *(LA)* exceeds the pressure in the left ventricle *(LV)* during diastole, producing a diastolic pressure gradient *(shaded area)*. (Modified from Bashore TM: *Invasive cardiology: principles and techniques,* Philadelphia, 1990, BC Decker, p. 264.) *ECG,* Electrocardiogram.

6. **Is there effective medical management for MS?**
   Yes. Patients with mild symptoms and normal PA pressure can be treated with diuretics to reduce LA pressure and relieve pulmonary congestion. The combination of LA enlargement and continued inflammation from a smoldering rheumatic process predisposes patients with MS to develop atrial fibrillation (AF). AF with rapid heart rate affects the MS patient gravely because it diminishes transit time for blood flow from LA to LV, further increasing LA pressure and diminishing cardiac output. Rate control with beta-adrenergic blocking agents (β-blockers), calcium channel blockers, or digoxin is imperative. If these agents fail to control heart rate, cardioversion is indicated. Once AF has developed in the MS patient, the risk of stroke approaches 10% per year. Thus, anticoagulation to an international normalized ratio (INR) of 2.5 to 3.5 is mandatory unless a grave contraindication exists.

7. **What is the definitive management for severe MS?**
   If symptoms cannot be controlled easily medically or if asymptomatic pulmonary hypertension develops, this mechanical lesion must be treated by mechanical relief of the stenosis, because either condition worsens MS prognosis. In most cases, mitral balloon valvotomy is the preferred therapy. In

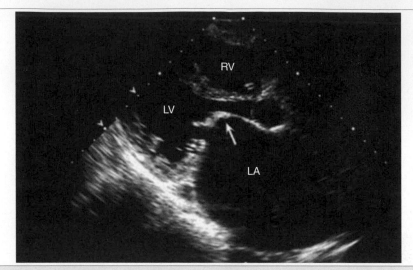

Figure 31-2. Two-dimensional echocardiogram of the parasternal long-axis view during diastole of a patient with mitral stenosis. The mitral valve leaflets are thickened and have the typical hockey-stick appearance *(arrow)*. Note also that the left atrium *(LA)* is enlarged. *LV,* Left ventricle; *RV,* right ventricle. (Modified from Libby P, Bonow RO, Mann DL, Zipes DP: *Braunwald's heart disease: a textbook of cardiovascular medicine,* ed 8, Philadelphia, 2008, Saunders.)

TABLE 31-1. ECHOCARDIOGRAPHIC CRITERIA FOR THE ASSESSMENT OF THE SEVERITY OF MITRAL STENOSIS

	Mild	Moderate	Severe
Mean gradient	<5 mm Hg	5-10 mm Hg	>10 mm Hg
PA systolic pressure	<30 mm Hg	30-50 mm Hg	>50 mm Hg
Valve area	>1.5 cm^2	1.0-1.5 cm^2	<1.0 cm^2

Modified from Bonow RO, Carabello BA, Chatterjee K, et al: ACC/AHA 2006 guidelines for the management of patients with valvular heart disease. *J Amer Coll Cardiol* 48:e1-e148, 2006.
PA, Pulmonary artery.

this procedure, a balloon is passed percutaneously from the femoral vein across the atrial septum (by needle puncture) through the mitral valve, where it is inflated (Fig. 31-3). Balloon inflation ruptures the adhesions at the commissures caused by the rheumatic process, allowing as much as doubling of the mitral valve area and normalizing cardiac output, LA pressure, and PA pressure, in turn, relieving symptoms.

Criteria have been established to determine whether balloon valvotomy should be performed or the patient referred for surgery. These four criteria are valve mobility, subvalvular thickening, leaflet thickening, and degree of valvular calcification. In addition to these characteristics, the degree of mitral regurgitation (MR) is assessed, because balloon valvotomy can worsen the degree of mitral regurgitation. Balloon valvotomy is ineffective when mitral annular calcification is the cause of MS.

Class I indications for percutaneous mitral balloon valvotomy include the following:

- Symptomatic (New York Heart Association [NYHA] class II to IV) patients with moderate to severe MS with favorable valve characteristics, in the absence of LA thrombus or moderate to severe MR (class I; level of evidence A)
- Asymptomatic patients with moderate to severe MS and pulmonary hypertension (PA systolic pressure greater than 50 mm Hg at rest or more than 60 mm Hg with exercise) and valve morphology favorable for balloon valvotomy, in the absence of LA thrombus or moderate to severe MR (class I; level of evidence C)

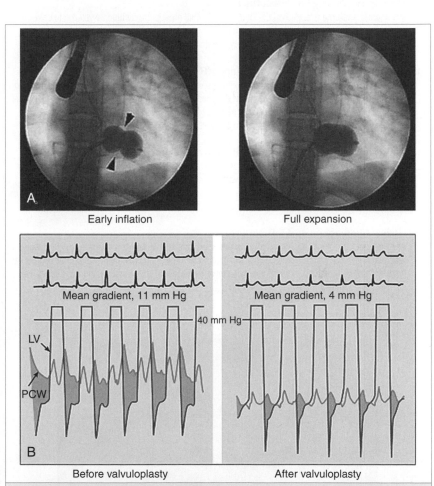

Figure 31-3. Percutaneous balloon mitral valvotomy (BMV) for mitral stenosis using the Inoue technique. **A,** The catheter is advanced into the left atrium via the transseptal technique and guided antegrade across the mitral orifice. As the balloon is inflated, its distal portion expands first and is pulled back so that it fits snugly against the orifice. With further inflation, the proximal portion of the balloon expands to center the balloon within the stenotic orifice *(left, arrowheads)*. Further inflation expands the central *waist* portion of the balloon *(right)*, resulting in commissural splitting and enlargement of the orifice. **B,** Successful BMV results in significant increase in mitral valve area, as reflected by reduction in the diastolic pressure gradient between left ventricle *(LV)* and pulmonary capillary wedge *(PCW)* pressure, as indicated by the *shaded area*. (From Delabays A, Goy JJ: Images in clinical medicine: percutaneous mitral valvuloplasty, *N Engl J Med* 345:e4, 2001.)

8. **What are the causes of MR?**
   There are two broad categories of MR, primary and secondary. In primary MR, disease of the mitral valve causes it to leak, imparting a volume overload on the LV. In secondary MR, disease of the LV causes wall motion abnormalities, ventricular dilation, and annular dilation, rendering the mitral valve incompetent. The most common causes of primary MR include myxomatous degeneration and mitral valve prolapse, infective endocarditis, rheumatic heart disease, and collagen vascular disease. Causes of secondary MR include coronary artery disease and subsequent myocardial infarction, and dilated cardiomyopathy.

9. **How does primary MR affect the LV?**
   MR imparts a volume overload on the LV because the LV must pump additional volume to compensate for that lost to regurgitation. In some way, MR causes sarcomeres to lengthen, increasing end-diastolic volume, enabling the LV to increase its total stroke volume.

10. **What are the other effects of primary MR on the heart and lungs?**
    MR also causes volume overload on the LA, increasing LA pressure. Increased LA pressure leads to pulmonary congestion and the symptoms of dyspnea, orthopnea, and paroxysmal nocturnal dyspnea. Eventually MR may also lead to pulmonary hypertension, RV pressure overload, and RV failure. LA enlargement also predisposes the patient to atrial fibrillation.

11. **What are the clues to MR on physical examination?**
    The typical murmur of MR is holosystolic, radiating to the axilla. It may be accompanied by a systolic apical thrill; the apical beat is displaced downward and to the left, indicating LV enlargement. In severe MR, an S3 is usually heard. Here the S3 may not indicate heart failure but rather is caused by the increased LA volume emptying into the LV at higher than normal pressure.

12. **How is the diagnosis of MR confirmed?**
    Although both the chest radiograph and the electrocardiogram (ECG) may indicate LV enlargement, as with other valvular heart diseases, echocardiography is the diagnostic modality of choice (Fig. 31-4). It demonstrates LA and LV size and volume, allows assessment of LV function and PA pressure, and can reliably quantify the amount of MR present.

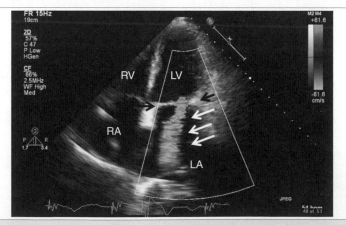

Figure 31-4. Mitral regurgitation. Apical four-chamber view with color Doppler revealing severe mitral regurgitation *(white arrows)*. *Black arrows* point to the mitral valve. Note that in actuality, the regurgitant jet is displayed in color, corresponding to the flow of blood. *LA*, left atrium; *LV*, left ventricle; *RA*, right atrium; *RV*, right ventricle.

Echocardiographic findings suggestive of severe MR include enlarged LA or LV, the color Doppler MR jet occupying a large proportion (more than 40%) of the LA, a regurgitant volume 60 ml or more, a regurgitant fraction 50% or greater, a regurgitant orifice 0.40 cm^2 or greater, and a Doppler vena contracta width 0.7 cm or larger.

Severity of MR is established using the criteria in Table 31-2. Magnetic resonance imaging may be used to establish or confirm the severity of MR and its attendant volume overload.

13. **Are there effective medical therapies for chronic primary MR?**
No. The asymptomatic patient will not benefit from medical therapy, and once symptoms develop, MR should be treated surgically. It should be noted that some patients with MR also have systemic hypertension, which should be treated in the same manner in which hypertension is routinely treated.

14. **What is the definitive therapy for primary MR, and when should it be employed?**
As with all primary valve disease, MR is a mechanical problem requiring a mechanical solution. Here, however, the therapy for MR departs from that of other valve lesions. Unlike the aortic valve, the mitral valve serves to do more than just direct forward cardiac flow. The mitral valve is also an integral part of the LV, coordinating LV contraction and maintaining LV shape. When the valve is destroyed at the time of surgery, there is a precipitous fall in LV function postoperatively, which does not occur when the valve apparatus is conserved. Further, operative mortality is lower with valve repair than with valve replacement. Thus, every attempt should be made to repair rather than replace the valve at the time of surgery.

Because the onset of symptoms worsens prognosis for patients with MR, mitral valve repair should be performed at that time. However, some patients fail to develop symptoms even though LV dysfunction has ensued. To guard against permanent LV dysfunction, mitral surgery should be performed before ejection fraction falls to 60% or less, or before the LV can no longer contract to an end-systolic dimension of 40 mm. The onset of atrial fibrillation or pulmonary hypertension is also an indication for surgery. It should be noted that not all mitral valves can be repaired. In such cases, mitral valve replacement is performed.

TABLE 31-2. ANGIOGRAPHIC AND ECHOCARDIOGRAPHIC CRITERIA FOR THE ASSESSMENT OF THE SEVERITY OF MITRAL REGURGITATION

	Mild	Moderate	Severe
Angiographic grade	1+	2+	3-4+
Color Doppler jet area	Small central jet (<4 cm^2 or <20% LA area)		Vena contracta width >0.7 cm with large central MR jet (area >40% LA), any wall-impinging jet, or any swirling in LA
Doppler vena contracta width	<0.3 cm	0.3-0.69 cm	≥0.7 cm
Regurgitant volume	<30 ml	30-59 ml	≥60 ml
Regurgitant fraction	<30%	30-49%	≥50%
Regurgitant orifice	<0.20 cm^2	0.20-0.39 cm^2	≥0.40 cm^2
Chamber size			Enlarged LA or LV

Modified from Bonow RO, Carabello BA, Chatterjee K, et al: ACC/AHA 2006 guidelines for the management of patients with valvular heart disease. *J Amer Coll Cardiol* 48:e1-e148, 2006.
LA, Left atrium; *LV*, left ventricle; *MR*, mitral regurgitation.

Class 1 indications for mitral valve repair or replacement include the following:

- Symptomatic acute severe MR
- Development or presence of NYHA class II to IV symptoms in patients with chronic severe MR in the absence of severe LV dysfunction (ejection fraction less than 30% or end-systolic dimension greater than 55 mm)
- Asymptomatic patients with chronic severe MR and mild to moderate LV dysfunction (ejection fraction of 30%-60% or end-systolic dimension 40 mm or more)

15. How is secondary MR managed?

This area is one of substantial uncertainty. In virtually all cases of secondary MR, there is also severe LV dysfunction and heart failure. As such, standard therapy for heart failure is indicated. When mitral surgery should be undertaken is unclear, but it is usually reserved for those patients who have failed medical therapy for heart failure, including cardiac resynchronization therapy when appropriate. The last decade has produced substantial interest in percutaneous approaches to MR. While none are yet approved for general use in the US, a percutaneously deployed device that clips the two mitral leaflets together may be effective in treating functional MR and in inoperable patients with primary MR. Results from Europe, where the device is commercially available, are promising.

16. What is mitral valve prolapse?

Mitral valve prolapse (MVP) is the condition in which there is systolic billowing of one or both mitral leaflets into the LA (Fig. 31-5), with or without resulting MR. It is usually diagnosed by

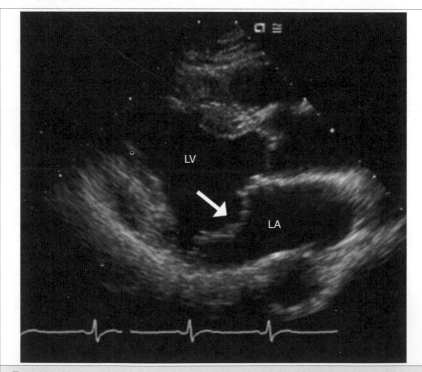

Figure 31-5. Mitral valve prolapse. The mitral leaflets prolapse across the plain of the mitral valve, into the left atrium *(arrow)*. *LA,* Left atrium; *LV,* left ventricle. (Modified from Libby P, Bonow RO, Mann DL, Zipes DP: *Braunwald's heart disease: a textbook of cardiovascular medicine,* ed 8, Philadelphia, 2008, Saunders.)

echocardiography, according to established criteria (valve prolapse of 2 mm or more beyond the mitral annulus, as seen in the parasternal long-axis view). Its prevalence is 1% to 2.5%.

17. What is the classic auscultatory finding in MVP?

The classic finding is a midsystolic click and late systolic murmur, although the click may actually vary somewhat within systole, depending on changes in LV dimension. There may actually be multiple clicks. The clicks are believed to result from the sudden tensing of the mitral valve apparatus as the leaflets prolapse into the LA during systole.

18. What is the natural history of asymptomatic MVP?

The course of patients with MVP can range from benign, with a normal life expectancy, to worsening MR and progressive LA dilation and LV dysfunction and congestive heart failure.

BIBLIOGRAPHY, SUGGESTED READINGS, AND WEBSITES

1. Bonow RO, Carabello BA, Chatterjee K, et al: ACC/AHA 2006 guidelines for the management of patients with valvular heart disease, *J Amer Coll Cardiol* 48:e1–e148, 2006.

2. Carabello BA: The pathophysiology of mitral regurgitation, *J Heart Valve Dis* 9:600–608, 2000.

3. Carabello BA: Modern management of mitral stenosis, *Circulation* 112:432–437, 2005.

4. Carabello BA: The current therapy for mitral regurgitation, *J Am Coll Cardiol* 52:319–326, 2008.

5. Gaasch WH: Overview of the Management of Chronic Mitral Regurgitation. In Basow, DS, editor: UpToDate, Waltham, MA, 2013, UpToDate. Available at: http://www.uptodate.com/contents/overview-of-the-management-of-chronic-mitral-regurgitation. Accessed March 26, 2013.

6. Feldman T, Foster E, Glower DD, et al: Percutaneous repair or surgery for mitral regurgitation, *N Engl J Med* 364:1395–1406, 2011.

7. I Hanson: Mitral regurgitation. Available at: http://www.emedicine.com. Accessed March 26, 2013.

8. CM Otto, Pathophysiology and Clinical Features of Mitral Stenosis. In Basow, DS, editor: UpToDate, Waltham, MA, 2013, UpToDate. Available at: http://www.uptodate.com/contents/pathophysiology-clinical-features-and-evaluation-of-mitral-stenosis. Accessed March 26, 2013.

9. Dima C: Mitral stenosis. Available at http://www.emedicine.com. Accessed March 26, 2013.

10. Vahanian A, Baumgartner H, Bax J, et al: Guidelines on the management of valvular heart disease: the Task Force on the Management of Valvular Heart Disease of the European Society of Cardiology, *Eur Heart J* 28:230–268, 2007.

CHAPTER 32

PROSTHETIC HEART VALVES

Stephan M. Hergert, MD, and Ann Bolger, MD, FACC, FAHA

Heart valve diseases are common and may result from congenital, inflammatory, infectious, or degenerative causes. The decisions regarding how to surgically correct these valvular problems, how to follow the patients after surgery, and what problems to anticipate are addressed in this chapter.

1. **What are important considerations in the preoperative evaluation and planning of patients who are to undergo valve repair or replacement?**
   Patients who are advised to have valve surgery require careful preoperative planning and assessment. Cardiac catheterization to rule out coronary artery obstructions that might require bypass is advised in adults more than 40 years old. Dental evaluation to identify abscesses or other potential sources of postoperative valvular infection is advisable. Carotid ultrasound to exclude significant stenosis in patients with bruits or neurologic symptoms is often requested. Visualization of the aorta, often with computed tomography (CT) scan, to assess atherosclerosis at potential cannulation sites and root dimensions, may occasionally be required before valve replacement.

2. **What types of prosthetic valves are used for valve replacement, and which ones are most commonly used in current practice?**
   Representative bioprosthetic and mechanical heart valve types are shown in Figure 32-1 and discussed here.

   A *stentless bioprosthesis* is a bovine or porcine heart valve implanted without a frame. In the aortic position, the aortic root is used to attach the valve. The major advantage is that the size of the

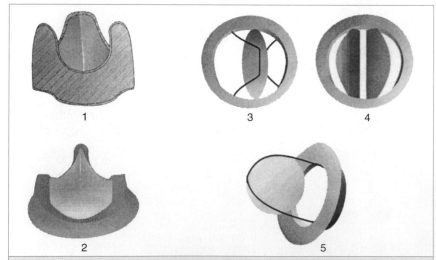

Figure 32-1. Bioprosthetic and mechanical heart valves. *(1)* Biologic nonstented and *(2)* stented valves; *(3)* mechanical single tilting disc valve, *(4)* mechanical bileaflet valve, and *(5)* ball-in-cage valve.

implanted valve can be larger, because no space is required for a supporting frame. Data suggest that left ventricular function is better protected by nonstented compared with stented valves. Anticoagulation is recommended for the first 3 months after implantation.

A *stented bioprosthesis* has a wire frame that provides the structure for the biologic material. The biologic material is usually bovine or porcine pericardium, which is specially treated to reduce antigenicity. Anticoagulation is recommended for the first 3 months after implantation.

A *single tilting disc mechanical valve* opens with a minor and major orifice. The disc material is polycarbonate. The first successful valve was the Bjork-Shiley valve, introduced in 1969. These valves are rarely used in current practice.

A *bileaflet mechanical valve* has two semicircular discs. The disc material is polycarbonate. The first bileaflet valve was introduced in 1977 by St. Jude Medical. Bileaflet valves are the most common mechanical heart valves used in current practice.

Transcatheter aortic valve implantation (TAVI) or *transcatheter aortic valve replacement* (TAVR) has been performed at investigational sites for nearly 10 years, mostly commonly in Europe. In the United States, it has recently been approved, though programs that can implant such valves must meet strict standards. It is intended for patients with severe aortic stenosis who are not good surgical candidates for conventional valve replacement. The valve is implanted via a transarterial (femoral or axillary) or transapical approach. In Europe, the valve may also be implanted by a direct aortic approach. Significant risks of serious adverse events, such as valve displacement, cardiac tamponade, myocardial infarction, stroke, or injury of the aorta or femoral or axillary artery, are associated with this procedure. The procedure is illustrated in Figure 32-2.

The *ball-in-cage model* is an older type of valve that is still encountered in some patients today. The Starr-Edwards mechanical valve prosthesis was introduced by Professor Albert Starr in 1961. It was the first mechanical heart valve. Some patients still have functioning Starr-Edwards prostheses after more than 30 years. The main drawback of this valve is its high-pressure gradient and the nonphysiologic streaming of flow through the valve. For these reasons, as well as the need for higher degrees of anticoagulation, the valve is no longer used in clinical practice.

3. **What is a heterograft, and what is an allograft (homograft), and what is a Ross procedure?**
A *heterograft* is a biologic valve derived from an animal. An *allograft* (also called a homograft) is a heart valve taken from a human cadaver. Allografts have the advantage of natural configuration

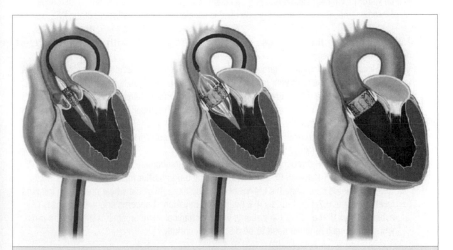

Figure 32-2. Transcatheter aortic valve replacement. After balloon valvuloplasty of the stenotic aortic valve, the prosthetic valve is positioned at the level of the aortic annulus. The balloon is inflated, deploying the stented valve in position.

and the fact that they include a portion of the aortic root that can be incorporated in the valve replacement procedure if necessary (e.g., aortic root abscess). Careful matching of allograft size to the patient is critical to the performance and durability of the valve. The Ross procedure uses the patient's own pulmonic valve to replace their aortic valve. The pulmonic valve is then replaced with a bioprosthesis. Advantages are a lack of antigenicity and the potential for growth of the valve over time, as required in children.

4. How does one choose between bioprosthetic and mechanical valves?

A bioprosthesis is preferred in older patients and in patients in whom lifetime anticoagulation poses important risks. This includes persons with high trauma risk, clotting disorders, gastrointestinal problems with the potential for bleeding, and persons who may not be able to comply with required anticoagulant medication and follow-up testing. The major disadvantage of biologic prostheses is primary valve failure as a result of leaflet degeneration, which limits their functional life span. Mechanical heart valves, which have greater durability than bioprosthetic valves, are usually preferred in patients younger than 65 years and without contraindications to long-term anticoagulation.

5. What are the anticoagulation strategies for patients with prosthetic valves, and what are the risks for thromboembolic or hemorrhagic events?

The degree and type of anticoagulation depends on the valve type and location, and the overall risk of thrombosis. Guidelines on anticoagulation of prosthetic heart valves have been published by both the American College of Cardiology/American Heart Association (ACC/AHA) and the American College of Chest Physicians (ACCP). Suggested anticoagulation regimens are given in Table 32-1.

6. How does one handle anticoagulation issues in patients with mechanical valve prostheses before elective surgery or invasive procedures?

When warfarin must be discontinued for elective procedures, the patient can be treated with unfractionated heparin (UFH) (target activated partial thromboplastin time [aPTT] 55-70 seconds) while the international normalized ratio (INR) decreases. Low-molecular-weight heparin (LMWH) is not approved for protection against thromboembolism from mechanical valve prostheses; a recent ACCP practice guidelines does discuss the use of therapeutic-dose LMWH for bridging patients off and back on warfarin. Vitamin K administration can create a hypercoagulable state, which increases the risk of thromboembolism, and should not be used to accelerate the normalization of the INR.

7. How are anticoagulation issues managed when patients with mechanical heart valves become pregnant?

Female patients who anticipate pregnancy may initially opt for valve prostheses that avoid the need for anticoagulation. For patients with mechanical prostheses, anticoagulation must be continued during pregnancy, but the risk of adverse fetal effects from warfarin mandates a different anticoagulation strategy. The ACCP's Conference on Antithrombotic and Thrombolytic Therapy recommends one of the following three regimens:

- Treatment with LMWH or UFH between weeks 6 and 12 and close to term; warfarin during the rest of the pregnancy
- Treatment with UFH throughout the whole pregnancy (subcutaneous UFH 17,500-20,000 U twice a day; aPTT between 55 and 70 seconds by 6 hours after injection)
- Weight-adjusted subcutaneous LMWH twice a day throughout the whole pregnancy (plasma level of anti-Xa 0.7-1.2 U/mL by 4-6 hours after injection). Concerns about the efficacy of subcutaneous UFH or LMWH in patients with mechanical valve prosthesis persist; the pros and cons of each regimen need to be discussed carefully.

8. How should prosthetic valve thrombosis be treated?

Patients with thrombosis of a right-sided prosthetic valve should be considered for fibrinolytic therapy if there are no contraindications. The treatment for patients with left-sided valve thrombosis depends

TABLE 32-1. SUGGESTED ANTICOAGULATION REGIMENS AFTER AORTIC AND MITRAL VALVE REPLACEMENT

	Aortic Position			Mitral Position	
	Bioprosthetic Valve	Mechanical Valve	Transcatheter (Biological) Valve	Bioprosthetic Valve	Mechanical Valve
No other risk factors for thrombosis	Vitamin K antagonist INR 2-3 for the first 3 months, *then* aspirin 50-100 mg/d	Vitamin K antagonist INR 2-3	Aspirin 50-100 mg/d (lifelong) *and* clopidogrel 75 mg/d (3 months)	Vitamin K antagonist INR 2-3 (at least 3 months)	Vitamin K antagonist INR 2.5-3.5 (lifelong)
With risk factors for thrombosis*	Vitamin K antagonist INR 2-3	Vitamin K antagonist INR 2.5-3.5	Vitamin K antagonist INR 2-3 *and* aspirin 50-100 mg/d or clopidogrel 75 mg/d (at least one year)	Vitamin K antagonist INR 2-3 (lifelong) *and* aspirin 50-100 mg/d or clopidogrel 75 mg/d	Vitamin K antagonist INR 2.5-3.5 (lifelong) *and* aspirin 50-100 mg/d or clopidogrel 75 mg/d
Very high risk for thrombosis	Vitamin K antagonist INR 2-3 *and* aspirin 50-100 mg/d or clopidogrel 75 mg/d	Vitamin K antagonist INR 2.5-3.5 *and* aspirin 50-100 mg/d or clopidogrel 75 mg/d If aspirin or clopidogrel cannot be used, INR 3.5-4.5 may be indicated.	Vitamin K antagonist INR 2-3 *and* aspirin 50-100 mg/d or clopidogrel 75 mg/d	Vitamin K antagonist INR 2.5-3.5 (lifelong) *and* aspirin 50-100 mg/d or clopidogrel 75 mg/d	Vitamin K antagonist INR 3.5-4.5 (lifelong) may be indicated by risk level, or if aspirin or clopidogrel cannot be used.

INR, International normalized ratio.
*Risk factors such as atrial fibrillation, left ventricular dysfunction, or hypercoagulable state

on the size of the thrombus. If the cross-sectional area is smaller than 0.8 cm², fibrinolytic therapy is favored. For larger valve thrombosis, a surgical approach should be considered.

9. **How does one prevent, diagnose, or treat prosthetic valve endocarditis?**
Endocarditis on a prosthetic valve is a potentially catastrophic event that may require repeat surgery to cure the infection. Such infections usually originate on the prosthetic sewing ring and rapidly extend into perivalvular tissues. The risk of endocarditis is approximately the same for mechanical and biologic valve prostheses, although some studies have suggested slightly higher risks for biologic valves. The AHA published new prophylaxis guidelines in 2007 suggesting that patients with prosthetic heart valves should be considered for endocarditis prophylaxis for procedures likely to create bacteremia with an endocarditis-causing organisms. In the UK, the National Institute of Clinical

Excellence Guidelines now do not recommend antibiotic prophylaxis before dental procedures for any patient.

Because artificial valves often create artifacts that complicate valve imaging, transesophageal echocardiography (TEE) is almost always required to adequately assess prosthetic heart valves for endocarditis, and to rule out perivalvular extension of infection. In cases of mechanical heart valve endocarditis, early surgery and re-replacement is often required, especially in the presence of perivalvular extension of infection, and may improve patient survival. Attempted medical treatment of prosthetic valve endocarditis requires at least 4 to 6 weeks of antibiotic therapy.

10. How does one use echocardiography to follow patients after heart valve surgery?

All prosthetic valves are stenotic compared with natural valves, because of the extra space required for their sewing ring. As a result, the transvalvular flow velocity is expected to be higher than normal across prostheses; each valve type and size has an expected range of velocities and pressure gradients defined by the manufacturer. Flow patterns at closure are also valve specific; mechanical prostheses normally have multiple regurgitation jets (an exception to this being the ball-in-cage prosthesis).

In evaluating prosthetic valves, it is important to know the valve type and size. The forward flow across the valve is measured with Doppler imaging, and used to calculate the peak and mean gradients for comparison to normal values. The gradients will increase with higher heart rate and with increased flow volume. Unexplained increases in valve gradients may indicate obstruction from endocarditis, thrombosis, leaflet calcification, or tissue overgrowth.

During phases of the cardiac cycle when the valve is closed, spectral and color Doppler are used to identify valvular insufficiency. Some mild valvular insufficiency may be normally seen with mechanical valves due to leaflet closure and hinge points. With biologic prostheses, transvalvular insufficiency jets indicate valve dysfunction. Eccentric regurgitation in any type of prosthesis may result from paravalvular leaks caused by suture dehiscence, with or without endocarditis.

Other echocardiographic clues to prosthetic valve dysfunction are progressive chamber enlargement, abnormal pulmonary vein flow patterns (for mitral regurgitation), diastolic reversal of aortic flow (aortic prosthetic regurgitation), and pulmonary hypertension (as estimated from the tricuspid insufficiency jet).

11. What can cause recurrent symptoms when the prosthetic valve appears normal?

A mitral prosthesis that extends into the left ventricle (high profile) may crowd the outflow tract and cause signs and symptoms of outflow obstruction. This can also be seen after mitral valve repair, where redundant components of the native valve oppose the septum in systole. Intraventricular pressure gradients in the outflow tract can be identified with Doppler echocardiography. Low-profile valves have largely addressed this problem. All prostheses are smaller than the natural valves that they replace because of the space required for their sewing ring. Undersized valves relative to patient requirements can result in relative valvular stenosis. This can be investigated with Doppler studies.

12. Should magnetic resonance imaging (MRI) be used after valve replacement?

According to a recent AHA scientific statement, the majority of prosthetic heart valves that have been tested have been labeled as *MR safe*; the remainder of heart valves and rings that have been tested have been labeled as *MR conditional*. On the basis of various studies and findings, the presence of a prosthetic heart valve that has been formally evaluated for MR safety should not be considered a contraindication to an MR examination at 3 Tesla or less (and possibly even 4.7 Tesla in some cases) any time after implantation. In cases where there is any doubt as to the safety of MRI scanning of a specific valve, the safety of the study should be discussed with an MRI specialist.

BIBLIOGRAPHY, SUGGESTED READINGS, AND WEBSITES

1. Ali A, Halstead JC, Cafferty F, et al: Are stentless valves superior to modern stented valves? A prospective randomized trial, *Circulation* 114:1535–1540, 2006.

2. Aurigemma GP, Gaasch WH: Routine Management of Patients with Prosthetic Heart Valves. In Basow, DS, editor: UpToDate, Waltham, MA, 2013, UpToDate. Available at: http://www.uptodate.com/contents/management-of-patients-with-prosthetic-heart-valves. Accessed March 26, 2013.

3. Bates SM, Greer IA, Hirsh J, et al: Use of antithrombotic agents during pregnancy: the Seventh ACCP Conference on Antithrombotic and Thrombolytic Therapy, *Chest* 126:627S–644S, 2004.

4. Bonow RO, Carabello B, Chatterjee K, et al: ACC/AHA 2006 guidelines for the management of patients with valvular heart disease: executive summary, *Circulation* 114:e84–e231, 2006.

5. Douketis JD, et al: Perioperative management of antithrombotic therapy: Antithrombotic Therapy and Prevention of Thrombosis, 9th ed: American College of Chest Physicians Evidence-Based Clinical Practice Guidelines, *Chest* 141:e326S–e350S, 2012.

6. Edwards MB, Taylor KM, Shellock FG, et al: Prosthetic heart valves: evaluation of magnetic field interactions, heating, and artifacts at 1.5 T, *J Magn Reson Imaging* 12:363–369, 2000.

7. Elkayam U, Bitar F: Valvular heart disease and pregnancy: part II: prosthetic valves, *J Am Coll Cardiol* 46:403–410, 2005.

8. Gott VL, Alejo DE, Cameron DE: Mechanical heart valves: 50 years of evolution, *Ann Thorac Surg* 76:S2230–S2239, 2003.

9. Hammermeister K, Sethi GK, Henderson WG, et al: Outcomes 15 years after valve replacement with a mechanical versus a bioprosthetic valve: final report of the Veterans Affairs randomized trial, *J Am Coll Cardiol* 36:1152–1158, 2000.

10. Kovacs MJ, Kearon C, Rodger M, et al: Single-arm study of bridging therapy with low-molecular-weight heparin for patients at risk of arterial embolism who require temporary interruption of warfarin, *Circulation* 110:1658–1663, 2004.

11. Kulik A, Be´dard P, Lam B-K, et al: Mechanical versus bioprosthetic valve replacement in middle-aged patients, *Eur J Cardiothorac Surg* 30:485–491, 2006.

12. Levine GN, Arai A, Bleumke D, et al: Safety of MRI/MRA in patients with cardiovascular devices; a scientific statement: statement by the AHA Council on Clinical Cardiology, *Circulation* 116:2878–2921, 2007.

13. Mohty D, Orszulak TA, Schaff HV, et al: Very long-term survival and durability of mitral valve repair for mitral valve prolapse, *Circulation* 104:I1–I7, 2001.

14. Stein PD, Alpert JS, Bussey HI, et al: Antithrombotic therapy in patients with mechanical and biological prosthetic heart valves, *Chest* 119:220S–227S, 2001.

15. Whitlock RP, et al: Antithrombotic and thrombolytic therapy for valvular disease: Antithrombotic Therapy and Prevention of Thrombosis, 9th ed: American College of Chest Physicians Evidence-Based Clinical Practice Guidelines, *Chest* 141:e576S–e600S, 2012.

16. Wilson W, Taubert KA, Gewitz M, et al: Prevention of infective endocarditis: guidelines from the American Heart Association, *J Am Dent Assoc* 138:739–745, 2007. 747–60.

CHAPTER 33

ENDOCARDITIS AND ENDOCARDITIS PROPHYLAXIS

Julia Ansari, MD, and Glenn N. Levine, MD, FACC, FAHA

1. **What are believed to be the first steps in the development of infective endocarditis (IE)?**

   IE is believed to occur only after one first develops what is termed nonbacterial thrombotic endocarditis (NBTE). According to the most recent American Heart Association (AHA) statement on endocarditis, it is believed that turbulent blood flow produced by certain types of congenital or acquired heart disease traumatizes the endothelium. This turbulent blood flow may be the result of flow from a high- to a low-pressure chamber or across a narrowed orifice. This trauma of the endothelium then creates a predisposition for deposition of platelets and fibrin on the surface of the endothelium, resulting in what is called NBTE. If bacteremia (or fungemia) occurs, the organisms may then colonize this site, resulting in IE.

2. **How often does routine tooth brushing and flossing cause transient bacteremia?**

   Transient bacteremia occurs 20% to 68% of the time with routine tooth brushing and flossing. It occurs 20% to 40% of the time with use of wooden toothpicks, and 7% to 71% of the time with chewing food. This is part of the rationale of the latest AHA guidelines deemphasizing antibiotic prophylaxis during certain dental and other procedures—namely, that the vast majority of the time bacteremia is due to daily activities and not to the occasional or rare dental or other procedure. The emphasis now is more on maintaining good oral hygiene and access to routine dental care.

3. **True or false: Prospective randomized placebo-controlled trials have demonstrated that antibiotic prophylaxis before a dental or other procedure reduces the risk of IE?**

   False. Despite the fact that for 50 years antibiotic prophylaxis has been recommended, there has never been a prospective randomized placebo-controlled trial to support this recommendation. In fact, the data on whether antibiotic prophylaxis even significantly affects bacteremia is contradictory, with some studies showing some reduction and others showing no reduction.

4. **What are the four conditions identified as having the highest risk of adverse outcome from endocarditis for which prophylaxis with dental procedures is still recommended?**
   - Prosthetic cardiac valve
   - Previous IE
   - Certain cases of congenital heart disease (CHD), such as:
     - Unrepaired cyanotic CHD
     - Repaired CHD with prosthetic material or devices during the first 6 months after the procedure
     - Repaired CHD with residual defects
   - Cardiac transplantation recipients who develop cardiac valvulopathy

5. **Which of the above AHA criteria for endocarditis prophylaxis is not recommended for prophylaxis in the 2009 European Society of Cardiology (ESC) guidelines?**

   Cardiac transplant recipients with valvulopathy. The 2009 ESC guidelines take an approach that is generally similar to that of the 2007 AHA guidelines on which conditions and which procedures

---

Box 33-1 SUMMARY OF THE MAJOR CHANGES IN THE UPDATED AMERICAN HEART ASSOCIATION'S SCIENTIFIC STATEMENT ON INFECTIVE ENDOCARDITIS PROPHYLAXIS

- Bacteremia resulting from daily activities is much more likely to cause infective endocarditis (IE) than bacteremia associated with a dental procedure.
- Only an extremely small number of cases of IE might be prevented by antibiotic prophylaxis, even if prophylaxis is 100% effective.
- Antibiotic prophylaxis is not recommended based solely on an increased lifetime risk of acquisition of IE.
- Recommendations for IE prophylaxis are limited to only the four conditions identified as having the highest risk of adverse outcome from endocarditis (see text).
- Antibiotic prophylaxis is no longer recommended for any other form of congenital heart disease, except for the conditions listed in the text.
- Antibiotic prophylaxis is recommended for all dental procedures that involve manipulation of gingival tissues or periapical region of teeth or perforation of oral mucosa only for patients with underlying cardiac conditions associated with the highest risk of adverse outcome from IE (see text).
- Antibiotic prophylaxis is recommended for procedures on respiratory tract or infected skin, skin structures, or musculoskeletal tissue only for patients with underlying cardiac conditions associated with the highest risk of adverse outcome from IE (see text).
- Antibiotic prophylaxis solely to prevent IE is not recommended for genitourinary (GU) or gastrointestinal (GI) tract procedures.

Modified from Wilson W, Taubert KA, Gewitz M, et al: Prevention of infective endocarditis guidelines from the American Heart Association. *Circulation* 116:1736-1754, 2007.

---

should be considered for endocarditis prophylaxis. However, the ESC guidelines do not list cardiac transplant recipients with valvulopathy as a population that should receive prophylaxis, noting that prophylaxis in this group is not supported by strong evidence, and that the probability of IE from dental origin is extremely low in such patients.

6. **In the new AHA guidelines, for those patients with conditions listed in Question 4, which dental procedures carry a recommendation of endocarditis prophylaxis?**
The guidelines emphasize that *all dental procedures* that involve the manipulation of gingival tissue or the periapical region of teeth or perforation of the oral mucosa should receive endocarditis prophylaxis. Procedures that do not require prophylaxis include routine anesthetic injections through noninfected tissue, dental radiographs, placement of removable prosthodontic or orthodontic appliances, bleeding from trauma to the lips or oral mucosa, and select other procedures and manipulations. The guidelines emphasize that prophylaxis for the former mentioned procedures "may be reasonable for these patients," although "its effectiveness is unknown" (and this prophylaxis recommendation is given a class IIb recommendation, with level of evidence C). New changes in the AHA guidelines on IE are summarized in Box 33-1.

7. **For those patients with conditions for which antibiotic prophylaxis is recommended, undergoing dental procedures for which prophylaxis is recommended, what regimens are recommended?**
Antibiotic treatment should be administered as a single dose before the procedure, with antimicrobial therapy directed against viridians group streptococci. Amoxicillin (2 g orally [PO]), administered 30 to 60 minutes before the procedure, is the first-line recommendation. Those unable to take oral medication can be treated with ampicillin (2 g intramuscularly [IM] or intravenously [IV]) or cefazolin

or ceftriaxone (1 g IM or IV). For those allergic to the penicillins or ampicillin, potential agents to use include cephalexin, clindamycin, azithromycin, clarithromycin, cefazolin, and ceftriaxone.

8. **For what other procedures may prophylaxis be considered in patients with high-risk lesions?**

The new AHA guidelines deemphasize prophylaxis for most other procedures. Antibiotic prophylaxis solely to prevent IE is not recommended for genitourinary (GU) or gastrointestinal (GI) tract procedures. Among those procedures where prophylaxis may be considered (class IIb, level of evidence C) are:

- Invasive procedures of the respiratory tract that involve incision or biopsy of the respiratory mucosa (e.g., tonsillectomy, adenoidectomy)
- Bronchoscopy with incision of the respiratory tract mucosa (but not otherwise for bronchoscopy)
- Invasive respiratory tract procedures to treat an established infection (e.g., drainage of an abscess or empyema)
- Surgical procedures that involve infected skin, skin structures, or musculoskeletal tissue

9. **Is endocarditis prophylaxis recommended in patients treated with coronary stents, pacemakers, or defibrillators, those undergoing transesophageal echocardiography (TEE), or those who have undergone coronary artery bypass grafting (CABG) (without valve replacement)?**

No. Note, however, that some electrophysiologists will pretreat or post-treat patients undergoing pacemaker or defibrillator implantation with antibiotics to prevent local infection (but not endocarditis).

10. **What factors (discussed in detail in the ESC guidelines on endocarditis) should raise the suspicion for endocarditis?**

- Bacteremia or sepsis of unknown cause
- Fever
- Constitutional symptoms such as unexplained malaise, weakness, arthralgias, and weight loss
- Hematuria, glomerulonephritis, and suspected renal infarction
- Embolic event of unknown origin
- New heart murmur (primarily regurgitant murmurs)
- Unexplained new atrioventricular (AV) nodal conduction abnormality (prolonged PR interval, heart block)
- Multifocal or rapidly changing pulmonic infiltrates
- Peripheral abscesses
- Cutaneous lesions (Osler nodes, Janeway lesions)
- Ophthalmic manifestations (Roth spots)

11. **When should cardiac echo (echocardiography) be obtained in cases of suspected endocarditis?**

As soon as possible. Transthoracic echocardiography (TTE) has a sensitivity of 60% to 75% in the detection of native valve endocarditis. It can detect 70% of vegetations larger than 6 mm but only 25% of vegetations less than 5 mm. In cases where the clinical suspicion of endocarditis is low, a good-quality TTE is usually adequate. In cases where the suspicion of endocarditis is higher, a negative TTE should be followed by transesophageal echocardiography, which has a sensitivity of 88% to 100% and a specificity of 91% to 100% for native valves. TTE is not considered a sensitive test for prosthetic valve endocarditis, and a TEE is routinely obtained in such cases. TEE is also considerably more sensitive for detecting myocardial abscesses. Figure 33-1 demonstrates a mitral valve vegetation visualized by TEE.

12. **What is the procedure for obtaining blood cultures in cases of suspected endocarditis?**

Three separate sets of blood cultures should be obtained, each at least 1 hour apart from the others (different authorities differ on the exact timing recommendations, but this is a reasonable ballpark

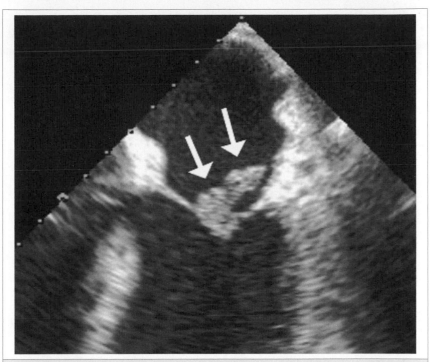

Figure 33-1. A vegetation *(arrows)* on the mitral valve, as visualized by transesophageal echocardiography. (Courtesy Dr. Kumudha Ramasubbu.)

figure). For what is called *subacute* IE, some experts recommend the cultures be drawn over a period of 24 hours. These blood cultures should not be obtained from intravenous lines (although some may recommend additional blood cultures be obtained from indwelling lines). At least 5 mL, and ideally 10 mL, of blood should be added to each culture bottle. In patients treated for a short period with antibiotics, one should wait, if possible, for at least 3 days after antibiotic discontinuation before obtaining new blood cultures.

13. **What is the most common overall organism reported to cause endocarditis?**
Staphylococcus aureus is the most common cause of IE, followed by viridians group streptococci, and then enterococci, and coagulase-native staphylococci.

14. **What is the most common organism causing subacute native valve endocarditis?**
Viridans group *Streptococcus.*

15. **What is the most common organism causing endocarditis in intravenous drug abusers (IVDA)?**
Staphylococcus aureus.

16. **What is the most common organism causing early prosthetic valve endocarditis?**
Staphylococcus infection, particularly *S. epidermidis* and *S. aureus.*

17. What is _Enterococcus faecalis_ endocarditis often associated with?

E. faecalis endocarditis is often associated with malignancy or manipulation of the gastrointestinal or genitourinary tract.

18. What is the most common cause of culture-negative endocarditis?

The most common cause of culture-negative endocarditis is prior use of antibiotics. Other causes include fastidious organisms (HACEK group, _Legionella, Chlamydia, Brucella_, certain fungal infections, etc.) and noninfectious causes. The HACEK group of organisms may cause large vegetations and large-vessel embolism.

19. How does one diagnose endocarditis caused by fastidious and nonculturable agents?

Techniques using the polymerase chain reaction (PCR) can detect and identify nonculturable organisms. Limitations of PCR include lack of reliable application to whole blood samples, risk of contamination, false negatives due to the presence of PCR inhibitors in clinical samples, inability to provide information concerning bacterial sensitivity to antimicrobial agents, and persistent positivity despite clinical remission.

20. What is the mortality rate from IE?

The in-hospital mortality rate of patients with IE varies from 9.6 to 26%, but individual response to IE and its treatment differs considerably from patient to patient.

21. Has the incidence or mortality from endocarditis decreased over the last three decades?

No. The 2009 ESC guidelines point out that neither the incidence of endocarditis nor mortality from endocarditis has decreased in the past 30 years.

22. What are the Duke criteria for the diagnosis of endocarditis?

The Duke criteria is a set of criteria proposed for the _definite_ and _possible_ diagnosis of IE, published in 1994 (see Bibliography), based on both pathologic and clinical criteria. These criteria were a modification of previously proposed criteria (the _Von Reyn criteria_). These criteria were then themselves slightly modified in 2000, with the criteria incorporating the value of TEE, special recognition of _Coxiella burnettii_, and several other issues (see Bibliography). These revisions became known as the "modified Duke criteria" and are presented in Boxes 33-2 and 33-3.

23. What are some of the complications of endocarditis?

- Valve destruction and development of regurgitant lesions (aortic insufficiency [AI] or mitral regurgitation [MR])
- Abscess formation
- AV node heart block (as a result of abscess formation and extension to the area of the AV node and/or the bundle of His)
- Prosthetic valve dehiscence and perivalvular leaks
- Peripheral embolization (brain, kidneys, spleen, lungs, etc.)

24. What are generally accepted indications for surgery in patients with active IE?

Decisions regarding surgery will depend both on the indications for surgery and the patient's overall status and risks of surgery. Recommendations vary among the ACCF/AHA guidelines on valvular disease, the ESC guidelines on IE, and other experts who have weighed in on the topic. In general, accepted indications include acute AI or AR (or valvular stenosis) leading to heart failure, infection caused by fungi or other organisms not likely to be successfully treated with antibiotics, complications such as abscess formation, or recurrent embolism. Other potential indications for surgery include pseudoaneurysm, perforation, fistula, valve aneurysm, and dehiscence of a prosthetic valve.

Box 33-2 THE MODIFIED DUKE CRITERIA DEFINITIONS OF DEFINITE, POSSIBLE, AND REJECTED ENDOCARDITIS

Definite Infective Endocarditis

Pathologic Criteria

1. Microorganisms demonstrated by culture or histologic examination of a vegetation, a vegetation that has embolized, or an intracardiac abscess specimen; or
2. Pathologic lesions; vegetation or intracardiac abscess confirmed by histologic examination showing active endocarditis

Clinical Criteria (see Box 33-3)

1. Two major criteria; or
2. One major criterion and three minor criteria; or
3. Five minor criteria

Possible Infective Endocarditis (see Box 33-3)

1. One major criterion and one minor criterion; or
2. Three minor criteria

Rejected

1. Firm alternate diagnosis explaining evidence of infective endocarditis; or
2. Resolution of infective endocarditis syndrome with antibiotic therapy for 4 days or less; or
3. No pathologic evidence of infective endocarditis at surgery or autopsy, with antibiotic therapy for 4 days or less; or
4. Does not meet criteria for possible infective endocarditis, as above

Modified from Li JS, Sexton DJ, Mick N, et al: Proposed modifications to the Duke criteria for the diagnosis of infective endocarditis. *Clin Infect Dis* 30:633-638, 2000.

ACCF/AHA guidelines for surgery in cases of IE are summarized in Table 33-1; ESC guidelines for surgery are summarized in Table 33-2.

25. **Are patients with mechanical prosthetic heart valves more likely to develop endocarditis than those with bioprosthetic heart valves?**
    No. The incidence for patients with both types of prosthetic heart valves is approximately 1% per year of follow-up.

26. **What are Osler nodes?**
    Osler nodes are small, tender red-purple nodules. They most commonly occur in the fingers, hands, toes, and feet. They may be caused by circulating immune complexes.

27. **What are Janeway lesions?**
    Janeway lesions are irregular macules located on the hands and feet (Fig. 33-2). As opposed to Osler nodes, they are painless.

28. **What is marantic endocarditis?**
    Marantic endocarditis is the term previously used for what is now referred to as nonbacterial thrombotic endocarditis. The term reportedly derived from the Greek *marantikos,* meaning "wasting away." The vegetations in NBTE are sterile and believed to be composed of platelets and fibrin. The finding of such sterile vegetations occurs in the setting of chronic wasting diseases, chronic infections (e.g., tuberculosis [TB], osteomyelitis), certain cancers, and disseminated intravascular coagulation. These often large vegetations may embolize to the brain, the coronary arteries, or the periphery.

29. What is Libman-Sacks endocarditis?

Libman-Sacks endocarditis is a form of NBTE seen in patients with systemic lupus erythematosus (SLE). Described in 1924, the vegetations most commonly occur on the mitral valve, although they can affect all four cardiac valves. The lesions are due to accumulations of immune complexes, fibrin, and mononuclear cells. Most lesions do not cause symptoms, although valvular regurgitation or stenosis can occasionally occur because of the lesions. Embolization of the lesions is rare.

Box 33-3 THE MODIFIED DUKE CRITERIA FOR THE DIAGNOSIS OF ENDOCARDITIS

Major Criteria
- Blood culture positive for infective endocarditis (IE)
  - Typical microorganisms consistent with IE from 2 separate blood cultures:
    - Viridans streptococci; *Streptococcus bovis*, HACEK group, *Staphylococcus aureus*; or
    - Community-acquired enterococci, in the absence of a primary focus; or
  - Microorganisms consistent with IE from persistently positive blood cultures, defined as follows:
    - At least two positive blood cultures of blood samples drawn >12 h apart; or
    - All of three or a majority of four or more separate cultures of blood (with first and last sample drawn at least 1 h apart)
  - Single positive blood culture for *Coxiella burnetii* or anti–phase I IgG antibody titer >1:800
- Evidence of endocardial involvement
- Echocardiogram positive for IE (TEE recommended in patients with prosthetic valves, rated at least "possible IE" by clinical criteria, or complicated IE [paravalvular abscess]; TTE as first test in other patients), defined as follows:
  - Oscillating intracardiac mass on valve or supporting structures, in the path of regurgitant jets, or on implanted material in the absence of an alternative anatomic explanation; or
  - Abscess; or
  - New partial dehiscence of prosthetic valve
- New valvular regurgitation (worsening or changing or preexisting murmur not sufficient)

Minor Criteria
- Predisposition, predisposing heart condition or injection drug use
- Fever, temperature >38°C
- Vascular phenomena, major arterial emboli, septic pulmonary infarcts, mycotic aneurysm, intracranial hemorrhage, conjunctival hemorrhages, or Janeway lesions
- Immunologic phenomena: glomerulonephritis, Osler nodes, Roth spots, or rheumatoid factor
- Microbiological evidence: positive blood culture but does not meet a major criterion as noted above (excluding single positive cultures for coagulase-negative staphylococci and organisms that do not cause endocarditis) or serological evidence of active infection with organism consistent with IE
- Echocardiographic minor criteria eliminated

Modified from Li JS, Sexton DJ, Mick N, et al: Proposed modifications to the Duke criteria for the diagnosis of infective endocarditis. *Clin Infect Dis* 30:633-638, 2000.
TEE, Transesophageal echocardiography; *TTE*, transthoracic echocardiography.

TABLE 33-1. SUMMARY OF THE AMERICAN COLLEGE OF CARDIOLOGY FOUNDATION/AMERICAN HEART ASSOCIATION RECOMMENDATIONS FOR SURGERY FOR INFECTIVE ENDOCARDITIS

	Native Valve Endocarditis	Prosthetic Valve Endocarditis
Class I (surgery is indicated)	IE with valvular regurgitation (or stenosis) resulting in heart failure or hemodynamic evidence of elevated left ventricular end-diastolic or left atrial pressure IE caused by fungal or other highly resistant organisms IE complicated by heart block, annular or aortic abscess, or destructive penetrating lesions	IE with heart failure IE with valve dehiscence IE with evidence of increasing obstruction or worsening regurgitation IE with complications (e.g., abscess formation)
Class IIa (surgery is reasonable)	IE with recurrent emboli and persistent vegetations despite appropriate antibiotic therapy	IE with persistent bacteremia or recurrent emboli despite appropriate antibiotic treatment
Class IIb (surgery may be considered)	IE with mobile vegetations >10 mm with or without emboli	IE with relapsing infection
Class III (routine surgery is not indicated)		Routine surgery is not indicated for patients with uncomplicated IE caused by first infection with a sensitive organism

Table created from text in RO Bonow, BA Carabello, C Kanu, et al: 2008 Focused update incorporated into the ACC/AHA 2006 guidelines for the management of patients with valvular heart disease. *J Am Coll Cardiol* 52:e1-e142, 2008.
IE, Infective endocarditis.

TABLE 33-2. RECOMMENDATIONS FROM THE 2009 EUROPEAN SOCIETY OF CARDIOLOGY GUIDELINES ON THE PREVENTION, DIAGNOSIS, AND TREATMENT OF INFECTIVE ENDOCARDITIS: INDICATIONS AND TIMING OF SURGERY IN LEFT-SIDED NATIVE VALVE INFECTIVE ENDOCARDITIS

Recommendations: Indications for Surgery	Timing	Class of Recommendation	Level of Evidence
Heart Failure			
Aortic or mitral IE with severe acute regurgitation of valve obstruction causing refractory pulmonary edema or cardiogenic shock	Emergency	I	B
Aortic or mitral IE with fistula into a cardiac chamber or pericardium causing refractory pulmonary edema or shock	Emergency	I	B
Aortic or mitral IE with severe acute regurgitation or valve obstruction and persisting heart failure or echocardiographic signs of poor hemodynamic tolerance (early mitral closure or pulmonary hypertension)	Urgent	I	B
Aortic or mitral IE with severe regurgitation and no heart failure	Elective	IIa	B
Uncontrolled Infection			
Locally uncontrolled infection (abscess, false aneurysm, fistula, enlarging vegetation)	Urgent	I	B
Persisting fever and positive blood cultures >7-10 days	Urgent	I	B
Infection caused by fungi or multiresistant organisms	Urgent/ elective	I	B
Prevention of Embolism			
Aortic or mitral IE with large vegetations (>10 mm) following one or more embolic episodes despite appropriate antibiotic therapy	Urgent	I	B
Aortic or mitral IE with large vegetations (>10 mm) and other predictors of complicated course (heart failure, persistent infection, abscess)	Urgent	I	C
Isolated very large vegetations (>15 mm)	Urgent	IIb	C

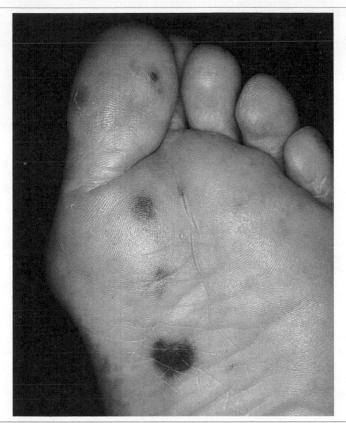

Figure 33-2. Janeway lesions in a patient with *Staphylococcus aureus* endocarditis. (From Sande MA, Strausbaugh LJ: Infective endocarditis. In Hook EW, Mandell GL, Gwaltney JM Jr, et al, editors: *Current concepts of infectious diseases*, New York, 1977, Wiley Press.)

BIBLIOGRAPHY, SUGGESTED READINGS, AND WEBSITES

1. Bonow RO, Carabello BA, Kanu C, et al: 2008 Focused update incorporated into the ACC/AHA 2006 guidelines for the management of patients with valvular heart disease, *J Am Coll Cardiol* 52:e1–e142, 2008.

2. Brusch JL: *Infective Endocarditis*. Available at: http://emedicine.medscape.com/article/216650-overview. Accessed March 26, 2013.

3. Durack DT, Lukes AS, Bright DK: New criteria for diagnosis of infective endocarditis: utilization of specific echocardiographic findings. Duke Endocarditis Service, *Am J Med* 96:200–209, 1994.

4. Horstkotte D, Follath F, Gutschik E, et al: Guidelines on prevention, diagnosis and treatment of infective endocarditis executive summary; the task force on infective endocarditis of the European Society of Cardiology, *Eur Heart J* 25:267–276, 2004.

5. Li JS, Sexton DJ, Mick N, et al: Proposed modifications to the Duke criteria for the diagnosis of infective endocarditis, *Clin Infect Dis* 30:633–638, 2000.

6. Mylonakis E, Calderwood SB: Infective endocarditis in adults, *N Engl J Med* 345:1318–1330, 2001.

7. Sexton DJ: *Infective Endocarditis*. In Basow, DS, editor: UpToDate, Waltham, MA, 2013, UpToDate. Available at: http://www.uptodate.com/contents/infective-endocarditis-historical-and-duke-criteria. Accessed March 26, 2013.

8. The Task Force on the Prevention: Diagnosis, and Treatment of Infective Endocarditis of the European Society of Cardiology (ESC). Guidelines on the prevention, diagnosis, and treatment of infective endocarditis (new version 2009), *Eur Heart J* 30:2369–2413, 2009.

9. Wilson W, Taubert KA, Gewitz M, et al: Prevention of infective endocarditis: guidelines from the American Heart Association, *Circulation* 116:1736–1754, 2007.

CHAPTER 34

ATRIAL FIBRILLATION

Jose L. Baez-Escudero, MD, FHRS, and Miguel Valderrábano, MD

1. **How common is atrial fibrillation (AF)?**

   AF is the most commonly encountered arrhythmia in clinical practice, accounting for one-third of cardiac hospitalizations annually. Its incidence rises with increasing age for men and women, with an estimated prevalence of 5% at age 75 and 15% at age 85. As many as 2.3 million Americans and 4.5 million people in the European Union are estimated to have AF.

2. **What cardiovascular diseases are likely to coexist in patients with AF?**

   Hypertensive heart disease is the most common preexisting condition. However, systolic dysfunction, coronary artery disease (CAD), rheumatic valve disease, nonrheumatic valvular heart disease, chronic lung disease, and hyperthyroidism are common comorbidities. Patients without identifiable cardiovascular disease or other conditions associated with AF are said to have *lone AF*. These patients have a favorable prognosis with respect to thromboembolism and mortality.

3. **What arrhythmias are related to AF?**

   AF may occur in association with other arrhythmias, most commonly atrial flutter or atrial tachycardia. Atrial flutter may degenerate into AF and AF may organize to atrial flutter, particularly during treatment with antiarrhythmic agents prescribed to prevent recurrent AF. The electrocardiogram (ECG) pattern may fluctuate between atrial flutter and AF, reflecting changing activation of the atria. Focal atrial tachycardias, atrioventricular (AV) reentrant tachycardias, and AV nodal reentrant tachycardias may also trigger AF.

4. **What are the main anatomic and physiologic substrates for the initiation of AF?**

   Available data support both a *focal* triggering mechanism involving automaticity or multiple reentrant wavelets. The pulmonary veins (PVs) are the most common source of these rapid atrial impulses. Other known contributing factors in the genesis of AF include atrial electrical remodeling, sympathetic and parasympathetic stimuli, the renin-angiotensin-aldosterone system, and inflammation.

5. **Which agents are effective in slowing the ventricular response in acute AF?**

   In the absence of an accessory bypass tract and preexcitation syndrome (such as in patients with Wolff-Parkinson-White [WPW] syndrome), intravenous (IV) administration of beta-adrenergic blocking agents (β-blockers; esmolol, metoprolol, or propranolol) or nondihydropyridine calcium channel antagonists (verapamil, diltiazem) is recommended to slow the ventricular response to AF in the acute setting, exercising caution in patients with hypotension or systolic heart failure. In patients with AF and systolic dysfunction who do not have an accessory pathway, IV digoxin or amiodarone is recommended. However, digoxin should not be used as a sole agent.

6. **How do you decide which antithrombotic therapy is most appropriate?**

   Several schemes for stratification of stroke risk can identify patients who benefit most and least from anticoagulation. The most commonly used tool as outlined in the current guidelines is the $CHADS_2$ score for AF stroke risk scheme (Fig. 34-1), in which patients are stratified for risk according to the presence of moderate risk factors (1 point) and high risk factors (2 points). The use of appropriate anticoagulation is then decided according to the sum of points, as outlined in Table 34-1. A recently updated and modified CHA_2DS_2-VASc scoring system (Table 34-2) has been validated and used in

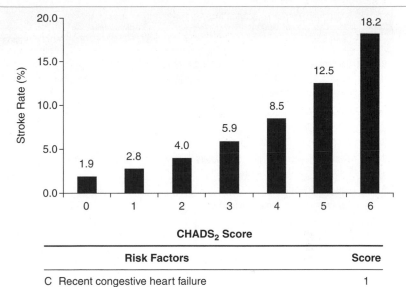

Risk Factors	Score
C Recent congestive heart failure	1
H Hypertension	1
A Age ≥75 yrs	1
D Diabetes mellitus	1
S₂ History of stroke or transient ischemic attack	2

Figure 34-1. CHADS₂ stroke risk scheme. The more risk factors, the higher the risk of stroke. (Modified from Rockson SG, Albers GW: Comparing the guidelines: anticoagulation therapy to optimize stroke prevention in patients with atrial fibrillation. *J Am Coll Cardiol* 43:929-935, 2004.)

TABLE 34-1.	AMERICAN COLLEGE OF CARDIOLOGY/AMERICAN HEART ASSOCIATION/EUROPEAN SOCIETY OF CARDIOLOGY 2006 GUIDELINES: RECOMMENDED THERAPIES ACCORDING TO CHADS₂ STROKE RISK
Risk Category	**Recommended Therapy**
No risk factors	Aspirin, 81-325 mg daily
One moderate risk factor	Aspirin, 81-325 mg daily, or warfarin (INR 2-3, target 2.5) (depending on patient preference)
Any high risk factor or >1 moderate risk factor	Warfarin (INR 2-3, target 2.5)

INR, international normalized ratio.

patients who fall in the intermediate risk category. CHA₂DS₂-VASc assigns points for risk factors not included in the CHADS₂ score, such as female gender, age 65 to 75, and vascular disease.

7. **Why is antithrombotic therapy so important in AF?**
   AF is an independent risk factor for stroke. The rate of ischemic stroke in patients with nonvalvular AF is about two to seven times that of people without AF, and the risk increases dramatically as

TABLE 34-2.	THE CHA$_2$DS$_2$-VASC SCORING SYSTEM	
	Condition	**Points**
C	Congestive heart failure (or left ventricular systolic dysfunction)	1
H	Hypertension: blood pressure consistently above 140/90 mm Hg (or treated hypertension on medication)	1
A$_2$	Age ≥ 75 years	2
D	Diabetes mellitus	1
S$_2$	Prior stroke or TIA or thromboembolism	2
V	Vascular disease (e.g., peripheral artery disease, myocardial infarction, aortic plaque)	1
A	Age 65-74 years	1
Sc	Sex category (i.e., female gender)	1

TIA, Transient ischemic attack.

patients grow older. Paroxysmal and chronic AF are associated with a similar risk of thromboembolism. Anticoagulation therapy is essential in patients with AF to reduce the risk of embolic stroke. Aspirin (81 or 325 mg/day) reduces the risk of thromboembolism by approximately 35%. Warfarin reduces the risk by 65%. Full-dose warfarin is also superior to low-dose (international normalized ratio [INR] 1.2-1.5) warfarin plus aspirin. The risk of a serious bleeding complication while on warfarin therapy (with an INR goal of 2-3) is 1.3% to 2.5% per year. Although the elderly may have a greater risk of bleeding, they also carry a greater risk of stroke and therefore benefit the most from warfarin therapy.

8. **What are some alternatives to warfarin for anticoagulation?**
   A narrow therapeutic range and the need for regular monitoring of its anticoagulatory effect impair the effectiveness and safety of warfarin, creating a need for alternative anticoagulant drugs. Interactions of warfarin with food and other drugs also hamper its use. Recently developed and FDA approved oral anticoagulants include direct thrombin antagonists such as dabigatran and factor Xa inhibitors such as rivaroxaban. Dabigatran is at least noninferior to warfarin in all AF patients at low, moderate, or high risk of stroke. It is given twice a day and does not require monitoring. The once-daily drug rivaroxaban has also been shown to be noninferior to warfarin for the prevention of stroke or systemic embolism, without additional risk of major bleeding. Antidotes have not been developed yet for these drugs, although strategies for overdose treatment and bleeding (e.g., charcoal therapy and hemodialysis in dabigatran overdose) have been proposed.

9. **When should cardioversion be considered to convert a patient from AF to sinus rhythm?**
   Cardioversion (CV) may be achieved by means of drugs or direct-current electrical shocks when the patient has new-onset AF that is less than 48 hours in duration. If the duration is more than 48 hours or unknown, the patient should be treated with anticoagulation therapy for 3 weeks before and 4 weeks after CV to prevent thromboembolism. Alternatively, a patient can undergo transesophageal echocardiography (TEE) to rule out left atrial thrombus and, if negative, proceed with CV while receiving appropriate anticoagulation. In cases of early relapse of AF after CV, repeated direct-current cardioversion attempts may be made after administration of antiarrhythmic medication. Administration of flecainide, dofetilide, propafenone, or ibutilide is recommended for pharmacologic cardioversion of AF.

10. **How do you approach rate versus rhythm control issues?**

Two landmark studies, the Atrial Fibrillation Follow-up Investigation of Rhythm Management (AFFIRM) and the Rate Control versus Electrical Cardioversion (RACE) trials, found that treating AF with a rhythm-control strategy, involving CV and antiarrhythmic drug (AAD) therapy, offers no survival or clinical advantages over a simpler rate-control strategy. However, these studies primarily enrolled older patients (older than age 65 years) with persistent AF who were mildly symptomatic. Moreover, in the AFFIRM study, fewer than two-thirds of those in the rhythm control arm were actually able to stay in sinus rhythm. Thus, the results cannot be extrapolated to many subgroups of patients, including younger patients; those with new, first-onset AF who may benefit from early conversion to sinus rhythm; patients with persistent AF who are highly symptomatic; and patients with significant systolic heart failure who have a hemodynamic benefit from the atrial kick.

11. **Which antiarrhythmic drugs are most commonly used to maintain long-term sinus rhythm and prevent AF recurrence?**

Before initiating any AADs, treatment of precipitating or reversible causes of AF is recommended. The AADs most commonly used have been sotalol, amiodarone, dronedarone, propafenone, dofetilide, and flecainide. Quinidine and procainamide are no longer used because of safety concerns. Flecainide and propafenone should be used in conjunction with an AV nodal blocker agent. These two antiarrhythmics are contraindicated in patients with CAD. Dronedarone is contraindicated in patients with systolic congestive heart failure and should not be used in patients with chronic persistent AF. Dofetilide and amiodarone are most suited for patients with AF and systolic dysfunction. Dofetilide and sotalol prolong the QT interval and are both excreted by the kidney. Their dosing requires titration according to the patient's creatinine clearance and their administration is usually initiated in a hospital setting with periodic ECG monitoring.

12. **When is catheter ablation of AF indicated, and who is the ideal candidate?**

Pulmonary vein isolation (PVI) with radiofrequency catheter ablation (RFA) is the most common ablation procedure performed in current practice. Because it has been shown to be superior to antiarrhythmics therapy alone, PVI appears in the new guidelines as a first-line option for treatment of paroxysmal or persistent AF in patients who have failed an AAD regimen. Patient selection, optimal set of ablation lesions, absolute rates of treatment success, and the frequency of complications remain incompletely defined. The ideal candidate for PVI is a person with nonvalvular paroxysmal AF, who has failed at least one AAD, and who is highly symptomatic. The patient's left atrium should be less than 5.5 cm in diameter, without other significant cardiac disease. The procedure has also been shown to be efficacious in some patients with chronic AF, as well as in patients with congestive heart failure. Some new technologies, such as balloon cryoablation, balloon laser ablation, and multielectrode catheter RFA, have been recently developed and are currently being studied as alternatives to conventional open-irrigated catheter RFA.

13. **What are potential complications of PVI?**

A worldwide survey on AF catheter ablation showed an overall incidence of major complications of 6%. Potential complications include bleeding, hematoma, or fistula at the site of femoral access, periprocedural thromboembolism, cardiac perforation or tamponade, esophageal injury including atrioesophageal fistula, pulmonary vein stenosis, phrenic nerve injury, and radiation-induced skin injury. Development of reentrant and focal left atrial tachycardias, often more symptomatic than the initial AF, may be seen after the procedure and may be transient.

14. **What is the role of AV nodal ablation followed by permanent pacing in treating AF?**

The guidelines specifically state that AV node ablation followed by permanent pacing should be used only as a fallback treatment rather than as a primary strategy, because of the risk of long-term right ventricular (RV) pacing. In general, patients most likely to benefit from this strategy are those with symptoms or tachycardia-mediated cardiomyopathy related to rapid ventricular rate during AF that cannot be controlled adequately with AADs or negative chronotropic medications. Biventricular pacing is often used with or without a defibrillator in patients that are candidates for AV nodal ablation and have a history of cardiomyopathy. Although the symptomatic benefits of AV nodal ablation are clear, limitations include the persistent need for anticoagulation, loss of AV synchrony, and lifelong pacemaker dependency.

15. **What is the role of left atrial appendage (LAA) occluders in the prevention of stroke in AF patients?**

Percutaneously placed LAA closure devices can decrease the risk of ischemic stroke in patients with AF, without the need for long-term oral anticoagulation, and may be a useful strategy in patients with contraindications to long-term oral anticoagulation. These devices are deployed in the LAA and occlude the LAA, preventing blood from entering the appendage and hence avoiding thrombus formation. The Watchman closure device (Atritech, Inc., Plymouth, Minn.) was studied in the randomized trial Embolic Protection in Patients with Atrial Fibrillation (PROTECT-AF), in which patients with the device took warfarin for at least the first six weeks. PROTECT-AF found the device noninferior to standard warfarin therapy for protection against stroke, cardiovascular death, or systemic embolism in patients with AF and a CHADS$_2$ score >1. This study led to the approval of the Watchman device in Europe. A larger randomized trial comparing the device to warfarin (Prospective Randomized Evaluation of the WATCHMAN LAA Closure Device in Patients with Atrial Fibrillation versus Long Term Warfarin Therapy [PREVAIL]) is currently underway.

BIBLIOGRAPHY, SUGGESTED READINGS, AND WEBSITES

1. Gage BF, Waterman AD, et al: Validation of clinical classification schemes for predicting stroke: results from the National Registry of Atrial Fibrillation, *JAMA* 285:2864–2870, 2001.

2. Heart Rhythm Society: 2012 HRA/ECAS expert concensus statement on catheter and surgical ablation of atrial fibrillation (AFib). Available at: http://www.hrsonline.org/Practice-Guidance/Clinical-Guidelines-Documents/Expert-Consensus-Statement-on-Catheter-and-Surgical-Ablation-of-Atrial-Fibrillation-AFib/2012-Catheter-and-Surgical-Ablation-of-AFib. Accessed February 11, 2013.

3. Hsu L-F, Jaïs P, Sanders P, et al: Catheter ablation for atrial fibrillation in congestive heart failure, *N Engl J Med* 351:2373–2383, 2004.

4. Kalman J, Kim Y-H, Klein G, et al: Worldwide survey on the methods, efficacy, and safety of catheter ablation for human atrial fibrillation, *Circulation* 111:1100–1105, 2005.

5. Oral H, Pappone C, Morady F, et al: Circumferential pulmonary-vein ablation for chronic atrial fibrillation, *N Engl J Med* 354:934–941, 2006.

6. Schirmer SH, Baumhäkel M, Neuberger HR, et al: Novel anticoagulants for stroke prevention in atrial fibrillation: current clinical evidence and future developments, *J Am Coll Cardiol* 56:2067–2076, 2010.

7. StopAfib.org: Atrial fibrillation: For patients by patients. Available at: http://www.stopafib.org. Accessed February 11, 2013.

8. Van Gelder IC, Hagens VE, Bosker HA, et al: A comparison of rate control and rhythm control in patients with recurrent persistent atrial fibrillation, *N Engl J Med* 347:1834–1840, 2002.

9. Wolf PA, Abbott RD, Kannel WB: Atrial fibrillation as an independent risk factor for stroke: the Framingham Study, *Stroke* 22:983–988, 1991.

10. Wyse DG, Waldo AL, DiMarco JP, et al: The atrial fibrillation follow-up investigation of rhythm management (AFFIRM Investigators). A comparison of rate control and rhythm with atrial fibrillation, *N Engl J Med* 347:1825–1833, 2002.

CHAPTER 35

SUPRAVENTRICULAR TACHYCARDIA

Glenn N. Levine, MD, FACC, FAHA

1. **What does the term supraventricular tachycardia (SVT) mean?**
   By strict definition, a *supraventricular tachycardia* is any tachycardia whose genesis is not in the ventricles. Thus, the term can encompass atrial fibrillation and flutter, atrial tachycardia and multifocal atrial tachycardia, and reentrant tachycardias. Others will use the terms *SVT* or *paroxysmal SVT* to more specifically refer to the reentrant tachycardias of atrioventricular (AV) nodal reentrant tachycardia (AVNRT) and AV reentrant tachycardia (AVRT), as well as atrial tachycardia and several uncommon supraventricular arrhythmias. For the purposes of this chapter, we will use the term *SVT* to refer to any tachycardia not caused by ventricular tachycardia, and the term *paroxysmal SVT* to refer to tachycardias resulting from AVNRT, AVRT, and atrial tachycardia (although the reader should recognize that this is somewhat arbitrary and not universally accepted, and we will not discuss in detail other rare causes of paroxysmal SVT).

2. **What is the most common cause of paroxysmal SVT?**
   AVNRT accounts for 60% to 70% of paroxysmal SVTs, followed by AVRT.

3. **What factors are part of the *generic* workup for supraventricular tachycardia?**
   - History, including type and duration of symptoms (palpitations, lightheadedness, chest pains, dyspnea, presyncope, precipitating factors)
   - Questions regarding the intake of alcohol, caffeine, and illicit drugs
   - Cardiac history (myocardial infarction, valvular disease, cardiac surgery)
   - Physical examination (although often unrevealing)
   - 12-lead electrocardiogram (ECG) (looking for signs of chamber enlargement, preexcitation, etc.)
   - Echocardiogram (often unrevealing because paroxysmal SVT can occur in the absence of structural heart disease, although atrial arrhythmias will often occur in the setting of dilated atria)
   - Laboratory tests (electrolyte abnormalities, hyperthyroidism)

4. **What are the causes of narrow complex regular tachycardias (regular referring to fixed R-R intervals—the time or *distance* between QRS complexes)?**
   ECGs of the more common SVTs that cause narrow complex regular tachycardias are shown in Figure 35-1.
   - Sinus tachycardia (not really an arrhythmia, but still in the differential diagnosis)
   - Atrial flutter
   - Atrial tachycardia
   - AVNRT
   - AVRT
   - Rare causes of narrow complex QRS, especially in adults, that are often difficult to diagnose and are more suited for discussion at the cardiology fellow or attending level, include sino-atrial (SA) nodal reentrant tachycardia and focal junctional tachycardia.

5. **What are the causes of narrow complex irregular tachycardias (tachycardias with irregular R-R intervals)?**
   ECGs of SVTs that cause narrow complex irregular tachycardias are shown in Figure 35-2.
   - Multifocal atrial tachycardia (MAT)
   - Atrial flutter with "variable conduction"
   - Atrial fibrillation

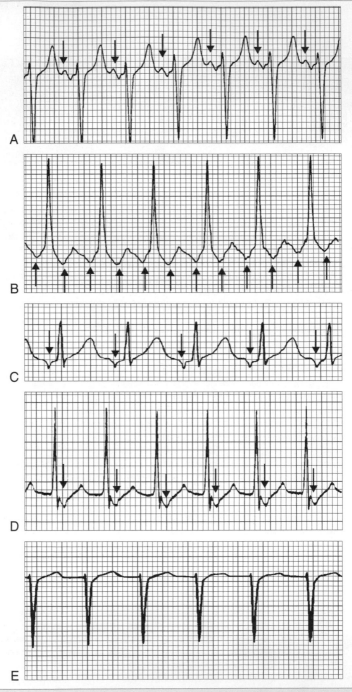

Figure 35-1. SVTs that cause a narrow complex regular tachycardia. **A,** Sinus tachycardia. Normal appearing P waves *(arrows)* are present before each QRS complex. **B,** Atrial tachycardia. Abnormal, inverted P waves *(arrows)* are present before each QRS complex. **C,** Atrial flutter. Flutter waves *(arrows)* are present. There is 2:1 conduction. **D,** Atrioventricular nodal reentrant tachycardia (AVNRT). No P waves are present before the QRS complexes. Retrograde, inverted P waves *(arrows)* are visible immediately after the QRS complexes. **E,** Atrioventricular reentrant tachycardia (AVRT). No P waves are present before the QRS complexes. Although retrograde P waves are sometimes seen in the ST-T segment with AVRT, none are visible in this particular rhythm strip.

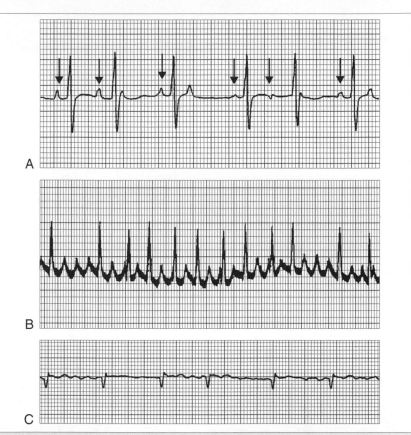

Figure 35-2. Supraventricular tachycardia (SVTs) that cause a narrow complex irregular tachycardia. **A,** Multifocal atrial tachycardia (MAT). P waves of differing morphologies *(arrows)* are present before the QRS complexes. **B,** Atrial flutter with variable block. Flutter waves are intermittently visible between the QRS complexes. **C,** Atrial fibrillation. No organized atrial activity is present.

6. **How should one determine the correct diagnosis of a narrow complex tachycardia?**
   This can be done in two simple steps. First, decide if the rhythm is regular or irregular. Second, look for P waves or atrial activity. Figure 35-3 demonstrates how this simple two-step process will lead to the correct diagnosis.

7. **What drug is most commonly implicated in cases of drug-induced atrial tachycardia?**
   Digoxin. Digoxin toxicity can cause many arrhythmias, including *paroxysmal atrial tachycardia with block*. In paroxysmal atrial tachycardia (PAT) with block, there is atrial tachycardia but also AV nodal block, leading to a slow ventricular response rate (Fig. 35-4). In cases of PAT with block, digoxin toxicity should be suspected.

8. **What is the most common ventricular response rate in patients who develop atrial flutter?**
   Atrial flutter most commonly occurs at a rate of 300 beats/min, although the rate can be somewhat slower in patients on antiarrhythmic agents that slow ventricular conduction (such

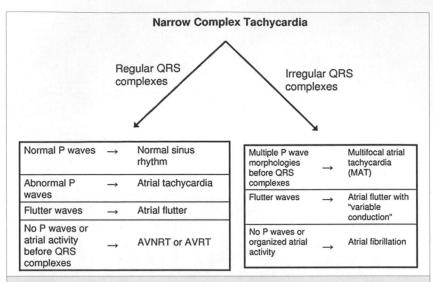

Figure 35-3. Simple algorithm for the diagnosis of narrow complex tachycardias. Step one is to decide if the rhythm is regular or irregular (are the QRS complexes occurring at regular or irregular intervals). Step two is to search for the presence of P waves or organized atrial activity.

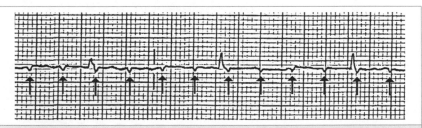

Figure 35-4. Atrial tachycardia with block. The arrows point to P waves generated by the atrial tachycardia. Most of these P waves are not conducted in to the ventricle. The finding of atrial tachycardia with significant atrioventricular (AV) node block is highly suggestive of digoxin toxicity.

as amiodarone) or in cases of massively dilated atria. Most commonly, there is 2:1 AV block, meaning that only every other atrial impulse is conducted down to the ventricles. Thus, the most common ventricular response rate is 150 beats/min (see Fig. 35-1, *C*). The finding of a regular narrow complex tachycardia at exactly 150 beats/min should raise suspicion of atrial flutter as the causative arrhythmia.

9. **Which is more common, AVNRT or AVRT?**
   AVNRT is more common in the general population. In patients with known preexcitation syndrome (Wolff-Parkinson-White [WPW] syndrome), AVRT, which requires an accessory circuit, is more common. Thus, statistically, the cause of a narrow complex regular tachycardia is more likely to be AVNRT than AVRT, unless the patient has known WPW (or evidence of it on a baseline ECG).

10. **What is the most common cause of atrial tachycardia?**

Atrial tachycardia (see Fig. 35-1, *B*) is most commonly caused by a discrete autonomic focus, although a microreentrant circuit causes a small percentage of atrial tachycardias. Precipitating factors and causes of atrial tachycardia include:

- Diseased atrial tissue (fibrosis, inflammation, etc.)
- Increased sympathetic stimulation (hyperthyroidism, caffeine, etc.)
- Excessive alcohol consumption
- Digoxin toxicity
- Electrolyte abnormalities
- Hypoxemia

Although textbooks describe the rate of atrial tachycardia as anywhere between 100 and 220 beats/min, a rate of approximately 160 to 180 beats/min is most common. AV conduction is usually 1:1 unless the tachycardia is very rapid, in which case 2:1 conduction may occur. Because most cases of atrial tachycardia are due to an autonomic focus and not a reentrant pathway, the arrhythmia most commonly does not terminate with cardioversion. Adenosine usually (but not always) will not terminate the arrhythmia, but adenosine administration may be useful in cases in which the cause of regular SVT is unclear (see Question 12).

11. **What is concealed conduction?**

In many patients with preexcitation syndrome (e.g., WPW), conduction from the atrium to the ventricle will result in the appearance of a *delta wave* on the 12-lead ECG. However, in some patients with WPW, the accessory bypass tract does not conduct in such an antegrade direction but only in a retrograde direction (*up* from the ventricle to the atrium). No delta wave appears on the baseline ECG because there is no antegrade conduction, but the accessory pathway is capable of retrograde conduction and participating in the genesis of AVRT (impulses travel down the His-Purkinje system, into the ventricle, and then up the accessory pathway into the atrium).

12. **In cases of SVT in which the cause is not clear, what is generally considered first-line drug therapy?**

Adenosine is most commonly administered in cases of SVT of unclear origin. Adenosine will transiently block AV nodal conduction. In patients with atrial flutter or atrial tachycardia, it will slow the ventricular response rate and may allow identification of flutter waves or the abnormal P waves of atrial tachycardia. In cases of AVNRT and AVRT, it may break the arrhythmia by interrupting the reentrant circuit. The dosing is 6 mg, administered quickly through a large-bore intravenous (IV) line, followed, if unsuccessful in terminating the arrhythmia, by a first dose of 12 mg, followed in turn by a second dose of 12 mg. Lower doses of adenosine (such as 3 mg) are recommended by some authorities if adenosine is administered through a central line, and adenosine should be used with caution, if at all, and in lower doses, in heart transplant patients.

Although adenosine is a frontline agent for arrhythmia diagnosis and termination, it is not useful for more sustained ventricular rate control in patients with atrial fibrillation or atrial flutter because of its very short half-life. Patients who do not respond to adenosine can be treated acutely with IV beta-adrenergic blocking agents (β-blockers) or IV diltiazem or verapamil, both of which have onset of action within minutes and are good AV node blocking agents. IV digoxin is not considered a good choice for acute therapy because its onset of action is approximately 1 hour.

13. **For what arrhythmia should AV nodal blocking agents *not* be administered?**

In rare cases of atrial fibrillation in the setting of an accessory bypass tract (WPW syndrome), some conduction of impulses will occur down the AV node and His-Purkinje system into the ventricle, and some conduction will occur down the bypass tract. In such cases, administration of AV nodal blocking agents (adenosine, digoxin, β-blockers, calcium channel blockers) may lead to increased conduction down the accessory bypass tract, producing an increased ventricular response rate and possibly precipitating ventricular fibrillation.

14. **Do patients with atrial flutter require anticoagulation before cardioversion?**
Previously it was believed that the risk of embolization during cardioversion for atrial flutter was negligible. However, observational studies have reported rates of embolization with cardioversion of atrial flutter ranging between 1.7% to 7%. Although a collective review showed that the rate of embolization with cardioversion for atrial flutter was lower than for that with atrial fibrillation (2.2% vs. 5% to 7%), expert consensus is that this rate is sufficient to warrant anticoagulation (and/or transesophageal echocardiogram) similar to that used in patients with atrial fibrillation who are to undergo cardioversion.

15. **Can SVT cause a wide QRS complex tachycardia?**
Yes, SVT occurring in the setting of baseline bundle branch block will produce a wide complex (QRS width of 120 ms or more) tachycardia. At faster heart rates, patients can also develop what is called *rate-related* bundle branch block. Rarely, a wide complex SVT can also be caused by AVRT with antidromic conduction.

16. **What is AVRT with antidromic conduction?**
In approximately 90% of cases of AVRT, the reentrant circuit is composed of conduction *down* the AV node and His-Purkinje system, into the ventricle, and then *up* the bypass tract (this is called orthodromic conduction). However, in about 10% of cases of AVRT, the reentrant circuit is composed of conduction from the atrium *down* the bypass tract, into the ventricle, and then *up* the His-Purkinje system and AV node and into the atrium. This is termed *antidromic conduction.* Because ventricular depolarization occurs without the use of the His-Purkinje system and left and right bundle branches, the QRS complexes appear wide.

17. **What factors make the diagnosis of a wide QRS complex more likely to be ventricular tachycardia (VT) than SVT?**
    - **P-wave dissociation** (also called AV dissociation): In P-wave dissociation, the QRS complexes occur at a greater rate than the P waves and there is no fixed relationship between the QRS complexes and the P waves. This finding is highly suggestive of VT. Unfortunately, P-wave dissociation can only be clearly discerned in 30% of cases of VT.
    - **QRS complex width:** In the absence of antiarrhythmic agents or an accessory pathway, a QRS width of more than 140 ms with a right bundle branch block (RBBB) morphology or a QRS width of more than 160 ms with a left bundle branch block (LBBB) morphology favors the diagnosis of VT.
    - **Negative concordance:** Negative concordance is the finding of similar QRS morphologies in all the precordial leads, with QS complexes present. This finding is essentially diagnostic for VT.
    - **Ventricular fusion beats:** Fusion beats are QRS complexes that may be formed from the *fusion* of an impulse originating in the ventricle with an impulse originating in the atria and traveling down the AV node and His-Purkinje system. The finding of fusion beats indicates VT.
    Importantly, the presence of stable hemodynamics and no cardiac symptoms does not distinguish between SVT and VT.

BIBLIOGRAPHY, SUGGESTED READINGS, AND WEBSITES

1. Blomström-Lundqvist C, Scheinman MM, Aliot EM, et al: ACC/AHA/ESC guidelines for the management of patients with supraventricular arrhythmias, *J Am Coll Cardiol* 42:1493–1531, 2003.
2. Delacrétaz E: Clinical practice. Supraventricular tachycardia, *N Engl J Med* 354:1039–1051, 2006.

CHAPTER 36

VENTRICULAR TACHYCARDIA

Jose L. Baez-Escudero, MD, FHRS, and Miguel Valderrábano, MD

1. **What is the differential diagnosis of a wide complex tachycardia (WCT)?**
   The differential includes the following:
   - Ventricular tachycardia (VT) (monomorphic or polymorphic)
   - Supraventricular tachycardia (SVT) with aberrant conduction or underlying bundle branch block
   - Antidromic SVT using an accessory pathway for antegrade conduction (Wolff-Parkinson-White syndrome)
   - Toxicity related (hyperkalemia, digoxin, other drugs; Fig. 36-1)
   - Pacemaker-mediated tachycardia
   - Telemetry artifacts

   Of note, a wide-QRS tachycardia should always be presumed to be VT if the diagnosis is unclear. VT is defined as three or more consecutive QRS complexes arising from the ventricles. Sustained VT is that which causes symptoms or lasts more than 30 seconds.

2. **What is the pathophysiologic substrate of VT?**
   It depends on the clinical scenario, but the most common mechanism is reentry, followed by automaticity.

3. **What is the most common underlying heart disease predisposing to VT?**
   The most common conditions predisposing to VT are coronary artery disease and coronary ischemia. VT in the setting of acute ischemia and immediately after myocardial infarction (MI) is related to excess ventricular ectopy as a result of increased automaticity (Na^+,K^+-ATPase malfunction, increase in intracellular calcium, tissue acidosis, and locally released catecholamines). After completion of an infarct, patients with resultant ischemic cardiomyopathy can suffer from recurrent sustained mono-morphic VT. In this case, VT originates in scarred myocardium where islands of infarcted tissue surrounded by strands of functional myocytes provide the substrate for the creation of a reentrant circuit.

4. **Can VT occur in other nonischemic heart diseases?**
   Scar-related VT can occur in other nonischemic conditions whenever an inflammatory or infiltrative disorder damages the myocardium. Sarcoidosis or Chagas disease are typical examples in which VT can occur as a result of such nonischemic scars. Fatty infiltration of the right ventricle leads to

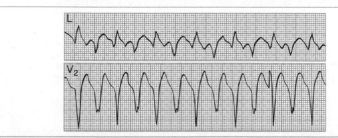

Figure 36-1. Bidirectional ventricular tachycardia in a patient with digitalis toxicity. (Modified from Marriott HJL, Conover MB: *Advanced concepts in arrhythmias,* ed 2, St Louis, 1989, Mosby.)

areas of unexcitable myocardium that can generate reentrant circuits in patients with arrhythmogenic right ventricular dysplasia. Myocardial scars leading to reentry also occur after surgical correction of congenital heart diseases. Dilated cardiomyopathies can lead to reentry within the diseased conduction system, the so-called bundle-branch reentry, where impulses use the right and left bundles as antegrade and retrograde pathways (less commonly in the opposite direction). Conceivably, any structural heart disease can lead to reentry.

5. **Can VT occur in the absence of structural heart disease?**

VT can occur in the structurally normal heart. Monomorphic VT occurs in two distinct clinical entities in the absence of heart disease. One is outflow tract VT. This condition leads to VT typically during or after exercise or in enhanced catecholamine states. It is thought to be generated by triggered activity in the form of delayed after-depolarizations, typically created in situations of calcium overload. It originates most commonly from the right ventricular outflow tract but occasionally can arise from the left ventricular outflow tract and even the aortic cusps. The second condition is idiopathic fascicular VT (also known as verapamil-sensitive or Belhassen VT). It typically occurs in young, healthy individuals with normal hearts, and most commonly involves a right bundle branch block (RBBB) and left anterior fascicular block pattern, because it arises from the left posterior fascicle. Both these forms are curable with mapping and ablation.

Primary electrical disorders can also lead to VT. Familial long QT syndromes typically lead to torsades des pointes, as does short QT syndrome. Brugada syndrome leads to primary ventricular fibrillation (Fig. 36-2). Catecholaminergic polymorphic ventricular tachycardia (CPVT) is the result of a mutation of the ryanodine receptor and typically causes exercise-induced bidirectional and polymorphic VT.

6. **What electrocardiogram (ECG) features favor VT as the cause of a wide complex tachycardia?**

VT rhythms have rates between 100 and 280 beats/min and can be monomorphic or polymorphic. Typical ECG clues that favor VT include the following:

- Presence of **fusion beats,** which identify simultaneous depolarization of the ventricle by both the normal conduction system and an ectopic impulse originating in the ventricle.
- **Capture beats,** which are normally conducted sinus beats with a narrow QRS complex that generally occur at a shorter interval than the tachycardia.
- **Atrioventricular (AV) dissociation,** the finding of independent atrial and ventricular activity at differing rates (30% of cases). Look for visible P waves that "march through" (scan and compare ST segments and T waves, look for subtle QRS changes). If there are more QRSs than Ps, it is likely to be VT. If AV dissociation is not obvious, it can be unmasked with carotid sinus massage or administration of adenosine.
- A **QRS width** more than 140 ms (RBBB morphology) or more than 160 ms (left bundle branch block [LBBB] morphology). These suggest VT, especially in the setting of a normal QRS during sinus rhythm.
- Limb lead concordance (identical QRS direction). If QRS is negative in I, II, and III (an extreme leftward or **northwest axis**), this strongly favors VT.

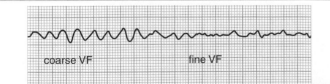

Figure 36-2. Coarse ventricular fibrillation *(VF)*, which then degenerates further into fine ventricular fibrillation. (From Goldberger E: *Treatment of cardiac emergencies,* ed 5, St Louis, 1990, Mosby.)

- **Precordial lead concordance** (V1 through V6), especially negative concordance. This is highly specific for the diagnosis of VT.
- Certain **QRS morphologic features** also may be helpful. Most aberrant conduction patterns have a precordial rS complex, whereas the absence of rS complexes suggests VT. An atypical right bundle pattern (R > R′), a monophasic or biphasic QRS in lead V1, and a small R wave coupled with a large deep S wave or a Q-S complex in V6 support the diagnosis of VT.
- **Presence of Q waves.** Remember that postinfarction Q waves are preserved in VT. Their presence in WCT is a sign of previous infarction; therefore, VT is more likely.

7. What is torsade de pointes?

Torsade de pointes, or *torsades,* is a French term that literally means "twisting of the points." It was first described by Dessertenne in 1966 and refers to a polymorphic intermediate ventricular rhythm between VT and ventricular fibrillation. It has a distinct morphology in which cycles of tachycardia with alternating peaks of QRS amplitude turn about the isoelectric line in a regular pattern (Fig. 36-3). Before the rhythm is triggered, a baseline prolonged QT interval and pathologic U waves are present, reflecting abnormal ventricular repolarization. A short-long-short sequence between the R-R interval (marked bradycardia or preceding pause) occurs before the trigger response. Drugs that prolong the QT (e.g., antiarrhythmics, some antibiotics and antifungals, and tricyclic antidepressants) and electrolyte disorders such as hypokalemia and hypomagnesemia are common triggers. When the ECG finding occurs, it should be treated as any life-threatening VT, and immediate efforts must be made to determine the underlying cause of QT lengthening.

8. What critical decisions must be made in the management of sustained VT?

The critical decision in the management of a patient with sustained VT is the urgency with which to treat the rhythm. In a hemodynamically stable and minimally symptomatic patient, treatment should be delayed until a 12-lead ECG can be obtained. The axis and morphology help to make the diagnosis of VT, as well as shed light on the potential mechanism and origin of the rhythm. During the delay, a brief medical history and baseline laboratory values can be obtained (especially serum levels of potassium and magnesium, as well as cardiac biomarkers). Specific attention should be paid to a history of myocardial infarction, systolic heart failure, history of structural heart disease, family history of sudden cardiac death, and potentially proarrhythmic drugs.

9. What methods are used to terminate sustained VT?

With any question of hemodynamic instability, termination should be done immediately with synchronized direct current electrical cardioversion. Hemodynamic instability is defined as hypotension resulting in shock, congestive heart failure, myocardial ischemia (infarction or angina), or signs or symptoms of inadequate cerebral perfusion. It is important to ensure that the energy is delivered in a synchronized fashion before cardioversion. Failure to do so may accelerate the rhythm or induce ventricular fibrillation. If the patient is conscious, adequate intravenous (IV) sedation should always be provided. Termination of hemodynamically stable VT may be attempted medically. Reasonable drugs

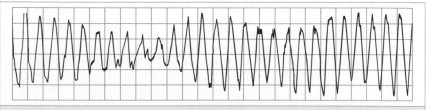

Figure 36-3. Torsades de pointes, in which the QRS axis seems to rotate about the isoelectric point. (Modified from Olgin JE, Zipes DP: Specific arrhythmias: diagnosis and treatment. In Libby P, Bonow RO, Mann DL, Zipes DP, editors: *Braunwald's heart disease: a textbook of cardiovascular medicine,* ed 8, Philadelphia, 2008, Saunders.)

of choice are IV procainamide (or ajmaline in some European countries), lidocaine, and IV amiodarone. For ischemic monomorphic VT, intravenous lidocaine is also a reasonable option. Pace termination (either through transvenous insertion of a temporary pacer or by reprogramming an implantable cardioverter-defibrillator [ICD]) can be useful to treat patients with sustained monomorphic VT that is refractory to cardioversion or is recurrent despite the use of the above-mentioned drugs. If VT is associated with acute ischemia, urgent angiography and revascularization are paramount.

10. **Once the acute episode is terminated, what are the next managing strategies?**
    This depends on the clinical situation and on the individual patient. Any potentially reversible cause—specifically, ischemia, heart failure, or electrolyte abnormalities—should be sought and treated aggressively. In general, beta-adrenergic blocking agents (β-blockers) are usually safe and effective and should be administered in most patients in whom concomitant antiarrhythmic drugs are indicated. Amiodarone and sotalol have been the mainstay of preventive therapy, especially in patients with left ventricle (LV) dysfunction. However, the long-term clinical success of medical regimens is low, and amiodarone carries a risk of serious side effects. All patients should be risk stratified for the likelihood of recurrence and subsequent risk of sudden cardiac death. Appropriate consultation with an electrophysiologist should be obtained to assess the need for ICD implantation (indications for ICDs are discussed in Chapter 38). Although cardiac device therapy has revolutionized treatment, providing excellent protection from sudden cardiac death, it does not prevent recurrences. Patients with defibrillators may remain symptomatic, with palpitations, syncope, and recurrent shocks for VT. Ablation of the reentrant circuits that cause VT also provides a nonpharmacologic option for the reduction of symptoms.

11. **How is catheter ablation of VT performed?**
    VT ablation remains challenging and is offered primarily at experienced centers. Endocardial mapping of VT to identify an optimal region for ablation can be time-consuming because of the complexity of the reentry circuits and the existence of certain circuit portions deep within the endocardium. Most ventricular reentry circuits have an exit somewhere along the border zone of the infarct scars. It is near such an exit that sinus rhythm pacing (pace mapping) is expected to produce a QRS morphology similar to that of VT. This approach, combined with modern three-dimensional voltage-mapping technologies that reconstruct and relate electrophysiologic characteristics to specific anatomy, have greatly facilitated the ablation procedure. Ablation can be achieved using traditional radiofrequency, or with other technologies, such as cryoablation or laser. When endocardial circuits are resistant to ablation, the technique of transthoracic pericardial access with epicardial mapping of VT is used. This approach facilitates localization and ablation of deep and epicardial circuits and requires the insertion of a sheath into the pericardial space, using a needle and guidewire under fluoroscopic control. If a separate indication for heart surgery is present (e.g., need for surgical revascularization, LV aneurysmectomy, mitral valve repair or replacement), surgical ablation may be considered.

12. **When is catheter ablation used to treat VT?**
    Ablation has traditionally been used for secondary prevention after an ICD-terminated VT and as an alternative to chronic antiarrhythmic therapy. It may also be considered as an option for reducing ICD therapies in patients with recurrent appropriate shocks and as an alternative to drug therapy for idiopathic VT. The probability of success varies, depending on an individual's substrate for the arrhythmia. A patient with a VT arising from the right ventricular outflow tract in a structurally normal heart will have a much higher likelihood of success when compared with a patient with a severely reduced ejection fraction from a large anterior wall MI with multiple VT morphologies. The target endpoint of any VT ablation is always lack of inducible VT.

BIBLIOGRAPHY, SUGGESTED READINGS, AND WEBSITES

1. Brugada P, Brugada J, Mont L, Smeets J, Andries EW: A new approach to the differential diagnosis of a regular tachycardia with a wide QRS complex, *Circulation* 83:1649–1659, 1991.

2. Marchlinski FE, Callans DJ, Gottlieb CD, Zado E: Linear ablation lesions for control of unmappable ventricular tachycardia in patients with ischemic and nonischemic cardiomyopathy, *Circulation* 101:1288–1296, 2000.

3. Reddy VY, Reynolds MR, Neuzil P, et al: Prophylactic catheter ablation for the prevention of defibrillator therapy, *N Engl J Med* 357:2657–2665, 2007.

4. Zipes DP, Camm AJ, Borggrefe M, et al: ACC/AHA/ESC 2006 guidelines for management of patients with ventricular arrhythmias and the prevention of sudden cardiac death: a report of the American College of Cardiology/American Heart Association Task Force and the European Society of Cardiology Committee for Practice Guidelines, *Circulation* 114:e385–e484, 2006.

CHAPTER 37

CARDIAC PACEMAKERS AND RESYNCHRONIZATION THERAPY

Jose L. Baez-Escudero, MD, and Miguel Valderrábano, MD

1. **What are the components of a pacing system?**
Pacing systems consist of a pulse generator and pacing leads, which can be placed in either the atria or the ventricles. Pacemakers provide an electrical stimulus to cause cardiac depolarization during periods when intrinsic cardiac electrical activity is inappropriately slow or absent. The battery most commonly used in permanent pacers has a life span of 5 to 9 years.

2. **What is the accepted pacing nomenclature for the different pacing modalities?**
The North American Society of Pacing and Electrophysiology and the British Pacing and Electrophysiology Group have developed a code to describe various pacing modes. It usually consists of three letters, but some systems use four or five:
   - Letter 1: chamber that is paced (*A* = atria, *V* = ventricles, *D* = dual chamber)
   - Letter 2: chamber that is sensed (*A* = atria, *V* = ventricles, *D* = dual chamber, *O* = none)
   - Letter 3: response to a sensed event (*I* = pacing inhibited, *T* = pacing triggered, *D* = dual, *O* = none)
   - Letter 4: rate-responsive features (an activity sensor), for example, an accelerometer in the pulse generator that detects bodily movement and increases the pacing rate according to a programmable algorithm (*R* = rate-responsive pacemaker)
   - Letter 5: Antitachycardia features

   A pacemaker in VVI mode denotes that it paces and senses the ventricle and is inhibited by a sensed ventricular event. The DDD mode denotes that both chambers are capable of being sensed and paced.

3. **What is the most important clinical feature that establishes the need for cardiac pacing?**
The most important clinical feature consists of symptoms clearly associated with bradycardia. Symptomatic bradycardia is the cardinal feature in the placement of a permanent pacemaker in acquired atrioventricular (AV) block in adults. Reversible causes, such as drug toxicity (digoxin, beta-adrenergic blocking agents [β-blockers], and calcium channel blockers), electrolyte abnormalities, Lyme disease, transient increases in vagal tone, and sleep apnea syndrome, should be sought, and the offending agents should be discontinued. The clinical manifestations of symptomatic bradycardia include fatigue, lightheadedness, dizziness, presyncope, syncope, manifestations of cerebral ischemia, dyspnea on exertion, decreased exercise tolerance, and congestive heart failure.

4. **What are the three types of acquired AV block?**
There are three degrees of AV block: first, second, and third (complete). This classification is based on both the electrocardiogram (ECG) and the anatomic location of the conduction disturbance.
   First-degree block refers to a stable prolongation of the PR interval to more than 200 ms and represents delay in conduction at the level of the AV node. There are no class I indications for pacing in isolated asymptomatic first-degree block.
   Second-degree block is divided into two types. Mobitz type I (Wenckebach) exhibits progressive prolongation of the PR interval before an atrial impulse fails to stimulate the ventricle. Anatomically, this form of block occurs above the bundle of His in the AV node. Type II exhibits no prolongation of the PR interval before a dropped beat and anatomically occurs at the level of the bundle of His. This rhythm may be associated with a wide QRS complex.

Third-degree or *complete block* defines the absence of AV conduction and refers to complete dissociation of the atrial and ventricular rhythms, with a ventricular rate less than the atrial rate. The width and rate of the ventricular escape rhythm help to identify an anatomic location for the block: narrow QRS is associated with minimal slowing of the rate, generally at the AV node, and wide QRS is associated with considerable slowing of rate at or below the bundle of His. Permanent pacemaker implantation is indicated for third-degree and advanced second-degree AV block at any anatomic level associated with bradycardia with symptoms (including heart failure) or ventricular arrhythmias presumed to be due to AV block.

5. **What is the anatomic location of bifascicular or trifascicular block?**
Bifascicular block is located below the AV node and involves a combination of block at the level of the right bundle with block within one of the fascicles of the left bundle (left anterior or left posterior fascicle).

Trifascicular block refers to the presence of a prolonged PR interval in addition to a bifascicular block. Based on the surface ECG, it is impossible to tell whether the prolonged PR interval is due to delay at the AV node (suprahisian) or in the remaining conducting fascicle (infrahisian, hence the term *trifascicular block*). Pacing is indicated when bifascicular or trifascicular block is associated with the following:
   - Complete block and symptomatic bradycardia
   - Alternating bundle branch block
   - Intermittent type II second-degree block with or without related symptoms
   - Symptoms suggestive of bradycardia and an HV interval greater than 100 ms on invasive electrophysiology study

6. **When is pacing indicated for asymptomatic bradycardia?**
There are few indications for pacing in patients with bradycardia who are truly asymptomatic:
   - Third-degree AV block with documented asystole lasting 3 or more seconds (in sinus rhythm) or escape rates below 40 beats/min in patients while awake
   - Third-degree AV block or second-degree AV Mobitz type II block in patients with chronic bifascicular and trifascicular block
   - Congenital third-degree AV block with a wide QRS escape rhythm, ventricular dysfunction, or bradycardia markedly inappropriate for age

Potential (class II) indications for pacing in asymptomatic patients include the following:
   - Third-degree AV block with faster escape rates in patients who are awake
   - Second-degree AV Mobitz type II block in patients without bifascicular or trifascicular block
   - The finding on electrophysiologic study of block below or within the bundle of His or an HV interval of 100 ms or longer

When bradycardia, even if extreme, is present only during sleep, pacing is not indicated.

7. **What is sick sinus syndrome?**
Sinus node dysfunction (SND), also referred to as *sick sinus syndrome*, is a common cause of bradycardia. Its prevalence has been estimated to be as high as 1 in 600 patients over the age of 65 years, and the syndrome accounts for approximately 50% of pacemaker implantations in the United States. SND may be due to replacement of nodal tissue with fibrous tissue at the sinus node itself, or it may be due to extrinsic causes (e.g., drugs, electrolyte imbalance, hypothermia, hypothyroidism, increased intracranial pressure, or excessive vagal tone). Abnormal automaticity and conduction in the atrium predispose patients to atrial fibrillation and flutter, and the bradycardia-tachycardia syndrome is a common manifestation of sinus node dysfunction. Therapy to control the ventricular rate during tachycardia by blocking AV conduction with β-blockers, calcium-channel blockers, or digitalis may not be possible, because it may further depress the sinus node. Permanent pacemaker implantation is indicated for SND with documented symptomatic bradycardia, including frequent sinus pauses that produce symptoms. It is also indicated for symptomatic chronotropic incompetence and for symptomatic sinus bradycardia that results from required drug therapy for

medical conditions (e.g., rate control for atrial tachyarrhythmias, chronic stable angina, or systolic heart failure).

8. **Is pacing indicated for neurocardiogenic syncope?**
    Neurocardiogenic syncope occurs when triggering of a neural reflex results in a usually self-limited episode of systemic hypotension characterized by both bradycardia and peripheral vasodilation. Many of these patients have a prominent vasodepressor component to their syndrome, and implantation of a pacemaker may not completely relieve symptoms. Hence, the role of pacing in patients with neurocardiac syncope and confirmed bradycardia is controversial. When bradycardia occurs only in specific situations, patient education, pharmacologic trials, and prevention strategies are indicated before pacing in most patients.

9. **What are the indications for pacing after myocardial infarction (MI)?**
    Indications in this setting do not require the presence of symptoms. The indications, in large part, are to treat the intraventricular conduction defects that result from infarction. Pacing is indicated in the setting of acute MI for the following:
    - Complete third-degree block or advanced second-degree block that is associated with block in the His-Purkinje system (wide-complex ventricular rhythm)
    - Transient advanced (second- or third-degree) AV block with a new bundle branch block.
    Pacing in the setting of an acute MI may be temporary rather than long-term or permanent.

10. **What are potential complications associated with pacemaker implantation?**
    Complications in the hands of experienced operators are rare (approximately 1% to 2%) and include bleeding, infection, pneumothorax, hemothorax, cardiac arrhythmias, cardiac perforation causing tamponade, diaphragmatic (phrenic) nerve pacing, pocket hematoma, coronary sinus trauma, and prolonged radiation exposure. Late complications include erosion of the pacer through the skin (requires pacer replacement, lead extraction, and systemic antibiotics), and lead malfunction (e.g., lead fracture, break in lead insulation, or dislodgement).

11. **What is pacemaker syndrome?**
    Historically, *pacemaker syndrome* refers to progressive worsening of symptoms, particularly congestive heart failure, after single-chamber ventricular pacing. This was due to asynchronous ventricular pacing, leading to inappropriately timed atrial contractions, including those occurring during ventricular systole. Dual-chamber pacing and appropriate pacing mode selection prevent the occurrence of pacemaker syndrome. *Pseudo–pacemaker syndrome* occurs when a patient without a pacemaker has PR prolongation so severe that the P waves are closer to the preceding R waves than to the following ones, leading to atrial contractions during the preceding ventricular systole.

12. **What is twiddler's syndrome?**
    Twiddler's syndrome is a rare complication of pacemaker implantation caused by repetitive and often unintentional twisting of the generator in the pacemaker pocket, producing lead dislodgement or fracture and subsequent pacemaker failure. It is most commonly observed in patients with behavioral disorders.

13. **What is pacemaker-mediated tachycardia?**
    Pacemaker-mediated tachycardia (PMT) is a form of reentrant tachycardia that can occur in patients who have a dual-chamber pacemaker. If the AV node retrogradely conducts a ventricular-paced beat or a premature ventricular contraction (PVC) back to the atrium and depolarizes the atrium before the next atrial-paced beat, this atrial activation will be sensed by the pacemaker atrial lead and interpreted as an intrinsic atrial depolarization. Consecutively, the pacemaker will then pace the ventricle after the programmed AV delay and perpetuate the cycle of ventricular pacing → retrograde ventriculoatrial (VA) conduction → atrial sensing → ventricular pacing (the pacemaker forms the antegrade limb of the circuit, and the AV node is the retrograde limb). Consider PMT in patients with a

dual-chamber pacemaker who experience palpitations, rapid heart rates, lightheadedness, syncope, or chest discomfort. It is corrected by programming the pacemaker with a postventricular atrial refractory period (PVARP) so that atrial events occurring shortly after ventricular events are ignored by the pacemaker.

14. **What is cardiac resynchronization therapy?**

Cardiac resynchronization therapy (CRT) refers to simultaneous pacing of both ventricles (biventricular [Bi-V] pacing). The rationale for CRT is based on the observation that the presence of a bundle branch block or other intraventricular conduction delay can worsen systolic heart failure by causing ventricular dyssynchrony, thereby reducing the efficiency of contraction. Pacing of the left ventricle (LV) is achieved either by placing a transvenous lead in the lateral venous system of the heart through the coronary sinus (preferred approach; Fig. 37-1) or by placement of an epicardial LV lead (requires a limited thoracotomy and general anesthesia). The rationale for CRT is that ventricular dyssynchrony can further impair the pump function of a failing ventricle. Potential mechanisms of benefit include improved contractile function (improvement in ejection fraction [EF], increase in cardiac index and blood pressure, decrease in pulmonary capillary wedge pressure) and reverse ventricular remodeling (reductions in LV end-systolic and end-diastolic dimensions, severity of mitral regurgitation, and LV mass).

15. **When is CRT indicated?**

CRT is indicated in patients with advanced heart failure (usually New York Heart Association [NYHA] class III or IV), severe systolic dysfunction (LV ejection fraction 35% or less), and intraventricular conduction delay (QRS more than 120 ms), who are in sinus rhythm and have been on optimal medical

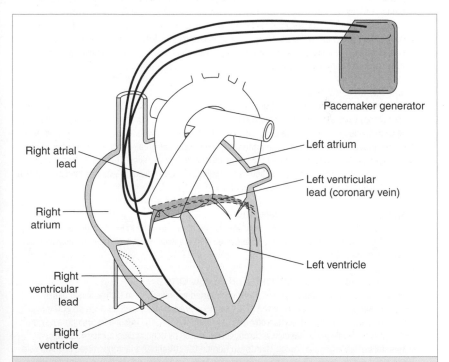

Figure 37-1. Biventricular (Bi-V) pacemaker. Note the pacemaker lead in the coronary sinus vein that allows pacing of the left ventricle simultaneously with the right ventricle. Bi-V pacing is used in selected patients with congestive heart failure with left ventricular conduction delays to help resynchronize cardiac activation and thereby improve cardiac function. (From Goldberger AL: *Clinical electrocardiography: a simplified approach*, ed 7, Philadelphia, 2006, Mosby.)

therapy. CRT can be achieved with a device designed only for pacing or can be combined with a defibrillator (many patients who are candidates for an implantable cardioverter-defibrillator [ICD] are also candidates for CRT). CRT has been shown not only to improve quality of life and decrease heart failure symptoms (improvement in NYHA class by one class or increased 6-minute walk distance) but also to reduce mortality and improve survival.

16. **Do all patients with dyssynchrony respond to CRT?**
Not all patients who undergo CRT have a clinical response to it. In general, responders have lower mortality, fewer heart failure events, and fewer symptoms than nonresponders. The incidence of nonresponders is about 25% and is similar among patients with ischemic and nonischemic cardiomyopathy.

17. **What are some additional benefits seen in responders to CRT?**
CRT allows patients to tolerate more aggressive medical therapy and neurohormonal blockade, particularly with β-blockers. It also improves diastolic function. CRT reduces frequency of ventricular arrhythmias and ICD therapies among patients previously treated with an ICD who were upgraded to a CRT device. It may also reduce frequency and duration of atrial tachyarrhythmias, including atrial fibrillation.

18. **Is a CRT defibrillator (CRT-D) useful in minimally symptomatic patients with heart failure?**
Until recently, it was unknown if CRT would benefit patients with NYHA class I-II heart failure symptoms. Many patients with NYHA class I-II symptoms meet criteria for placement of an ICD as primary prevention. Many of these patients eventually progress to NYHA class III-IV symptoms over time. Two recently completed trials—Multicenter Automatic Defibrillator Implantation Trial with Cardiac Resynchronization Therapy (MADIT-CRT) and Resynchronization Reverses Remodeling in Systolic Left Ventricular Dysfunction (REVERSE)—evaluated the effect of CRT on patients with minimal or mild congestive heart failure (CHF) symptoms (NYHA class I-II). The larger MADIT-CRT trial randomized more than 1800 patients with EF less than 30%, QRS wider than 130 ms, and NYHA class I-II, to CRT-D or to standard ICD alone. Patients in the CRT-D group had a significant reduction in the combined endpoint of death or heart failure hospitalization (25% for the ICD group vs. 17% for the CRT-D group; $P = 0.001$). Based on these results, the U.S. Food and Drug Administration approved a new indication for CRT-D for ischemic cardiomyopathy patients with NYHA class I or greater heart failure or for non-ischemic cardiomyopathy with NYHA class II or greater, including all patients with EF less than 30%, QRS wider than 130 ms, and left bundle branch block. The requirement of left bundle branch block was based on subgroup analysis. This new indication expands the use of CRT-D to patients with less symptomatic heart failure.

19. **Can ventricular pacing be deleterious?**
In patients with LV dysfunction, right ventricular pacing alone can lead to intraventricular dyssynchrony, precipitate heart failure, and lead to overall worse outcomes. In such patients, consideration should be given to CRT.

20. **Can CRT help patients with CHF and narrow QRS?**
Initial single-center, nonrandomized case series reported improvement in LV function in patients with CHF and narrow QRS who received CRT. The theory was that the QRS duration on ECG may not accurately detect electrical dyssynchrony that may benefit from CRT. This theory was primarily driven by the perception of ventricular dyssynchrony as measured by echocardiographic tissue velocity parameters. The Resynchronization Therapy in Normal QRS (RethinQ) trial randomized patients with NYHA class III symptoms, EF less than 35%, narrow QRS (<130 ms), and echocardiographic evidence of dyssynchrony, to receive an ICD alone or CRT-D. There was no significant difference in the primary endpoint of improvement in peak oxygen consumption at 6 months. At this time, there is no conclusive evidence to support the use of CRT in patients with a narrow QRS duration of less than 120 ms.

BIBLIOGRAPHY, SUGGESTED READINGS, AND WEBSITES

1. Abraham WT, Fisher WG, Smith AL, et al: Cardiac resynchronization in chronic heart failure, *N Engl J Med 346* 1845–1853, 2002.

2. Beshai JF, Grimm RA, Nagueh SF, et al: Cardiac-resynchronization therapy in heart failure with narrow QRS complexes, *N Engl J Med* 357:2461–2471, 2007.

3. Bristow MR, Saxon LA, Boehmer J, et al: Cardiac-resynchronization therapy with or without an implantable defibrillator in advanced chronic heart failure, *N Engl J Med 350* 2140–2150, 2004.

4. Ellenbogen KA, Wilkoff BL, Kay GN, et al: *Clinical cardiac pacing, defibrillation and resynchronization therapy*, ed 3, Philadelphia, 2006, Saunders.

5. Epstein AE, DiMarco JP, Ellenbogen KA, et al: ACC/AHA/HRS 2008 guidelines for device-based therapy of cardiac rhythm abnormalities: executive summary: a report of the American College of Cardiology/American Heart Association Task Force on Practice Guidelines (Writing Committee to Revise the ACC/AHA/NASPE 2002 Guideline Update for Implantation of Cardiac Pacemakers and Antiarrhythmia Devices), *J Am Coll Cardiol* 51:2085–2105, 2008.

6. Jarcho JA: Resynchronizing ventricular contraction in heart failure, *N Engl J Med* 352:1594–1597, 2005.

7. Linde C, Abraham WT, Gold MR, et al: Randomized trial of cardiac resynchronization in mildly symptomatic heart failure patients and in asymptomatic patients with left ventricular dysfunction and previous heart failure symptoms, *J Am Coll Cardiol* 52:1834–1843, 2008.

8. Moss AJ, Hall WJ, Cannom DS, et al: Cardiac-resynchronization therapy for the prevention of heart-failure events, *N Engl J Med* 361:1329–1338, 2009.

CHAPTER 38

IMPLANTABLE CARDIOVERTER-DEFIBRILLATORS

Jose L. Baez-Escudero, MD, and Miguel Valderrábano, MD

1. **What are the components of an implantable cardioverter-defibrillator (ICD) system?**

   ICDs are composed of a pulse generator (typically implanted in the left pectoral region) and one or more intracardiac leads. Typically the right ventricular (RV) lead contains two distal electrodes (tip and ring) that are used to sense local electrical ventricular signals and to pace if necessary. This lead also contains one or two defibrillation coils (one sits in the RV and the other in the superior vena cava) specifically designed to deliver high voltages. Additional leads may include an atrial lead (for pacing, sensing, and arrhythmia discrimination) or a left ventricular (LV) lead for cardiac resynchronization (Fig. 38-1). All transvenous defibrillators are also capable of pacemaker functions.

2. **How does an ICD deliver shocking energy?**

   ICDs use lithium-vanadium batteries that are reliable energy sources with predictable discharge curves. An ICD is able to deliver a charge larger than its battery voltage because of a system of internal capacitors. These hold a charge and then release it all at once when it is needed. Shocking energy travels around a circular circuit, usually formed between the defibrillator lead coils and the device titanium-housed can.

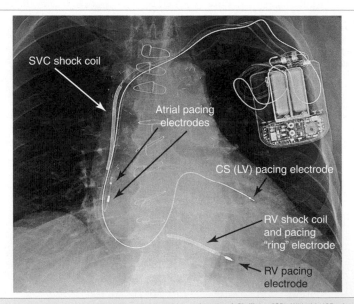

Figure 38-1. A radiograph of a patient with an implantable cardioverter-defibrillator (ICD). With this ICD, shock coils are present in both the right ventricle *(RV)* and the superior vena cava *(SVC)*. There is also a coronary sinus *(CS)* lead present for biventricular pacing. (From Miller R, Eriksson L, Fleisher L, et al: *Miller's anesthesia*, ed 7, Philadelphia, 2009, Churchill Livingstone.) *LV*, left ventricle.

3. How does the ICD detect and define a rhythm?

The ICD collects intracardiac electrical signals (a process called *sensing*) and then processes them with dedicated software to classify the rhythm (a process called *detection*). The ICD identifies an arrhythmia by counting intervals between successive electrograms sensed by the intracardiac leads. In the ventricular lead, beat-to-beat intervals are counted and assigned into a category, usually called a *zone*. For example, normal sinus rhythm is expected to be slower than approximately 160 beats/min, which corresponds to beat-to-beat intervals longer than 375 ms. Shorter intervals would fall in the ventricular tachycardia (VT) zone and even shorter ones in the ventricular fibrillation (VF) zone. The ICD diagnoses an abnormally fast rhythm when a sufficient number of consecutive beat-to-beat intervals fall into either the VT or VF zone. This rate-based detection scheme can be adjusted to meet the individual patient's needs by programming for different categories and therapies (e.g., antitachycardia pacing as appropriate therapy for slow VT). Also, detection algorithms can take into account onset of tachycardia (abrupt in VT, versus gradual in sinus tachycardia), stability (regular in VT, versus irregular in atrial fibrillation), the relationship with the atrial activation timings, and even the morphology of the ventricular signal, to maximize accuracy of detection and minimize inappropriate therapies. After therapy is delivered, the ICD monitors the following intervals to redetect sinus rate (which means the therapy was successful) or redetect the arrhythmia (which results in additional therapy).

4. How does ICD therapy improve survival?

ICD therapy, compared with conventional or traditional antiarrhythmic drug therapy, has been associated with mortality reductions from 23% to 55%, depending on the risk group participating in each trial, with the improvement in survival due almost exclusively to a reduction in sudden cardiac death (SCD). The trials are subcategorized into two types: *primary prevention* (prophylactic) trials, in which the subjects have not experienced life-threatening sustained VT, VF, or resuscitated cardiac arrest but are at risk; and *secondary prevention* trials, involving subjects who have had an abortive cardiac arrest, a life-threatening VT, or ventricular tachyarrhythmia as the cause of syncope.

5. What are the key clinical trials that evaluated the benefit of ICD for primary prevention?

Clinical trials have evaluated the risks and benefits of ICDs in prevention of sudden death and have improved survival in multiple patient populations, including those with prior myocardial infarction (MI) and heart failure caused by either coronary artery disease or nonischemic dilated cardiomyopathy (DCM). Table 38-1 summarizes the important trials that evaluated the mortality benefit of ICDs for primary prevention.

6. What are the current class I indications for ICD implantation for primary prevention of SCD?

Assuming patients are receiving chronic optimal medical therapy and have a reasonable expectation of survival with good functional status for more than 1 year, the following are the current indications for ICD therapy:

- Patients with left ventricular ejection fraction (LVEF) less than 35% as a result of prior MI, who are at least 40 days post-MI, and are in New York Heart Association (NYHA) functional class II or III.
- Patients with LV dysfunction as a result of prior MI who are at least 40 days post-MI, have an LVEF less than 30%, and are in NYHA functional class I.
- Patients with nonischemic DCM who have an LVEF 35% or less and who are in NYHA functional class II or III.
- Patients with nonsustained VT as a result of prior MI, LVEF less than 40%, and inducible VF or sustained VT at electrophysiologic study.
- Patients with syncope of undetermined origin with clinically relevant, hemodynamically significant sustained VT or VF induced at electrophysiologic study.
- Patients with structural heart disease and spontaneous sustained VT, whether hemodynamically stable or unstable.

TABLE 38-1. TRIALS THAT EVALUATED THE BENEFIT OF IMPLANTABLE CARDIOVERTER-DEFIBRILLATORS FOR PRIMARY PREVENTION OF SUDDEN CARDIAC DEATH

Trial	# of Points	Age (Years)	LVEF (%)	Follow-up (Months)	Control Therapy	Mortality (%) Control	Mortality (%) ICD	P
MUSTT (Multicentre Unstable Tachycardia Trial)	704	67 ± 12	30	39	No EP-guided therapy	48	24	.06
MADIT (Multicentre Automatic Defibrillator Implantation Trial)	196	63 ± 9	26	27	Conventional	38.6	15.7	.009
MADIT II (Multicentre Automatic Defibrillator Implantation Trial)	1232	64 ± 10	23	20	Optimal medical therapy	19.8	14.2	.007
DEFINITE (Defibrillators in Non-Ischemic Cardiomyopathy Treatment Evaluation)	458	58	21	29.0 ± 14.4	Optimal medical therapy	14.1	7.9	.08
SCD-HeFT (Sudden Cardiac Death in Heart Failure)	2521	60.1	25	45.5	Optimal medical therapy	36.1	28.9	.007

EP, Electrophysiologic; *ICD,* implantable cardioverter-defibrillator.

7. **What are the current class I indications for ICD implantation for secondary prevention of SCD?**

Secondary prevention refers to prevention of SCD in those patients who have survived a prior sudden cardiac arrest or sustained VT. Evidence from multiple randomized controlled trials supports the use of ICDs for secondary prevention of SCD regardless of the type of underlying structural heart disease. In patients resuscitated from cardiac arrest, the ICD is associated with clinically and statistically significant reductions in SCD total mortality compared with antiarrhythmic drug therapy in prospective randomized controlled trials. Hence, ICDs are indicated for secondary prevention of SCD in patients who survived VF or hemodynamically unstable VT or experienced VT with syncope and have an LVEF 40% or less, after evaluation to define the cause of the event and to exclude any completely reversible causes.

8. **What other special populations may also benefit from ICD therapy?**

Certain patients with less common forms of cardiomyopathy, as well as patients with inherited conditions who share genetically determined susceptibility to VT and SCD, also benefit from ICD therapy (especially when a history of arrhythmia or syncope is present, or for primary prevention in patients with a very strong family history of early mortality). These patients meet class II indications for ICD implantation that are outlined in the current guidelines in detail, including the following:

- Patients with congenital heart disease who are survivors of cardiac arrest, after evaluation to define the cause of the event and exclude any reversible causes
- Hypertrophic cardiomyopathy (HCM) with one or more risk factor for SCD (VF, VT, family history of SCD, unexplained syncope, LV thickness 30 mm or more, abnormal blood pressure response to exercise)
- Brugada syndrome with a history of previous cardiac arrest, documented sustained VT, or classic electrocardiogram (ECG) phenotype with unexplained syncope
- Idiopathic VF and/or VT
- Noncompaction of the LV
- Long- and short-QT syndromes with previous cardiac arrest or unexplained syncope
- Catecholaminergic polymorphic VT
- Arrhythmogenic RV dysplasia and/or cardiomyopathy
- Infiltrative cardiomyopathies such as sarcoidosis, amyloidosis, Fabry disease, hemochromatosis, giant cell myocarditis, or Chagas disease
- Certain muscular dystrophies

9. **What is defibrillator threshold testing?**

The *defibrillation threshold* (DFT) is defined as the amount of energy required to reliably defibrillate the heart during an arrhythmia. During implant, the electrophysiologist may elect to perform DFT testing, in which VF is induced, detected, and then terminated by the device in a step-down sequence to find the minimal reliable level of energy needed to achieve defibrillation. Defibrillation efficacy traditionally has been performed with successive attempts to determine the DFT using approximately 20 J in a device that could deliver 25 to 30 J. A safety margin of 10 J was required for the implantation of the earliest defibrillators. Because DFT testing involves inducing potentially fatal VF several times and requires deep conscious sedation, some electrophysiologists forego DFT testing at implant and program the device to the highest output settings. Additionally, an ICD can be potentially tested without inducing VF, using upper limit of vulnerability (ULV) testing.

10. **What is antitachycardia pacing?**

Antitachycardia pacing (ATP) has long been recognized as a way to pace-terminate certain types of arrhythmias, particularly slow monomorphic VT involving a reentry circuit. The idea is to deliver a few seconds of pacing stimuli to the heart at a rate faster than the tachycardia. The basic principle is that in most reentrant circuits there an excitable gap—that is, a time between successive activations, when the myocardium is available to respond to excitations. Pacing in a reentrant circuit during the excitable gap introduces new activation wave fronts that collide with the one of the preexisting tachycardia and can terminate it. Advantages offered by ATP include the following:

- ATP is not painful (sometimes barely noticed by some patients).
- ATP may reduce battery drainage by terminating the arrhythmia without the need for shocks.
- It is an easily programmable feature on most ICDs.

On the other hand, ATP has potential disadvantages. If ineffective, it can delay defibrillation therapies and prolong the time during which the patient is in tachycardia, which may lead to syncope. ATP can also accelerate VT into faster rhythms and even VF.

For this reason, it is mostly used in patients that remain stable and asymptomatic during episodes of slow VT, generally below 200 beats/min. However, more aggressive ATP programming has been shown to decrease ICD shocks, and newer ICDs incorporate ATP while charging for a shock.

11. **How common are inappropriate shocks in patients with ICDs?**

Inappropriate shocks occur when a device delivers therapy for a fast supraventricular rhythm or for abnormal sensing in the ventricle. They occur in up to 11% of patients with ICDs and can constitute up to a third of all shock episodes a patient experiences. The most common rhythm triggering an inappropriate shock is atrial fibrillation with rapid ventricular response, followed by other supraventricular tachycardias (SVTs), including sinus tachycardia. Smoking, atrial fibrillation, diastolic hypertension, young age, nonischemic cardiomyopathy, and prior appropriate shocks increase the chance of receiving an inappropriate shock. They are associated with increased mortality in patients with ICDs and have important psychologic effects in this population. ICD programming options currently available should be used to reduce the risk of inappropriate shocks.

12. **What is the totally subcutaneous defibrillator?**

The totally *subcutaneous ICD* (S-ICD) is a newly developed device that is capable of providing the same proven defibrillation protection as conventional ICDs, but without the serious complications associated with the presence of a transvenous endocardial defibrillator lead. The S-ICD electrode is implanted in the parasternal area in the subcutaneous space and then connected to an active high-voltage can. Defibrillation is delivered between the coil on the electrode and the active can. Sensing is accomplished using both or any one of the proximal and distal ring electrodes and the electrically conductive pulse generator enclosure. This device may potentially reduce or eliminate problems such as failure to achieve vascular access, intravascular injury, and lead failure requiring difficult procedures for extraction and replacement. Additional potential benefits of such a device include the preservation of venous access for other uses and the avoidance of radiation exposure during fluoroscopy, which is required for transvenous ICD implantation. These benefits would be especially important for young patients with no pacing indications, in whom leads may fail during the decades that therapy is needed.

13. **What are ICD lead failures?**

Although conceptually simple, ICD leads are complicated devices with manufacturer-specific designs that vary from model to model. These design differences may include variations in insulation, cable/conductor, length, diameter, and fixation mechanism. Over time, ICD leads can fail due to several mechanisms, most of them related to lead design and time after implant. The clinical presentation of ICD lead failure varies. A lead failure is rare and most of the time can be diagnosed through routine monitoring of the ICD. A high impedance is a frequent presentation consistent with a lead fracture. However, lead failures can result in significant clinical events, including failure to pace and/or defibrillate, inappropriate shocks, and even death. Most lead failures are managed with lead extraction and replacement.

BIBLIOGRAPHY, SUGGESTED READINGS, AND WEBSITES

1. Bardy GH, Lee KL, Mark DB, et al: Amiodarone or an implantable cardioverter-defibrillator for congestive heart failure, *N Engl J Med* 352:225–237, 2005.

2. Bardy GH, Smith WM, Hood MA, et al: An entirely subcutaneous implantable cardioverter-defibrillator, *N Engl J Med* 363:36–44, 2010.

3. Daubert JP, Zareba W, Cannom DS, et al: Inappropriate implantable cardioverter-defibrillators shocks in the MADIT II study: frequency, mechanisms, predictors, and survival impact. *J Am Coll Cardiol* 51 1357–1365, *J Am Coll Cardiol* 51:1357–1365, 2008.

4. DiMarco JP: Implantable cardioverter-defibrillators, *N Engl J Med* 349:1836–1847, 2003.

5. Epstein AE, DiMarco JP, Ellenbogen KA, et al: ACC/AHA/HRS 2008 guidelines for device-based therapy of cardiac rhythm abnormalities: executive summary: a report of the American College of Cardiology/American Heart Association Task Force on Practice Guidelines (Writing Committee to Revise the ACC/AHA/NASPE 2002 Guideline Update for Implantation of Cardiac Pacemakers and Antiarrhythmia Devices), *J Am Coll Cardiol* 51:2085–2105, 2008.

6. Hohnloser SH, Kuck KH, Dorian P, et al: Prophylactic use of an implantable cardioverter-defibrillator after acute myocardial infarction, *N Engl J Med* 351:2481–2488, 2004.

7. Kadish A, Dyer A, Daubert JP, et al: Prophylactic defibrillator implantation in patients with nonischemic dilated cardiomyopathy, *N Engl J Med* 350:2151–2158, 2004.

8. Moss AJ, Zareba W, Hall WJ, et al: Prophylactic implantation of a defibrillator in patients with myocardial infarction and reduced ejection fraction, *N Engl J Med* 346:877–883, 2002.

CHAPTER 39

BASIC LIFE SUPPORT AND ADVANCED CARDIAC LIFE SUPPORT

Vissia S. Pinili, MSN, RN, CPAN, CCRN, Nicole R. Keller, PharmD, BCNSP, and Glenn N. Levine, MD, FACC, FAHA

1. Why was the A-B-C (airway, breathing, compression) sequence of cardiopulmonary resuscitation (CPR) changed to C-A-B (compression, airway, breathing)?

According to American Heart Association (AHA) guidelines for CPR and emergency cardiovascular care (ECC), chest compression were often delayed while the rescuer opened the airway to give mouth-to-mouth breaths, retrieved a barrier device, or gathered and assembled ventilation equipment. Starting the resuscitation sequence with chest compressions is also hoped to encourage more persons to initiate CPR.

2. What factors constitute "high-quality CPR"?

Components of high-quality CPR include:

- Chest compressions at least 100 times per minute
- Depth of chest compressions for adults of at least 2 inches (5 cm), for children compressions of 2 inches, and for infants compressions of 1.5 inches (4 cm)
- Allowing for complete chest recoil after each compression
- Minimizing interruptions in chest compressions
- Avoiding excessive ventilation

3. What is your first step if you are alone and come across an unresponsive adult victim with no signs of breathing?

Activate the emergency response system and get an automated external defibrillator (AED), if available in the area, then return to the victim. If you return with an AED, turn it on and follow the prompt. If no AED is available, check for a pulse and begin CPR until emergency medical services (EMS) arrives to take over.

Figure 39-1 is an algorithm for adult basic life support (BLS) decisions and actions. A summary of key BLS components for treating adults, children, and infants is given in Table 39-1.

4. For patients with respiratory arrest (but with a perfusing heart rhythm), how often should breaths be delivered?

For respiratory arrest with a perfusion cardiac rhythm, breaths should be delivered every 5 to 6 seconds (10-12 breaths/min).

5. What is the most common cause of airway obstruction in the unconscious adult patient?

In adults the most common cause of airway obstruction in an unconscious patient is loss of tone in the throat muscles, leading to airway occlusion by the tongue. This may be treated by head tilt–chin lift, jaw thrust, or insertion of an oropharyngeal airway.

6. How many joules of energy are indicated for the treatment of ventricular fibrillation (VF) or pulseless ventricular tachycardia (VT) when using a biphasic defibrillator?

Biphasic defibrillators are now used at many institutions, replacing the older monophasic defibrillators. The amount of energy will often be device specific, ranging from 120 to 200 J. If

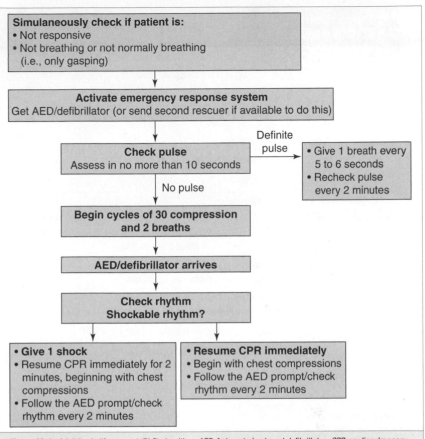

Figure 39-1. Adult basic life support (BLS) algorithm. *AED*, Automated external defibrillator; *CPR*, cardiopulmonary resuscitation.

the appropriate setting is unknown, use 200 J. Additional shocks should be equivalent or higher energy. This contrasts to the older monophasic defibrillators, for which a setting of 360 J is recommended.

7. **In order, what are the preferred routes of drug administration?**
   - Intravenous (IV) is the preferred route of drug administration. The guidelines emphasize that resuscitation attempts should not be delayed by trying to achieve central IV access when peripheral IV access can be easily achieved.
   - When IV access is not possible, intraosseous (IO) is preferred over endotracheal (ET). The IO route can be used in both children and adults.
   - Absorption of drugs given via the ET route is considered to be less reliable and predictable. In addition, the optimal dose of most drugs given via the ET route is unknown; the typical dose of drugs administered via the ET route is reported to be 2 to 2.5 times that of the IV route. Drugs delivered via the ET route should be diluted in 5 to 10 mL of water or normal saline. Advanced cardiac life support (ACLS) drugs that can be given via the ET route are naloxone, atropine, vasopressin, epinephrine, and lidocaine (NAVEL).

TABLE 39-1.   SUMMARY OF KEY BASIC LIFE SUPPORT COMPONENTS FOR ADULTS, CHILDREN, AND INFANTS

Component	Recommendations		
	Adult	Children	Infants
Recognition	Unresponsive		
	No breathing or no normal breathing (i.e., only gasping)	No breathing or only gasping	
	No pulse palpated within 10 seconds for all ages		
CPR sequence	C-A-B (Compressions, Airway, Breathing)*		
Compression rate	At least 100/min		
Compression depth	At least 2 inches (5 cm)	At least 1/3 AP diameter About 2 inches (5 cm)	At least 1/3 AP diameter About 1.5 inches (4 cm)
Chest wall recoil	Allow complete recoil between compressions HCPs rotate compressions every 2 minutes		
Compression interruptions	Minimize interruptions in chest compressions Attempt to limit interruptions to <10 seconds		
Airway	Head tilt-chin lift (if suspected trauma, use jaw thrust)		
Compression to ventilation ratio (until advanced airway placed)	1 or 2 rescuers: 30:2	Single rescuer: 30:2 2 rescuers: 15:2	
Ventilations: when rescuer is either untrained or trained but not proficient	Compressions only		
Ventilations with advanced airway	1 breath every 6-8 seconds (8-10 breaths/min). Asynchronous with chest compressions. About 1 second per breath. Visible chest rise		
Defibrillation	Attach and use AED as soon as available. Minimize interruptions in chest compressions before and after shock. Resume CPR beginning with compressions immediately after each shock.		

From American Heart Association: *Highlights of the 2010 American Heart Association Guidelines for CPR and ECC.* Available at : http://www.heart.org/idc/groups/heart-public/@wcm/@ecc/documents/downloadable/ucm_317350.pdf. Accessed March 26, 2013.
AED, Automated external defibrillator; *AP,* anterior-posterior; *CPR,* cardiopulmonary resuscitation; *HCP,* health care provider.
*Excluding the newly born, in whom the etiology of an arrest is nearly always asphyxia.

8. **After the first unsuccessful shock of a patient with VF or pulseless VT, which two drugs should be considered?**
   - Epinephrine 1 mg IV or IO is the traditional medication to be considered. Additional similar doses of epinephrine can be administered every 3 to 5 minutes. If ET administration is necessary,

the suggested dose is epinephrine 2 to 2.5 mg diluted in 5 to 10 mL of water or normal saline, injected directly into the ET tube. Although a mainstay of the AHA's ACLS VT/VF algorithm, it is acknowledged that there is actually very little data to support the use of epinephrine in this situation.

- One dose of vasopressin 40 units IV or IO can be used to replace the first or second dose of epinephrine. Vasopressin is a nonadrenergic peripheral vasoconstrictor that causes coronary and renal vasoconstriction.

9. **After several unsuccessful shocks, and treatment with epinephrine or vasopressin, what other drugs (and their doses) should be considered?**
Amiodarone (or lidocaine if amiodarone is not available) should be considered. Soberingly, no antiarrhythmic has ever actually been shown to improve survival to hospital discharge, although amiodarone has been shown to increase rates of survival to hospital admission.
   - The dose of amiodarone is 300 mg IV or IO once, with consideration of a subsequent 150 mg IV or IO, if indicated, 3 to 5 minutes after the first 300-mg dose.
   - The dose of lidocaine is 1 to 1.5 mg/kg IV or IO, with subsequent doses of 0.5 to 0.75 mg/kg IV or IO given over 5- to 10-minute intervals, to a maximum total lidocaine dose of 3 mg/kg.

10. **If the patient is in torsades de pointes, in addition to defibrillation, what medication can be considered?**
Magnesium can be given at a dose of 1 to 2 g IV or IO. It is recommended that it be diluted in 10 mL of 5% dextrose in water (D5W) and administered over 5 to 20 minutes.

11. **After administering a drug via a peripheral IV, what steps should be taken to promote delivery of the drug to the central circulation?**
After administering a drug via a peripheral IV, a 20-mL bolus of IV fluid should be administered and the extremity should be elevated for 10 to 20 seconds.

12. **Can one shock a hypothermic patient who is in VF or VT?**
Yes, but there is a caveat. For the hypothermic patient (temperature less than 30° C [86° F]) in VF or VT, a single defibrillation is deemed appropriate.

13. **If a person who was in VF or VT is successfully defibrillated, and amiodarone is to be started to prevent further VF or VT, what is the dosing (assuming he or she has not already received any amiodarone)?**
The following regimen is what is given in the ACLS booklet and is the "classical" loading of amiodarone. An initial bolus of 150 mg IV is given over 10 minutes. This is followed by an infusion of 1 mg/min for 6 hours (total 360 mg), then an infusion of 0.5 mg/min over the next 18 hours (540 mg).

14. **What are the treatable causes of pulseless electrical activity?**
Because pulseless electrical activity (PEA) has such a poor prognosis unless a reversible cause of the rhythm is quickly identified and addressed, it is important to commit to memory the treatable causes of PEA. The *H's* and *T's* of PEA are given in Table 39-2. Hypovolemia and hypoxemia are reported to be the two most common and easily reversible causes of PEA.
   An algorithm for ACLS of adult cardiac arrest (including patients exhibiting PEA) is given in Figure 39-2.

15. **What drugs can be considered in a patient with PEA?**
Epinephrine and vasopressin can be used, as described earlier for the treatment of VF or VT, although no vasopressors has been shown to increase survival in PEA. Atropine is no longer recommended for asystole or PEA.

TABLE 39-2. POTENTIALLY TREATABLE CAUSES OF PULSELESS ELECTRICAL ACTIVITY	
H's	**T's**
Hypovolemia	Toxins
Hypoxia	Tamponade (cardiac)
Hydrogen ion (acidosis)	Tension pneumothorax
Hyper- or hypokalemia	Thrombosis (coronary and pulmonary)
Hypoglycemia	Trauma
Hypothermia	

Modified from American Heart Association: *Advanced cardiovascular life support provider manual*, Dallas, 2011, American Heart Association.

16. **In bradycardic patients, such as those with hears block, what are the primary treatments if they are symptomatic and suffering from poor perfusion?**
The immediate use of transcutaneous pacing is now emphasized for patients with symptomatic bradycardia. While preparations are being made for transcutaneous pacing, the following pharmaceutical interventions should be considered:
   - Atropine 0.5 mg IV, which may be repeated every 3 to 5 minutes to a total dose of 3 mg. The use of atropine should not be relied on in patients with Mobitz II second-degree atrioventricular (AV) block or third-degree (complete) AV block. Some have considered the use of atropine in Mobitz II or third-degree heart block ("infrahisian" heart block) contraindicated, although this is not explicitly stated in the latest ACLS guidelines.
   - Epinephrine 2 to 10 mcg/min
   - Dopamine 2 to 10 mcg/kg/min

17. **Is transcutaneous pacing recommended for the treatment of a patient in asystole?**
As noted in the ACLS algorithm, several randomized controlled trials have failed to show benefit from attempted transcutaneous pacing in patients in asystole. Thus, it is not currently recommended in this situation.

18. **In a symptomatic yet stable patient with a regular narrow complex tachyarrhythmia, what drug is recommended as a first-line agent?**
Adenosine has become the drug of choice for a *symptomatic yet stable* patient with a narrow complex tachyarrhythmia. The distinction between *stable* and *unstable* is subjective, but the symptomatic yet stable patient might be described as one who is slightly lightheaded (systolic blood pressure [SBP] of approximately 80 mm Hg) or having mild shortness of breath or chest discomfort. Patients experiencing more severe symptoms would be those with altered mentation because of low blood pressure, or with moderate to severe shortness or breath or chest discomfort. Note that although adenosine, which blocks AV conduction, may terminate some narrow complex tachycardias, such as AV nodal reentrant tachycardia (AVNRT) or AV reentrant tachycardia (AVRT), it will not terminate rhythms such as atrial flutter or atrial tachycardia (although it may lead to a transient decrease in conduction through the AV node and slower ventricular response rate, allowing identification of the rhythm). Adenosine would not be expected to terminate an irregular narrow complex tachycardia, because the genesis of these rhythms does not involve the AV node.

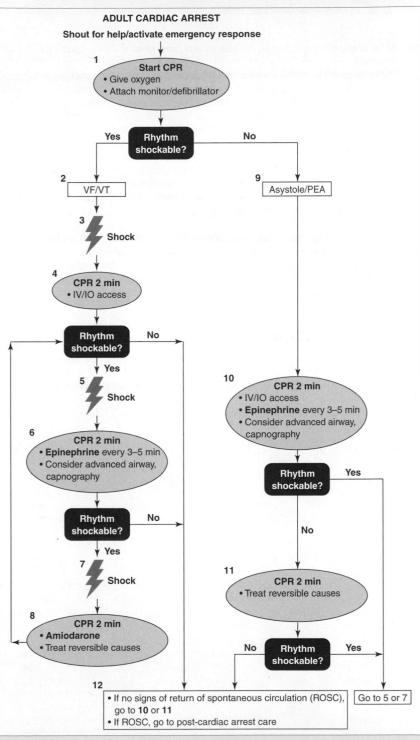

Figure 39-2. Advanced cardiac life support (ACLS) adult cardiac arrest algorithm. *CPR*, Cardiopulmonary resuscitation; *IO*, intraosseous; *IV*, intravenous; *PEA*, pulseless electrical activity; *VF*, ventricular fibrillation; *VT*, ventricular tachycardia.

19. **What is the dosing regimen for adenosine, and what are its primary side effects?**

The adenosine dosing regimen is a 6 mg rapid IV push, followed (if no rhythm conversion) by a 12 mg rapid IV push. The half-life of adenosine is only several seconds, so every effort must be made to administer it quickly and ensure its quick delivery to the central circulation (see Question 11). The effects of adenosine may be potentiated by dipyridamole or carbamazepine (consider a starting dose of 3 mg) and blocked by theophylline or caffeine. Adenosine may cause the patient to experience flushing, shortness of breath, or chest discomfort. Because it can cause bronchospasm, it should be avoided in patients with significant reactive airway disease. The practitioner should also be aware that because of its profound effects on AV nodal conduction, it may result in asystole for several seconds or more, an often disconcerting occurrence to the practitioner watching the telemetry monitor. Prolonged asystole has been reported in patients with transplanted hearts and following central venous administration; a lower dose of 3 mg should be considered in such situations.

20. **After return of spontaneous circulation (ROSC), what intervention has been shown to improve neurologic recovery in comatose patients?**

Therapeutic hypothermia improves neurologic recovery in comatose patients. Patients are cooled to 32° to 34° C for 12 to 24 hours via surface cooling devices (ice bags and/or cooling blankets) and cold , non–dextrose containing, isotonic fluids (30 mL/kg). Decisions on percutaneous coronary intervention (PCI) are not affected by therapeutic hypothermia.

BIBLIOGRAPHY, SUGGESTED READINGS, AND WEBSITES

1. American Heart Association: *American Heart Association Guidelines for CPR and ECC*, 2010. Available at: http://www.heart.org. Accessed March 26, 2013.

2. American Heart Association: *Advanced cardiovascular life support provider manual*, Dallas, 2011, American Heart Association.

HYPERTENSION

Gabriel B. Habib, Sr., MD, MS, FACC, FAHA, FCCP

1. **Define hypertension. What is the prevalence of hypertension in the United States, Mexico, and worldwide?**

   The Joint National Committee on Detection, Evaluation, and Treatment of High Blood Pressure, in its seventh report (JNC 7), defined *hypertension* as an average of two or more diastolic readings more than 90 mm Hg on at least two consecutive visits, or an average of multiple systolic readings more than 140 mm Hg. Isolated systolic hypertension is diagnosed if systolic blood pressure (SBP) is more than 140 mm Hg with a diastolic blood pressure less than 90 mm Hg. A new category called *prehypertension* is now defined as a blood pressure less than the arbitrary cutoff of 140/90 mm Hg for hypertension but greater than an *optimal* blood pressure of 120/80 mm Hg. Patients with prehypertension, unlike hypertensive patients, do not require antihypertensive drug therapy, but should be counseled to start health-promoting lifestyle modifications aimed at preventing the development of hypertension. Hypertension is classified into 2 stages: stage I: 140/90 to 159/99 mm Hg and stage II 160/100 or higher. In the latest National Health and Nutrition Examination Survey 2005-2008, about 33% of adults 20 years of age or older have hypertension (Table 40-1).

   Prevalence of hypertension worldwide varies from as low as 3% of men in rural India to 72% of men in Poland. Hypertension prevalence is about the same in the United States and Mexico, at about 33% of the adult population.

2. **What are the goals of hypertension treatment?**

   Reducing elevated blood pressure levels is an important strategy to prevent various complications of systemic hypertension, such as stroke, myocardial infarction (MI), heart failure, and renal disease. The best predictor of the efficacy in preventing various cardiorenal complications is the degree of reduction of blood pressure. The risk of death from ischemic heart disease or stroke in cohort longitudinal studies is lowest at a blood pressure of approximately 115/75 mm Hg and doubles beginning at 115/75 mm Hg with each 20 mm Hg increment in SBP.

   Although blood pressure less than 120/80 mm Hg is associated in observational cohort studies with the lowest risk of death from ischemic heart disease and stroke, the goal of blood pressure treatment recommended by JNC 7 (2001) is a blood pressure less than 140/90 mm Hg in patients

TABLE 40-1. JNC 7 CATEGORIES OF HYPERTENSION	
Category	**Blood Pressure**
Normal	<120/80 mm Hg
Prehypertension	120-130/80-89 mm Hg
Hypertension: Stage 1	140-159/90-99 mm Hg
Hypertension: Stage 2	≥160/100 mm Hg

Modified from Chobanian AV, Bakris GL, Black HR, et al: *Seventh report of the Joint National Committee on Prevention, Detection, Evaluation, and Treatment of High Blood Pressure (JNC-7)*, Bethesda, Md., 2003, National Institutes of Health, pp 54-55.

with uncomplicated hypertension, and less than 130/80 mm Hg in higher risk hypertensive patients with chronic kidney disease and/or diabetes mellitus.

The American Heart Association (AHA) Task Force released a scientific statement in 2007 for the treatment of hypertension in the prevention of coronary artery disease (CAD). This AHA Task Force recommended more aggressive control of blood pressure among those at high risk for CAD: individuals with diabetes mellitus, chronic kidney disease (as recommended in JNC 7), but also in patients with cardiovascular disease, congestive heart failure, or a 10-year Framingham risk score of 10% or more. These individuals are advised to maintain a blood pressure less than 130/80 mm Hg. Moreover, the AHA Task Force recommended a goal blood pressure of less than 120/80 in patients with congestive heart failure.

Targeting an SBP of less than 120 mm Hg, as compared with less than 140 mm Hg, in patients with type 2 diabetes mellitus did not reduce the rate of a composite outcome of fatal and nonfatal major cardiovascular events in the recently reported Action to Control Cardiovascular Risk in Diabetes (ACCORD) blood pressure trial. However, SBP less than 120 mm Hg did significantly reduce stroke risk, a secondary study endpoint. Thus, it is NOT recommended at this time to target SBP less than 120 mm Hg in type 2 diabetic patients.

3. **Is systolic or diastolic blood pressure more powerful as a predictor of cardiovascular complications of hypertension?**
Systolic and diastolic blood pressure levels are independently predictive of the risk of cardiovascular complications in hypertensive patients. However, SBP is more powerful in predicting cardiovascular complications, particularly in patients over the age of 50 years. *Pulse pressure*—the difference between systolic and diastolic blood pressure—is also an independent predictor of cardiovascular complications. A wide pulse pressure is usually indicative of a noncompliant stiff aorta with a reduced ability to distend and recoil back. Thus, during systolic ejection of blood from the left ventricle into the aorta and systemic circulation, the aorta does not distend and the force of ejection is transmitted more forcefully into the peripheral vessels, thus causing an exaggerated SBP level recording. During diastole, the elastic recoil of the aorta is more limited, contributing to a lower diastolic blood pressure. Thus, a noncompliant aorta would increase SBP and reduce diastolic blood pressure, resulting in a widened pulse pressure.

4. **You have diagnosed a new case of hypertension. What is your next step?**
Arterioles are the vessels that sustain the most damage from persistent elevation of blood pressure. Therefore, the first step is to do a *damage assessment* by evaluating the target organs of hypertension, keeping in mind that their involvement is an expression of arteriolar damage with subsequent ischemia and ischemia-induced changes.

- **Kidney:** Signs of involvement range from minimal proteinuria or slight increase of serum creatinine to end-stage renal disease. Kidney size is evaluated by a variety of imaging methods and has prognostic significance. Hypertension is the second leading cause of renal failure in the United States, particularly in African Americans.
- **Brain:** The eye fundus appearance is the mirror of the brain circulation. Findings range from minor atherosclerotic changes to papilledema and hemorrhages, which can be seen with severe hypertension and hypertensive crisis. A careful neurologic examination may reveal signs of previously undiagnosed strokes, and history may reveal previous transient ischemic attacks.
- **Heart:** The direct consequence is left ventricular hypertrophy (LVH) with increased left ventricular (LV) mass; this is easily documented by electrocardiogram (ECG), two-dimensional, and M-mode echocardiogram or cardiac magnetic resonance imaging (MRI). LVH is strongly associated with an increased risk of sudden death and MI, and constitutes the basis for decreased LV compliance and subsequent diastolic dysfunction. A thorough evaluation for the presence of CAD, guided by a skillful interview, is required. Holter monitoring may be necessary for evaluating LVH-associated arrhythmias. The last step in the natural history of the disease is LV dilation and pump failure, with the classical signs of congestive heart failure (CHF).

5. **What is resistant hypertension and how prevalent is it?**
Resistant hypertension is defined as blood pressure that remains above goal in spite of the concurrent use of three antihypertensive agents of different classes. Ideally, one of the three agents should

be a diuretic and all agents should be prescribed at optimal dose amounts. Resistant hypertension identifies patients who are at risk of having reversible causes of hypertension or patients who, by virtue of persistently elevated blood pressure levels, may benefit from special diagnostic and therapeutic considerations. In a recent analysis of the National Health and Nutrition Examination Survey (NHANES), only 53% of hypertensive patients were controlled to less than 140/90; the majority of the remaining 47% of these patients probably have resistant hypertension. While the exact prevalence of resistant hypertension is unknown, it is estimated from published hypertension clinical trials, including the Antihypertensive and Lipid-Lowering Treatment to Prevent Heart Attack (ALLHAT) trial, that about 20% to 30% of hypertensive patients have resistant hypertension.

Factors recognized to be associated with resistant hypertension include older age, high baseline blood pressure, obesity, excessive dietary salt ingestion, chronic kidney disease, diabetes mellitus, LVH, African American race, female gender, and residence in southeastern U.S. regions (Box 40-1). Medications that interfere with blood pressure control (Box 40-2), such as nonsteroidal antiinflammatory drugs (NSAIDs), should be specifically inquired about in hypertensive poorly controlled patients.

Box 40-1 PATIENT CHARACTERISTICS ASSOCIATED WITH RESISTANT HYPERTENSION

- Older age
- High baseline blood pressure
- Obesity
- Excessive dietary salt ingestion
- Chronic kidney disease
- Diabetes
- Left ventricular hypertrophy
- Black race
- Female sex
- Residence in southeastern United States

From Calhoun D, Jones D, Textor D, et al: Resistant hypertension: diagnosis, evaluation, and treatment: a scientific statement from the American Heart Association Professional Education Committee of the Council for High Blood Pressure Research. *Hypertension* 51:1403-1419, 2008.

Box 40-2 MEDICATIONS THAT CAN INTERFERE WITH BLOOD PRESSURE CONTROL

- Nonnarcotic analgesics
- Nonsteroidal antiinflammatory agents, including aspirin
- Selective COX-2 inhibitors
- Sympathomimetic agents (decongestants, diet pills, cocaine)
- Stimulants (methylphenidate, dexmethylphenidate, dextroamphetamine, amphetamine, methamphetamine, modafinil)
- Alcohol
- Oral contraceptives
- Cyclosporine
- Erythropoietin
- Natural licorice
- Herbal compounds (ephedra or ma huang)

COX-2, cyclooxygenase-2.
From Calhoun D, Jones D, Textor D, et al: Resistant hypertension: diagnosis, evaluation, and treatment: a scientific statement from the American Heart Association Professional Education Committee of the Council for High Blood Pressure Research. *Hypertension* 51:1403-1419, 2008.

6. **What is secondary hypertension?**

Up to 5% of all hypertension cases are *secondary*, meaning that a specific cause can be identified. Most of these causes are treatable (e.g., surgery for an adrenal tumor, stenting of a renal artery stenosis, or correction of an aortic coarctation). Given the low prevalence of secondary hypertension, routine screening for secondary hypertension is not usually recommended. A targeted approach is much more cost-effective, and clinical and laboratory clues are critically important in evaluating patients for specific causes of secondary hypertension. Signs, symptoms, and findings suggestive of secondary hypertension are discussed later and in Table 40-2.

7. **When should one suspect secondary hypertension?**

The following scenarios should trigger a search for possible causes of secondary hypertension (see Table 40-2):

- Onset at a young age (younger than 35 years) in female patients raises the suspicion of renal artery medial fibromuscular dysplasia.
- Onset at a late age (older than 55 years) suggests atherosclerotic renal vascular disease (renal artery stenosis).
- Unexplained hypokalemia—sometimes manifested by generalized weakness—either in the absence of diuretic use or an exaggerated hypokalemia following low doses of diuretics suggests primary hyperaldosteronism.
- Paroxysmal episodes of palpitations, sweating, and headaches suggest a pheochromocytoma.
- Abdominal/lumbar trauma may result in a perirenal hematoma with subsequent small unilateral kidney.

TABLE 40-2.   CLINICAL SIGNS, SYMPTOMS, AND FINDINGS SUGGESTIVE OF SECONDARY CAUSES OF HYPERTENSION

Signs, Symptoms, and Findings	Suggested Secondary Cause
Onset at young age (<35 years) in female patient	Renal artery medial fibromuscular dysplasia
Onset at a late age (>55 years), especially in a patient with atherosclerosis Exaggerated drop in blood pressure and/or kidney function with initiation of ACEI Abdominal bruit	Renal artery stenosis
Unexplained hypokalemia	Primary hyperaldosteronism
Paroxysmal episodes of palpitations, sweating, and headaches	Pheochromocytoma
Use of birth control pills, laxatives, or licorice	Drug-induced due to mineralocorticoid effects
Renal calculi, elevated calcium level	Hyperparathyroidism
Reduced femoral pulses with high blood pressure values only in the upper extremities	Aortic coarctation
Abdominal striae, truncal obesity	Cushing disease
Loud snoring, witnessed apnea	Obstructive sleep apnea
Worsening renal function, polycystic kidneys or small kidneys on ultrasound	Renal parenchymal disease

ACEI, Angiotensin-converting enzyme inhibitor.

- A transient episode of periorbital swelling and dark-colored urine that went untreated may point to a chronic glomerulonephritis.
- Multiple episodes of cystitis or urinary infection left untreated or with incomplete treatment will lead to and suggest chronic pyelonephritis.
- Use of birth control pills by young women and laxative use by elderly people or licorice use, which has a mineralocorticoid effect, suggest mineralocorticoid-induced hypertension.
- A history of chronic pain may be the clue for analgesic nephropathy.
- Renal calculi may be the sign of hyperparathyroidism or the cause of obstructive nephropathy.
- Reduced femoral pulses with high blood pressure values only in the upper extremities suggests aortic coarctation.
- Abdominal bruits suggest renal artery stenosis. The cause may be either atherosclerosis in an elderly patient or fibromuscular dysplasia in a young woman. Renal artery stenosis is also suggested by an exaggerated drop in blood pressure following initiation of treatment with angiotensin-converting enzyme (ACE) inhibitors or angiotensin-receptor blockers.
- Bilateral abdominal palpable masses commonly are due to polycystic kidney disease. Typically the history reveals the presence of hypertension with renal failure in other family members.
- Abdominal striae are the sign of Cushing disease, along with the typical truncal obesity.
- Resistance to a multiple drug regimen can point to a secondary cause of hypertension. In fact, in clinical practice, resistant hypertension with failure to control blood pressure to recommended goals despite at least three antihypertensive agents in optimal dosages is the most important clue that should lead to a thorough evaluation for secondary causes of hypertension.

8. **What is the recommended initial diagnostic workup for a hypertensive patient?**
Any newly diagnosed patient with hypertension should have measurements of serum creatinine, sodium, potassium, calcium, and hematocrit, full fasting lipid profile, 12-lead ECG, and chest radiograph. Because essential hypertension accounts for the large majority—more than 95%—of all hypertension, a thorough and costly diagnostic workup for secondary causes of hypertension is not routinely recommended unless there are clinical or laboratory clues suggesting secondary hypertension.

9. **What are the most common causes of secondary hypertension among patients with treatment-resistant or uncontrolled hypertension, when do you suspect them, and how do you confirm them?**
Secondary hypertension is common among patients with resistant hypertension. The most common causes of secondary hypertension among patients with resistant hypertension are obstructive sleep apnea, renal parenchymal and vascular disease, and, possibly, primary aldosteronism. Rare causes of secondary hypertension include pheochromocytoma, Cushing syndrome, hyperparathyroidism, aortic coarctation, and intracranial tumors. Following are important clinical or laboratory clues to these secondary hypertension causes:

- **Obstructive sleep apnea:** Untreated obstructive sleep apnea is an increasingly recognized cause of secondary hypertension. Clues include loud snoring, witnessed apnea, and excessive daytime somnolence. Diagnosis is confirmed with a sleep study.
- **Renal artery stenosis:** This is suspected in patients with atherosclerotic peripheral or coronary vascular disease, early age (younger than 35 years) or late age (older than 55 years) at onset of hypertension, abnormal renal function or worsening renal function with the use of an ACE inhibitor or in patients with a unilateral small kidney. Renal ultrasonography is not recommended and magnetic resistance angiography is the most specific and reliable noninvasive diagnostic imaging modality. Contrast angiography is also useful for the diagnosis and for possible renal angioplasty. It is important to recognize that the anatomic diagnosis of a renal artery stenosis, independent of its cause, does not imply that the stenosis is the cause of hypertension. Causation can be confirmed by documenting the *functionality* of the lesion by measuring renal vein renin activity and documenting a renin activity ratio greater than 1.5 between the

two sides. Fibromuscular dysplasia is a type of renal artery stenosis that most commonly occurs in younger women

- **Primary hyperaldosteronism:** This is suspected in hypertensive patients with unexplained hypokalemia. Diagnosis is suspected by a suppressed renin activity and a high 24-hour urinary aldosterone excretion in the course of a high dietary sodium intake and is confirmed radiographically with a localizing imaging procedure such as computed tomography (CT) or MRI with a specific adrenal protocol.
- **Renal parenchymal disease:** This is suspected in patients with chronic kidney disease and impaired renal function, but causation of the hypertension is often difficult to confirm because longstanding untreated hypertension may also cause renal parenchymal disease. Imaging techniques that evaluate kidney size, presence of hydronephrosis and obstructive nephropathy, calculi, polycystic kidney disease, or congenital malformations are useful to detect specific causes of renal parenchymal disease.
- **Pheochromocytoma:** A rare secondary cause of hypertension that often presents with paroxysmal and postural hypotension, usually in a younger adult, with intermittent episodes of headache, palpitation, and sweating. The best screening test is plasma-free metanephrines (normetanephrine and metanephrine).

10. **A 32-year-old man complains of intermittent episodes of headaches, palpitations, and profuse sweating. Over the last year, he has been treated three times in the emergency department for hypertensive crisis. He does not remember what his blood pressure was, but he felt lightheaded when trying to stand, even before reaching the emergency department (ED). In your office, he always has a blood pressure below 120/70 mm Hg. He has noticed low-grade fever at times and has lost a few pounds. After you examine him, he feels funny, so you measure his blood pressure again. This time it is 165/110 mm Hg, with a heart rate of 115 beats/min. Laboratory studies only show a slightly elevated serum glucose and white blood cell count (WBC) of 18,000/mL with a normal differential. What is your diagnosis?**
This is a typical presentation for a pheochromocytoma. The clues given by the patient's history are invaluable for diagnosis: Many patients with pheochromocytoma have a normal baseline blood pressure, with high blood pressure values only on occasion. *Postural hypotension* is a classical feature. High serum catecholamine levels explain the sweating and palpitations and the low fever, elevation of serum glucose, and leukocytosis. Gentle palpation of the abdomen during physical examination may sometimes trigger a crisis. Because of the general and metabolic manifestations of the disease, it may mimic a large variety of conditions (e.g., vasculitis, diabetes), and a high level of suspicion is always necessary.

Some patients present with a high blood pressure that is constant rather than paroxysmal. A *rule of 10* may be applied: 10% of all cases are familial, 10% are bilateral, 10% are due to a malignant adrenal tumor, 10% recur, 10% are extra-adrenal, 10% occur in children, 10% are associated with a multiple endocrine neoplasia (MEN) syndrome, and 10% present with a stroke as the inaugural symptom.

Diagnosis of a pheochromocytoma is rewarding because this very sick patient who is prone to life-threatening complications can be virtually cured. The current recommendation for biochemical diagnosis of pheochromocytoma is urine testing for metanephrines and fractionated catecholamines. These tests only certify the presence of a catecholamine-secreting tumor; therefore, the next step is to localize it (90% are in the adrenal medulla; the other 10% are scattered where chromaffin tissue is found). The preferred treatment is laparoscopic adrenalectomy.

11. **How important are nonpharmacologic strategies in hypertension treatment?**
Hypertension treatment is a lifelong commitment regardless of the recommended treatment modality. Thus, compliance to treatment is critically important in achieving the expected clinical benefits of treatments. Hypertensive patients should be appropriately educated about the natural history and

complications of hypertension and the critical importance of compliance with any treatment recommendation. Goal blood pressure attainment is much more likely achieved with earlier initiation of combination antihypertensive drug therapies—particularly in stage 2 hypertension, characterized by blood pressure levels greater than 160/100 mm Hg—and by frequent monitoring of blood pressure at home and in the doctor's office and appropriate uptitration of antihypertensive medications to reach accepted goals of blood pressure treatments.

Patients and some physicians tend to be skeptical about the importance of lifestyle changes. Often the skepticism of the physician may be communicated to the patient even without the physician's conscious effort. It is critically important that patients and their physicians believe in the benefit of lifestyle changes. Current hypertension guidelines describe lifestyle changes as *therapeutic* to emphasize their proven benefit. Therapeutic lifestyle changes—weight loss; reduced intake of saturated fat and salt; reduced dietary calorie intake; regular exercise and moderation of alcohol intake; consumption of adequate amounts of calcium, potassium, magnesium, and fiber; and smoking cessation—are at the top of the JNC 7 treatment algorithm recommended for all patients. Therapeutic lifestyle changes have been proven to be effective in reducing blood pressure levels by 10 to 20 mm Hg, changes that are at times similar to the efficacy of one additional antihypertensive drug. In patients with prehypertension—with blood pressure levels between 120/80 and 140/90 mm Hg—therapeutic lifestyle changes, but not pharmacologic treatment, are generally recommended to prevent hypertension development, with the exception of diabetics and/or patients with chronic kidney disease. Pharmacologic treatment is generally recommended not solely, but in addition to and as an adjunct to, therapeutic lifestyle changes in *hypertensive* patients—that is, patients with blood pressure levels greater than 140/90 mm Hg. Antihypertensive drug therapy is recommended at lower levels of blood pressure (more than 130/80 mm Hg) in higher-risk patients with diabetes mellitus and chronic kidney disease, and the goal of blood pressure treatment is also lower, namely less than 130/80 mm Hg. In patients with uncomplicated hypertension, goal blood pressure levels are less than 140/90 mm Hg.

12. **True or false: Beta-adrenergic blocking agents (β-blockers) are preferred initial antihypertensive agents in hypertensive patients with no known hypertensive complications.**

False. In large placebo-controlled prospective clinical trials, diuretics and β-blockers as a group have been shown to reduce cardiovascular complications of hypertension. However, the evidence of these cardioprotective effects of thiazide diuretics in hypertensive patients is more compelling, and in clinical trials comparing diuretic and β-blockers, such as the Medical Research Council (MRC) trial, diuretics were more effective than β-blockers. Thus, the JNC 7 report recommends thiazide diuretics, not β-blockers, as preferred initial treatments in patients with uncomplicated hypertension—that is, patients with no compelling comorbid conditions that may favor specific antihypertensive agents.

Compelling indications in hypertensive patients for the use of a β-blocker as an antihypertensive agent include a history of MI, compensated heart failure, and CAD. Contraindications to β-blockers must be carefully weighed against their potential therapeutic benefits. For example, a β-blocker should be avoided in a patient admitted to the hospital with acutely decompensated heart failure, but may be started at lower doses then gradually uptitrated in patients with well-compensated and stable heart failure. Withdrawal of β-blockers, particularly in patients with CAD, should be performed gradually to avoid rebound increase in anginal symptoms upon their discontinuation.

13. **Are alpha-adrenergic blocking agents (α-blockers) effective in preventing cardiovascular complications of hypertension, and when is it appropriate to use them in hypertensive patients?**

α-Blockers are effective antihypertensive agents but have not been shown in either placebo-controlled or active-controlled clinical prospective trials to be effective in preventing cardiovascular complications of hypertension. In the ALLHAT trial, the largest hypertensive clinical trial that randomized hypertensive patients to an ACE inhibitor, a calcium channel blocker, or an α-blocker versus a thiazide diuretic, the α-blocker arm of the trial was prematurely terminated because of an almost doubling of the risk of heart failure and a 25% excess cardiovascular death rate among patients treated with an α-blocker compared with a thiazide diuretic. Thus, α-blockers are *not* recommended as initial antihypertensive agents.

However, α-blockers may be used as a second- or third-line antihypertensive agent to treat hypertension and may be used because of a compelling and specific reason for the use of an α-blocker to minimize obstructive urinary symptoms in older men with benign prostatic hyperplasia.

14. **When are ACE inhibitors specifically recommended in hypertensive patients?**
The JNC 7 report recommends a thiazide as an initial antihypertensive agent in patients with uncomplicated hypertension. Compelling indications for the selection of an ACE inhibitor include heart failure, previous MI, diabetes mellitus, chronic kidney disease, high CAD risk, and for recurrent stroke prevention. These recommendations are based on several randomized, prospective, controlled clinical trials confirming the benefits of ACE inhibitors in preventing cardiovascular or renal complications in these patients. ACE inhibitors prevent myocardial remodeling, heart failure progression, progressive ventricular enlargement after a recent MI, MIs, and stroke in patients with cardiovascular disease, and have also been proven to prevent progression of renal disease among diabetics with established diabetic renal disease.

15. **What are the goals for hypertension treatment in African Americans recommended by the International Society of Hypertension in Blacks (ISHIB)?**
African Americans have a significantly higher prevalence of hypertension than any other racial ethnic group in the United States and suffer a much higher risk of hypertensive complications. Unlike the JNC 7 report, the ISHIB Consensus report recommend lower blood pressure goals in African Americans, specifically:

- Goal blood pressure is less than 135/85 mm Hg for primary prevention of cardiovascular disease in African Americans without target organ damage, diabetes mellitus, cardiovascular disease, or peripheral vascular disease (including systolic or diastolic heart failure), or cardiovascular disease (CVD) including heart failure (systolic or diastolic)
- Goal blood pressure is less than 130/80 mm Hg in African Americans with target organ damage, or with preclinical or clinical CVD.

ISHIB also recommended *earlier* initiation of a two-drug combination at a blood pressure 15/10 mm Hg above goal blood pressure, rather than 20/10 mm Hg above goal (as recommended by the JNC 7 report).

16. **What is the prevalence of hypertension among African Americans and Hispanic Americans compared to non-Hispanic whites?**
Hypertension affects about 33% of all adults aged 20 years or older in the United States (according to the NHANES [2005-2008] and the AHA Statistical Update on Cardiovascular Disease and Stroke [2012]). African Americans have a significantly higher prevalence of hypertension, at approximately 44%. This percentage has been rising in the last 20 years, more so than in whites. Hispanics have a lower hypertension prevalence, at approximately 25%.

BIBLIOGRAPHY, SUGGESTED READINGS, AND WEBSITES

1. ACCORD Study Group: Effects of Intensive Blood Pressure Control in Type 2 Diabetics, *N Engl J Med* 362: 1575–1585, 2010.
2. Agency for Healthcare Research and Quality: 2009 National Healthcare Disparities Report, Table 2_1_3.2b. Available at http://www.ahrq.gov/qual/qrdr09/2_diabetes/T2_1_3-2b.htm. Accessed March 20, 2013.
3. ALLHAT Officers and Coordinators for the ALLHAT Collaborative Research Group: Major cardiovascular events in hypertensive patients randomized to doxazosin vs. chlorthalidone: the Antihypertensive and Lipid-Lowering Treatment to Prevent Heart Attack Trial (ALLHAT), *JAMA* 2831967–1975, 2000.
4. ALLHAT Officers and Coordinators for the ALLHAT Collaborative Research Group: Major outcomes in high-risk hypertensive patients randomized to angiotensin-converting enzyme inhibitor or calcium channel blocker vs diuretic: the Antihypertensive and Lipid-Lowering Treatment to Prevent Heart Attack Trial (ALLHAT), *JAMA* 288:2981–2997, 2002.

5. Calhoun D, Jones D, Textor D, et al: Resistant hypertension: diagnosis, evaluation, and treatment: a scientific statement from the American Heart Association Professional Education Committee of the Council for High Blood Pressure Research, *Hypertension* 51:1403–1419, 2008.

6. Chobanian AV, Bakris GL, Black HR, et al: Seventh report of the Joint National Committee on Prevention, Detection, Evaluation, and Treatment of High Blood Pressure: the JNC 7 report, *JAMA* 289:2560–2572, 2003, Erratum, *JAMA* 290:197, 2003.

7. Chobanian AV, Bakris GL, Black HR, et al: Seventh report of the Joint National Committee on Prevention, Detection, Evaluation, and Treatment of High Blood Pressure. Available at http://www.nhlbi.nih.gov/guidelines/hypertension/express.pdf (PDF file). Accessed March 19, 2013.

8. Cusham WC, Ford CE, Cutler JA, et al: Success and predictors of blood pressure control in diverse North American settings: the antihypertensive and lipid-lowering treatment to prevent heart attack trial (ALLHAT), *J Clin Hypertens (Greenwich)* 4:393–404, 2002.

9. Cutler JA, Davis BR: Thiazide-type diuretics and ^{2}-adrenergic blockers as first-line drug treatments for hypertension, *Circulation* 117:2691–2705, 2008.

10. Flack JM, Sica DA, Bakris G, et al: on behalf of the International Society on Hypertension in Blacks: ISHIB consensus statement. Management of high blood pressure in Blacks. An update of the International Society on Hypertension in Blacks Consensus Statement, *Hypertension* 56:780–800, 2010.

11. Hajjar I, Kotchen TA: Trends in prevalence, awareness, treatment, and control of hypertension in the United States, 1998-2000, *JAMA* 290:199–206, 2003.

12. Heart Outcomes Prevention Evaluation Study Investigators: Effects of an angiotensin-converting-enzyme inhibitor, ramipril, on cardiovascular events in high-risk patients, *N Engl J Med* 342:145–153, 2000.

13. Kearney PM, Whelton M, Reynolds K, et al: Worldwide prevalence of hypertension: a systematic review, *J Hypertens* 1:11–19, 2004.

14. Lloyd-Jones DM, Evans JC, Larson MG, et al: Differential control of systolic and diastolic blood pressure: factors associated with lack of blood pressure control in the community, *Hypertension* 36:594–599, 2000.

15. ONTARGET Investigators: Telmisartan, ramipril or both in patients at high risk for vascular events, *N Engl J Med* 358:1547–1559, 2008.

16. Roger VL, Go AS, Lloyd-Jones DM, et al: Heart disease and stroke statistics—2012 update. a report from the American Heart Association, *Circulation* 125:e2–e220, 2012.

17. Rosendorff C, Black HR, Cannon CP, et al: Treatment of hypertension in the prevention and management of ischemic heart disease: a scientific statement from the American Heart Association Council for High Blood Pressure Research and the Councils on Clinical Cardiology and Epidemiology and Prevention, *Circulation* 115:2761–2788, 2007.

18. Sorlie PD, Backlund E, Johnson NJ, et al: Mortality by Hispanic status in the United States, *JAMA* 270:2464–2468, 1993.

19. TRANSCEND Investigators: Effects of the angiotensin-receptor blocker telmisartan on cardiovascular events in high-risk patients intolerant to angiotensin-converting enzyme inhibitors: a randomized controlled trial, *Lancet* 372:1174–1183, 2008.

CHAPTER 41

HYPERCHOLESTEROLEMIA

Glenn N. Levine, MD, FACC, FAHA

1. **Who should be screened for hypercholesterolemia?**
   The National Cholesterol Education Program (NCEP) Adult Treatment Panel III (ATP III) recommends that all adults age 20 years or older should undergo fasting lipoprotein profile every 5 years. Testing should include total cholesterol, low-density lipoprotein (LDL) cholesterol, high-density lipoprotein (HDL) cholesterol, and triglycerides.

2. **True or false: Coronary atherosclerosis is common in persons in their 20s and 30s.**
   True. Autopsy and intravascular ultrasound (IVUS) studies have demonstrated detectable atheromas and/or atherosclerosis in 50% to 69% of asymptomatic young persons.

3. **What are the ATP III classifications of LDL cholesterol, total cholesterol, HDL cholesterol, and triglyceride levels based on measured values?**
   The values, as denoted in ATP III, are given in Table 41-1. Note that since publication of this classification in 2001, a goal of LDL less than 70 mg/dL has emerged as desirable in some very high-risk populations and thus an LDL of significantly less than 100 mg/dL would now be considered optimal in such patients. To convert the values in the table to mmol/L, divide by 88.6.

4. **What are important secondary causes of hypercholesterolemia?**
   - Diabetes
   - Hypothyroidism
   - Obstructive liver disease
   - Chronic renal failure or nephrotic syndrome
   - Drugs (e.g., progestins, anabolic steroids, or corticosteroids)

5. **What is a lipoprotein?**
   A lipoprotein is the particle that transports cholesterol and triglycerides. Lipoproteins are composed of proteins (called apolipoproteins), phospholipids, triglycerides, and cholesterol (Fig. 41-1).

6. **What is lipoprotein (a)?**
   Lipoprotein (a), often represented as Lp(a), is an LDL-like particle that contains apolipoprotein B (apo B). It has independently been correlated with an increased risk of adverse cardiovascular event in certain patient populations. According to a 2008 consensus report from the American Diabetes Association and American College of Cardiology Foundation, "the clinical utility of routine measurement of Lp(a) is unclear, although more aggressive control of other lipoprotein parameters may be warranted in those with high concentrations of Lp(a)."

7. **What is the minimal LDL goal for secondary prevention?**
   The minimal LDL goal for secondary prevention in patients with established coronary artery disease (CAD) is an LDL less than 100 mg/dL. This is also now the goal in patients with coronary heart disease risk equivalents (see Question 8). In an update to ATP III, it was emphasized that an LDL less than 100 mg/dL is a *minimal* goal of therapy. In light of more recent studies (Pravastatin or Atorvastatin Evaluation and Infection Therapy [PROVE-IT], Heart Protection Study [HPS], and Treating to New Targets [TNT]), a goal of LDL less than 70 mg/dL should be considered in patients with

TABLE 41-1.	NCEP-ATP III CLASSIFICATION OF LDL, TOTAL CHOLESTEROL, HDL CHOLESTEROL, AND TRIGLYCERIDE LEVELS*	
VALUE (mg/dL)	**CLASSIFICATION**
LDL Cholesterol	
<100	Optimal
100-129	Near or above optimal
130-159	Borderline high
160-189	High
≥190	Very High
Total Cholesterol	
<200	Desirable
200-239	Borderline high
≥240	High
HDL Cholesterol	
<40	Low
≥60	High
Triglycerides	
<150	Normal
150-199	Borderline high
200-499	High
≥500	Very high

To convert mg/dL to mmol/L, divide by 88.6.
Modified from Expert Panel on Detection, Evaluation, and Treatment of High Blood Cholesterol in Adults: Executive Summary of The Third Report of The National Cholesterol Education Program (NCEP) Expert Panel on Detection, Evaluation, and Treatment of High Blood Cholesterol in Adults (Adult Treatment Panel III). *JAMA* 285:2486-2497, 2001.
*Note that since publication of this classification, a goal of LDL less than 70 mg/dL has emerged as desirable in some very-high risk populations.

coronary heart disease at *very high* risk. Patients with coronary heart disease classified as *very high* risk include those with the following:
- Multiple major coronary risk factors (especially diabetes)
- Severe and poorly controlled risk factors (especially continued cigarette smoking)
- Multiple risk factors of metabolic syndrome (see Question 9)
- Acute coronary syndrome

8. **What is a coronary heart disease risk equivalent?**
Patients with established coronary heart disease (those being treated for secondary prevention) have been recommended for the most aggressive treatment for elevated LDL levels. ATP III established *coronary heart disease risk equivalents* to denote those at high risk for cardiovascular disease and events, who would warrant equivalently aggressive lipid therapy as provided to those with established CAD. ATP III recommends that patients with these risk equivalents should have LDL levels lowered to below 100 mg/dL *at a minimum*. These coronary heart disease risk equivalents include the following:
- Diabetes
- Other clinical forms of atherosclerosis (e.g., peripheral arterial disease, abdominal aortic aneurysm, and symptomatic carotid artery disease)

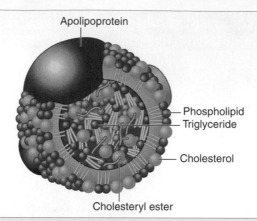

Figure 41-1. A lipoprotein particle. The polar surface coat is composed of apoproteins, phospholipids, and free cholesterol. The nonpolar lipid core is composed of cholesterol esters and triglycerides. (From Genest J, Libby P: Lipoprotein disorders and cardiovascular disease. In Libby P, Bonow RO, Mann DL, Zipes DP, editors: *Braunwald's heart disease: a textbook of cardiovascular medicine,* ed 8, Philadelphia, 2008, Saunders.)

- Multiple cardiac risk factors that confer a 10-year risk for CAD greater than 20% (based on the Framingham risk table)

9. **What factors make up metabolic syndrome?**
   - Abdominal obesity (waist circumference in men more than 40 inches [102 cm] or in women more than 35 inches [88 cm])
   - Triglycerides 150 mg/dL or more
   - Low HDL cholesterol (less than 40 mg/dL in men or less than 50 mg/dL in women)
   - Blood pressure 135/85 mm Hg or higher
   - Fasting glucose 110 mg/dL or more

10. **What medications should be used to lower LDL levels?**
    Statins are the first-line agents to lower LDL levels. If adequate LDL lowering is not achieved, a more potent statin can be considered. If adequate LDL is still not achieved, either a bile acid sequestrant, fibrate, or nicotinic acid should be added. Note that patients may need to be followed more carefully for side effects, such as liver function test (LFT) elevation and myopathy, with certain combination therapies. At the time of this writing, and likely until the results of the Improved Reduction of Outcomes: Vytorin Efficacy International Trial (IMPROVE-IT) are presented, ezetimibe should only be used as a secondary agent if the agents listed here are not tolerated or do not lead to adequate LDL reduction. Table 41-2 summarizes the drugs used to treat hypercholesterolemia, their effects, and their side effects.

11. **Is there an age cutoff for secondary prevention therapy with statins?**
    No. Older secondary prevention trials with statins included many patients in their 60s and 70s and demonstrated benefit in older and younger patients. Thus, for secondary prevention, according to ATP III, "no hard-and-fast age restrictions appear necessary when selecting persons with established coronary heart disease for LDL-lowering therapy." Since publication of ATP III, the Prospective Study of Pravastatin in the Elderly at Risk (PROSPER), and several other trials were published. In PROSPER, subjects age 70 to 82 with a history of vascular disease or risk factors were randomized to treatment with pravastatin or placebo. After an average of 3.2 years of follow-up, the composite ischemic endpoint was reduced by 15%. The results of PROSPER, HPS, and Anglo-Scandinavian Cardiac Outcomes Trial (ASCOT) reinforce that statin therapy should be used in elderly patients for secondary prevention and should be seriously considered in elderly patients for primary prevention.

TABLE 41-2. DRUGS USED IN THE TREATMENT OF HYPERCHOLESTEROLEMIA

DRUG CLASS	LIPID/LIPOPROTEIN EFFECTS	SIDE EFFECTS	CONTRAINDICATIONS
Statins	LDL ↓ 18%-55% HDL ↑ 5%-15% TG ↓ 7%-30%	Myopathy Increased LFTs	Absolute: active or chronic liver disease Relative: concomitant use of certain drugs
Bile acid sequestrants	LDL ↓ 15%-30% HDL ↑ 3%-5% TG—no change or increase	Gastrointestinal distress Constipation Decreased absorption of other drugs	Absolute: dysbetalipoproteinemia or TG > 400 mg/dL Relative: TG > 200 mg/dL
Nicotinic acid	LDL ↓ 5%-25% HDL ↑ 15%-35% TG ↓ 20%-50%	Flushing Hyperglycemia Hyperuricemia (or gout) Upper GI distress Hepatotoxicity	Absolute: chronic liver disease or severe gout Relative: diabetes, hyperuricemia, or peptic ulcer disease
Fibric acids	LDL ↓ 5%-20% HDL ↑ 10%-20% TG ↓ 20%-50%	Dyspepsia Gallstones Myopathy	Absolute: severe renal disease or severe hepatic disease
Ezetimibe	LDL ↓ 18%-20% HDL ↑ 1% TG ↓ 5%-11%	Approximately 1% higher rate of LFT elevations when used with statin vs. statin alone	Absolute: active liver disease when used with a statin

Modified from Expert Panel on Detection, Evaluation, and Treatment of High Blood Cholesterol in Adults: Executive summary of the third report of the National Cholesterol Education Program (NCEP) Expert Panel on Detection, Evaluation, and Treatment of High Blood Cholesterol in Adults (Adult Treatment Panel III). *JAMA* 285:2486-2497, 2001.
GI, Gastrointestinal; *HDL*, high-density lipoprotein; *LDL*, low-density lipoprotein; *LFT*, liver function test; *TG*, triglyceride.

12. **What is non-HDL cholesterol?**

The non-HDL cholesterol level is the total cholesterol level minus HDL cholesterol level. It is an approximation of very-low-density lipoprotein (VLDL) plus LDL levels. VLDL cholesterol is felt in clinical practice to be the most readily available measure of atherogenic remnant lipoproteins. Reduction of non-HDL cholesterol is considered a secondary target of therapy in persons with high triglycerides (200 mg/dL or more). The goals for non-HDL cholesterol are generally 30 mg/dL higher than those for LDL cholesterol (Box 41-1). For example, in patients with coronary heart disease and coronary heart disease risk equivalents, the LDL goal is less than 100 mg/dL and the non-HDL goal is less than 130 mg/dL.

13. **What factors and conditions are believed to be associated with or cause low HDL cholesterol?**
   - Elevated triglycerides
   - Overweight and obesity
   - Physical inactivity

> **Box 41-1 RECOMMENDATIONS ON LIPID THERAPY FROM THE AMERICAN HEART ASSOCIATION AND AMERICAN COLLEGE OF CARDIOLOGY FOUNDATION (AHA/ACCF) SECONDARY PREVENTION AND RISK REDUCTION THERAPY FOR PATIENTS WITH CORONARY AND OTHER ATHEROSCLEROTIC VASCULAR DISEASE: 2011 UPDATE**
>
> **Class I**
> 1. A lipid profile in all patients should be established, and for hospitalized patients, lipid-lowering therapy as recommended below should be initiated before discharge. (Level of Evidence: B)
> 2. Lifestyle modifications including daily physical activity and weight management are strongly recommended for all patients. (Level of Evidence: B)
> 3. Dietary therapy for all patients should include reduced intake of saturated fats (to <7% of total calories), trans fatty acids (to <1% of total calories), and cholesterol (to <200 mg/d). (Level of Evidence: B)
> 4. In addition to therapeutic lifestyle changes, statin therapy should be prescribed in the absence of contraindications or documented adverse effects. (Level of Evidence: A)
> 5. An adequate dose of statin should be used that reduces LDL-C to <100 mg/dL *and* achieves at least a 30% lowering of LDL-C. (Level of Evidence: C)
> 6. Patients who have triglycerides ≥200 mg/dL should be treated with statins to lower non–HDL-C to <130 mg/dL. (Level of Evidence: B)
> 7. Patients who have triglycerides >500 mg/dL should be started on fibrate therapy in addition to statin therapy to prevent acute pancreatitis. (Level of Evidence: C)
>
> **Class IIa**
> 1. If treatment with a statin (including trials of higher-dose statins and higher-potency statins) does not achieve the goal selected for a patient, intensification of LDL-C–lowering drug therapy with a bile acid sequestrant* or niacin† is reasonable. (Level of Evidence: B)
> 2. For patients who do not tolerate statins, LDL-C–lowering therapy with bile acid sequestrants* and/or niacin† is reasonable. (Level of Evidence: B)
> 3. It is reasonable to treat very high-risk‡ patients with statin therapy to lower LDL-C to <70 mg/dL. (Level of Evidence: C)
> 4. In patients who are at very high risk‡ and who have triglycerides ≥200 mg/dL, a non–HDL-C goal of <100 mg/dL is reasonable. (Level of Evidence: B)
>
> **Class IIb**
> 1. The use of ezetimibe may be considered for patients who do not tolerate or achieve target LDL-C with statins, bile acid sequestrants,* and/or niacin.† (Level of Evidence: C)
> 2. For patients who continue to have an elevated non–HDL-C while on adequate statin therapy, niacin† or fibrate§ therapy (Level of Evidence: B) or fish oil (Level of Evidence: C) may be reasonable.
> 3. For all patients, it may be reasonable to recommend omega-3 fatty acids from fish‖ or fish oil capsules (1g/d) for cardiovascular disease reduction. (Level of Evidence: B)
>
> Modified from Smith SC Jr, Benjamin EJ, Bonow RO, Braun LT, et al: AHA/ACCF secondary prevention and risk reduction therapy for patients with coronary and other atherosclerotic vascular disease: 2011 update: a guideline from the American Heart Association and American College of Cardiology Foundation endorsed by the World Heart Federation and the Preventive Cardiovascular Nurses Association. *J Am Coll Cardiol* 58:2432-2446, 2011.
> *The use of bile acid sequestrants is relatively contraindicated when triglycerides are ≥200 mg/dL and is contraindicated when triglycerides are ≥500 mg/dL.
> †Dietary supplement niacin must not be used as a substitute for prescription niacin.
> ‡Presence of established CVD plus (1) multiple major risk factors (especially diabetes), (2) severe and poorly controlled risk factors (especially continued cigarette smoking), (3) multiple risk factors of the metabolic syndrome (especially high triglycerides ≥200 mg/dL plus non–HDL-C ≥130 mg/dL with low HDL-C <40 mg/dL), and (4) patients with ACSs.
> §The combination of high-dose statin plus fibrate (especially gemfibrozil) can increase risk for severe myopathy. Statin doses should be kept relatively low with this combination.
> ‖Pregnant and lactating women should limit their intake of fish to minimize exposure to methylmercury.

- Type 2 diabetes mellitus
- Cigarette smoking
- Very high carbohydrate intakes (more than 60% of energy intake)
- Certain drugs (e.g., beta-adrenergic blocking agents [β-blockers], anabolic steroids, and progestational agents)

14. **What is the difference between myopathy, myalgia, myositis, and rhabdomyolysis?**
    - **Myopathy:** general term referring to any disease of muscles
    - **Myalgia:** muscle ache or weakness without creatine kinase (CK) elevation
    - **Myositis:** muscle symptoms with increased CK levels
    - **Rhabdomyolysis:** muscle symptoms with marked CK elevation (more than 10 times the upper limit of normal [ULN])

15. **What is the incidence of nonspecific muscle aches or joint pains in patients treated with statins?**
    In placebo-controlled trials, the incidence of nonspecific muscle aches (myalgia) or joint pains in patients treated with statins is approximately 5%. Interestingly, the rates of these complaints are similar in these trials between active treatment and placebo groups. Nevertheless, it is generally accepted that some patients will have a temporal development of such symptoms after initiation of statin therapy that is likely due to such therapy. The incidence of severe myopathy or overt rhabdomyolysis (CK elevation greater than 10 times ULN) is approximately 1 in 1000 with currently available statins.

BIBLIOGRAPHY, SUGGESTED READINGS, AND WEBSITES

1. Baylor College of Medicine: Lipids Online website. Available at, http://www.lipidsonline.org. Accessed February 27, 2013.
2. Brunzell JD, Davidson M, Furberg CD, et al: Lipoprotein management in patients with cardiometabolic risk, *J Am Coll Cardiol* 51:1512–1524, 2008.
3. Genest J, Libby P: Lipoprotein disorders and cardiovascular disease. In Libby P, Bonow RO, Mann DL, Zipes DP, editors: *Braunwald's heart disease: a textbook of cardiovascular medicine*, ed 8, Philadelphia, 2008, Saunders.
4. Grundy SM, Cleeman JI, Merz CN, et al: Implications of recent clinical trials for the National Cholesterol Education Program Adult Treatment Panel III guidelines, *J Am Coll Cardiol* 44:720–732, 2004.
5. Pasternak RC, Smith SC Jr, Bairey-Merz CN, et al: ACC/AHA/NHLBI clinical advisory on the use and safety of statins, *Circulation* 106:1024–1028, 2002.
6. Rosenson RS: Overview of Treatment of Hypercholesterolemia. Available at: http://www.utdol.com.
7. Rosenson RS: Screening Guidelines for Dyslipidemia. In Basow, DS, editor: UpToDate, Waltham, MA, 2013, UpToDate. Available at: http://www.uptodate.com/contents/screening-guidelines-for-dyslipidemia. Accessed March 26, 2013.
8. Smith SC Jr, Allen J, Blair SN, et al: AHA/ACC guidelines for secondary prevention for patients with coronary and other atherosclerotic vascular disease: 2006 update: endorsed by the National Heart, Lung, and Blood Institute, *Circulation* 113:2363–2372, 2006.
9. Smith SC Jr, Benjamin EJ, Bonow RO, Braun LT, et al: AHA/ACCF secondary prevention and risk reduction therapy for patients with coronary and other atherosclerotic vascular disease: 2011 update: a guideline from the American Heart Association and American College of Cardiology Foundation endorsed by the World Heart Federation and the Preventive Cardiovascular Nurses Association, *J Am Coll Cardiol* 58:2432–2446, 2011.

CHAPTER 42

DIABETES AND CARDIOVASCULAR DISEASE

Ashish Aneja, MD, and Michael E. Farkouh, MD, MSc, FACC

1. **What is the current global burden of diabetes, and what is its impact on the epidemiology of cardiovascular disease (CVD)?**
    The global burden of diabetes mellitus (DM) in 1985 was an estimated 30 million people. By 2003, it was estimated that there were around 194 million people with diabetes, and this figure is expected to rise to almost 350 million by 2025. At present, the prevalence of DM is much higher in developed countries, but because of urbanization and adoption of western diets and lifestyles, developing countries are rapidly catching up with their developed counterparts. The disease affects a disproportionately higher number of young people in the developing world. The lifetime risk of diabetes is estimated at 32.8% for U.S. males and 38.5% for U.S. females.

    Knowledge of the epidemiology of DM is important to place the expected contribution of DM to the global CVD burden into perspective. The relationship between DM type 1 and type 2 and CVD is well established. In particular, DM is a very strong risk factor for the development of coronary artery disease (CAD) and stroke. The hazard ratio for CAD death in diabetic patients is considered as high as 2.03 (95% confidence interval [CI], 1.60 to 2.59) for men and 2.54 (95% CI, 1.84 to 3.49) for women. Atherosclerosis accounts for 80% of all deaths in diabetic persons, compared with about 30% among nondiabetic persons. Atherosclerotic disease also accounts for greater than 75% of hospitalizations for diabetes-related complications. Patients with diabetes but without previous myocardial infarction (MI) carry the same level of risk for subsequent acute coronary events as nondiabetic patients with previous MI. These results have prompted the Adult Treatment Panel III of the National Cholesterol Education Program to establish diabetes as a CAD risk equivalent, mandating aggressive antiatherosclerotic therapy.

2. **What is the impact of diabetes on CVD outcomes?**
    In addition to its salutary effects on stable atherosclerotic disease, diabetic patients experience an increased rate of early and late complications following acute coronary syndrome (ACS). Diabetic patients with non–ST segment elevation ACS also experience more in-hospital MIs, associated complications and higher death rates. Diabetic patients also respond less optimally to fibrinolytic therapy, an effect that is sex-dependent—diabetic women fare worse than men. In patients with ACS complicated by hypotension and cardiogenic shock, diabetes is an independent risk variable for adverse outcomes, including death. In the short and long terms, diabetic patients with ACS experience higher rates of heart failure, death, and repeat infarction and require more frequent coronary revascularization.

3. **What effect, if any, does diabetes have on the clinical manifestations and prognosis of peripheral arterial disease (PAD) and cerebrovascular disease?**
    Diabetes increases the risk of PAD about two- to fourfold. It is more commonly associated with femoral bruits and absent pedal pulses and with a high rate of abnormal ankle-brachial indices, ranging from 11% to 16% in different studies. The duration and severity of diabetes correlates with the incidence and extent of PAD. The pattern of PAD in diabetic patients is characterized by a preponderance of infrapopliteal occlusive disease and vascular calcification. Clinically, PAD in diabetic patients manifests more commonly with claudication and also a higher rate of amputation—the most common cause of nontraumatic amputations.

Diabetic patients also have a higher rate of intracranial and extracranial cerebrovascular atherosclerosis and calcifications. Patients with a history of stroke have a threefold higher likelihood of being diabetic than do controls, with a risk of stroke that may be up to three- to fourfold higher than that of nondiabetic patients. Compared with nondiabetic subjects, the mortality from stroke in diabetic patients is almost threefold higher. Diabetes also results in a disproportionately higher stroke rate in younger patients and increases the risk of severe carotid disease. In patients younger than 55 years, diabetes increases the risk of stroke about 10 times according to one study. Diabetic patients also suffer worse poststroke outcomes, including a higher mortality rate and recurrence risk and a greater probability of vascular dementia.

4. **What is the overall impact of diabetes on the vascular tree?**
Cardiovascular (CV) complications in diabetic patients can be the result of macrovascular disease, including CAD, peripheral arterial disease, and cerebrovascular disease, or can be due to microvascular disease that can result in nephropathy, retinopathy, and neuropathy. Many regard diabetic cardiomyopathy as a distinct entity that is thought to result primarily from hyperglycemia-induced myocardial adverse effects.

5. **What is the burden of additional CV risk factors in diabetic patients, and what is their cumulative impact on the atherosclerosis morphology and burden?**
Diabetic patients are known to bear a higher burden of CV risk factors, including twice the prevalence of hypertension, and a higher prevalence of dyslipidemia, including lower high-density lipoprotein (HDL) cholesterol, higher triglycerides, and higher small, dense low-density lipoprotein (LDL) cholesterol levels. The clustering of CV risk factors appears to have a multiplicative effect in diabetic patients, who experience a threefold higher CV mortality than do nondiabetic persons for each risk factor present. In addition, CAD in diabetic patients involves a greater number of coronary vessels and more diffuse atherosclerotic lesions, including significantly more severe proximal and distal CAD.
Atherosclerotic plaque ulceration and thrombosis also occur more often in diabetic patients. Atherosclerotic plaques in diabetic patients are considered high-risk because of a greater propensity for erosion or rupture, which accounts for a higher incidence of ACS in this population. Diabetic plaques are characterized by high levels of inflammatory cell infiltration, large lipid cores, thin fibrous caps, the presence of new vessel formation (neovascularization) and hemorrhage within the plaque.

6. **What characteristics of the atherosclerotic plaque in diabetic patients make it unstable compared with plaque in nondiabetic patients?**
Diabetic patients harbor a proinflammatory and prothrombotic milieu with greater C-reactive protein (CRP), matrix metalloproteinase 3 and 9 (MMP-3 and MMP-9), intercellular adhesion molecule (ICAM), nuclear factor kappa-light-chain-enhancer of activated B cells (NF-κB), monocyte chemotactic protein-1 (MCP-1), plasminogen activator inhibitor-1 (PAI-1), and superoxide concentrations. In addition to its adverse effects on the endothelium, diabetes promotes processes that lead to monocyte transmigration across the endothelium into the vessel wall and uptake of oxidized LDLs into these cells, resulting in foam cell and fatty streak formation. In addition to plaque initiation, diabetes renders the atherosclerotic plaque unstable. Endothelial cells in diabetic patients release cytokines and enzymes (MMPs) that impair collagen synthesis by vascular smooth muscle cells and also accelerate its breakdown. Because collagen is an essential component of the plaque fibrous cap, weakening it renders the plaque unstable. Plaque rupture or erosion triggers an intense local prothrombotic milieu, resulting in thrombus formation. In addition, following plaque rupture, platelets of diabetic patients aggregate more aggressively and are more likely to disaggregate with more efficacious antiplatelet agents (especially prasugrel and ticagrelor, when compared to clopidogrel), as demonstrated in the diabetic cohorts of the Trial to Assess Improvement in Therapeutic Outcomes by Optimizing Platelet Inhibition with Prasugrel Thrombolysis in Myocardial Infarction 38 (TRITON-TIMI 38) and Platelet Inhibition and Patient Outcomes (PLATO) trials. Diabetes also results in elevated factor VII levels (procoagulant) and reduced protein C and antithrombin III levels (naturally occurring anticoagulants). Finally, diabetic endothelial cells produce more tissue factor, the major procoagulant found in atherosclerotic plaques.

7. **What broad management strategy is advocated for diabetic patients with CVD?**
A multidisciplinary approach is the cornerstone in the successful management of diabetes and CVD. Since the presence of diabetes is considered equivalent to having CAD, aggressive management of all potential risk factors, including hypertension, dyslipidemia, and the hypercoagulable state, are recommended. In addition to measures to promote weight loss by dietary modification and exercise, diabetic patients benefit from aggressively managing conventional risk factors. The strongest evidence supporting a multifaceted and comprehensive approach in the management of diabetic patients comes from the Steno-2 trial. It demonstrated that a strategy including lifestyle and pharmacologic interventions intended to reduce CV risk in type 2 diabetic patients with microalbuminuria was significantly more effective in reducing CV events and mortality than was usual care in the long term.

8. **How does the treatment of hyperglycemia and insulin resistance impact outcomes in diabetic patients with CVD?**
Tight glycemic control has been shown to improve microvascular complications, including diabetic nephropathy. The current American Diabetes Association target for HbA_{1C} is less than 7% and for the American College of Clinical Endocrinology less than 6.5%. Diabetic nephropathy occurs in 40% of patients with type 1 and type 2 diabetes, and the main risk factors for its development include poor glycemic control, hypertension, and ethnicity. The Diabetes Control and Complications Trial (DCCT) and the United Kingdom Prospective Diabetes Study group trial (UKPDS) demonstrated that the development and progression of microalbuminuria can be prevented through strict glycemic control. This was also demonstrated for type 2 patients in the Action in Diabetes and Vascular Disease: Preterax and Diamicron MR Controlled Evaluation (ADVANCE) trial.

   Despite epidemiologic evidence linking poor glycemic control with CVD, aggressive glucose control for reduction of CV risk is controversial and potentially harmful in susceptible populations. This has recently been an area of considerable debate because of the results of two recent large randomized controlled trials: Action to Control Cardiovascular Risk in Diabetes (ACCORD) and ADVANCE. The means used to attain glycemic control have also recently received much scrutiny because of reports suggesting increased risk of CVD, including mortality, MI, and fluid retention and/or heart failure, with thiazolidinediones (TZD), in particular rosiglitazone. Another TZD, pioglitazone, which is believed to have a relatively benign CV profile, has recently been associated with a higher incidence of bladder carcinoma and bone fractures.

   For these reasons, metformin remains the first-line treatment option in most type 2 diabetes patients and seems to have a beneficial effect on insulin resistance without an adverse effect on CVD. The Bypass Angioplasty Revascularization Investigation 2 Diabetes (BARI 2D) trial has demonstrated that an insulin-sensitizing strategy led by metformin was superior to an insulin provision strategy in reducing CV events in diabetic patients with established coronary disease. This landmark study also demonstrated the efficacy of medical management in diabetic patients with less extensive coronary disease.

9. **What are the currently recommended strategies for the management of diabetic dyslipidemia?**
The lipid abnormalities in diabetes improve with lifestyle modifications, including weight loss, exercise, smoking cessation, and dietary changes, which are the first line of treatment. The most effective intervention in the management of diabetic patients with CAD is the use of statin medications, which have proven especially useful in this population. In the Scandinavian Simvastatin Survival Study (4S) and Cholesterol and Recurrent Events (CARE) trials and the Heart Protection Study (HPS), simvastatin demonstrated a significantly greater benefit in mortality and MI of diabetic subjects compared with nondiabetic subjects. The goal for LDL cholesterol is less than 100 mg/dL for patients without CAD and less than 70 mg/dL for those with CAD.

   In addition to statins, fibric acid derivatives may be especially beneficial in diabetic patients because of their effects in lowering triglycerides and raising HDL levels. Treatment with gemfibrozil significantly reduced the risk of MI in the Veterans Affairs High-Density Lipoprotein Cholesterol Intervention Trial (VA-HIT). In addition to the lipid-lowering effect, fibric acid derivatives may have antiatherogenic, antithrombogenic, and antiinflammatory effects. However, the role of fibric acid derivatives has been questioned in diabetic patients recently, following the results of the ACCORD lipid study in which adding a fibrate to a statin did not confer additional CV protection. Nicotinic acid also produces a similar favorable effect on the lipid profile in diabetic patients but needs investigation in a large study, following disappointing results from the Atherothrombosis Intervention in Metabolic Syndrome with Low HDL/High Triglycerides: Impact on Global Health Outcomes (AIM-HIGH) trial. In addition, diabetic patients on niacin may require close monitoring of their glucose levels.

10. What do the current guidelines recommend for management of hypertension in diabetic patients?

The goal blood pressure in diabetic patients is less than 130/80 mm Hg. Those with a blood pressure 140/90 mm Hg or more should be given drug therapy in addition to lifestyle and behavioral therapy. However, the effect of blood pressure reduction below 120/70 mm Hg remains unclear. It is not uncommon for diabetic patients to require multiple agents for optimal blood pressure control. Unless contraindicated or not tolerated, either an angiotensin-converting enzyme (ACE) inhibitor or an angiotensin-receptor blocker (ARB) should be included in all blood pressure regimens for diabetic patients. Diuretics, beta-adrenergic blocking agents (β-blockers), ACE inhibitors, ARBs, and calcium channel antagonists all effectively decrease blood pressure in diabetic patients.

Regardless of the agent chosen, evidence from prior randomized clinical trials overwhelmingly favors good blood pressure control. The recommendations given here are based on the results of trials of hypertension or CV prevention. In the Heart Outcomes and Prevention Evaluation (HOPE) study, ramipril significantly decreased the rates of MI, stroke, and death in patients with diabetes and one additional CV risk factor. The Losartan Intervention for Endpoint Reduction in Hypertension (LIFE) study demonstrated that losartan was more effective than atenolol for reducing CV mortality in diabetic patients with hypertension and left ventricular hypertrophy (LVH).

11. What are the principles of management of chronic CAD in diabetic patients?

Diabetic patients are more likely to experience painless cardiac ischemia and suffer more silent MIs and sudden cardiac death. Evidence from observational studies and randomized trials has shown significant mortality benefit with β-blockers in diabetic patients. β-Blockers are well tolerated in diabetic patients; masking or prolongation of hypoglycemic symptoms is infrequent, particularly with cardioselective agents. Recommendations include continuing antiplatelet therapy; ACE inhibitors and ARBs should be used as appropriate for blood pressure control, and β-blockers are recommended in diabetic patients after an MI. However, routine screening for CAD in diabetic patients is not recommended, as demonstrated in the Detection of Ischemia in Asymptomatic Diabetics (DIAD) trial. The multifaceted approach to the diabetic patient is illustrated in Figure 42-1.

12. What strategies for coronary revascularization are currently recommended for the management of multivessel CAD in diabetic patients?

The optimal revascularization strategy in stable diabetic patients with multivessel coronary disease has been debated extensively in recent years. The Bypass Angioplasty Revascularization Investigation (BARI) trial substudy of diabetic patients indicated that coronary artery bypass grafting (CABG) offered a clinically meaningful and statistically significant survival advantage in diabetic patients when compared to balloon angioplasty. Even in nondiabetic patients, the need for future revascularization has been traditionally higher in the angioplasty group compared with CABG, and these differences are even more pronounced in diabetic patients. However, BARI was conducted in an era when stents were not available. The Bypass Angioplasty Revascularization Investigation 2 Diabetes (BARI-2D) trial suggested that diabetic patients with three-vessel and severe coronary disease should preferably be managed with open revascularization. Because BARI-2D did not compare percutaneous coronary intervention (PCI) and CABG in patients with multivessel disease, the question was being addressed in the Future Revascularization Evaluation in Patients with Diabetes Mellitus: Optimal Management of Multivessel Disease (FREEDOM) trial. FREEDOM revealed that in diabetic patients with advanced coronary artery disease, CABG was superior to PCI with drug-eluting stents in reducing death and myocardial infarction rates, albeit with a higher stroke risk.

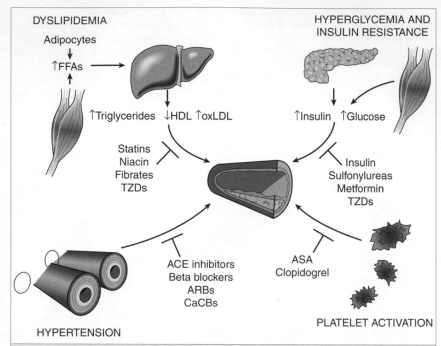

Figure 42-1. Diabetes requires therapy for each metabolic abnormality to stem the onset and progression of atherosclerosis. Statins improve the lipid profile and decrease the risk of MI and death. Treatment of hypertension decreases the rate of myocardial infarction (MI) and stroke in patients with diabetes. Therapy should include angiotensin-converting enzyme *(ACE)* inhibitors or angiotensin II receptor blockers *(ARBs)* for their microvascular and possible atherosclerosis benefits. The heightened thrombotic potential of the diabetic state supports the use of platelet antagonists, such as aspirin or clopidogrel. Although strict treatment of hyperglycemia does not significantly reduce the incidence of MI or death, the improvement in microvascular outcomes itself warrants vigorous pursuit of rigorous glycemic control in diabetes. (Modified from Libby P, Plutzky J: Diabetic macrovascular disease: the glucose paradox? *Circulation* 106:2760, 2002.) *ASA,* Aspirin; *CaCBs,* calcium channel blockers; *FFAs,* free fatty acids; *HDL,* high-density lipoprotein; *oxLDL,* oxidized low-density lipoprotein; *TZDs,* thiazolidinediones.

BIBLIOGRAPHY, SUGGESTED READINGS, AND WEBSITES

1. ADVANCE Collaborative Group, Patel A, MacMahon S, et al: Intensive blood glucose control and vascular outcomes in patients with type 2 diabetes, *N Engl J Med* 358:2560–2572, 2008.

2. American Diabetes Association: Standards of medical care in diabetes—2006, *Diabetes Care* 29(Suppl 1):S4–S42, 2006.

3. Aneja A, Tang WH, Bansilal S, et al: Diabetic cardiomyopathy: insights into pathogenesis, diagnostic challenges, and therapeutic options, *Am J Med* 121(9):748–57.

4. Beckman JA, Creager MA, Libby P: Diabetes and atherosclerosis: epidemiology, pathophysiology, and management, *JAMA* 287:2570–2581, 2002.

5. Berry C, Tardif JC, Bourassa MG: Coronary heart disease in patients with diabetes. Part I: Recent advances in prevention and noninvasive management, *J Am Coll Cardiol* 49:631–642, 2007.

6. Effects of ramipril on cardiovascular and microvascular outcomes in people with diabetes mellitus: results of the HOPE study and MICRO-HOPE substudy, *Lancet* 355:253–259, 2000.

7. Farkouh ME, Domanski M, Sleeper LA, et al: FREEDOM Trial Investigators: Strategies for multivessel revascularization in patients with diabetes, *N Engl J Med* 367(25):2375–84, 2012 Dec 20.

8. Gaede P, Lund-Andersen H, Parving HH, et al: Effect of a multifactorial intervention on mortality in type 2 diabetes, *N Engl J Med* 358:580–591, 2008.

9. Gerstein HC, Miller ME, Byington RP, et al: Effects of intensive glucose lowering in type 2 diabetes, *N Engl J Med* 358:2545–2559, 2008.

10. Goldberg RB, Mellies MJ, Sacks FM, et al: Cardiovascular events and their reduction with pravastatin in diabetic and glucose-intolerant myocardial infarction survivors with average cholesterol levels: subgroup analyses in the cholesterol and recurrent events (CARE) trial: the CARE investigators, *Circulation* 98:2513–2519, 1998.

11. Grundy SM, Cleeman JI, Merz CN, et al: Implications of recent clinical trials for the National Cholesterol Education Program Adult Treatment Panel III Guidelines, *J Am Coll Cardiol* 44:720–732, 2004.

12. Gu K, Cowie CC, Harris MI: Diabetes and decline in heart disease mortality in US adults, *JAMA* 281:1291–1297, 1999.

13. Khardori R: *Diabetes mellitus, type 2*, Available at http://emedicine.medscape.com/article/117853-overview. Accessed February 27, 2013.

14. Malmberg K, Yusuf S, Gerstein HC, et al: Impact of diabetes on long-term prognosis in patients with unstable angina and non-Q-wave myocardial infarction: results of the OASIS (Organization to Assess Strategies for Ischemic Syndromes) registry, *Circulation* 102:1014–1019, 2000.

15. McCullock DK: *Overview of medical care in adults with diabetes mellitus*. In Basow, DS, editor: UpToDate, Waltham, MA, 2013, UpToDate. Available at http://www.uptodate.com/contents/overview-of-medical-care-in-adults-with-diabetes-mellitus. Accessed March 26, 2013.

16. Nesto RW: *Coronary artery revascularization for angina in patients with diabetes mellitus and multivessel coronary artery disease*. In Basow, DS, editor: UpToDate, Waltham, MA, 2013, UpToDate. Available at http://www.uptodate.com/contents/coronary-artery-revascularization-in-patients-with-diabetes-mellitus-and-multivessel-coronary-artery-disease. Accessed March 26, 2013.

17. Pyorala K, Pedersen TR, Kjekshus J, et al: Cholesterol lowering with simvastatin improves prognosis of diabetic patients with coronary heart disease, *Diabetes Care* 20:614–620, 1997.

18. Smith SC Jr, Allen J, Blair SN, et al: ACC/AHA guidelines for secondary prevention for patients with coronary and other atherosclerotic vascular disease: 2006 update: endorsed by the National Heart, Lung, and Blood Institute, *Circulation* 113:2363–2372, 2006.

19. Skyler JS, Bergenstal R, Bonow RO, et al: Intensive glycemic control and the prevention of cardiovascular events: implications of the ACCORD, ADVANCE, and VA Diabetes Trials: a position statement of the American Diabetes Association and a Scientific Statement of the American College of Cardiology Foundation and the American Heart Association, *J Am Coll Cardiol* 53:298–304, 2009.

CHAPTER 43

SMOKING CESSATION: A PRIORITY FOR THE CARDIAC PATIENT

Andrew Pipe, CM, MD

1. **Why is smoking cessation of fundamental importance in the management of the cardiac patient?**

   Smoking cessation is the most important of the modifiable risk factors for cardiovascular disease. The products of tobacco smoke contribute directly, and distinctly, to the development of atherosclerosis and the adverse consequences that follow (Box 43-1). The benefits of smoking cessation cannot be exaggerated. A rapid and sustained reduction in the likelihood of cardiac disease or a cardiac event occurs in those who successfully stop smoking; those with established cardiac disease experience a dramatic reduction in the likelihood of recurrence, complication, or death following cessation. In both instances, the benefits of smoking cessation accrue rapidly and reflect the elimination, rather than the ongoing management, of a major risk factor (Table 43-1). Smoking cessation should be accorded a priority in those with cardiac disease—in every professional setting—to do otherwise should be seen as reflective of substandard care.

2. **Why have cardiologists neglected the treatment of tobacco addiction in the past?**

   For too long, a variety of dogmas and misconceptions have surrounded the management of the patient who smokes; prominent among which was the perception that smoking was a "habit" or a "lifestyle choice" and that successful smoking cessation required little more than "grit and determination." These outdated beliefs have impeded our ability to address this fundamental, major cardiovascular risk factor. Assumptions and misconceptions have also clouded clinicians' understanding of the role that pharmacotherapy can play in aiding cessation. Misplaced concerns regarding the safety of nicotine replacement therapy in the cardiac setting, for example, have sometimes precluded the use of this effective cessation pharmacotherapy.

3. **What should every health care professional know about smoking?**

   Nicotine is the most addictive substance encountered in ones community. It takes only a few days to establish nicotine addiction once inhalation has been "mastered." Thereafter, brain function,

---

Box 43-1 SMOKING AND THE GENESIS OF CARDIOVASCULAR DISEASE AND CARDIAC EVENTS

The Products of Tobacco Smoke:
1. Contribute to a proinflammatory state
2. Damage endothelial surfaces
3. Induce endothelial dysfunction
4. Distort the lipid profile and oxidize lipoproteins
5. Facilitate platelet aggregation and activation
6. Elevate fibrinogen levels
7. Potentiate the development of atheroma
8. Contribute to plaque "instability"
9. Produce elevated levels of carboxyhemoglobin and impair oxygen transport

TABLE 43-1. MORTALITY RISK REDUCTION IN THOSE WITH CORONARY HEART DISEASE	
Smoking Cessation	36%
Statin Therapy	29%
β-Blocker Therapy	23%
ACE-I Therapy	23%
ASA Therapy	15%

See: Critchley JA, Capewell S: Mortality risk reduction associated with smoking cessation in patients with coronary heart disease. A systematic review. *JAMA* 290:86-97, 2003.
ACE, Angiotensin-converting enzyme; *ASA,* aspirin.

structure, and neurochemistry become transformed. Smokers smoke to ensure constant levels of nicotine—and the elevated levels of dopamine, and other neurotransmitters, whose release follows the stimulation of nicotine receptors. The cigarette is a perversely engineered drug-delivery device constructed to deliver a precise aliquot of nicotine as rapidly as possible. Following the inhalation of tobacco smoke, nicotine is delivered very rapidly via the arterial system to the brainstem where it initiates a cascade of neurotransmitter activity and dopamine release. Most smokers know why they shouldn't smoke; most smokers do not want to be smokers; and many smokers will make one or two unassisted quit attempts each year—most of which will fail. Smokers generally do not need more education or lectures. They want help. Optimal cessation strategies involve the following:

- Provision of pharmacotherapy to eliminate or curb the symptoms of withdrawal and craving that lead to the use of a cigarette
- Communication of strategic, tactical advice regarding the management of those circumstances, settings, and situations that typically accompany and stimulate smoking

4. **How might smokers with cardiac disease be better assisted with cessation?**
A systematic approach to the identification and documentation of the smoking status of all patients, in every clinical setting, permits the provision of advice regarding the fundamental importance of cessation in the management of any cardiac condition and, more importantly, prompts the delivery of specific cessation assistance and appropriate follow-up. Serendipitous considerations of smoking status, offhand advice regarding the need for cessation, or the assumption that this is the responsibility of others (typically the family physician) have contributed in the past to substandard care of the cardiac patient who smokes.

The management of tobacco addiction can be addressed in exactly the same way as other cardiovascular risk factors: a risk factor is identified; a strategy for its management is outlined; and, medication is provided, monitored, and titrated for as long as is necessary until a desired end point is reached. Contemporary approaches to smoking cessation reflect exactly the same approach. They involve the provision of tactical advice and counseling in association with the use of appropriately prescribed (and often titrated) cessation pharmacotherapy, until a patient—free of the discomfort of cravings and withdrawal symptoms—acquires a repertoire of nonsmoking behaviors and is able to comfortably tolerate all the circumstances and situations which were previously associated with smoking.

In hospitals and other settings, clinical protocols, care maps, and other systematized approaches to the identification and treatment of smokers are becoming the norm and greatly facilitate and enhance the care of patients addicted to tobacco (Box 43-2).

5. **What is a good starting point for smoking cessation?**
In the past, approaches to smoking cessation have placed an emphasis on patient preparation and planning prior to reaching a "quit date." There is increasing evidence that asking about willingness to embark on a quit attempt at the time of a patient encounter can be very helpful, capitalizing on

---

Box 43-2 A SYSTEMATIC APPROACH TO SMOKING CESSATION IN EVERY CARDIAC SETTING

Identify. Identify the smoking status of all patients: "Have you used any form of tobacco in the past 6 months?" "Have you used any form of tobacco in the past 7 days?"

↓

Document. Ensure that smoking status and history is documented in the medical record and prompts an appropriate cessation intervention.

↓

Advise. Ensure that the patient is advised of the importance of cessation in an unambiguous, nonjudgmental, personally relevant manner.

↓

Act. Provide cessation pharmacotherapy and strategic cessation advice as appropriate.

↓

Follow-up. Arrange appropriate follow-up (smoking cessation clinic, primary care practitioner, community services, quit lines, etc.)

---

any recent clinical event and a patient's interest in cessation. Even among those disinclined to make a quit attempt, the provision of smoking cessation pharmacotherapy, which will induce a decline in cigarette consumption, has been demonstrated to be effective in stimulating a quit attempt and cessation. This approach mirrors our initial prescription of lipid-lowering or antihypertensive medications: their effectiveness is evaluated in the weeks that follow, when retitration of therapy may be necessary. This reduce-to-quit (RTQ) paradigm may be particularly appropriate in the cardiac setting, where further follow-up is likely to occur. Both the patient and clinician will be pleasantly surprised to note that cigarette consumption has fallen appreciably, serving as an appropriate entree to a more carefully planned cessation attempt with specific focus on titration of pharmacotherapy and ongoing follow-up (perhaps in association with the family physician).

6. **How can one best use pharmacotherapy to optimize the likelihood of cessation?**
   The appropriate use of pharmacotherapy, its monitoring and titration, and follow-up, will substantially increase the likelihood of successful cessation. Three generations of pharmacotherapy are currently available: nicotine replacement therapy (NRT), bupropion, and varenicline. Patient experience or preference may be the fundamental determinant of choice of therapy. Combination NRT (patch plus short-acting NRT) and varenicline have demonstrated the greatest overall effectiveness, tripling the likelihood of successful cessation. In all cases, the titration of therapy may be necessary to ensure effectiveness or to mitigate certain side effects.

7. **Can NRT be initiated in the in-patient setting in patients with cardiac disease?**
   Yes. NRT may be offered to smokers within hours of patient admission—nicotine withdrawal will occur rapidly in many smokers, producing discomfort, a variety of behavioral challenges for clinical staff, and complicating compliance with treatment of their cardiac condition. Evidence has been accumulating for years attesting to the safety of NRT in cardiac patients. Nicotine in this setting is delivered slowly via the venous system (not the arterial system, as is the case with smoking); achieves steady state levels that will always be far less than those to which a smoker has been accustomed; is not accompanied by carbon monoxide and countless other toxins; and, is being provided to patients who have developed marked tolerance to the cardiovascular effects of nicotine. A standardized order template may be useful (Table 43-2).

8. **What if a smoker reports that NRT has not decreased their desire to smoke?**
   Many smokers will report that the use of NRT is not associated with any decrease in the desire to smoke—a classic indication of underdosing. It has been calculated that the standard doses of NRT,

TABLE 43-2.	UNIVERSITY OF OTTAWA HEART INSTITUTE STANDARD ORDERS FOR NICOTINE REPLACEMENT THERAPY, BUPROPION, AND VARENICLINE
Standard Orders for Nicotine Replacement Therapy (NRT)*	
20 Cigarettes per day	21-mg NRT Patch +/× Short Acting NRT
30 Cigarettes per day	21 + 7-mg NRT Patches +/× Short Acting NRT
40 Cigarettes per day	2 × 21-mg NRT Patches +/− Short Acting NRT
Standard Orders for Bupropion*	
Day 1 to 3	150 mg qd
Day 4 to Week 12	150 mg bid
Standard Orders for Varenicline*	
Day 1 to 3	0.5 mg qd
Day 4 to 7	0.5 mg bid
Week 2 to 12	0.5-1.0 mg bid (initial course may be repeated)

Short Acting NRT, is an NRT inhaler, NRT lozenge, NRT spray, or NRT gum.
*In each case, be prepared to titrate therapy to ensure control of withdrawal and craving or to address dose-related side effects. Therapy may be prolonged as is necessary in order to prevent relapse to smoking. Consideration may be given to combining therapies in those in whom single-agent treatment is insufficient to address symptoms of withdrawal and craving and/or in whom total cessation has not been achieved.

for example, will not meet the nicotine "needs" of a majority of current smokers. Smokers are able to titrate nicotine intake with considerable precision; thus, the use of a nicotine inhaler in association with a nicotine patch will allow the emerging nonsmoker to titrate nicotine to meet particular needs—usually at times of more intense cravings or withdrawal. Use of NRT, as with every cessation pharmacotherapy can be continued until its discontinuation is not accompanied by an urge to smoke or a lapse to smoking in response to certain stimuli or surroundings. It is exceptionally rare for patients to become NRT dependent.

9. **Can bupropion be useful for smoking cessation?**
An antidepressant, bupropion was found to be efficacious in smoking cessation. It stimulates noradrenergic and dopaminergic centers in the brain associated with withdrawal and craving, respectively, and may also act as a nicotine antagonist. It is contraindicated in those with a history of, or propensity for, seizures. Like all smoking cessation medications, it may cause transient insomnia or sleep disturbance and can be associated with dose-related side effects (dry mouth, skin rash, tremor, among others) that will respond to titration of therapy—in this case, a reduction in dose. Its use begins with a 7-day period during which doses are gradually increased to achieve therapeutic levels prior to a quit date.

10. **Can varenicline be useful for smoking cessation?**
Varenicline acts as an $\alpha_4\beta_2$ nicotinic acetylcholine receptor partial agonist and partial antagonist. As such, it stimulates this receptor, triggering a degree of dopamine release in the forebrain while occupying, and blocking, the receptor site, preventing nicotine from exerting any effect if smoking occurs. Most patients receiving varenicline experience little or no craving for nicotine and, if a cigarette is smoked, derive no sensation or "benefit" typically associated with smoking. It has been shown to be the most effective single agent in inducing cessation and has demonstrated effectiveness in those with stable cardiovascular disease. Concerns have been raised about an increase in cardiovascular events among those using this medication. However, no clear evidence of a causal relationship

has been identified, nor has a biologically plausible reason for any such effects been identified, and the publication of a recent meta-analysis has dispelled those concerns. The risks of any smoking cessation pharmacotherapy must always be considered against the risks of continued smoking. The principal side effect of varenicline is nausea, which can typically be managed by taking the medication with meals and a full glass of water, or by reducing the dose.

BIBLIOGRAPHY, SUGGESTED READINGS, AND WEBSITES

1. Aboyans V, Thomas D, Lacroix P: The cardiologist and smoking cessation, *Curr Opin Cardiol* 25:469–477, 2010.

2. Ambrose J, Barua R: The pathophysiology of cigarette smoking and cardiovascular disease: an update, *J Am Coll Cardiol* 43:1731–1737, 2004.

3. Benowitz N, Gourlay S: Cardiovascular toxicity of nicotine: implications for nicotine replacement therapy, *J Am Coll Cardiol* 29:1422–1431, 1997.

4. Benowitz NL: Cigarette smoking and cardiovascular disease: pathophysiology and implications for treatment, *Prog Cardiovasc Dis* 46:91–111, 2003.

5. Benowitz NL: Neurobiology of Nicotine Addiction: Implications for Smoking Cessation Treatment, *Am J Med* 121(4A):S3–S10, 2008.

6. Critchley JA, Capewell S: Mortality risk reduction associated with smoking cessation in patients with coronary heart disease: a systematic review, *JAMA* 290:86–97, 2003.

7. Ebbert JO, Burke MV, Hays JT, et al: Combination treatment with varenicline and nicotine replacement therapy, *Nicotine Tob Res* 11:572–576, 2009.

8. Erhardt L: Cigarette smoking: an undertreated risk factor for cardiovascular disease, *Atherosclerosis* 205:23–32, 2009.

9. Fiore MC, Jaen CR, Baker TB, et al: *Treating tobacco use and dependence: 2008 update clinical practice guideline*, Rockville, Md, 2008, U.S. Department of Health and Human Services, Public Health Service.

10. Hubbard R, Lewis S, Smith C, et al: Use of nicotine replacement therapy and the risk of acute myocardial infarction, stroke, and death, *Tob Control* 14:416–421, 2005.

11. Hurt RD, Dale LC, Offord KP, et al: Serum nicotine and cotinine levels during nicotine-patch therapy, *Clin Pharmacol Ther* 54:98–106, 1993.

12. Hurt RD, Sachs DP, Glover ED, et al: A comparison of sustained-release bupropion and placebo for smoking cessation, *N Engl J Med* 337:1195–1202, 1997.

13. Jorenby DE, Hays JT, Rigotti NA, et al: Efficacy of varenicline, and $\alpha_4 \beta_2$ nicotinic acetylcholine receptor partial agonist, vs placebo or sustained-release bupropion for smoking cessation: a randomized controlled trial, *JAMA* 296:56–63, 2006.

14. Pipe A: Tobacco and cardiovascular disease: achieving smoking cessation in cardiac patients. In Yusuf S, editor: *Evidence based cardiology*, ed 3, Oxford, England, 2010, Blackwell Publishing.

15. Prochaska JJ, Hilton JF: Risk of cardiovascular serious adverse events associated with varenicline use for tobacco cessation: systematic review and meta-analysis, *BMJ* 344:e2856, 2012.

16. Rigotti NA, Pipe AL, Benowitz NL, et al: Efficacy and safety of varenicline for smoking cessation in patients with cardiovascular disease: a randomized trial, *Circulation* 121:221–229, 2010.

CHAPTER 44

EXERCISE AND THE HEART

Eric H. Awtry, MD, and Gary J. Balady, MD

1. What is the difference between physical activity and exercise?

Physical activity refers to the contraction of skeletal muscle that produces bodily movement and requires energy. *Exercise* is physical activity that is planned and is performed with the goal of attaining or maintaining physical fitness. *Physical fitness* is a set of traits that allows an individual to perform physical activity.

2. What is the difference between isometric and isotonic exercise?

Isotonic muscle contraction produces limb movement without a change in muscle tension, whereas *isometric* muscle contraction produces muscle tension without a change in limb movement. Most physical activities involve a combination of both forms of muscle contraction, although one form usually predominates. Isotonic exercise (also referred to as aerobic, dynamic, or endurance exercise) involves high-repetition movements against low resistance and includes such activities as walking, running, swimming, and cycling. Isometric exercise (also referred to as resistance exercise or strength training) consists of low-repetition movements against high resistance and includes such activities as weight lifting and body building.

3. What is the training effect?

Regular isotonic exercise results in improved exercise capacity, whereas regular resistance exercise results in increased strength. These changes allow an individual to exercise at a higher intensity and for a longer duration while attaining a lower heart rate (HR) for a given submaximal level of exercise. This is referred to as the *training effect.*

4. What are the acute cardiovascular changes that occur with exercise?

Isotonic exercise results in an increase in HR and stroke volume that produces a four- to sixfold increase in cardiac output in healthy individuals. The increase in HR relates both to a withdrawal of vagal tone and an increase in sympathetic tone. HR gradually rises during exercise to a maximal level that can be predicted by the following formula:

$$\text{Maximum predicted heart rate} = 220 - \text{age in years}$$

Stroke volume increases by 20% to 50% as a result of both increased venous return from exercising muscles and more complete left ventricular emptying (owing to enhanced myocardial contractility and to decreased peripheral vascular resistance due to vasodilation in exercising muscle). Vascular beds other than in the heart, brain, and exercising muscle undergo vasoconstriction during exercise. This, in conjunction with the increase in cardiac output, results in a rise in systolic blood pressure. The diastolic blood pressure remains unchanged or falls slightly.

Isometric exercise results in a moderate increase in cardiac output, predominantly as a result of an increase in heart rate. Contracting muscle produces a rise in peripheral vascular resistance and may result in an increase in both systolic and diastolic blood pressure.

5. What are the chronic cardiovascular changes that occur with exercise?

The increase in cardiac output associated with isotonic exercise creates a volume load that results in left ventricular dilation with minimal increase in wall thickness. The vasoconstriction and increased afterload associated with isometric exercise produces a pressure load that results in left ventricular hypertrophy without dilation.

6. **How is exercise intensity defined?**
   Exercise intensity is defined by the amount of energy required for the performance of the physical activity per unit of time. This can be measured directly using respiratory gas analysis to quantify oxygen uptake during exercise or can be approximated using standard regression models to estimate energy expenditure per a given work rate of exercise. Exercise intensity can also be expressed in terms of resting oxygen requirement (metabolic equivalents [METs]), where one MET equals the amount of oxygen consumed by a resting, awake individual, and is equivalent to 3.5 mL O_2/kg of body weight/min. Light exercise denotes those activities requiring less than 3 METs, moderate activity denotes activities requiring 3 to 6 METs, and vigorous activity denotes activities requiring more than 6 METs.

7. **How much exercise is necessary to maintain cardiovascular fitness?**
   Current guidelines from the American Heart Association (AHA) and the American College of Sports Medicine (ACSM) recommend that all healthy adults perform moderate-intensity aerobic exercise (e.g., brisk walking) for at least 30 minutes on at least 5 days of the week, or perform vigorous-intensity aerobic exercise (e.g., jogging) for at least 20 minutes on at least 3 days of the week. In addition, resistance exercise should be performed on at least 2 days of the week. Individuals who wish to improve their level of fitness or achieve substantial weight loss may need to perform significantly greater amounts of exercise. Importantly, exercise need not be performed all at one sitting; 10- or 15-minute periods of exercise can be accumulated throughout the day and applied to the daily exercising goal.

8. **What is the effect of exercise on cardiac risk factors?**
   Exercise has beneficial effects on hypertension, diabetes, hyperlipidemia, and obesity. In addition, exercise has favorable effects on endothelial function, thrombosis, inflammation, and autonomic tone (Table 44-1).

TABLE 44-1.	BENEFICIAL EFFECTS OF ENDURANCE EXERCISE ON ATHEROSCLEROTIC RISK FACTORS
FACTOR	**EFFECT OF EXERCISE**
Hypertension	Modest ↓ in both SBP (approximately 4 mm Hg) and DBP (approximately 3 mm Hg)
Diabetes	↑ Insulin sensitivity, ↓ hepatic glucose production, preferential use of glucose over fatty acids by exercising muscle
Hyperlipidemia	Significant ↓ in TG, modest ↑ in HDL, minimal change in LDL
Obesity	Modest weight loss (2-3 kg), ↓ in body fat necessary to maintain weight loss
Thrombosis	↓ Fibrinogen, ↓ platelet activation
Endothelial function	Improved vasodilation, possibly through ↑ NO synthesis
Autonomic tone	↑ Vagal tone, ↓ sympathetic tone
Inflammation	↓ Inflammatory markers (CRP, TNF-α, IL-6)

CRP, C-reactive protein; *DBP*, diastolic blood pressure; *HDL*, high-density lipoprotein; *IL*, interleukin; *LDL*, low-density lipoprotein; *NO*, nitric oxide; *SBP*, systolic blood pressure; *TG*, triglycerides; *TNF*, tumor necrosis factor.

9. **Do endurance training and resistance training have similar benefits?**
    Endurance and resistance training have some similar effects and some complementary effects. Both improve insulin resistance, bone mineral density, and body composition. Endurance training improves peak measured exercise capacity, whereas resistance training improves muscle strength. Endurance training expends a greater amount of calories during exercise, whereas resistance training increases resting energy expenditure because of increased muscle mass.

10. **What is the effect of exercise on mortality?**
    Observational studies demonstrate an inverse linear relationship between the amount of physical activity performed and all-cause mortality. This is true for healthy individuals and for those with chronic diseases including diabetes and cardiovascular disease. A person who adheres to current exercise recommendations may benefit from a 30% to 50% reduction in all-cause mortality, when compared with inactive individuals; however, this benefit has not yet been demonstrated in adequately powered randomized controlled trials. In addition, exercise capacity (as measured in METs) is a strong predictor of the risk of death in patients with and without cardiovascular disease. Greater exercise capacity is associated with longer survival.

11. **Is it ever too late to obtain the benefits of exercise?**
    There does not appear to be an age limit after which exercise confers no benefit, and available data suggest that exercise is associated with a reduction in mortality even in the elderly. Additionally, individuals who are inactive but subsequently become physically active have a decreased risk of cardiovascular events and a lower mortality than those persons who remain inactive. Exercise attenuates, but does not prevent, the gradual decline in exercise capacity that occurs with aging; however, it does increase a person's maximal exercise capacity at any given age. Importantly, exercise that is performed at a young age but is not continued throughout adulthood does not appear to improve long-term survival.

12. **Is it safe for patients with known coronary artery disease (CAD) to exercise?**
    Yes. Exercise is not only safe in patients with known CAD, but it confers multiple benefits. Meta-analyses demonstrate that patients with CAD who are enrolled in cardiac rehabilitation (CR) programs have a 20% lower risk of death and a 25% lower risk of cardiac death compared with patients who are not enrolled in an exercise program. In addition, in patients following percutaneous coronary intervention (PCI), participation in CR is associated with a 43% reduction in all-cause mortality. Furthermore, patients who undergo exercise training have improvement in various cardiac risk factors, have less angina and less ischemia at a given level of exertion, and have increased exercise capacity. Importantly, there is a direct relationship between the number of CR sessions attended and the magnitude of the benefit obtained. In a recent analysis of 30,161 persons in the Medicare database who had suffered a recent myocardial infarction (MI), acute coronary syndrome, or had undergone recent coronary artery bypass surgery, those who attended all 36 CR sessions had an incrementally lower risk of both death and MI than patients who attended 24 sessions (14% and 12% reduction, respectively), 12 sessions (22% and 23% reduction, respectively), or only one session (47% and 31% reduction, respectively). Unfortunately, only a minority of patients attend the full course of CR; addressing barriers to participation in these programs is paramount to their success.

13. **How long after MI can a patient begin an exercise program?**
    Patients who are clinically stable after MI can begin an exercise program as part of inpatient CR within 1 to 2 days of their infarction. Initial activity may be limited to range-of-motion exercises, but is rapidly increased to assisted walking. Activity is then gradually increased so that most patients can independently perform activities of daily living at the time of hospital discharge. Current AHA/American College of Cardiology (ACC) guidelines suggest that after MI all stable patients should be referred to formal outpatient CR programs. This is especially true for patients with multiple cardiac risk factors and for moderate- or high-risk patients (e.g., patients with residual CAD, patients with depressed

left ventricular [LV] systolic function) for whom a supervised exercise program is appropriate. Stable patients can usually enroll in these programs 2 to 3 weeks after MI.

14. Is exercise safe for patients with heart failure?

Yes, providing that the patient is compensated and not congested. The hemodynamic effects associated with isotonic exercise (increased stroke volume, decreased systemic vascular resistance [SVR]) are beneficial in patients with depressed LV systolic function. In a recent large trial of patients with stable heart failure, exercise training resulted in improved exercise capacity, reduced heart failure symptoms, and improved quality of life scores. Importantly, these benefits were not associated with an increase in adverse cardiac events, including no significant increase in device discharges in patients with implantable cardioverter-defibrillators. Although isometric exercise was previously avoided in patients with heart failure, recent data suggest that light to moderate levels of resistance training are well tolerated by patients with heart failure and may yield similar benefits as in healthy individuals.

15. Does exercise benefit patients who are limited by leg claudication?

Yes. Supervised exercise programs (usually walking) are currently recommended as first-line therapy for the treatment of intermittent claudication. Recent studies demonstrate that exercise training in patients with claudication results in improved exercise capacity, reduction in claudication symptoms, and improved quality of life scores. These benefits may be of a similar magnitude to those achievable with surgical or percutaneous peripheral revascularization. Furthermore, in patients with peripheral arterial disease (PAD) but without claudication, exercise training improves exercise capacity and leg strength. Patients with symptomatic PAD should be encouraged to exercise to the point of mild to moderate claudication, and then to rest; exercise should be resumed when symptoms have resolved. Because PAD is strongly associated with CAD, an aggressive risk-factor modification regimen is an essential adjunct to exercise training in patients with PAD.

16. What is an exercise prescription?

An *exercise prescription* is a recommended exercise regimen that is individualized for a particular patient and takes into account the patient's physical abilities, cardiac status, and medical comorbidities. The exercise prescription has four components: *intensity, duration, frequency*, and *modality*.

17. How is an exercise prescription developed after MI?

Upon entry into a CR program, patients undergo formal exercise testing to quantify their exercise capacity, assess for inducible ischemia, and derive an exercise intensity that is both safe and effective. Exercise *intensity* is generally prescribed using a range of HRs derived from the exercise test that represents 50% to 85% of heart rate reserve, where *heart rate reserve* is the difference between resting HR and peak exercise HR. For patients who develop ischemia during the exercise test (manifested by symptoms or electrocardiogram [ECG] changes), the peak training HR should be set at 10 beats/min below the rate at which the ischemia occurred. Exercise should then be performed for a minimum *duration* of 20 to 30 minutes and a *frequency* of 3 to 5 days per week. *Modalities* for endurance training commonly include walking and/or jogging (treadmill), rowing, cycling, and stair climbing.

18. Should patients with heart disease perform resistance training exercise?

Yes. Resistance training is now a standard part of a comprehensive exercise regimen for patients with cardiovascular disease, and appears to be particularly beneficial in the elderly, patients with stable heart failure, and those with diabetes. The improvement in muscular strength and endurance that accompanies resistance training aids in the performance of activities of daily living and may facilitate return to the workplace. Resistance training is prescribed at an *intensity* of 10 to 15 repetitions per set, using a load that is based on the maximum load (ML) that the patient can lift a single time (upper body: 30% to 40% ML; lower body: 50 to 60% ML). Patients should perform 1 to 3 sets of 8 to 10 different upper- and lower-body exercises at a frequency of 2 to 3 times per week. Common modalities for resistance training include free weights, weight machines, wall pulleys, elastic bands, and calisthenics.

19. What is aerobic interval training?

Standard exercise training involves a period of continuous moderate intensity exercise. *Aerobic interval training* (AIT) refers to a regimen that alternates 3- to 4-minute periods of high-intensity exercise (90% to 95% peak exercise HR) with similar periods of moderate intensity exercise (60% to 70% peak exercise HR). When compared to a standard exercise regimen, AIT appears to result in greater improvement in measurements of cardiovascular fitness in patients with heart failure and following coronary artery bypass graft (CABG). Nonetheless, at this time, the limited safety and efficacy data with this regimen precludes the routine recommendation for AIT in patients with cardiac disease.

20. What are the cardiovascular risks of exercise?

Overall, the risk of adverse cardiovascular events related to exercise in healthy individuals is extremely low and varies depending on an individual's age, gender, level of physical fitness, and medical condition. Most adverse events relate to structural or congenital heart disease in young athletes (e.g., hypertrophic cardiomyopathy, coronary anomalies, right ventricular dysplasia) or CAD in older individuals. The performance of vigorous exercise is associated with a transient increase in MI and sudden cardiac death, especially in sedentary individuals with underlying CAD.

21. Should patients be screened before enrolling in an exercise program?

The AHA recommends screening of high school and college athletes by obtaining a personal and family history and performing a cardiovascular physical examination before competing in sports, and every 2 to 4 years thereafter. Further testing is not suggested in the absence of abnormal findings. In general, healthy individuals without symptoms of cardiovascular disease can embark on low- to moderate-intensity exercise programs without preexercise screening. However, preexercise stress testing should be considered in asymptomatic men older than age 45 years and asymptomatic women older than age 55 years (particularly those with multiple cardiovascular risk factors or diabetes) who plan to participate in vigorous exercise, in patients with established CAD, and in those who have exercise-related symptoms that suggest the possibility of CAD.

22. What are the contraindications to participation in an exercise program?

Absolute contraindications to exercise include unstable coronary heart disease, decompensated heart failure, symptomatic valvular stenosis, severe systemic hypertension (blood pressure more than 180/110 mm Hg), and uncontrolled arrhythmias. Detailed recommendations regarding athletic competition are provided in the 36th Bethesda Conference on Eligibility Recommendations for Competitive Athletes with Cardiovascular Abnormalities.

BIBLIOGRAPHY, SUGGESTED READINGS, AND WEBSITES

1. Maron BJ, Zipes DP. 36th Bethesda Conference: eligibility recommendations for competitive athletes with cardiovascular abnormalities. *J Am Coll Cardiol*, 45:2–64, 2005.

2. American Association of Cardiovascular and Pulmonary Rehabilitation: *The AACVPR website* Available at: http://www.aacvpr.org. Accessed March 13, 2013.

3. American College of Sports Medicine: *The ACSM website* Available at: http://www.acsm.org. Accessed March 13, 2013.

4. American Diabetes Association: Physical activity/exercise and diabetes, *Diabetes Care* 29:1433–1438, 2006.

5. American Heart Association: *The AHA website (search Exercise)* Available at: http://www.heart.org. Accessed March 13, 2013.

6. Awtry EA, Balady GJ: Exercise and physical activity. In Topol EJ, editor: *Textbook of cardiovascular medicine*, ed 3, Philadelphia, 2007, Lippincott Williams and Wilkins.

7. Balady GJ, Ades PA: Exercise and Sports Cardiology. In Bonow RO, Mann DL, Zipes DP, Libby P, editors: *Braunwald's Heart Disease: A Textbook of Cardiovascular Medicine*, ed 9, Philadelphia, 2012, Saunders, pp 1784–1792.

8. Balady GJ, Ades PA, Bittner VA, et al: Referral, enrollment, and delivery of cardiac rehabilitation/secondary prevention programs at clinical centers and beyond: a presidential advisory from the American Heart Association, *Circulation* 124:2951–2960, 2011.

9. Balady GJ, Williams MA, Ades PA, et al: Core components of cardiac rehabilitation/secondary prevention programs: 2007 update. A statement from the American Heart Association, *Circulation* 115:2675–2682, 2007.

10. Downing J, Balady GJ: The role of exercise training in heart failure, *J Am Coll Cardiol* 58:561–569, 2011.

11. Hamburg NM, Balady GJ: Exercise rehabilitation in peripheral artery disease: functional impact and mechanisms of benefits, *Circulation* 123:87–97, 2011.

12. Hammill BG, Curtis LH, Schulman KA, et al: 2010 Relationship between cardiac rehabilitation and long-term risks of death and myocardial infarction among elderly Medicare beneficiaries, *Circulation* 121:63–70, 2010.

13. Haskell WL, Lee I-M, Pate RP, et al: Physical activity and public health: updated recommendation for adults from the American College of Sports Medicine and the American Heart Association, *Circulation* 116:1081–1093, 2007.

14. Maron BJ, Thompson PD, Ackerman MJ, et al: Recommendations and considerations related to preparticipation screening for cardiovascular abnormalities in competitive athletes: 2007 update. A scientific statement from the American Heart Association Council on Nutrition, Physical Activity, and Metabolism, *Circulation* 115:1643–1655, 2007.

15. Murphy TP, Cutlip DE, Regensteiner JG, et al: Supervised exercise versus primary stenting for claudication resulting from aortoiliac peripheral artery disease: six-month outcomes from the Claudication: Exercise Versus Endoluminal Revascularization (CLEVER) study, *Circulation* 125:130–139, 2012.

16. O'Connor CM, Whellan DJ, Lee KL, et al: Efficacy and safety of exercise training in patients with chronic heart failure: HF-ACTION randomized controlled trial, *JAMA* 301:1439–1450, 2009.

17. Thompson PD: Exercise prescription and proscription for patients with coronary artery disease, *Circulation* 112:2354–2363, 2005.

18. Thompson PD, Franklin BA, Balady GJ, et al: Exercise and acute cardiovascular events: placing the risks into perspective: a scientific statement from the American Heart Association Council on Nutrition, Physical Activity, and Metabolism and the Council on Clinical Cardiology, *Circulation* 115:2358–2368, 2007.

19. Thompson WR, editor: *American College of Sports Medicine Guidelines for Exercise Testing and Prescription*, ed 8, Philadelphia, 2010, Lippincott, Williams and Wilkins.

20. Williams MA, Haskell WL, Ades PA, et al: Resistance exercise in individuals with and without cardiovascular disease: 2007 update. A scientific statement from the American Heart Association Council on Clinical Cardiology and Council on Nutrition, Physical Activity, and Metabolism, *Circulation* 116:572–584, 2007.

21. Wisløff U, Støylen A, Loennechen JP, et al: Superior cardiovascular effect of aerobic interval training versus moderate continuous training in heart failure patients: a randomized study, *Circulation* 115:3086–3094, 2007.

ADULT CONGENITAL HEART DISEASE

Luc M. Beauchesne, MD, FACC

1. **Which patients with adult congenital heart disease require antibiotic prophylaxis?**

   The indications for antibiotic prophylaxis for endocarditis changed in 2007 with the new American Heart Association guidelines. A more restricted use of antibiotic prophylaxis in congenital heart disease is proposed, with increased emphasis on oral health. Prophylaxis is now suggested only in the following circumstances:
   - Unrepaired cyanotic heart disease
   - Prosthetic valves
   - Residual defects after repair with prosthetic material
   - The first 6 months after repair with a device or prosthesis
   - Patients with a history of prior endocarditis

   The new guidelines have also eliminated indications for prophylaxis for genitourinary (GU) or gastrointestinal (GI) procedures. (See also Chapter 33 on endocarditis and endocarditis prophylaxis.)

2. **What are the three main types of atrial septal defects (ASDs), and what are their associated anomalies?**

   The three main types of ASDs are secundum (70%), primum (20%), and sinus venosus (10%). The *secundum ASD* is a defect involving the floor of the fossa ovalis of the atrial septum. It usually presents as an isolated anomaly. The *primum ASD* is a defect at the base of the atrial septum adjacent to the atrioventricular valves. It is invariably part of an atrioventricular septal defect (endocardial cushion defect), and a cleft mitral valve is almost always present. The *sinus venosus ASD* is a defect of the posterior part of the septum, usually located in the superior part. In the majority of cases, a sinus venosus ASD is associated with anomalous connections or drainage of the right-sided pulmonary veins (Fig. 45-1).

3. **When should an ASD be closed? Which ASDs cannot be closed by a percutaneous device?**

   ASDs vary in size. If the ASD is large enough, the associated left to right shunt will lead to right-sided volume overload and pulmonary overcirculation. Chronic right-sided volume overload leads to pulmonary hypertension, right ventricular dysfunction, tricuspid regurgitation, and right atrial dilation. Patients with ASDs also often develop atrial arrhythmias. Hemodynamically significant ASDs are usually 10 mm or larger, have a shunt ratio greater than 1.5, and are associated with right ventricular enlargement on imaging. It is recommended that only hemodynamically significant ASDs be closed. Most secundum ASDs can be closed percutaneously. Primum and sinus venosus ASDs *cannot* be closed percutaneously and require surgical closure.

4. **List the four types of ventricular septal defects (VSDs).**

   Different classifications for VSDs have been used; one common approach divides VSDs into four types:
   - Membranous or perimembranous VSDs involve the membranous ventricular septum, a small localized area of the normal ventricular septum that is fibrous. This is the most common type of VSD seen in the adult.
   - Muscular VSDs involve the trabecular portion of the septum.

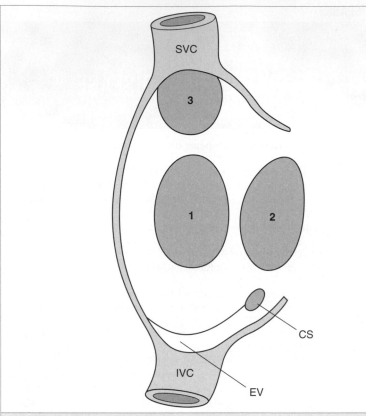

Figure 45-1. Atrial septal defects: *1*, secundum; *2*, primum; *3*, sinus venosus. (Modified from Gatzoulis MA, Webb GD, Daubeney PEF, et al: *Diagnosis and management of adult congenital heart disease*, Edinburgh, 2003, Churchill Livingstone, p 163.) *CS*, Coronary sinus; *EV*, eustachian valve; *SVC*, superior vena cava; *IVC*, inferior vena cava.

- Inlet VSDs involve the part of the ventricular septum that is adjacent to the tricuspid and mitral valves. Inlet VSDs are always associated with atrioventricular septal defects.
- Outlet VSDs (also known as supracristal VSD) involves the portion of the ventricular septum that is just below the aortic and pulmonary valve (Fig. 45-2).

5. **What are the long-term complications of a small VSD in the adult patient?**
   In the adult, there are two groups of patients with unrepaired VSD. The smallest group consists of patients with a large VSD that has been complicated by severe pulmonary hypertension (Eisenmenger syndrome). However, the vast majority of adult patients with VSDs have small defects that are hemo-dynamically insignificant (i.e., do not cause left ventricular dilation or pulmonary hypertension). As a rule these patients have a benign natural history. Rarely, some patients develop complications such as endocarditis, atrial arrhythmias, tricuspid regurgitation, aortic regurgitation, and double-chamber right ventricle.

6. **What are the complications of a bicuspid aortic valve?**
   A bicuspid aortic valve is present in 0.5% to 1% of the population. The main complications are progressive aortic stenosis, aortic regurgitation, or a combination of both. Other complications include endocarditis and aortopathy. Although infrequent (<10%), aortic coarctation is also a well-described

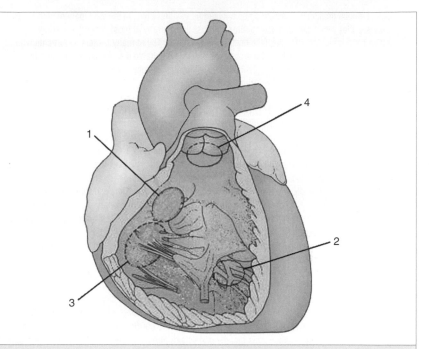

Figure 45-2. Ventricular septal defects: *1*, perimembranous; *2*, muscular; *3*, inlet; *4*, outlet. (Modified from Gatzoulis MA, Webb GD, Daubeney PEF, et al: *Diagnosis and management of adult congenital heart disease*, Edinburgh, 2003, Churchill Livingstone, p 171.)

association and must be ruled out in these patients. Patients in whom the bicuspid valve demonstrates signs of valve degeneration on echocardiography are at an increased risk of cardiovascular events and need close regular follow-up.

7. **How is hemodynamic severity of coarctation of the aorta assessed in the adult patient?**

    In coarctation of the aorta, the narrowing is typically in the proximal portion of the descending aorta, just distal to the left subclavian artery. Adult patients can be divided into two groups: those with *native* (i.e., unrepaired) coarctation and those who are postrepair (some of which have residual stenosis). Some coarctations are mild and not hemodynamically significant. Findings suggestive of a hemodynamically significant coarctation include small luminal diameter (less than 10 mm or less than 50% of reference normal descending aorta at the diaphragm), presence of collaterals, and elevated gradient (more than 20 mm Hg clinically, by catheterization, or by echocardiogram). The clinical gradient can be measured by comparing the highest arm systolic pressure (left or right) to the systolic pressure in the leg (typically measured by palpation of the pedal pulses while inflating a cuff at the calf level). Patients with hemodynamically significant coarctations are at risk of a number of complications, including refractory hypertension, accelerated atherosclerosis, cerebrovascular disease, and aortopathy.

8. **In coarctation of the aorta in the adult patient, when should percutaneous stenting be considered?**

    Most clinicians think that adult patients with hemodynamically significant coarctation of the aorta should be considered for intervention. Although surgery has been available for several decades, percutaneous dilation with stenting has evolved as an alternative. In the adult patient with residual stenosis after repair, stenting has become the first-line therapy at most centers. For adults with native coarctation, stenting has also become first-line therapy at many centers. In patients who undergo percutaneous stenting, the anatomy needs to be suitable (i.e., no significant arch hypoplasia). In adult patients who undergo surgery, the usual procedure is placement of an interposition graft which is done through a left-sided thoracotomy approach.

9. **Which adult patients with patent ductus arteriosus (PDA) require percutaneous device closure?**
   A PDA connects the proximal part of the left pulmonary artery to the proximal descending aorta, just distal to the left subclavian artery. The unrepaired ductus in an adult is usually small in diameter and the resultant left to right shunt is hemodynamically insignificant. However, in some patients the ductus diameter is large and results in severe pulmonary hypertension (Eisenmenger syndrome) if not repaired in childhood. Occasionally, some adults have moderate-size ducts resulting in shunting that is not hemodynamically negligible, but not significant enough to cause severe pulmonary hypertension. In these patients the left ventricle will be dilated and the pulmonary pressure may be mildly elevated. Clinically they will have a continuous murmur, a large pulse pressure, and signs of ventricular dilation. This latter group should undergo percutaneous closure in an attempt to prevent long-term complications. Although controversial, some centers advocate routine closure of small PDAs to prevent endarteritis.

10. **How is Marfan syndrome diagnosed?**
    The criteria for the diagnosis of Marfan syndrome have evolved over the years. The latest iteration was published in 2010 and has put more emphasis on gene testing, presence of aortic dilation, and abnormalities of the corneal lens. The main role of the cardiologist is to carefully assess the patient for aortic abnormalities. This usually consists of performing an echocardiogram and an MRI of the aorta. Patients with suspected Marfan syndrome should be referred to a geneticist, as the clinical phenotype overlaps with multiple other systemic disorders and the role of genetic testing is continuously evolving.

11. **When should Marfan patients with aortic root dilation be referred for surgery?**
    Although any part of the aorta can be involved in Marfan syndrome, the root is usually affected. Surgery (for root dilation) is done to prevent aortic dissection or rupture and is generally recommended when the aortic diameter is 50 mm or more. For patients with rapid progression (more than 5 mm/year) or a family history of dissection, intervention is recommended by some specialists at 45 mm or more. Traditionally, a Bentall procedure was performed in which the native aortic valve and root were replaced with a composite conduit (a tube graft attached to a prosthetic valve). If technically possible, the preferred first-line approach now consists of a valve-sparing procedure (David procedure) in which the root is replaced by a prosthetic conduit and the native valve is kept in place.

12. **What is tetralogy of Fallot, and what is the main complication seen in the adult?**
    Tetralogy of Fallot (TOF) consists of four features: right ventricular outflow tract (RVOT) obstruction, a large VSD, an overriding ascending aorta, and right ventricular hypertrophy. The RVOT obstruction is the clinically important lesion and may be subvalvular, valvular, or supravalvular, or may be at multiple levels. Repair, done in infancy, involves closing the VSD and relieving the RVOT obstruction. In many patients, to relieve the RVOT obstruction, surgery on the pulmonary annulus and valve leaflets is required and is usually complicated by severe residual pulmonary insufficiency. In the adult, over time, chronic severe pulmonary insufficiency often leads to right ventricular dysfunction and exercise intolerance, for which a pulmonary valve replacement (PVR) may be necessary. When PVR is performed, a tissue prosthesis is usually placed (homograft, porcine, or bovine prosthesis). The problem with tissue prostheses in young adults is that they require replacement at 10- to 15-year intervals. A percutaneous pulmonary valve prosthesis approach is increasingly being used to manage these patients with severe pulmonary insufficiency. Other complications in TOF include residual RVOT obstruction, residual VSD leak, right ventricular dysfunction, aortic root dilation, and arrhythmias.

13. **What are the three Ds of Ebstein anomaly?**
    Ebstein anomaly is characterized by an apically *displaced* tricuspid valve that is *dysplastic*, with a right ventricle that may be *dysfunctional*. The displacement affects predominantly the septal and posterior leaflets of the valve. The leaflets are usually diminutive and tethered to the ventricular wall. Typically, the anterior leaflet is unusually elongated. The right ventricle is often thin and can have both diastolic and systolic dysfunction. Half of patients have an interatrial communication, either patent foramen ovale (PFO) or ASD. Fifteen percent of patients have accessory pathways, which will manifest clinically as Wolf-Parkinson-White syndrome. The primary complication of Ebstein anomaly is tricuspid regurgitation and right-sided heart failure. If significant enough, placement of a tissue prosthesis or valve repair (if the valve anatomy is suitable) is indicated.

14. **What drug therapy should now be considered in all patients with Eisenmenger syndrome?**
    Eisenmenger syndrome refers to markedly elevated pulmonary pressures caused by a longstanding left to right shunt between the systemic and pulmonary artery circulations because of a congenital defect. Initially, *left to right* shunting leads to increased pulmonary vascular flow, which over time induces changes in the pulmonary vasculature leading to increased pulmonary vascular resistance. When the pulmonary vascular resistance is near, or exceeds, the systemic vascular resistance, the shunt reverses. The resultant *right to left* shunting results in hypoxia and cyanosis. The most common defect causing Eisenmenger syndrome is a VSD. Other causes include, among others, PDAs, atrioventricular septal defects, and ASDs. Traditionally these patients have been treated with supportive measures. However, studies have shown the beneficial use of oral pulmonary vasodilators, bosentan (an endothelin blocker), and sildenafil (a nitric oxide promoter). These agents decrease pulmonary artery pressure, improve functional capacity and have a mortality benefit. However, these medications are costly and it remains unclear which patients benefit most. Regardless, all Eisenmenger patients should be assessed by an appropriate specialist regarding the use of pulmonary vasodilator.

15. **When should an Eisenmenger patient be phlebotomized?**
    In Eisenmenger syndrome, hypoxia resulting from the right to left shunt stimulates marrow production of red blood cells and leads to an elevated hematocrit. Historically, Eisenmenger patients were phlebotomized routinely because an elevated hematocrit was thought to predispose to a thrombotic event, as with patients with the hematologic condition polycythemia vera. However, in recent years, data suggest that prophylactic phlebotomy in Eisenmenger patients may be more harmful than beneficial (i.e., it causes iron deficiency, decreases exercise tolerance, potentially increases the risk of stroke). As such, the use of phlebotomy has become more restrictive and should only be considered in two situations:
    - In patients with symptoms of hyperviscosity (headaches, dizziness, fatigue, achiness), who have a hematocrit more than 65% with no evidence of iron deficiency
    - Preoperatively, to improve hemostasis (goal hematocrit less than 65%)
      In modern practice, only a minority of Eisenmenger patients should undergo phlebotomy.

16. **Which types of congenital heart disease lesions have particularly poor outcomes in pregnancy?**
    Very high risk congenital heart disease lesions include the following:
    - Unrepaired cyanotic heart disease
    - Eisenmenger syndrome
    - Severe aortic stenosis
    - Marfan syndrome with a dilated aortic root (greater than 40 mm)
    - Mechanical valve prosthesis
    - Significant systemic ventricular dysfunction (ejection fraction 40% or less).
    These patients should be counseled accordingly about the significant maternal risks and poor fetal outcomes that are associated with pregnancy.

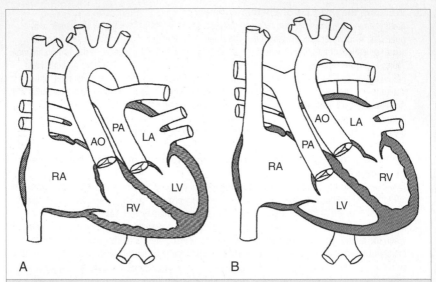

Figure 45-3. A, D-TGA. **B,** L-TGA. (Modified from Mullins CE, Mayer DC: *Congenital heart disease, a diagrammatic atlas,* New York, 1988, Wiley-Liss, pp 164, 182.) *AO,* Aorta; *D-TGA,* dextro-transposition of the great arteries; *L-TGA,* levo-transposition of the great arteries; *LA,* left atrium; *LV,* left ventricle; *PA,* pulmonary artery; *RA,* right atrium; *RV,* right ventricle.

17. **What are the two types of transpositions?**

Transposition complexes can be divided into two groups. In complete transposition of the great arteries (dextro- or D-TGA), the anomaly can be simplistically conceptualized as an *inversion of the great vessels* (Fig. 45-3, *A*). The aorta comes out of the right ventricle, and the pulmonary artery comes out of the left ventricle. Desaturated blood is pumped into the systemic circulation, whereas oxygenated blood is pumped into the pulmonary circulation. Without intervention, this condition is associated with very poor outcomes in early infancy.

Congenitally corrected transposition of the great arteries (levo- or L-TGA) can be conceptualized as an *inversion of the ventricles* (see Fig. 45-3, *B*). Desaturated blood and oxygenated blood are thus pumped in the appropriate arterial circulations. In many cases, associated anomalies, such as a VSD, pulmonary stenosis, an abnormal tricuspid valve, and heart block, are present. These patients can survive or present de novo in adulthood without surgical intervention.

18. **What is meant by a systemic right ventricle?**

A *systemic right ventricle* refers to a heart anomaly where the *morphologic* right ventricle pumps blood into the aorta. Ventricular morphology is determined by anatomic features typical to each ventricle. For example, the morphologic right ventricle has a tricuspid atrioventricular valve (with attachments to the septum and apical displacement compared with the mitral valve) and coarse apical trabeculations. L-TGA (see Question 17) is a congenital heart defect in which there is a systemic right ventricle. In the first few decades of life, the right ventricle is able to handle pumping into the high-pressure systemic circulation; however, in adulthood, the right ventricular function begins to deteriorate in the majority of patients. This is usually associated with tricuspid regurgitation and manifests clinically as heart failure.

19. **What is the difference between an atrial and an arterial switch?**

An *atrial* switch is a surgical procedure that was previously done for patients born with D-TGA (Fig. 45-4, *A*). The Mustard and Senning procedures are both examples of an atrial switch and

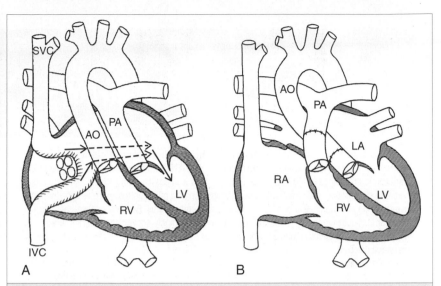

Figure 45-4. A, Atrial switch for D-TGA (Mustard or Senning procedure). The arrows show how a baffle shunts blood from the superior vena cava (SVC) and inferior vena cava (IVC) into the left ventricle (LV). Oxygenated blood from the pulmonary veins is shunted in to the right ventricle (RV). **B,** Arterial switch for D-TGA. The aorta (AO) and pulmonary artery (PA) are surgically "switched." (Modified from Mullins CE, Mayer DC: *Congenital heart disease, a diagrammatic atlas,* New York, 1988, Wiley-Liss, pp. 296, 300.) *D-TGA,* Dextro-transposition of the great arteries; *RA,* right atrium; *LA,* left atrium.

involve rerouting systemic and pulmonary venous flow to the respective pulmonary and systemic ventricles. These procedures were replaced by the *arterial* switch, which consists of "switching" the great arteries and reimplanting the coronary arteries to the *new* aorta (see Fig. 45-4, *B*). The arterial switch is performed in the first few weeks after birth and has been the standard of care for patients born with D-TGA for more than two decades.

BIBLIOGRAPHY, SUGGESTED READINGS, AND WEBSITES

1. Baumgartner H, Bonhoeffer P, De Groot NM, et al: ESC Guidelines for the management of grown-up congenital heart disease, *Eur Heart J* 31:2915–2957, 2010.

2. Canadian Adult Congenital Heart Network: *The CACH Network website.* Available at: http://www.cachnet.org. Accessed February 27, 2013.

3. Galiè N, Beghetti M, Gatzoulis MA, et al: Bosentan therapy in patients with Eisenmenger Syndrome. A multicenter, double-blind, randomized, placebo-controlled study, *Circulation* 114:48–54, 2006.

4. Gatzoulis MA, Webb GD, Daubeney PEF: *Diagnosis and management of adult congenital heart disease,* ed 2, Philadelphia, 2011, Churchill Livingstone.

5. Maron BJ, Zipes DP, Ackerman MJ, et al: Bethesda Conference report: 36th Bethesda Conference. Eligibility recommendations for competitive athletes with cardiovascular abnormalities, *J Am Coll Cardiol* 45:1312–1375, 2005.

6. National Marfan Foundation: *The NFM website.* Available at: http://www.marfan.org. Accessed February 27, 2013.

7. Nevil Thomas Adult Congenital Heart Library: *The Nevil Thomas Adult Congenital Heart Library website.* Available at: http://www.achd-library.com. Accessed February 27, 2013.

8. Silversides CK, Marelli A, Beauchesne L, et al: Canadian Cardiovascular Society 2009 Consensus Conference on the management of adults with congenital heart disease: executive summary, *Can J Cardiol* 26:143–150, 2010.

9. Warnes CA, Williams RG, Bashore TM, et al: ACC/AHA 2008 guidelines for the management of adults with congenital heart disease: a report of the American College of Cardiology/American Heart Association Task Force on Practice Guidelines, *J Am Coll Cardiol* 52:e143–e263, 2008.

CHAPTER 46

CARDIAC MANIFESTATIONS OF HIV/AIDS

Anu Elizabeth Abraham, MD, and Sheilah Bernard, MD

1. **How have the cardiac manifestations of human immunodeficiency virus/ acquired immunodeficiency syndrome (HIV/AIDS) changed over the years?**
   Cardiac manifestations of AIDS up until the early 1990s would not infrequently include pericardial disease, myocarditis, dilated and infiltrative cardiomyopathy, pulmonary disease with pulmonary hypertension, arrhythmias, and marantic or infectious endocarditis. Because patients tended to be younger, very little coronary atherosclerosis was noted. As highly active antiretroviral therapy (HAART) has emerged as an effective treatment for HIV, HIV has transformed from a fatal infection to a chronically managed disease.

   Cardiovascular disease is now the second most common cause of death in antiretroviral therapy (ART)-treated patients worldwide. HIV patients have a higher incidence of traditional cardiovascular risk factors, such as male gender, smoking, advanced age, glucose intolerance, insulin resistance, and dyslipidemia. They also have a higher incidence of nontraditional cardiac risk factors, including polysubstance abuse, lifestyle choices, immune dysregulation, and effects of ART.

   Over the next decades, children born with vertically transmitted HIV will survive to adulthood, with attendant cardiac complications from chronic inflammation, drug therapy, and immunosuppression.

2. **What are HIV-related cardiac complications?**
   Since the advent of ART in the 1990s, the incidence of HIV-related complications has significantly decreased, but cardiac complications include:
   - Pericardial effusion/tamponade
   - Dilated cardiomyopathy (systolic and diastolic dysfunction)
   - Myocarditis
   - Marantic (thrombotic) or infectious endocarditis
   - Cardiac tumors (Kaposi sarcoma, lymphoma)
   - Pulmonary arterial hypertension

3. **How common is pericardial effusion?**
   Pericardial effusion is an incidental finding in about 11% of HIV-infected patients and up to 30% of AIDS patients with CD4+ T cell counts (CD4 counts) less than 400 cells/μL who have cardiac echocardiograms. The effusions are typically small and patients are usually asymptomatic. The presence of an effusion is an independent predictor of mortality in these patients. It only rarely progresses to tamponade, which is more common in end-stage, cachectic patients who develop elevated intrapericardial pressures caused by low right-sided filling pressures *(low-pressure tamponade)*. The effusion is mostly transudative. *Mycobacterium tuberculosis* and *M. avium* are the principal causes of infectious pericarditis. Rarely, Kaposi sarcoma can bleed into the pericardium, causing tamponade physiology.

4. **Is HIV myocarditis or cardiomyopathy common?**
   In different series, one-third to one-half of patients in the pre-HAART era (or where HAART therapy was not available) dying of AIDS had lymphocytic infiltration at autopsy. Of these patients, 80% had no other pathogens identified. Additionally, up to 10% of endomyocardial specimens in HIV patients have evidence of other infections (e.g., Coxsackie B, Epstein-Barr virus, adenovirus, and cytomegalovirus).

The initiation of HAART therapy has significantly reduced the incidence of cardiomyopathy, likely due to both reduction in HIV itself and reduction in the presence of opportunistic infections.

HIV is thought to cause myocarditis from direct action of HIV on myocytes or indirectly through toxins. Patients with HIV and cardiomyopathy have a worse prognosis than those with cardiomyopathy due to other causes of cardiomyopathy (Fig. 46-1). Heart failure caused by HIV-associated left ventricular dysfunction is most commonly found in patients with the lowest CD4 counts and is a marker of poor prognosis. Despite the association of HIV and myocarditis and cardiomyopathy, in patients with HIV and with cardiomyopathy, other possible causes of heart failure (e.g., ischemic, valvular, and toxin-related heart failure) should be excluded.

5. How is HIV cardiomyopathy treated?
A standard heart failure regimen should be used as tolerated, including angiotensin-converting enzyme (ACE) inhibitors or angiotensin receptor blockers (ARBs), beta-adrenergic blocking agents (β-blockers), aldosterone antagonists, diuretics for volume overload, and digoxin for advanced disease. Additionally, nutritional and electrolyte deficiencies should be replenished.

6. Why is infective valvular endocarditis a rarity in AIDS?
Valvular devastation usually seen with bacterial infections does not occur in HIV patients because of impairment of autoimmune response. Patients who have hemodynamically significant valvular disease warrant valve replacement if their HIV is well controlled. Fulminant infective endocarditis can occur in late AIDS with high mortality. Patients with AIDS rarely will develop marantic (noninfectious) endocarditis, with large, friable, sterile thrombotic vegetations. These can be associated with disseminated intravascular coagulation (DIC) and systemic embolization.

7. What malignancies can affect the heart in AIDS/HIV?
Kaposi sarcoma is associated with herpesvirus 8 in homosexual AIDS patients. This tumor is often found in the subepicardial fat around surface coronary arteries. About 25% of AIDS patients with systemic Kaposi sarcoma had incidental cardiac involvement, with death as a result of underlying

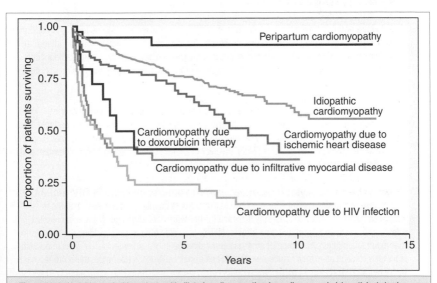

Figure 46-1. Variable survival in patients with dilated cardiomyopathy, depending on underlying etiologic basis. (From Felker GM, Thompson RE, Hare JM, et al: Underlying causes and long-term survival in patients with initially unexplained cardiomyopathy. *N Engl J Med* 342:1077, 2000.) *HIV*, Human immunodeficiency virus.

opportunistic infections. Non-Hodgkin lymphoma is more common in HIV-positive patients, with a poor prognosis. Leiomyosarcoma is rarely associated with Epstein-Barr virus in AIDS patients.

8. **Can nutritional deficiencies be responsible for HIV myopathy?**
   HIV infection leads to immune impairment and malnutrition, which can contribute to rapid progression to AIDS. Malnutrition can be linked to poor appetite (perhaps due to inability to eat foods due to infections such as oral thrush or esophagitis) and poor absorption in the gastrointestinal (GI) tract. Nutritional deficiencies are seen in late-stage, untreated AIDS. This may ultimately lead to electrolyte losses. Selenium deficiency increases the virulence of Coxsackie virus to cardiac tissue and is reversed by replenishing selenium. Low levels of B_{12}, carnitine, growth hormone, and thyroxine (T_4) can cause a reversible myopathy.

9. **How common is HIV-associated pulmonary arterial hypertension (PAH)?**
   The prevalence of PAH was estimated to be 0.5% of HIV-infected patients in 1997, before the advent of ART. Since that time, despite the increase of ART, the prevalence of PAH remains stable, based on more recent studies. PAH can be diagnosed in any stage and is not thought to be related to CD4 count. A recent case study showed median survival of 3.6 years and 84% of patients survived to 1 year. On histology, HIV-infected PAH patients do not differ from uninfected patients and exhibit concentric laminar fibrosis, medial hypertrophy, and plexiform lesions. It is not known whether HIV infects the pulmonary vascular system, but HIV proteins can lead to abnormal endothelial function. Therapy includes those used for primary pulmonary hypertension, including intravenous epoprostenol and endothelin antagonists. The benefit of ART on the progression of PAH is still controversial.

10. **How should HIV patients be screened for coronary artery disease?**
    The Framingham Risk Score (age, gender, blood pressure, total cholesterol, high-density lipoprotein [HDL], diabetes, and smoking) has been applied to HIV patients on therapy and reasonably predicts coronary artery disease (CAD) events. It has been shown to underestimate the risk of cardiovascular disease (CVD) in HIV patients who are also smokers. The Data Collection on Adverse Events of Anti-HIV Drugs (DAD) group has tried to incorporate HIV-specific risks (such as exposure to protease inhibitors or PIs) in addition to traditional risk factors, but these risk models are not yet validated. The Infectious Disease Society of America (IDSA) recommends fasting lipid panels and fasting glucose levels before and 4 to 6 weeks after initiation of HAART. Use of diagnostic stress testing is performed in these patients according to the current guidelines for the general population. Carotid intimal medial thickening, coronary artery calcium scores, highly sensitive C-reactive protein (CRP), adiponectin and other markers of CVD are also being investigated in the HIV patient population to predict early disease.

11. **What is the pathology of accelerated atherosclerosis in HIV patients?**
    Histopathologically, atherosclerosis in HIV patients is distinct from that in noninfected patients. Based on autopsy studies, these lesions have features of both atherosclerosis and transplant vasculopathy. These lesions reveal diffuse circumferential involvement with smooth muscle cell proliferation and elastic fibers, leading to endoluminal projections.

12. **What is the pathophysiology of accelerated atherosclerosis in HIV patients?**
    The relative risk of myocardial infarction (MI) in HIV patients compared to non-HIV patients is increased by 1.7- to 1.8-fold, and may increase further with increasing age. There is a complex relationship between HIV-related side effects, ART-related side effects, and traditional risk factors that result in a higher prevalence of atherosclerotic disease in HIV patients. ART is associated with increased visceral adiposity, insulin resistance, and abnormal glucose tolerance, therefore increasing the risk of CVD. Traditional risk factors such as hypertension (which may be associated with ART use) and tobacco use are highly prevalent in this population. HIV infection is known to lead to a state of increased inflammation, which has been identified as a factor for early atherosclerosis. HIV infection directly leads to endothelial dysfunction and HIV envelope proteins have been linked to higher levels

of endothelin-1 concentrations. In fact, the level of viremia and CD4 counts are predictive of cardiovascular disease.

13. What dyslipidemias occur with HIV disease?

Before therapy, in early HIV infection, triglycerides increase and HDL and low-density lipoprotein (LDL) levels decline. After ART is initiated, LDL and total cholesterol levels appear to increase. This may be due to general improvement in health or due to medication effects. The prevalence of hyperlipidemia in HIV patients is between 28% and 80% in various studies.

14. What are the effects of ART on cardiovascular risk?

Many ARTs have been associated with dyslipidemia (Table 46-1). Protease inhibitors (PIs) are associated with a small to moderate increase in total cholesterol and LDL and a significant rise in triglyceride levels. Non-nucleoside reverse transcriptase inhibitors (NNRTIs) are associated with dyslipidemia, but less so than are PIs. They typically result in a small increase in total cholesterol, LDL, as well as HDL (which is potentially beneficial). In general, the nucleoside reverse transcriptase inhibitors (NRTIs) have been associated with insulin resistance and the lipid profile changes are less severe than with PIs and NNRTIs. While PIs and NNRTIs have well-established effects on lipid profiles, the new agents such as fusion inhibitors, chemokine inhibitors, or integrase inhibitors have not shown these changes.

15. What is acquired lipodystrophy?

This is a disorder characterized by selective loss of adipose tissue from subcutaneous areas of the face, arms, and legs, with redistribution to the posterior neck *(buffalo hump)* and visceral abdomen. Visceral adiposity is associated with increased inflammatory markers. Lipodystrophy is also associated with attendant development of diabetes mellitus (DM), dyslipidemia, hepatic steatosis, hypertension, and acanthosis nigricans. It can occur in 20% to 40% of HIV patients taking PIs for more than 1 to 2 years. Exercise, with or without treatment with metformin, has been reported to improve body composition in patients with lipodystrophy.

TABLE 46-1. ANTIRETROVIRAL THERAPIES AND THEIR EFFECTS ON LIPID PROFILES AND CARDIOVASCULAR RISK		
Protease Inhibitors (PIs)	**Non-Nucleoside Reverse Transcriptase Inhibitors (NNRTIs)**	**Nucleoside Reverse Transcriptase Inhibitors (NRTIs)**
TC, LDL ↑; TG ↑↑	TC, LDL, HDL sl ↑	Insulin resistance, TC, LDL sl ↑
Atazanavir	Efavirenz	Stavudine
Ritonavir	Nevirapine	Tenofovir
Tipranavir	Etravirine	Abacavir
Darunavir		
Lopinavir		
Saquinavir		
Fosamprenavir		
Nelfinavir		

HDL, High-density lipoprotein; *LDL*, low-density lipoprotein; *TC*, total cholesterol: *TG*, triglycerides: *sl*, slight.

16. **How are these dyslipidemias treated?**

In an effort to improve cardiovascular risk profiles, treatment of dyslipidemia should also include attempts to improve diet, increase exercise, lose weight, promote smoking cessation, and manage hypertension and diabetes. Physicians can consider transitioning to a different class of antiretroviral drugs, such as replacing PIs with NNRTIs and/or NRTIs if the new regimen has the same ability to suppress viral replication. Several statins are degraded by cytochrome P-450 isoform 3A4 (CYP3A4), which is inhibited by PIs. Therefore, simvastatin is contraindicated with PI use, but others, such as atorvastatin and rosuvastatin, are less affected and still used to treat HIV-associated dyslipidemia. Pravastatin and ezetimibe, which are not metabolized by the cytochrome P-450 pathway, are also safe to use in this setting. Niacin has been shown to reduce triglyceride levels, but also increases insulin resistance. As a result, its benefit is unclear. Fish oil (omega-3 fatty acids) is well tolerated and has been shown to decrease triglyceride levels. Unfortunately, some studies have also noted an increase in LDL, so its overall clinical benefit is unclear.

17. **Can cardiothoracic surgery be performed safely in HIV patients?**

HIV patients can undergo cardiothoracic surgery (e.g., valve replacement, coronary artery bypass grafting [CABG]) with similar mortality to non-HIV patients, but with slightly higher morbidity (as a result of sepsis, sternal infection, bleeding, prolonged intubation, and readmission). There have not been large surgical series, but smaller studies have shown 81% event-free survival at 3 years for HIV patients undergoing CABG. CD4 counts do not drop postoperatively. Needlestick injuries of care givers remain a health care issue with all HIV patients.

18. **What oral hypoglycemics are recommended?**

Metformin is an attractive agent to use for glucose control because it reduces appetite, induces weight loss, and treats steatosis. The nucleoside analog abacavir and metformin can both cause lactic acidosis, so this combination of agents should be used cautiously. Insulin is used for more difficult diabetes management.

19. **What other drugs used in AIDS/HIV treatment can have cardiac complications?**

The nucleoside analogue abacavir can cause hypotension and lactic acidosis, and zidovudine can cause skeletal myopathy. The antiparasitic pentamidine, antiviral ganciclovir, and antibiotic erythromycin have been associated with acquired QT prolongation and torsades de pointes (polymorphic ventricular tachycardia). Chemotherapeutic agents, such as vincristine, interferon, interleukin, and doxorubicin, can lead to cardiomyopathy.

20. **What is the risk of mother-to-child transmission (MTCT) of HIV?**

Worldwide, approximately 3 million infants are born to mothers infected with HIV per year, but only 530,000 infants develop HIV per year. Of these new pediatric infections, 95% occur in sub-Saharan Africa or in South- and Southeast Asia. MTCT can occur during gestation, intrapartum (during delivery), or postpartum via breast feeding. Maternal HIV load is a strong predictor of MTCT. In 1994, a randomized controlled trial showed reduction in MTCT rates from 25.5% to 8.3% with zidovudine therapy of mothers during pregnancy and during delivery. Therapy was also provided to infants within 24 to 48 hours of delivery. With ART therapy and avoidance of breast feeding, overall MTCT rates in developed countries have decreased to 2%.

BIBLIOGRAPHY, SUGGESTED READINGS, AND WEBSITES

1. Barbaro G: Heart and HAART: Two sides of the coin for HIV-associated cardiology issues, *World J Cardiol* 2:53–57, 2010.
2. Barbazo G, Lipshultz SE: Pathogenesis of HIV-associated cardiomyopathy, *Ann N Y Acad Sci* 946:57–81, 2001.
3. Cicallini S, Almodovar S, Grilli E, Flores S: Pulmonary hypertension and human immunodeficiency virus infection: epidemiology, pathogenesis, and clinical approach, *Clin Microbio Infect* 17:25–33, 2011.
4. Cotter BR: Epidemiology of HIV cardiac disease, *Progress Cardiovasc Dis* 45:319–326, 2003.

5. Duggal S, Chugh TD, Duggal AS: 2011 HIV and malnutrition, *Clinical and Developmental Immunology* 1–8, 2012.

6. Feeney E, Mallon PWG: HIV and HAART-associated Dyslipidemia, *The Open Cardiovascular Medicine Journal* 5:49–63, 2011.

7. Friis-Moller N, Reiss P, Sabin CA, et al: Class of antiretroviral drugs and the risk of myocardial infarction, *N Engl J Med* 356:1723–1735, 2007.

8. Green MI: Evaluation and management of dyslipidemia in patients with HIV infection, *J Gen Int Med* 17:797–810, 2002.

9. Grinspoon SK, Grunfeld C, Kotler DP, et al: State of the Science Conference: initiative to decrease cardiovascular risk and increase quality of care for patients living with HIV/AIDS, Executive summary, *Circulation* 118:198–210, 2008.

10. Hakeen A, Bhatti S, Cilingiroglu M: The Spectrum of Atherosclerotic Coronary Artery Disease in HIV Patients, *Curr Atheroscler Rep* 12:119–124, 2010.

11. Ho JE, Hsue PY: Cardiovascular manifestations of HIV infection, *Heart* 95:1193–1202, 2009.

12. Hsue PY, Waters DD: What a Cardiologist Needs to Know about Patients with Human Immunodeficiency Virus Infection, *Circulation* 112:3947–3957, 2005.

13. Janda S, Quon BS, Swiston K: HIV and pulmonary arterial hypertension: a systematic review, *HIV Medicine* 11:620–634, 2010.

14. Katz AS, Sadaniantz A: Echocardiography in HIV cardiac disease, *Progress Cardiovasc Dis* 45:285–292, 2003.

15. Luzuriaga K: Mother-to-child Transmission of HIV: A Global Perspective, *Current Infectious Disease Reports* 9:511–517, 2007.

16. Malvestuttom C, Aberg J: Coronary heart disease in people infected with HIV, *Cleveland Clinic Journal of Medicine* 77:547–556, 2010.

17. Nakazono R, Jeudy J, White C: *HIV-related cardiac complications: CT and MRI findings* 198:364–364, 2012.

CHAPTER 47

CARDIOVASCULAR MANIFESTATIONS OF CONNECTIVE TISSUE DISORDERS AND THE VASCULITIDES

Nishant R. Shah, MD

1. **What is the leading cause of death in rheumatoid arthritis (RA) and what are the most common cardiac manifestations of RA?**

   The leading cause of death in RA is ischemic heart disease. Risk factors attributable to RA include chronic proinflammatory and prothrombotic states, endothelial dysfunction, dyslipidemia, insulin resistance, increased oxidative stress, nonsteroidal antiinflammatory drug (NSAID) use, and corticosteroid use. Other cardiac manifestations of RA include increased risk of congestive heart failure (CHF), pericarditis, and conduction block caused by myocardial rheumatoid nodules.

2. **What are the cardiovascular manifestations of systemic lupus erythematosus (SLE)?**

   The most common cardiac complication of SLE is pericarditis. Clinically evident myocarditis also occurs in 8% to 25% of patients. Libman-Sacks endocarditis is discussed later. Finally, premature atherosclerosis, due to many of the same independent risk factors noted previously for RA, is now recognized as a major cause of morbidity and mortality.

3. **What are the cardiovascular consequences of NSAIDs with predominantly cyclooxygenase-2 (COX-2) inhibition?**

   COX-2 inhibitors cause a shift toward thrombosis through reduced endothelial production of prostacyclin (a COX-2–mediated anti-thrombotic process) and relative sparing of platelet production of thromboxane A_2 (a COX-1–mediated pro-thrombotic process). For this reason, concurrent low-dose aspirin is recommended for patients on COX-2 inhibitors. Secondly, COX-2 inhibitors increase sodium and water retention, predisposing patients to edema, CHF exacerbations, and hypertension. Finally, COX-2 inhibitors prevent protective COX-2 upregulation in the setting of myocardial ischemia and infarction, leading to larger infarct size and increased risk of myocardial rupture. Of note, NSAIDs with predominantly COX-1 inhibition are associated with increased risk of gastrointestinal (GI) bleeding. For this reason, concurrent proton-pump inhibitor therapy is recommended for patients on COX-1 inhibitors.

4. **What is the major cardiovascular concern associated with tumor necrosis factor (TNF)-α antagonists?**

   Results from the Anti-TNF Therapy Against Congestive Heart Failure (ATTACH) trial suggest that high-dose TNF-α antagonist therapy actually *increases* death from any cause and heart failure hospitalization in patients with New York Heart Association (NYHA) class III/IV CHF.

5. **What are the clinical manifestations of antiphospholipid antibody syndrome?**

   Antiphospholipid antibodies (APLAs) promote intravascular clotting and can be found in primary APLA syndrome or secondary to other conditions, most commonly SLE. Clinical manifestations of APLA syndrome include spontaneous venous and arterial thromboses, strokes and neurologic syndromes, digital and extremity ischemia, livedo reticularis, thrombocytopenia, and recurrent spontaneous abortions. From a cardiac standpoint, acute coronary thromboses and diffuse small-vessel clotting resulting in global myocardial dysfunction have been described. In addition, *Libman-Sacks endocarditis*, defined by sterile vegetations on the mitral > aortic/tricuspid > pulmonary valves, is thought to arise from organization of thrombi and can cause valvular regurgitation or stenosis requiring surgical correction. Treatment for APLA syndrome is warfarin (goal international normalized ratio [INR] of 2.0-3.0) +/− daily low-dose aspirin, +/− hydroxychloroquine. Drugs associated with drug-induced lupus are given in Table 47-1.

6. **Describe the characteristic myocardial lesions of scleroderma and systemic sclerosis and their clinical manifestations.**
   Scleroderma of the myocardium manifests as biventricular random patchy fibrosis. Evidence thus far suggests that fibrosis results from recurrent ischemia and reperfusion injury caused by transient recurrent vasospasm of intramural small arteries and/or arterioles (myocardial Raynaud phenomenon). For this reason, calcium channel blocker therapy is appropriate for these patients. Clinically, patients with scleroderma are at increased risk for exercise-induced arrhythmias and biventricular heart failure. Of note, although a septal pseudoinfarct pattern and other conduction abnormalities can be seen on electrocardiography (ECG), a normal ECG is the most common finding.

7. **What is the most common cardiac complication of scleroderma and systemic sclerosis?**
   Cor pulmonale is the most common complication. Intimal proliferation of the small pulmonary arteries causes pulmonary hypertension and subsequent right-sided heart failure. For this reason, pulmonary function testing (PFT) for diffusion lung capacity for carbon monoxide (DLCO) has become standard in the treatment of scleroderma. Prostacyclin analogues and bosentan have been shown to reduce pulmonary vascular resistance and improve outcomes. Lung transplantation is another treatment option when medical management fails.

8. **What are the most common cardiac findings associated with the seronegative spondyloarthropathies?**
   Aortic regurgitation (AR) occurs due to aortic root thickening and dilatation, thickening and shortening of the aortic valve cusps, and development of a fibrous "bump." Mitral regurgitation (MR) is less common, but is due to a similar thickening at the basal portion of the anterior mitral leaflet (or secondary to AR). Complete atrioventricular (AV) nodal or bundle branch block can develop when the fibrosing process extends into the muscular septum. Interestingly, the combination of lone AR and severe conduction system disease in patients not known to have seronegative spondylarthritis is highly correlated with the presence of human leukocyte antigen (HLA)-B27.

9. **Name the clinical manifestations of polyarteritis nodosa (PAN), including the most common cardiovascular complications.**
   Polyarteritis nodosa is a nongranulomatous, patchy, necrotizing vasculitis of medium-sized muscular arteries. Constitutional symptoms (e.g., fever, malaise, myalgias, arthralgias, and weight loss) are common. Focal tissue ischemia and infarction can cause one of four cutaneous findings (painful subcutaneous nodules, non-blanching livedo reticularis, skin ulceration, or digital ischemia), asymmetric mononeuritis multiplex, hyperreninemic hypertension or renal insufficiency, or mesenteric infarction or aneurysmal rupture. Vasculitis in the distal coronary arteries cause recurrent, small myocardial infarctions (Fig. 47-1) that variably manifest as angina, acute myocardial infarction, congestive heart failure, or arrhythmias. Treatment for PAN is high-dose corticosteroids and cytotoxic therapy (cyclophosphamide, azathioprine, or methotrexate).

10. **What are the most common findings in Takayasu arteritis and how should these patients be managed?**
    Takayasu arteritis is a granulomatous vasculitis of the aorta and its branches that is most common in young Asian women. Resultant arterial stenosis is much more common than aneurysm formation. Claudication, especially in the upper extremities, is the most common symptom. The most common

TABLE. 47-1. DRUGS ASSOCIATED WITH DRUG–INDUCED LUPUS	
Drugs *Definitively* Known to Cause Drug-Induced Lupus	**Cardiovascular Medications that *Probably* Cause Drug-Induced Lupus**
Procainamide	β-Blockers
Hydralazine	Captopril
Diltiazem	Hydrochlorothiazide
TNF-α antagonists	Amiodarone
Minocycline	
Chlorpromazine	
Quinidine	
D-Penicillamine	
Isoniazid	
Methyldopa	
Interferon-α	

β-Blockers, Beta-adrenergic blocking agents; *TNF*, tumor necrosis factor.

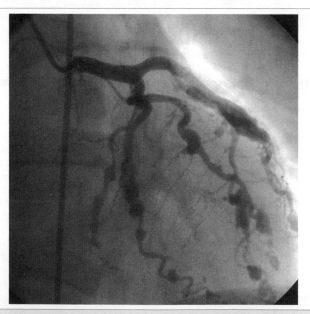

Figure 47-1. Numerous coronary artery aneurysms are present in this patient with polyarteritis nodosa (PAN). From Bonow RO, Mann DL, Zipes DP, Libby P, editors: *Braunwald's Heart Disease: A Textbook of Cardiovascular Medicine*, ed 9, Philadelphia, 2012, Saunders.

findings include bruits, hypertension, and upper extremity blood pressure and pulse asymmetry. Aneurysms, when they occur, are most common in the aortic root and can cause significant aortic regurgitation (AR). Angiographic evaluation of the entire aorta and its primary branches, to determine the distribution and severity of vascular lesions, is recommended. When contraindications to angiography exist, magnetic resonance (MR) or computed tomographic (CT) angiography are acceptable

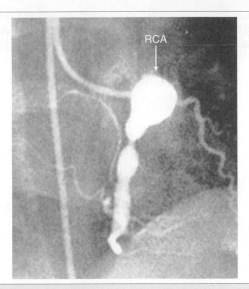

Figure 47-2. Coronary angiogram demonstrating giant aneurysm of the right coronary artery (RCA) in 6-year-old boy. (From Newburger JW, Takahashi M, Gerber MA, et al: Diagnosis, treatment, and long-term management of Kawasaki disease. *Pediatrics* 114:1708-1733, 2004.)

alternatives. High-dose corticosteroids and anatomical correction of clinically significant lesions are the treatments of choice. Cyclophosphamide, methotrexate, and anti-TNF agents are reserved for severe disease.

11. **What are the most common cardiac manifestations of Kawasaki disease?**
    Kawasaki disease is an acute systemic febrile illness most common in infants and young children. Defining symptoms include high-spiking fever, cervical lymphadenopathy (nontender, greater than 1.5 cm in diameter, usually unilateral), erythematous and/or desquamative skin rash, and mucous membrane lesions (oropharyngeal injection, strawberry tongue, bilateral nonexudative conjunctivitis). Typical lab abnormalities include leukocytosis, elevated erythrocyte sedimentation rate (ESR) and C-reactive protein (CRP), and late thrombocytosis. Thrombosis of coronary artery aneurysms (especially those greater than 8 mm) is the most common cause of death. For this reason, serial echocardiography to evaluate coronary artery anatomy and other parameters is crucial. Treatment consists of high-dose aspirin and intravenous immune globulin. A coronary angiogram from a patient with Kawasaki disease is shown in Figure 47-2.

12. **What is the most common cardiovascular complications of Marfan syndrome (MFS)?**
    MFS is caused by an autosomal dominant fibrillin gene defect. The most common cardiovascular complication is asymptomatic progressive aortic root enlargement beginning at the sinuses of Valsalva. The development of an ascending aortic aneurysm subsequently places patients at high risk for type A aortic dissection, aortic rupture, or aortic regurgitation (AR). Of note, mitral valve prolapse is present in 70% to 90% of MFS patients and progresses to mitral regurgitation in up to 50%.

13. **How should MFS be managed from a cardiovascular standpoint?**
    Annual imaging with transthoracic or transesophageal echocardiography (or with CT or MR angiography) is required to detect and assess aortic dilatation. When the aortic diameter reaches

5.0 cm, prophylactic aortic root replacement should be considered. Criteria for earlier consideration of surgery include more than 1 cm per year aortic diameter growth, family history of dissection at less than 5 cm, or moderate to severe AR. Finally, MFS patients should be on beta-adrenergic blocking agent (β-blocker) therapy, which has been shown to improve survival.

14. **How is Ehlers-Danlos Syndrome (EDS) type IV different from the other types?**
    EDS type IV patients have type III collagen defects, resulting in thin, translucent skin absent of the hyperextensibility characterizing other EDS patients. Additionally, EDS type IV patients are at high risk for life-threatening spontaneous arterial rupture, most commonly in the abdominal cavity and the gravid uterus. Bleeding should be managed as conservatively as possible, as these patients' tissues don't hold sutures well, and angiography should be avoided due to a high rate of complications.

BIBLIOGRAPHY, SUGGESTED READINGS, AND WEBSITES

1. Andrews J, Mason JC: Takayasu's arteritis—recent advances in imaging offer promise, *Rheumatology (Oxford)* 46(1):6–15, 2007.

2. Antman EM, Bennett JS, Daugherty A, et al: Use of nonsteroidal antiinflammatory drugs: an update for clinicians: a scientific statement from the American Heart Association, *Circulation* 115(12):1634–1642, 2007.

3. Arnett FC, Willerson JT: Connective tissue diseases and the heart. In Willerson JT, Cohn JN, Wellens HJJ, et al, editors: *Cardiovascular medicine*, ed 3, London, 2007, Springer-Verlag.

4. Chung ES, Packer M, Lo KH, et al: Randomized, double-blind, placebo-controlled, pilot trial of infliximab, a chimeric monoclonal antibody to tumor necrosis factor-alpha, in patients with moderate-to-severe heart failure: results of the anti-TNF Therapy Against Congestive Heart Failure (ATTACH) trial, *Circulation* 107(25):3133–3140, 2003.

5. Levine JS, Branch DW, Rauch J: The antiphospholipid syndrome, *N Engl J Med* 346(10):752–763, 2002.

6. Mandell BF, Hoffman GS: Rheumatic diseases and the cardiovascular system. In Libby P, Bonow R, Mann D, et al, editors: *Braunwald's heart disease: a textbook of cardiovascular medicine*, ed 8, Philadelphia, 2008, Saunders.

7. Milewicz DM: Inherited disorders of connective tissue. In Willerson JT, Cohn JN, Wellens HJJ, et al, editors: *Cardiovascular medicine*, ed 3, London, 2007, Springer-Verlag.

8. Milewicz DM: Treatment of aortic disease in patients with Marfan syndrome, *Circulation* 111:e150–e157, 2005.

9. Newburger JW, Takahashi M, Gerber MA, et al: Diagnosis, treatment, and long-term management of Kawasaki disease, *Circulation* 110:2747–2771, 2004.

10. Roman MJ, Salmon JE: Cardiovascular manifestations of rheumatologic diseases, *Circulation* 116:2346–2355, 2007.

11. Sattar N, McCarey DW, Capell H, McInnes IB: Explaining how "high-grade" systemic inflammation accelerates vascular risk in rheumatoid arthritis, *Circulation* 108:2957–2963, 2003.

12. Schur PH, Rose BD: Drug-Induced Lupus. In Basow DS, editor: UpToDate, Waltham, MA, 2013, UpToDate. Available at http://www.uptodate.com/contents/drug-induced-lupus. Accessed March 26, 2013.

13. Stone JH: Polyarteritis nodosa, *JAMA* 288:1632–1639, 2002.

CHAPTER 48

CARDIAC TUMORS

David Aguilar, MD, and Glenn N. Levine, MD, FACC, FAHA

1. Which are more common, primary cardiac tumors or metastatic tumors to the heart?

Metastatic tumors to the heart are markedly more common than primary cardiac tumors, with one source reporting metastatic involvement of the heart to be 20 to 40 times more prevalent than primary cardiac tumors. Primary cardiac tumors are extremely rare, occurring in one autopsy series in less than 0.1% of subjects.

2. What are the most common tumors that metastasize to the heart?

The most common tumors that spread to the heart are lung (bronchogenic) cancer, breast cancer, melanoma, thyroid cancer, esophageal cancer, lymphoma, and leukemia. Malignant melanoma has the greatest propensity to spread to the heart, with 50% to 65% of patients with malignant melanoma having cardiac metastases. Tumors may spread to the heart via direct extension, the circulatory system, or via lymphatics. Renal cell carcinoma may extend up the inferior vena cava all the way into the heart.

3. What are the most common primary cardiac tumors?

Benign tumors are more common than malignant tumors, occurring approximately three times as often as malignant tumors. In children, 90% of primary cardiac tumors are benign. The most common benign cardiac tumors in adults are myxomas, accounting for approximately half of all primary cardiac neoplasms; other common benign cardiac tumors are lipomas and papillary fibroelastomas. Rhabdomyomas are the most common benign tumor occurring in infants and children. Interestingly, rhabdomyomas usually regress over time and do not require specific treatment in asymptomatic individuals. Primary and secondary (metastatic) tumors involving the heart are listed in Table 48-1.

4. In what chamber do most myxomas occur?

Approximately 75% to 80% of myxomas occur in the left atrium (Fig. 48-1), with 15% to 20% occurring in the right atrium. Only 3% to 4% of myxomas arise in the left ventricle and 3% to 4% arise in the right ventricle. Myxomas are usually pedunculated and typically arise from the interatrial septum via a *stalk*. They are described on gross pathological examination as *gelatinous* in consistency. They most commonly occur between the third and sixth decades of life, and more frequently occur in women. They can cause effective obstruction of filling of the left or right ventricles, leading to left or right heart failure symptoms and findings, mimicking the symptoms and findings of mitral or tricuspid valve stenosis. Systemic embolism occurs in 30% to 40% of patients. Constitutional symptoms and findings (see Question 6) are also common. Most myxomas occur sporadically, but approximately 7% to 10% may be familial (see Question 10).

5. What are the most common primary malignant tumors?

The most common primary malignant tumors are sarcomas (Figs. 48-2 and 48-3). Such sarcomas include angiosarcomas (the most common), rhabdomyosarcomas, fibrosarcomas, and leiomyosarcomas. Upon imaging, sarcomas often appear as large heterogeneous, infiltrative masses that frequently occupy most of the affected chamber (see Fig. 48-3). The results of surgery or chemotherapy in the treatment of cardiac sarcomas have been generally poor, with mean survival of only 6 to 12 months.

TABLE 48-1.   PRIMARY AND SECONDARY (METASTATIC) TUMORS INVOLVING THE HEART

Primary Tumors

Myxoma
Lipoma
Papillary fibroelastoma
Rhabdomyoma
Fibroma
Angiosarcoma
Rhabdomyosarcoma
Lymphoma
Lipomatous hypertrophy

Secondary (Metastatic) Tumors

Lung (bronchogenic) cancer
Breast cancer
Esophageal cancer
Thyroid cancer
Melanoma
Lymphoma
Leukemia
Renal cell carcinoma

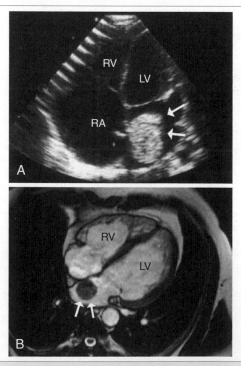

Figure 48-1. Left atrial myxoma *(arrows)*, as visualized on **(A)** transthoracic echocardiogram and **(B)** on cardiac MRI. **(A** modified from Erdol C, Ozturk C, Ocal A, et al: Contralateral recurrence of atrial myxoma—case report and review of the literature. *Images Paediatr Cardiol* 8:3-9, 2001.) *LV*, Left ventricle; *RA*, right atrium; *RV*, right ventricle.

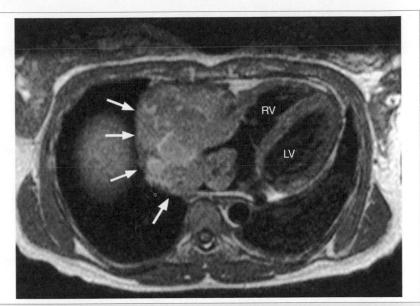

Figure 48-2. Massive angiosarcoma *(arrows)* arising from the right atrium, as visualized by MRI. (Modified from Sparrow PJ, Kurian JB, Jones TR, et al: MR imaging of cardiac tumors, *Radiographics* 25(5):1255-1276, 2005.) *LV*, Left ventricle; *RV*, right ventricle.

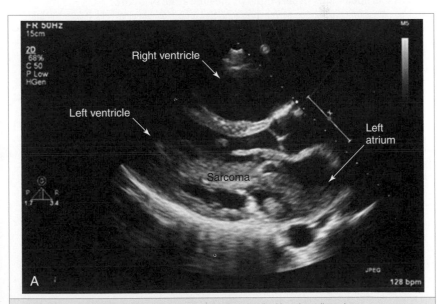

Figure 48-3. Large undifferentiated sarcoma in the left atrium visualized by echocardiography.

6. **What symptoms do cardiac tumors cause?**

   Symptoms of tumors often depend on the size and the location of the tumor, as well the histology of the tumor itself. Left-sided cardiac tumors may manifest with cardioembolic features such as stroke, visceral infarction, or peripheral emboli. Large cardiac tumors may also present with symptoms attributed to obstruction of flow or valvular dysfunction. Left atrial myxomas may cause effective mitral valve stenosis (or regurgitation). Tumors may also cause hemodynamic effects via compression or mass effects. Tumors may lead to atrial or ventricular arrhythmias. Tumors involving the pericardium can cause pericardial effusion and tamponade. Constitutional symptoms (fatigue, weight loss, fever) occur not infrequently, as well as anemia, elevated erythrocyte sedimentation rate, elevated C-reactive protein, and other nonspecific laboratory findings. In patients with known noncardiac cancer, the development of arrhythmias (particularly atrial fibrillation) or development of findings suggesting pericardial effusion or tamponade (distended neck veins, hypotension, paradoxical pulse, new low voltage on the electrocardiogram [ECG]) should prompt immediate evaluation for cardiac or pericardial metastasis.

7. **What is the workup for suspected cardiac tumors?**

   The initial workup is a transthoracic echocardiogram (echo). Many tumors will also be discovered incidentally or serendipitously by cardiac echo. Tumors may be further evaluated with transesophageal echo (TEE), cardiac magnetic resonance imaging (MRI), or cardiac computed tomography (CT). The role of positron emission tomography (PET) in the evaluation of cardiac tumors is evolving. Transvenous endomyocardial biopsy is generally not warranted for diagnosis but could be considered if the diagnosis cannot be established by noninvasive modalities (such as cardiac MRI) or less invasive (noncardiac) biopsy. Cytological analyses of pericardial effusion or pericardial biopsy may provide diagnostic information regarding metastatic cardiac tumors.

8. **What is a "tumor plop"?**

   A *tumor plop* is a sound heard in early diastole during auscultation. It is produced when a left atrial myxoma prolapses into the left ventricle during diastole (Fig. 48-4). The sound may be due to the tumor striking the left ventricular wall or to tension created on the tumor stalk.

9. **What is lipomatous hypertrophy of the interatrial septum?**

   Lipomatous hypertrophy is an abnormal, exaggerated growth of normal fat cells. It occurs in the interatrial septum, resulting in the appearance of a thickened atrial septum. The finding itself is benign.

10. **What is the most common valvular tumor?**

    The most common valvular tumor is papillary fibroelastoma. Papillary fibroelastomas are the second most common primary benign cardiac tumors and comprise 75% of valvular tumors. The most usual location is on the mitral and aortic valves, although they can occur on right-sided valves. Papillary fibroelastoma are often small (<1 cm) and appear flower-like or frond-like, with a narrow stalk. Most common symptoms related to papillary fibroelastomas are related to embolic events, such as strokes or transient ischemic attacks.

11. **What is the Carney complex?**

    Known by various names and acronyms, the Carney complex is an autosomal-dominant syndrome consisting of cardiac myxomas, cutaneous myxomas, spotty pigmentation of the skin, endocrinopathy, and other tumors. Myxomas occurring as part of the Carney complex are reported to account for 7% of all cardiac myxomas. Myxomas occurring as part of the Carney complex often present earlier in life, tend to be located in atypical locations, are often multiple, and often have a higher rate of recurrence after surgical resection compared with sporadic myxomas.

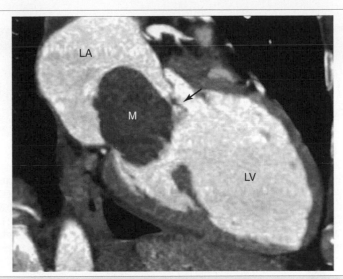

Figure 48-4. A left atrial myxoma *(M)* transiting across the mitral valve *(arrow)* in to the left ventricle. This may cause an audible "tumor plop." *LA*, Left atrium; *LV*, left ventricle. (From Haaga JR: CT and MRI of the Whole body, ed 5, Philadelphia, PA, 2008, Mosby, fig. 28-24.)

BIBLIOGRAPHY, SUGGESTED READINGS, AND WEBSITES

1. Basson CT: *Carney complex*. Available at: http://www.emedicine.com. Accessed March 23, 2013.
2. Bruce CJ: Cardiac tumours: diagnosis and management, *Heart* 97:151–160, 2011.
3. Meuller DK: *Benign cardiac tumors*. Available at: http://www.emedicine.com. Accessed March 25, 2013.
4. Goodkind MJ: *Cardiac tumors*. Available at: http://www.merck.com/mmpe. Accessed March 28, 2013.
5. Kapoor A: *Cancer of the heart*, New York, 1986, Springer Verlag.
6. Reardon MJ, Walkes JC, Benjamin R: Therapy insight: malignant primary cardiac tumors, *Nat Clin Pract Cardiovasc Med* 3:548–553, 2006.
7. Reynen K: Cardiac myxomas, *N Engl J Med* 333:1610–1617, 1995.
8. Reynen K, Kockeritz U, Strasser RH: Metastases to the heart, *Ann Oncol* 15:375–381, 2004.
9. Sharma GK: *Atrial myxoma*. Available at: http://www.emedicine.com. Accessed March 28, 2013.
10. Sparrow PJ, Kurian JB, Jones TR, et al: MR imaging of cardiac tumors, *Radiographics* 25:1255–1276, 2005.

CHAPTER 49

COCAINE AND THE HEART

Maria Elena De Benedetti, MD, and James McCord, MD

1. How common is cocaine use in the United States?

Cocaine is the second most commonly used illicit drug in the United States, with only marijuana being used more often. Between 1994 and 1998, the number of new cocaine users per year increased by 82%. In 2005, there were approximately 450,000 cocaine-related emergency department visits in the United States. In 2007, there were 2.1 million cocaine users age 12 or older, comprising 0.8% of the population. Users are more likely to be young, between 18 and 20 years of age. Males are more likely to be users than females by a 2:1 ratio. Cocaine-associated chest pain accounts for approximately 16% of all cocaine-related admissions, leading to the evaluation of approximately 64,000 patients annually. Of these, approximately 57% are admitted to the hospital for further evaluation.

2. What are the pharmacologic effects of cocaine?

Cocaine is a powerful sympathomimetic that acts by directly stimulating central sympathetic outflow and blocking presynaptic uptake of norepinephrine and dopamine (Fig. 49-1). This augmentation in postsynaptic catecholamines increases heart rate, mean arterial pressure, and left-ventricular contractility through stimulation of both α- and β-adrenergic receptors. Through enhanced α-adrenergic

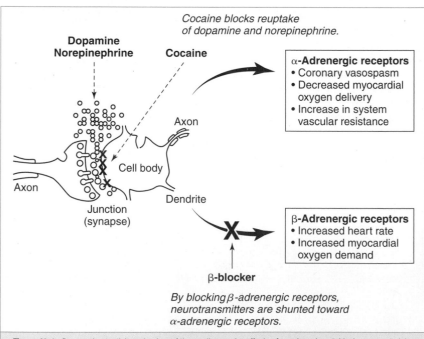

Figure 49-1. Proposed potential mechanism of the cardiovascular effects of cocaine when β-blockers are administered in cocaine-induced acute coronary syndrome.

receptor activation, increased endothelin production, and diminished nitric oxide generation, cocaine initiates coronary artery vasoconstriction. Cocaine may also enhance platelet aggregation and thrombus formation through heightened production of adenosine diphosphate, thromboxane A_2, and tissue plasminogen activator inhibitors, as well as reductions in protein C and antithrombin III. Cocaine causes toxic effects on cardiac muscle that arise primarily from Ca^{2+} overload during excessive β-adrenergic stimulation. Cocaine is well absorbed through all body mucous membranes and can be administered by nasal, sublingual, intramuscular, intravenous, and respiratory routes. The onset of action varies from 3 seconds to 5 minutes, depending on the administration route.

3. **What are the typical symptoms after cocaine ingestion?**
Cardiopulmonary complaints are the most commonly reported symptoms in patients after cocaine use, occurring in 56% of cases. Chest pain is the most common symptom and is typically described as a pressure sensation. Other common symptoms include dyspnea, anxiety, palpitations, syncope, dizziness, and nausea. The onset of symptoms usually occurs soon after ingestion, with two-thirds of patients presenting within 3 hours.

4. **What are the consequences of cocaine use?**
The cardiac and systemic effects of cocaine are complex. Cocaine-induced increase in sympathomimetic activity results in increased myocardial contractility, heart rate, blood pressure, and increased myocardial oxygen demand, while simultaneously decreasing myocardial oxygen supply due to vasoconstriction leading to hypertensive crises, acute myocardial infarction (AMI), aortic dissection, and stroke. Premature coronary atherosclerosis has been seen in young cocaine abusers, with obstructive coronary artery disease (CAD) seen in 35% to 40% of patients who undergo angiography for cocaine-associated chest pain. Cocaine may depress left ventricular function in the absence of acute coronary ischemia because of its direct negative inotropic effect on cardiac muscle, therefore leading to myocarditis and cardiomyopathy. Cocaine exhibits properties of a class I antiarrhythmic agent by Na-channel blockade. It also prolongs the duration of the QT interval by inhibiting myocyte repolarization that occurs by the efflux of potassium. Cocaine also increases intracellular calcium with resultant afterdepolarizations, reduces vagal activity, and increases myocyte irritability by inducing ischemia. Ischemia due to vasospasm and fatal ventricular arrhythmias due to ischemia are presumed to be important mechanisms of sudden death in these patients.

5. **How often does AMI occur after cocaine ingestion?**
Reported rates of AMI vary widely (1% to 31%); the variance in the incidence of AMI in studies likely relates to the difference in patient populations, AMI diagnostic criteria, and the use of newer, more sensitive troponin assays that can detect smaller levels of myocardial necrosis in patients that were previously classified as unstable angina. AMI occurs within minutes to days after cocaine exposure, independent of dose, length of use, or route of administration. However, the time during which individuals are at higher risk for developing AMI is within the first hour of cocaine use.

6. **What else should be considered in the differential diagnosis after cocaine use?**
Because patients who present to the emergency department after cocaine use are commonly hypertensive and tachycardic, aortic dissection needs to be considered in the differential diagnosis. Information concerning cocaine-induced aortic dissection is limited, but one study of 38 consecutive cases of aortic dissection demonstrated that a surprisingly high number (14, or 37%) were associated with cocaine use. However, among 921 patients in the International Registry of Aortic Dissection (IRAD), only 0.5% of aortic dissection cases were associated with cocaine use. In addition, an acute pulmonary syndrome, "*crack lung*," has been described after inhalation of freebase cocaine. The syndrome presents with hypoxemia, hemoptysis, respiratory failure, and diffuse pulmonary infiltrates. Chronic cocaine use can lead to decreased left ventricular systolic function and congestive heart failure. This may relate to accelerated atherosclerosis or myocarditis, both of which are associated with cocaine use.

7. **How does cocaine ingestion lead to AMI?**

   Cocaine can lead to AMI in a multifactorial fashion, including the following:
   - Increasing myocardial oxygen demand by increasing heart rate, blood pressure, and contractility
   - Decreasing oxygen supply as a result of vasoconstriction
   - Inducing a prothrombotic state by altering the balance between procoagulant and anticoagulant factors
   - Accelerating the atherosclerotic process

   Coronary vasospasm, rather than plaque rupture, likely constitutes the primary pathogenesis. In patients with preexisting high-grade coronary arterial narrowing, acute ischemia may be the result of increased myocardial oxygen demand associated with hypertension and tachycardia. In those present-ing with no underlying atherosclerotic obstruction, coronary occlusion may be due to vasospasm, thrombus formation, or both. For many years, the conventional assumption was that AMI after cocaine exposure was due solely to coronary vasospasm. Current knowledge suggests that vasospasm may only be the initiating pathophysiological event leading to thrombus formation rather than plaque rupture.

8. **Should younger patients with chest pain have a cocaine screening test?**

   The American Heart Association (AHA) recommends that establishing cocaine use should depend primarily on self-reporting. Because the use of cocaine influences treatment strategies, patients being evaluated for possible AMI should be queried about cocaine use; this applies especially to younger patients. Even if a young patient with chest pain denies cocaine use, the use of cocaine should be considered. Young patients with nontraumatic chest pain should be questioned regarding cocaine use.

9. **Are there any specific electrocardiogram findings in patients that use cocaine?**

   Abnormal electrocardiograms (ECGs) have been reported in 56% to 84% of patients with cocaine-associated chest pain. Many of these patients are younger and have the normal variant findings of early repolarization, namely, elevation of the J point as well as concave-up ST elevation and prominent T waves. In a study of 101 patients who had used cocaine, 42% manifested ST segment elevation on the ECG, but all of them ultimately had AMI excluded by serial cardiac marker testing. Left ventricular hypertrophy can also be noted on the ECG. In a series of 238 individuals who used cocaine, 33% had a normal ECG, 23% had nonspecific findings, 13% had left ventricular hypertrophy, 6% had left ventricular hypertrophy and early repolarization, and 13% had early repolarization alone.

10. **Should all patients with cocaine-associated chest pain be admitted to the hospital?**

    No. Most patients with cocaine-associated chest pain do not have ACS and can safely and efficiently be evaluated in a chest pain observation unit. In a prospective study of 344 patients with cocaine-associated chest pain, 42 (12%) high-risk patients with ST segment elevation or depression, elevated cardiac markers, or hemodynamic instability were directly admitted. The other 302 were evaluated in an observation unit over 9 to 12 hours with telemetry monitoring, serial troponin I measurement, and selective stress testing. Among the patients in the observation unit there were no cardiac deaths, 4 (2%) nonfatal AMIs, and 158 (52%) patients who underwent stress testing.

11. **Should all patients with cocaine-associated chest pain have a stress test?**

    No. The AHA states that stress testing is optional in patients who have an uneventful 9 to 12 hours of observation. Patients should be counseled about cessation of cocaine use. Patients can be followed in the outpatient setting and stress testing considered later, depending on cardiac risk factors and ongoing symptoms.

12. **How should patients with ST elevation myocardial infarction (STEMI) or non–ST elevation myocardial infarction (NSTEMI) be treated in the setting of cocaine use?**

    Rapid reperfusion by percutaneous coronary intervention (PCI) in a high-volume center by expe-rienced operators is preferred over fibrinolytic therapy in the setting of STEMI, and this is even more desirable after cocaine use. Many young patients will have early repolarization, and only a small percentage of these patients will actually be experiencing an AMI. Furthermore, hypertensive patients after cocaine use are at higher risk for significant bleeding complications. There have been case reports of intracranial hemorrhage after fibrinolytic therapy in the setting of STEMI associated with cocaine use. Fibrinolytic therapy should only be considered for patients who are clearly having a STEMI but cannot receive timely PCI. Patients with NSTEMI should be treated in similar fashion as patients without cocaine, with a notable exception regarding beta-adrenergic blocking agents (β-blockers; see Question 14).

13. **How should patients with cocaine-associated chest pain be treated?**
Patients who ingest cocaine are commonly hypertensive, tachycardic, and anxious. In patients who use cocaine, the AHA recommends the early use of intravenous benzodiazepines. Benzodiazepines decrease the central stimulating characteristics of cocaine and lessen anxiety. Their use has been shown to relieve chest pain and to have beneficial hemodynamic effects. Many times the hypertension and tachycardia will not need to be directly treated after the use of benzodiazepines. Aspirin should also be given. In patients who remain hypertensive, nitroglycerin or nitroprusside can be administered. Phentolamine is also an alternative. Calcium channel blockers have not been well studied in this population, but can be considered in patients who do not respond to benzodiazepines and nitroglycerin. However, short-acting nifedipine should not be used, and verapamil and diltiazem should be avoided in the setting of heart failure or decreased left ventricular systolic function (Fig. 49-2).

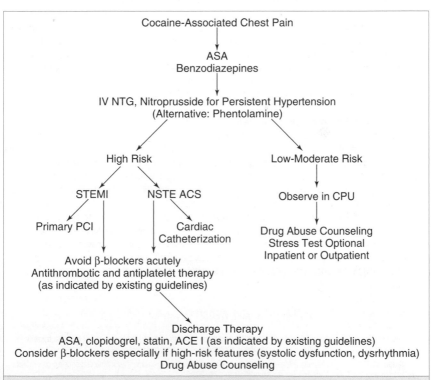

Figure 49-2. Therapeutic and diagnostic recommendations in cocaine-associated chest pain. *ACE,* Angiotensin-converting enzyme; *ACS,* acute coronary syndrome; *ASA,* aspirin; *β-blockers,* beta-adrenergic receptor blocking agents; *CPU,* chest pain unit; *IV,* intravenous; *NSTE,* non–ST segment elevation; *NTG,* nitroglycerin; *PCI,* percutaneous coronary intervention; *STEMI,* ST segment elevation myocardial infarction.

14. **Should β-blockers be given to patients with cocaine-associated chest pain?**

No. The AHA recommends that β-blockers not be administered acutely in patients with ACS or undifferentiated chest pain in the setting of cocaine use. After cocaine use, the administration of propranolol leads to worsening coronary vasoconstriction and increased systemic blood pressure because of the unopposed α-adrenergic effect. Multiple experimental animal models have shown in this setting that β-blockers elevate the coronary vascular resistance and decrease coronary blood flow, increase seizure activity, and increase mortality. There have been case reports of sudden cardiac death in humans shortly after the administration of β-blockers in the setting of cocaine use.

Although theoretically more attractive, the administration of labetalol in the setting of cocaine use is not recommended. Labetalol has substantially more β-blocking than α-blocking effects. In animal models, labetalol leads to increased seizure activity and death after cocaine administration and does not reverse coronary vasoconstriction in humans. The β_1-adrenoceptor–selective agent metoprolol has not been evaluated in the setting of cocaine, but the β_1-adrenoceptor–selective agent esmolol has been associated with an increase in systemic blood pressure after cocaine use. Compared to labetalol, carvedilol may be four times more effective at the α receptor and, unlike labetalol, carvedilol at recommended doses may attenuate the physiological and behavioral response to smoked cocaine. However, strong clinical evidence to change current guidelines recommendations is still lacking.

15. **How should tachyarrhythmias be treated after cocaine use?**

Sinus tachycardia and atrial tachyarrhythmias may respond to benzodiazepines. In cases of atrial tachyarrhythmias that do not respond to benzodiazepines, verapamil or diltiazem can be considered. Ventricular arrhythmias that occur immediately after cocaine use are thought to result from the Na-channel blocking effect of cocaine and may respond to the administration of sodium bicarbonate, similar to arrhythmias associated with type IA agents. Ventricular arrhythmias that occur several hours after cocaine use usually are due to ischemia, which should be treated as directed earlier. In case of persistent ventricular arrhythmias, lidocaine can be used.

16. **How should patients be managed after discharge?**

It is estimated that 60% of patients who present with cocaine-associated chest pain will continue to abuse cocaine after hospital discharge. Therefore, the cessation of cocaine use should be the primary goal. The combination of intensive group and individual drug counseling has been shown to be effective. The recurrence of chest pain is unlikely, and the prognosis is good in patients who discontinue cocaine use. Aggressive modification of risk factors is indicated for patients with AMI or CAD, similar to patients who do not use cocaine.

Although β-blockers should be avoided acutely, special consideration needs to be given in selected patients for chronic use. In patients with left ventricular systolic dysfunction, AMI, or ventricular arrhythmias, the long-term use of β-blockers should be strongly considered. The AHA recommends that this decision be individualized on the basis of risk-benefit assessment and recommends counseling the patient about the potential negative effects of the use of β-blockers and cocaine ingestion.

BIBLIOGRAPHY, SUGGESTED READINGS, AND WEBSITES

1. Chang AM, Walsh KM, Shofer FS, et al: Relationship between cocaine use and coronary artery disease in patients with symptoms consistent with an acute coronary syndrome, *Acad Emerg Med* 18:1–9, 2010.

2. Feldman JA, Fish SS, Beshansky JR, et al: Acute cardiac ischemia in patients with cocaine-associated complaints: results of a multicenter trial, *Ann Emerg Med* 36:469–476, 2000.

3. Hollander JE: The management of cocaine-associated myocardial ischemia, *N Engl J Med* 333:1267–1272, 1995.

4. Hollander JE, Hoffman RS, Burstein JL, et al: Cocaine-associated myocardial infarction. Mortality and complications. Cocaine-Associated Myocardial Infarction Study Group, *Arch Intern Med* 155:1081–1086, 1995.

5. Hollander JE, Hoffman RS, Gennis P, et al: Prospective multicenter evaluation of cocaine-associated chest pain. Cocaine Associated Chest Pain (COCHPA) Study Group, *Acad Emerg Med* 1:330–339, 1994.

6. Maraj S, Figueredo VM, Morris L, et al: Cocaine and the Heart, *Clin Cardiol* 33:264–269, 2010.

7. McCord J, Jneid H, Hollander JE, et al: Management of cocaine-associated chest pain and myocardial infarction, *Circulation* 117:1897–1907, 2008.

8. Weber JE, Shofer FS, Larkin GL, et al: Validation of a brief observation period for patients with cocaine-associated chest pain, *N Engl J Med* 348:510–517, 2003.

CHAPTER 50

DEEP VEIN THROMBOSIS

Alejandro Perez, MD, FSVM, RPVI, and Geno J. Merli, MD, FACP, FHM, FSVM

1. **What three primary factors promote venous thromboembolic (VTE) disease?**
   Development of venous thrombosis is promoted by the following (the *Virchow Triad*):
   - Venous blood stasis
   - Injury to the intimal layer of the venous vasculature
   - Abnormalities in coagulation or fibrinolysis

2. **List the risk factors for thromboembolic disease.**
   The numerous risk factors for thromboembolic disease include surgery, trauma, immobility, cancer, pregnancy, prolonged immobilization, estrogen-containing oral contraceptives or hormone replacement therapy, and acute medical illnesses. A more complete listing of these risk factors is given in Box 50-1.

3. **What is the natural history of venous thrombosis?**
   Resolution of fresh thrombi occurs by endogenous fibrinolysis and organization. *Fibrinolysis* results in actual clot dissolution. *Organization* reestablishes venous blood flow by restoring endothelial cells and incorporating into the venous wall residual clot not dissolved by fibrinolysis. Incomplete recanalization can cause postphlebitic syndrome in >20% of patients.

Box 50-1 RISK FACTORS FOR DEEP VENOUS THROMBOEMBOLISM

- Surgery
- Trauma (major or lower extremity)
- Immobility, lower extremity paresis
- Cancer (active or occult)
- Cancer therapy (hormonal, chemotherapy, angiogenesis inhibitors, or radiotherapy)
- Venous compression (tumor, hematoma, arterial abnormality)
- Previous history of thromboembolic disease
- Obesity
- Pregnancy and postpartum period
- Prolonged immobilization
- Lower-extremity or pelvic trauma or surgery
- Surgery with greater than 30 minutes of general anesthesia
- Congestive heart failure
- Nephrotic syndrome
- Estrogen-containing oral contraceptives or hormone replacement therapy
- Selective estrogen receptor modulators
- Inflammatory bowel disease
- Acute medical illness
- Myeloproliferative disorders
- Paroxysmal nocturnal hemoglobinuria
- Central venous catheter
- Inherited or acquired thrombophilia
- Increasing age

---

4. **Can patients with deep vein thrombosis (DVT) be accurately diagnosed clinically?**

No. The clinical diagnosis of DVT is neither sensitive nor specific. Less than 50% of patients with confirmed DVT present with the classic symptoms and signs of DVT, which include pain, tenderness, redness, swelling, and the *Homan sign* (calf pain with dorsiflexion of the foot). This sole use of clinical findings is artificial, because clinicians couple the medical and surgical history, concomitant medical problems, medications, and risk factors to decide on further testing to confirm DVT.

5. **Where is the most common origin for thrombi that result in pulmonary emboli?**

Thromboses in the deep veins of the lower extremities (Fig. 50-1) account for 90% to 95% of pulmonary emboli. Less common sites of origin include thromboses in the right ventricle, in upper extremity, prostatic, uterine, and renal veins; and, rarely, in superficial veins.

6. **How is the diagnosis of lower extremity DVT confirmed?**

Diagnostic evaluation of suspected DVT includes a clear correlation among clinical probability, test selection, and test interpretation.

Contrast venography is no longer appropriate as the initial diagnostic test in patients exhibiting DVT symptoms, although it remains the gold standard for confirmatory diagnosis of DVT. It is nearly 100% sensitive and specific and provides the ability to investigate the distal and proximal venous system for thrombosis. Venography is still warranted when noninvasive testing is inconclusive or impossible to perform, but its use is no longer widespread because of the need for administration of a contrast medium and the increased availability of noninvasive diagnostic strategies.

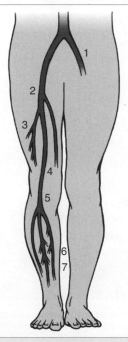

Figure 50-1. Common sites of deep venous thrombosis (DVT) in the lower body. *1,* Left iliac vein; *2,* common femoral vein; *3,* termination of deep femoral vein (profunda femoris); *4,* femoral vein; *5,* popliteal vein at adductor canal; *6,* posterior tibial vein; *7,* intramuscular veins of calf. (From Pfenninger JL, Fowler GC: *Pfenninger and Fowler's procedures for primary care,* ed 3, Philadelphia, 2010, Saunders.)

Ultrasound is safe and noninvasive and has a higher specificity than impedance plethysmography for the evaluation of suspected DVT. With color flow Doppler and compression ultrasound, DVT is diagnosed based on the inability to compress the common femoral and popliteal veins (Fig. 50-2). In patients with lower extremity symptoms, the sensitivity is 95% and specificity 96%. The diagnostic accuracy of ultrasound in asymptomatic patients, those with recurrent DVT, or those with isolated calf

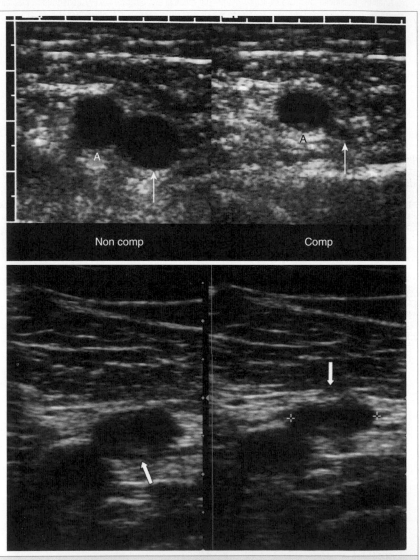

Figure 50-2. Normal and abnormal compression of the femoral vein with ultrasound examination. *Top Images:* Transverse image of the femoral artery *(A)* and vein *(thin white arrow)* before *(Non Comp)* and after *(Comp)* compression with the sonographic transducer, demonstrated normal vein collapse with compression. *Bottom Images:* There is minimum compression of the common femoral vein *(thick white arrow)* in this patient with deep vein thrombosis. (Top images from Rumack CM, Wilson SR, Charboneau JW, Levine D: *Diagnostic ultrasound,* ed 4, Philadelphia, 2010, Mosby. Bottom images from Mason RJ, Broaddus VC, Martin T, et al: *Murray and Nadel's textbook of respiratory medicine,* ed 5, Philadelphia, 2010, Saunders.)

DVT is less reliable. The sensitivity of ultrasound improves with serial testing in untreated patients. Repeat testing at 5 to 7 days will identify another 2% of patients with clots not apparent on the first ultrasound. Serial testing can be particularly valuable in ruling out proximal extension of a possible calf DVT. Because the accuracy of ultrasound in diagnosing calf DVT is acknowledged to be lower (81% for DVT below the knee versus 99% for proximal DVT), follow-up ultrasounds at 5 to 7 days are reasonable because most calf DVTs that extend proximally will do so within days of the initial presentation.

7. **When should prophylaxis of DVT be considered?**
   Two factors must be weighed in deciding to initiate prophylaxis of DVT: the degree of risk for thrombosis and the risk of prophylaxis. The risk factors for DVT are cumulative. The primary risk of pharmacologic prophylaxis is hemorrhage, which is generally uncommon if no coagulation defects or lesions with bleeding potential exist.

8. **What prophylactic measures are available?**
   Approaches to prophylaxis of DVT include antithrombotic drugs and pneumatic compression devices. Heparin, low-molecular-weight heparin (LMWH), fondaparinux, and warfarin are effective in preventing DVT. Subcutaneous heparin has been the mainstay of DVT prophylaxis, with efficacy in multiple surgical and medical scenarios. The LMWHs have been shown to be as effective or superior to unfractionated heparin (UFH) in different clinical circumstances. Warfarin dosing to maintain an international normalized ratio (INR) between 2 and 3 also has a low risk of bleeding and is effective in patients with total hip arthroplasty, total knee arthroplasty, and hip fracture surgery. However, warfarin takes several days to develop a full antithrombotic effect. Antiplatelet drugs such as aspirin are not effective in DVT prophylaxis in the general medical population, but aspirin has been used with efficacy in the orthopedic surgery population. Rivaroxaban can also be used for DVT prophylaxis in orthopedic surgeries.

   Intermittent pneumatic compression devices effect prophylaxis by maintaining venous flow in the lower extremities and are especially efficacious in patients who cannot receive anticoagulant medications. Modalities available include compressive devices applied to the feet alone, covering the calves, or extending to the thighs. No version has been shown to provide superior prophylaxis. There has been concern that compression stockings used for prophylaxis may cause unintended skin trauma without substantial benefit.

9. **What is the approach to DVT prophylaxis in the hospitalized, medically ill patient?**
   The acutely ill medical patient admitted to the hospital with congestive heart failure or severe respiratory disease, or who is confined to bed and has one or more additional risk factors, including active cancer, previous venous thromboembolism, sepsis, acute neurologic disease, or inflammatory bowel disease, should receive DVT prophylaxis with the following agents:
   - UFH: 5000 units subcutaneously (SC) every 8 or 12 hours
   - LMWH: dalteparin: 5000 IU SC every 24 hours or enoxaparin: 40 mg SC every 24 hours
   - Fondaparinux: 2.5 mg SC every 24 hours

10. **Should patients undergoing surgery receive DVT prophylaxis based on specific recommendations for each respective procedure?**
    Yes. Most surgical procedures have defined recommendations for preventing DVT in the postoperative period if age and other clinical comorbidities demonstrate an elevated risk based upon risk assessment models, such as that of the Rogers or Caprini score. The various prophylaxis regimens for different surgical procedures are listed in Box 50-2.

11. **Are there specific surgical groups that require extended DVT prophylaxis following hospital discharge?**
    For a patient undergoing total hip replacement, total knee replacement, and hip fracture surgery, extended DVT prophylaxis is recommended for up to 35 days after surgery, with LMWH, UFH, fondaparinux, warfarin, rivaroxaban, or aspirin.

Box 50-2 DEEP VEIN THROMBOSIS PROPHYLAXIS REGIMENS FOR VARIOUS SURGERIES

General Urologic, Gastrointestinal, Gynecologic, Bariatric, Vascular, Plastic, or Reconstructive Surgery

The following regimens are for patients undergoing major surgical procedures for benign or malignant disease and associated DVT risk factors:

- Unfractionated heparin: 5000 units SC every 8 hours
- LMWH: enoxaparin 40 mg SC every 24 hours, dalteparin 5000 IU SC every 24 hours
- External pneumatic compression sleeves plus one of the above regimens
- Fondaparinux: 2.5 mg SC, every 24 hours can be considered for patients with history of heparin associated thrombocytopenia.

Orthopedic Surgery

The following regimens are for patients undergoing orthopedic surgery:

Total Hip/Knee Surgery

- LMWH: enoxaparin 30 mg SC every 12 hours, dalteparin 5000 IU SC every 24 hours
- Unfractionated heparin: 5000 units SC every 8 hours
- Fondaparinux: 2.5 mg SC every 24 hours
- Rivaroxaban: 10 mg every 24 hours
- ASA: (optimal dose has yet to be determined)
- Intermittent pneumatic compression devices
- Warfarin: 5 mg the evening of surgery, then adjust dose to achieve an INR of 2 to 3.

Hip Fracture

- LMWH: enoxaparin 30 mg SC every 12 hours, dalteparin 5000 IU SC every 24 hours
- Unfractionated heparin: 5000 units SC every 8 hours
- Fondaparinux: 2.5 mg SC every 24 hours
- ASA: (optimal dose has yet to be determined)
- Intermittent pneumatic compression devices
- Warfarin: 5 mg the evening of surgery, then adjust dose to achieve an INR of 2 to 3.
- (Rivaroxaban is not approved for this indication at the time of this writing.)

Neurosurgery

The following regimens are for patients undergoing neurosurgery:

- External pneumatic compression sleeves are the prophylaxis of choice.
- Combination therapy with either unfractionated heparin (5000 units SC every 8 or 12 hours) or LMWH (enoxaparin 40 mg SC every 24 hours) can be used.

Coronary Artery Bypass Surgery

The following regimens are for patients undergoing coronary artery bypass surgery:

- LMWH (preferred over unfractionated heparin): enoxaparin 40 mg SC every 24 hours or dalteparin 5000 IU SC every 24 hours
- Unfractionated heparin: 5000 units, SC every 8 hours
- Fondaparinux: 2.5 mg, SC, every 24 hours for patients with history of heparin-induced thrombocytopenia
- External pneumatic compression sleeves for high–bleeding-risk patients

ASA, Aspirin; *DVT*, deep vein thrombosis; *INR*, international normalized ratio; *IU*, international units; *LMWH*, low-molecular-weight heparin; *SC*, subcutaneous.

For selected high-risk general surgery patients undergoing major cancer surgery or who have previously had venous thromboembolism, it is recommended that DVT prophylaxis be continued with LMWH: enoxaparin 40 mg SC every 24 hours or dalteparin 5000 IU SC every 24 hours for 35 days.

12. What treatment regimens are available for the treatment of DVT?
Several treatment regimens using UFH or a LMWH are available for the treatment of DVT. These are listed in Box 50-3.

13. Which LMWHs are renally excreted?
All the LMWHs are renally excreted. Enoxaparin is the only LMWH that has a recommended dose for creatinine clearance less than 30 mL/min (1 mg/kg SC every 24 hours). All other LMWHs listed here should not be used with creatinine clearance less than 30 mL/min.

14. When should warfarin be started with the regimens of treatment of DVT listed earlier?
In patients with acute DVT, warfarin should be administered on the first day of UFH or LMWH treatment at a dose of 5 to 10 mg.

15. When should these therapeutic regimens for treating DVT be discontinued and warfarin remain as the sole therapy?
These therapies must be used for at least 5 days and until the INR is more than 2 for 24 hours.

16. What is the target INR for treating patients with DVT?
The target INR for the treatment of DVT to prevent recurrent disease is 2 to 3.

17. How long should patients with acute DVT be treated with warfarin?
For patients with DVT secondary to a transient risk factor, 3 months of warfarin is appropriate. Idiopathic proximal DVT in patients without risk factors for bleeding should receive long-term warfarin therapy with a target INR of 2 to 3. Patients with DVT and cancer should receive LMWH for 3 to 6 months as the initial approach to management and long-term treatment with either warfarin or LMWH until the cancer is resolved or in remission.

Box 50-3 REGIMENS FOR THE TREATMENT OF DEEP VEIN THROMBOSIS

Unfractionated Heparin (UFH)
- Administer intravenous bolus of UFH (80 units/kg or 5000 units) followed by continuous infusion of 18 unit/kg/hr or 1000 units/hr. The activated partial thromboplastin time (aPTT) is checked every 6 hours to adjust the infusion to achieve the therapeutic aPTT of the hospital laboratory.
- Subcutaneous UFH at 333 units/kg is the initial dose, followed in 12 hours by 250 units/kg SC every 12 hours. Monitoring of the aPTT is not necessary.

Low-Molecular-Weight Heparin (LMWH)
- Enoxaparin 1 mg/kg subcutaneous (SC), every 12 hours or 1.5 mg/kg SC every 24 hours
- Dalteparin 200 units/kg SC every 24 hours
- Tinzaparin 175 anti-Xa units/kg SC every 24 hours

Fondaparinux
- Fondaparinux dosed by weight range: less than 50 kg, 5 mg SC every 24 hours; 50 to 100 kg, 7.5 mg SC every 24 hours; more than 100 kg, 10 mg SC every 24 hours

18. When can patients with acute DVT ambulate?

Patients can ambulate with acute DVT and should not be placed on bed rest unless the lower extremity is painful and cannot bear weight.

19. Can patients with acute DVT be treated as outpatients?

Yes. The LMWH regimens listed here can be used to treat patients in the outpatient setting. The same principles of management should be followed using these agents as with inpatient treatment.

20. When should catheter-directed thrombolysis be used to treat acute DVT?

In selected patients with extensive acute proximal iliofemoral DVT in which symptoms have been present for less than 14 days, who are functionally active, and who have a low bleeding risk, the use of pharmacomechanical thrombolysis is recommended if the appropriate expertise and resources are available.

21. Are inferior vena caval filters indicated for the initial treatment of acute DVT?

No. Vena caval filters are indicated when the patient cannot receive anticoagulation for the treatment of acute DVT. In certain cases (temporary contraindication to anticoagulant therapy), retrievable vena caval filters have been placed, with the plan to remove them in a defined time (2 to 4 weeks), after which anticoagulation therapy can be reinstituted.

22. When are gradient elastic stockings recommended as part of the treatment of acute DVT?

For patients with symptomatic DVT, the use of gradient elastic stockings with an ankle pressure of 30 to 40 mm Hg is recommended. The pressure may not be tolerated because of the degree of lower-extremity edema. Elastic bandages may be used because they can be adjusted to control swelling and the pain that is associated with increased external pressure. The elastic bandages can be used initially, but as the swelling recedes, gradient elastic stockings at 20 to 30 mm Hg or 30 to 40 mm Hg may be applied.

23. When is a low-intensity INR anticoagulant therapy indicated for the treatment of DVT?

For patients with idiopathic (unprovoked) DVT who have a strong preference for less frequent INR testing to monitor their therapy, it is recommended that after the first 3 months of therapy, low-intensity therapy at an INR of 1.5 to 1.9 with less frequent INR monitoring be employed instead of stopping warfarin anticoagulation.

24. Are there other INR ranges for DVT prophylaxis in orthopedic surgery?

Other target ranges such as 1.5-2.0 have been proposed for orthopedic surgery prophylaxis, but the INR range 2-3 has the most supportive clinical data.

25. Should compression ultrasound be used as routine screening in the total joint replacement surgery patient at the time of discharge?

Asymptomatic joint replacement surgery patients should not have compression ultrasound on discharge as screening test for DVT because the ultrasound is not as sensitive and specific in asymptomatic patients. Appropriate DVT prophylaxis should be the approach to management.

BIBLIOGRAPHY, SUGGESTED READINGS, AND WEBSITES

1. British Thoracic Society Standards of Care Committee: Pulmonary Embolism Guideline Development Group: British Thoracic Society guidelines for the management of suspected acute pulmonary embolism, *Thorax* 58:470–483, 2003.

2. Cardiovascular Disease Educational and Research Trust, Cyprus Cardiovascular Disease Educational and Research Trust, European Venous Forum, et al: Prevention and treatment of venous thromboembolism. International consensus statement (guidelines according to scientific evidence), *Int Angiol* 25:101–161, 2006.

3. Decousus H, Leizorovicz A, Parent F, et al: A clinical trial of vena caval filters in the prevention of pulmonary embolism in patients with proximal deep-vein thrombosis, *N Engl J Med* 338:409–415, 1998.

4. Gould MK, Garcia DA, Wren SM, et al: Prevention of VTE in Nonorthopedic Surgical Patients: Antithrombotic Therapy and Prevention of Thrombosis, 9th ed: American College of Chest Physicians Evidence-Based Clinical Practice Guidelines, *Chest* 141(Suppl 2):e227S–e277S, 2012.

5. Kahn SR, Lim W, Dunn AS, et al: Prevention of VTE in Nonsurgical Patients: Antithrombotic Therapy and Prevention of Thrombosis, 9th ed: American College of Chest Physicians Evidence-Based Clinical Practice Guidelines, *Chest* 141(Suppl 2):e195S–e226S, 2012.

6. Kearon C, Ginsberg JS, Julian JA, et al: Comparison of fixed-dose weight adjusted unfractionated heparin and low-molecular weight heparin for acute treatment of venous thromboembolism, *JAMA* 296:935–942, 2006.

7. Koopman MM, Prandoni P, Piovella F, et al: Treatment of venous thrombosis with intravenous unfractionated heparin administered in the hospital as compared with subcutaneous low-molecular-weight heparin administered at home, *N Engl J Med* 334:682–687, 1996.

8. Levine M, Gent M, Hirsh J, et al: A comparison of low-molecular-weight heparin administered primarily at home with unfractionated heparin administered in the hospital for proximal deep vein thrombosis, *N Engl J Med* 334:677–681, 1996.

9. The Matisse Investigators. Subcutaneous fondaparinux versus intravenous unfractionated heparin in the initial treatment of pulmonary embolism, *N Engl J Med* 349:1695–1702, 2003.

10. Merli GJ: Pathophysiology of venous thrombosis and the diagnosis of deep vein thrombosis-pulmonary embolism in the elderly, *Cardiol Clin* 26:203–219, 2008.

11. Merli G, Spiro T, Olsson CG, et al: Subcutaneous enoxaparin once or twice daily compared with intravenous unfractionated heparin for treatment of venous thromboembolic disease, *Ann Intern Med* 134:191–202, 2001.

12. Snow V, Qaseem A, Barry P, et al: Management of venous thromboembolism: a clinical practice guideline from the American College of Physicians and the American Academy of Family Physicians, *Ann Intern Med* 146(3):204–210, 2007.

13. Wells PS, Anderson DR, Rodger MA, et al: A randomized trial comparing 2 low-molecular-weight heparins for the outpatient treatment of deep vein thrombosis and pulmonary embolism, *Arch Intern Med* 165:733–738, 2005.

14. Falck-Ytter Y, Francis CW, Johanson NA, et al: Prevention of VTE in orthopedic surgery patients: Antithrombotic Therapy and Prevention of Thrombosis, 9th ed: American College of Chest Physicians Evidence-Based Clinical Practice Guidelines, *Chest* 141(Suppl 2):e278S–e325S, 2012.

CHAPTER 51

HEART DISEASE IN PREGNANCY

Rebecca M. LeLeiko, MD, and Sheilah Bernard, MD

1. What cardiac physiologic changes occur during pregnancy?

Hormonal changes cause an increase in both plasma volume (from water and sodium retention) and red blood cell volume (from erythrocytosis) during a normal pregnancy. A disproportionate increase in plasma volume explains the physiologic anemia of pregnancy. Maternal heart rate (HR) increases throughout the 40 weeks, mediated partially by increased sympathetic tone and heat production. Stroke volume subsequently continues to increase until the third trimester, when inferior vena cava (IVC) return may be compromised by the gravid uterus. Maternal cardiac output increases by 30% to 50% during a normal pregnancy. Systolic blood pressure drops during the first half of pregnancy and returns to normal levels by delivery. The physiologic changes related to cardiac output that occur during pregnancy are shown in Figure 51-1.

2. Are there independent vascular changes that occur during a normal pregnancy?

The vascular wall weakens during pregnancy as a result of estrogen and prostaglandin, leading to increased risk for vascular dissection. As the placenta develops, it creates a low-resistance circulation. These factors, in addition to heat production, contribute to the reduced systemic vascular resistance (SVR) that is a normal part of pregnancy.

3. What are normal cardiac signs and symptoms of pregnancy?

- *Hyperventilation* (as a result of increased minute ventilation)
- *Peripheral edema* (from volume retention and vena caval compression by the gravid uterus)
- *Dizziness/lightheadedness* (from reduced SVR and vena caval compression)
- *Palpitations* (normal HR increases by 10-15 beats/min)

4. What are pathologic cardiac signs and symptoms of pregnancy?

- *Anasarca* (generalized edema) and *paroxysmal nocturnal dyspnea* are not components of normal pregnancy and warrant workup.
- *Syncope* warrants evaluation for pulmonary embolism, tachy- or bradyarrhythmias, pulmonary hypertension, obstructive valvular pathology (aortic, mitral, or pulmonic stenosis), or hypotension.
- *Chest pain* may be due to aortic dissection, pulmonary embolism, angina, or even myocardial infarction. As more women delay childbearing, there is a higher incidence of preexisting cardiac disease and risk factors in pregnant women.
- *Hemoptysis* may be a harbinger of occult mitral stenosis, although rheumatic heart disease is becoming less common in developed countries.

5. What are normal cardiac examination findings during pregnancy?

- *Blood pressure* (BP) *will decline* and *HR will increase*.
- The *point of maximum impulse will be displaced laterally* as the uterus enlarges.
- *S_3 heart sound* is common because of increased rapid filling of the left ventricle (LV) in early diastole.
- A *physiologic pulmonic flow murmur* is common because of elevated stroke volume passing through a normal valve.

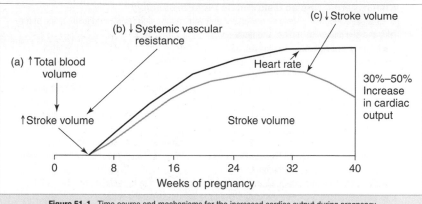

Figure 51-1. Time course and mechanisms for the increased cardiac output during pregnancy.

- A *mammary soufflé* (due to increased blood flow into the breasts) and *venous hum* (due to increased blood flow through jugular veins) are two continuous, superficial murmurs that can be obliterated by compressing the site with the diaphragm of the stethoscope. If the murmur does not change, consider patent ductus arteriosus or coronary arteriovenous (AV) fistula.

6. **What are pathologic cardiac exam findings during pregnancy?**
   - *Clubbing* and *cyanosis* are not a part of normal pregnancy; desaturation for any reason is abnormal and warrants investigation.
   - *Elevated jugular venous pressure* (JVP) is abnormal, reflecting elevated right atrial pressure. Although edema is common in this population, it is important to evaluate neck veins in any pregnant woman with peripheral edema.
   - *Pulmonary hypertension* (right ventricular heave, loud P_2, JVP elevation) findings should be investigated early. Women with preexisting pulmonary hypertension (pulmonary pressure greater than 75% of systemic pressure) should be counseled prior to pregnancy as to the risks.
   - *Systolic murmur 3/6 or louder* and any *diastolic murmur* audible in pregnancy are considered abnormal and warrant evaluation.
   - Audible S_4 is unusual during pregnancy and may reflect underlying hypertension.

7. **What are the cardiac changes that occur during labor and delivery?**
   With each contraction, 300 to 500 mL of blood are autotransfused from the uterus into the maternal circulatory system. Cardiac output (CO) drops less with vaginal delivery than with cesarean, so vaginal delivery is recommended more commonly in patients with cardiac disease. Vacuum-assisted delivery is used to shorten stage II of labor for women who may not tolerate pushing. After delivery, intravascular volume increases from release of the IVC compression, HR slows, and blood pressure, CO, and HR generally normalize postpartum; however, CO remains elevated in lactating women while they continue to breast-feed.

8. **Which women should undergo infective endocarditis (IE) prophylaxis at the time of delivery?**
   IE prophylaxis is *optional* in vaginal delivery for patients with prior IE, prosthetic valves, and congenital heart disease (CHD) within the first 6 months of repair, or after 6 months if there is residual shunting, surgically constructed systemic-to-pulmonary shunts or conduits, or posttransplantation valvulopathy. It is not indicated in cesarean section, per 2007 American Heart Association (AHA) guidelines, although it is often given.

9. **What maternal cardiac tests can be performed safely?**

    All tests using radiation should be performed only after a thorough review and justification of the risks and benefits to the mother and fetus.

    - Electrocardiograms and echocardiograms are safe, with no known risk to the fetus.
    - Chest radiographs can be performed with proper pelvic shielding.
    - MRI is considered safe (although there is little data during the first trimester).
    - Low-level exercise tolerance testing to 70% of maternal maximal HR is safe with low risk of fetal distress or bradycardia.
    - Transesophageal echocardiography (TEE) can be performed with appropriate sedation and monitoring.
    - Cardiac catheterization, balloon valvuloplasty, angioplasty, and percutaneous intervention are invasive diagnostic and therapeutic tests that may be life saving to the mother with appropriate pelvic shielding for the fetus.
    - Computerized tomography is relatively contraindicated due to radiation risk to the fetus.
    - Nuclear imaging is contraindicated due to radiation risk to the fetus.

10. **What are the highest-risk maternal cardiac conditions during pregnancy?**

    Moderate to severe mitral, aortic, and pulmonic stenosis are tolerated poorly during pregnancy. Patients should be counseled, with consideration of valvuloplasty or valve replacement before conception. These procedures can be performed during high-risk pregnancies if the patient decompensates. Pulmonary hypertension (pHTN) is also a high-risk condition, with historic maternal mortality rates of 30% to 56%. Although mortality remains unacceptably high, improvements in both the treatment of pHTN as well as the management of high-risk pregnancy have led to significant mortality reductions. Women with pHTN should be counseled regarding these risks. See Question 14 for discussion of CHD.

11. **Are regurgitant lesions equally risky?**

    Both mild to moderate aortic insufficiency and mitral regurgitation are tolerated well during pregnancy. The reduction in SVR can lessen the degree of regurgitation. Only patients with severe symptomatic regurgitation (New York Heart Association [NYHA] classes III or IV) should be considered for valve replacement before pregnancy. The only indication for valve replacement for regurgitant lesions during pregnancy is infective endocarditis.

12. **What are maternal complications seen in pregnant women with cardiac disease? What are some predictors of fetal complications?**

    Pulmonary edema, stroke, arrhythmia, and cardiac death are complications noted in a study of 599 such pregnancies. Fetal complications were seen more often in pregnancies with maternal cyanosis, left heart obstruction, anticoagulation, concomitant smoking, multiple gestations, and heart failure symptoms greater than NYHA class II.

13. **How are pregnant women anticoagulated during pregnancy?**

    Because warfarin is contraindicated during the first trimester and at term, 2012 American College for Chest Physicians (ACCP) guidelines recommend one of the following grade 1A strategies:

    - Aggressive adjusted-dose twice-daily low-molecular-weight heparin (LMWH) throughout pregnancy with doses adjusted to achieve target peak anti–activated factor X (anti-Xa) level 4 hours postinjection, or
    - Aggressive adjusted-dose twice-daily unfractionated heparin (UFH) throughout pregnancy administered subcutaneously to a therapeutic PTT, or
    - UFH or LMWH until week 13 of pregnancy with substitution by vitamin K antagonists (e.g., warfarin) until close to delivery. At that point UFH or LMWH is resumed.

    Long-term anticoagulants should be resumed postpartum with all regimens, as early as the same evening. Low-dose aspirin can be optionally added for high-risk patients with mechanical heart valves. Mothers taking warfarin may nurse after delivery.

14. **How are the common congenital lesions tolerated during pregnancy?**

In developed countries, congential heart disease (CHD) has superseded rheumatic heart disease as the most common preexisting heart disease in pregnancy. Repaired atrial septal defects (ASDs) and ventricular septal defects (VSDs) confer no increased cardiac risk. Unrepaired left-to-right intracardiac shunts (ASD and VSD) are well tolerated because of the reduction in SVR, which decreases left-to-right shunting during pregnancy. Patients are at an increased risk for paradoxical embolization if they develop deep vein thrombosis.

Right-to-left (cyanotic) shunting is poorly tolerated in pregnancy. Women with tetralogy of Fallot should undergo repair before contemplating pregnancy. Right-to-left shunting worsens during pregnancy because of reduction of SVR. Women with Eisenmenger syndrome risk a 30% to 50% maternal mortality with pregnancy. Women with such high risk are counseled to avoid pregnancy or undergo therapeutic termination.

15. **Which cardiac arrhythmias can complicate pregnancy?**

Patients may develop atrial and ventricular ectopy because of myocardial stretch. Reentrant pathways may emerge leading to atrial arrhythmias. These can be treated acutely with vagal maneuvers or adenosine if the mother is unstable. Recurrent supraventricular arrhythmias can be prevented with digitalis or beta-adrenergic blocking agents (β-blockers). Symptomatic ventricular arrhythmias are treated medically or with implantable cardioverter-defibrillators. If a pregnant woman suffers a cardiac arrest, the viable baby should be delivered after 15 minutes if there is no return of spontaneous maternal circulation.

16. **How do you treat a pregnant woman with an acute myocardial infarction?**

Pregnant women with ST segment elevation myocardial infarction (STEMI) should be taken to the catheterization laboratory for primary balloon angioplasty. Heparin can be used safely; however, there is little data on the use of stents, as clopidogrel has not been extensively studied in pregnancy. β-Blockers and low-dose aspirin can be used in pregnancy, but angiotensin-converting enzyme (ACE) inhibitors, angiotensin receptor blockers (ARBs), and statins should be avoided. Risk factors should be treated.

17. **How do women with hypertrophic cardiomyopathy (HCM) tolerate pregnancy?**

Management is similar to the nongravid state. Women with HCM will experience left ventricular end-diastolic pressure (LVEDP) elevations because of increased blood volume of pregnancy. If the LV is able to dilate, outflow obstruction may be reduced. At the time of delivery, anesthesia is critical to reduce sympathetic stimulation from pain; most anesthetic agents reduce myocardial contractility. Preload and afterload changes during delivery must be minimized to avoid increased outflow obstruction. Short-acting vasoconstrictors, diuretics, or volume adjustments may be necessary.

18. **What are the recommendations for patients with Marfan syndrome?**

Women with Marfan syndrome are at risk for aortic dissection because of the additional vascular changes of pregnancy. Genetic counseling should be performed before conception because of autosomal dominant transmission. Those with an aortic root diameter of more than 40 mm are at highest risk and are advised to avoid pregnancy. Management includes β-blockers, serial echocardiograms, and bed rest to avoid further root dilation. Type A dissection (involving the ascending aorta) should be managed surgically, with delivery of the viable fetus before repair. Type B dissection (descending aortic involvement) can be managed medically with labetalol or nitroprusside.

19. **Which commonly used cardiac medications should be avoided during pregnancy?**

Common cardiac medications that should be avoided during part or all of pregnancy are listed in Box 51-1.

Box 51-1 SAFETY OF CARDIAC MEDICATIONS IN PREGNANCY

- Women should be counselled that warfarin is a class X drug per US Food and Drug Administration. LMWH or UFHs should replace warfarin in the first trimester and after 36 weeks of pregnancy.
- Statins are also class X, although investigations on the use of statins in pregnancy are underway, with a recent meta-analysis suggesting that statin use may be safer than previously thought.
- ACE inhibitors, ARBs, atenolol, and amiodarone are class D.
- Hydralazine with nitrates should replace ACE inhibitors and ARBs in patients with heart failure.
- ACE inhibitors can be used in nursing mothers.
- Metoprolol, propranolol, or labetalol should be used instead of atenolol.

ACE, angiotensin-converting enzyme; *ARB*, angiotensin II receptor blocker; *LMWH*, low-molecular-weight heparin; *UFH*, unfractionated heparin.

---

20. **What is peripartum cardiomyopathy (PPCM)?**
    This is a syndrome of congestive heart failure diagnosed from the last month of pregnancy up to 5 months postpartum, with demonstration of reduced systolic function by echocardiogram, without identifiable or reversible cause. This is distinct from preexisting cardiac disease, which usually presents before the final month due to physiologic changes of pregnancy. Women with PPCM are treated with standard heart failure medications (hydralazine/nitrates while pregnant; ACE inhibitors after delivery). Prognosis is determined by degree of systolic function recovery. Maternal risk is higher during subsequent pregnancies if LV ejection fraction (EF) dysfunction (EF < 40%) persists. B-type natriuretic peptide (BNP) levels do not rise in a normal pregnancy; increased levels suggest cardiomyopathy, preeclampsia, eclampsia, and/or diabetes.

BIBLIOGRAPHY, SUGGESTED READINGS, AND WEBSITES

1. Bates SM, Greer IA, Middeldorp S, et al: VTE, thrombophilia, antithrombotic therapy, and pregnancy: antithrombotic therapy and prevention of thrombosis, ed 9: American College of Chest Physicians Evidence-Based Clinical Practice Guidelines, *Chest* 141:e691S–e736S, 2012.

2. Bédard E, Dimopoulos K, Gatzoulis MA: Has there been any progress made on pregnancy outcomes among women with pulmonary arterial hypertension? *Eur Heart J* 30:256–265, 2009.

3. Bonow RO, Carabello BA, Kanu C, et al: ACC/AHA Guidelines for management of patients with valvular heart disease, *Circulation* 114:493–496, 2006.

4. Drenthen W, Pieper P, Roos-Hesselink J, et al: Outcome of pregnancy in women with congenital heart disease: a literature review, *J Am Coll Cardiol* 49:2303–2311, 2007.

5. Elkayam U, Bitar F: Valvular heart disease in pregnancy, parts I (native) and II (prosthetic), *J Am Coll Cardiol* 46:223–230, 2005. 403-410.

6. James AH, Brancazio LR, Price T: Aspirin and reproductive outcomes, *Obstet Gynecol Surv* 63:49–57, 2008.

7. Kusters DM, Lahsinoui HH, van de Post JA: Statin use during pregnancy: a systematic review and meta-analysis, *Expert Rev Cardiovasc Ther* 10:363–378, 2012.

8. Reimold SC, Rutherford JD: Clinical practice: valvular heart disease in pregnancy, *N Eng J Med* 349:52–59, 2003.

9. Weiss BM, Zemp L, Seifert B, et al: Outcome of pulmonary vascular disease in pregnancy: a systematic overview from 1978 through 1996, *J Am Coll Cardiol* 31:1650–1657, 1998.

10. Wilson W, Taubert K, Gewitz M, et al: Prevention of infective endocarditis: Guidelines from the AHA, *Circulation* 116:1736–1754, 2007.

CHAPTER 52

HYPERTENSIVE CRISIS

*Anish K. Agarwal, MD, MPH, Christopher J. Rees, MD, and
Charles V. Pollack, MA, MD, FACEP, FAAEM, FAHA*

1. **What is a hypertensive crisis?**

   The term *hypertensive crisis* generally is inclusive of two different diagnoses, *hypertensive emergency* and *hypertensive urgency*. Distinguishing between the two is important because they require different intensities of therapy. It should be noted that older and less specific terminology, such as "malignant hypertension" and "accelerated hypertension," should no longer be used. The Seventh Report of the Joint National Committee on Prevention, Detection, Evaluation, and Treatment of High Blood Pressure (JNC-7) defines hypertensive emergency as being "characterized by severe elevations in blood pressure (more than 180/120 mm Hg), complicated by evidence of impending or progressive target organ dysfunction." JNC-7 defines hypertensive urgency as "those situations associated with severe elevations in blood pressure without progressive target organ dysfunction." There is no absolute value of blood pressure that defines a hypertensive urgency or emergency or separates the two syndromes. Instead, the most important distinction is whether there is evidence of impending or progressive end-organ damage, which defines an emergency, or other symptoms that are felt referable to the blood pressure.

2. **How commonly do these situations occur?**

   It is estimated that 50 to 75 million people have hypertension and that 1% to 2% of those will have a hypertensive emergency. In the elderly (>65 years of age), essential hypertension accounts for 424,000 emergency department (ED) visits per year, with an estimated 0.5% of all ED visits attributed to hypertensive crises.

3. **What are the causes of hypertensive crisis?**

   The most common cause of hypertensive emergency is an abrupt increase in blood pressure in patients with chronic hypertension. Medication noncompliance is a frequent cause of such changes. Blood pressure control rates for patients diagnosed with hypertension are less than 50%. The elderly and African Americans are at increased risk of developing a hypertensive emergency. Other causes of hypertensive emergencies include stimulant intoxication (cocaine, methamphetamine, and phencyclidine), withdrawal syndromes (clonidine, β-adrenergic blockers), pheochromocytoma, physiologic stress in the postoperative period (following cardiothoracic, vascular, or neurosurgical procedures), and adverse drug interactions with monoamine oxidase (MAO) inhibitors.

4. **What are the common clinical presentations of hypertensive crisis?**

   Typical presentations include severe headache, shortness of breath, epistaxis, faintness, or severe anxiety. Clinical syndromes typically associated with hypertensive emergency include hypertensive encephalopathy, intracerebral hemorrhage, acute myocardial infarction, acute heart failure, pulmonary edema, unstable angina, dissecting aortic aneurysm, or preeclampsia/eclampsia. Note that in hypertensive emergency presentations, there is evidence of impending or progressive target organ dysfunction and that the absolute value of the blood pressure is not pathognomonic.

5. **What historical information should be obtained?**

   A thorough history, especially as it relates to prior hypertension, is important to obtain and document, as most patients with a hypertensive emergency carry a diagnosis of hypertension and are either inadequately treated or are noncompliant with treatment.

   A thorough medication history is also essential. The patient's current medications need to be reviewed and updated to include timing, dosages, recent changes in therapy, last doses taken, and compliance. Patients should also be questioned about over-the-counter medication usage and recreational drug use because these agents may also affect blood pressure.

6. **How should the physical examination be focused?**
   Physical examination should start with recording the blood pressure in both arms with an appropriately sized blood pressure cuff. Direct ophthalmoscopy should be performed with attention to evaluating for papilledema and hypertensive exudates. A brief, focused neurologic examination to assess mental status and the presence or absence of focal neurologic deficits should be performed. The cardiopulmonary examination should focus on signs of pulmonary edema and aortic dissection, such as rales, elevated jugular venous pressure, or cardiac gallops. Peripheral pulses should be palpated and assessed. Abdominal examination should include palpation for abdominal masses and tenderness, and auscultation for abdominal bruits.

7. **What laboratory and ancillary data should be obtained?**
   All patients should have an electrocardiogram performed to assess for left ventricular hypertrophy, acute ischemia or infarction, and arrhythmias. Urinalysis should be performed to evaluate for hematuria and proteinuria as signs of acute renal failure. Women of child-bearing age should have a urine pregnancy test performed. Laboratory studies should include a basic metabolic profile with blood urea nitrogen (BUN) and creatinine, a urine or serum toxicology screen, and a complete blood cell count (CBC) with a peripheral smear to evaluate for signs of microangiopathic hemolytic anemia. If acute coronary syndrome is suspected, cardiac biomarkers should be assessed. Choice of radiographic studies, if any, should be based on the presentation and diagnostic considerations. A chest radiograph is often ordered to evaluate for pulmonary edema, cardiomegaly, and mediastinal widening. If there are any focal neurologic findings, a computed tomography (CT) scan of the brain should be performed to evaluate for hemorrhage.

8. **What are the cardiac manifestations of hypertensive emergencies?**
   Cardiac manifestations of hypertensive emergency include acute coronary syndromes, acute cardiogenic pulmonary edema, and aortic dissection. The latter deserves special attention because it has much higher short-term morbidity and mortality, requires more urgent and rapid reduction in blood pressure, and also requires specific inhibition of the reflex tachycardia often associated with blood pressure–lowering agents. It is recommended that patients with aortic dissection have their systolic blood pressure reduced to at least 120 mm Hg within 20 minutes, a much more rapid decrease than is recommended for other syndromes associated with hypertensive emergency.

9. **What are the central nervous system manifestations of hypertensive emergency?**
   Neurologic emergencies associated with hypertensive emergency include subarachnoid hemorrhage, cerebral infarction, intraparenchymal hemorrhage, and hypertensive encephalopathy. Patients with hemorrhage and infarction usually have focal neurologic findings and may have corresponding findings on head CT or magnetic resonance imaging (MRI) of the brain. Hypertensive encephalopathy is more difficult to diagnose; symptoms may include severe headache, vomiting, drowsiness, confusion, visual disturbances, and seizures; coma may ensue. Papilledema is often present on physical examination.

10. **What are the renal manifestations of hypertensive emergencies?**
    Renal failure can both cause and be caused by hypertensive emergency. Typically, hypertensive renal failure presents as nonoliguric renal failure, often with hematuria.

11. **What are the pregnancy-related issues with hypertensive emergency?**
    Preeclampsia is a syndrome that includes hypertension, peripheral edema, and proteinuria in women after the twentieth week of gestation. Eclampsia is the more severe form of the syndrome, with severe hypertension, edema, proteinuria, and seizures.

12. **What are general issues in the treatment of hypertensive urgency?**
Patients with hypertensive urgencies often have elevated blood pressure and nonspecific symptoms, but no evidence of progressive end-organ damage. These patients do not often require urgent treatment with parenteral antihypertensives. There is no evidence to suggest that urgent treatment of patients with hypertensive urgencies in an ED setting reduces morbidity or mortality. In fact, there is evidence that too-rapid treatment of asymptomatic hypertension has adverse effects. Rapidly lowering blood pressure below the autoregulatory range of an organ system (most importantly the cerebral, renal, or coronary beds) can result in reduced perfusion, leading to ischemia and infarction. It is usually appropriate in these situations instead to gradually reduce blood pressure over 24 to 48 hours. Most patients with hypertensive urgency can be treated as outpatients, but some may need to be admitted, as dictated by symptoms and situation and to ensure close follow-up and compliance. The most important intervention for hypertensive urgency is to ensure good follow-up, which helps to promote ongoing, long-term control of blood pressure. No guidelines and no evidence support a specific blood pressure *target* number that must be achieved in order to safely discharge a patient with hypertensive urgency.

13. **What are general issues in treating hypertensive emergencies?**
JNC-7 recommends that patients with hypertensive emergencies be treated as inpatients in an intensive care setting with an initial goal of reducing mean arterial blood pressure by 10% to 15%, but no more than 25%, in the first hour and then, if stable, to a goal of 160/100-110 mm Hg within the next 2 to 6 hours. This requires parenteral agents. Aortic dissection is a special situation that requires reduction of the systolic blood pressure to at least 120 mm Hg within 20 minutes. Treatment is also required to help blunt the reflex tachycardia associated with most antihypertensive agents. Ischemic stroke and intracranial hemorrhage are also special situations, and guidelines exist for the treatment of hypertension in these settings from multiple experts, including guidelines from the American Stroke Association/American Heart Association (ASA/AHA). These guidelines state that "there is little scientific evidence and no clinically established benefit for rapid lowering of blood pressure among persons with acute ischemic stroke." Too rapid a decline in blood pressure during the first 24 hours after presentation of an intracranial hemorrhage has been independently associated with increased mortality. The overall weight of evidence currently supports only judicious use of antihypertensive agents in the treatment of acute ischemic or hemorrhagic stroke. Expert guidance is recommended, especially if fibrinolytic therapy is being considered for acute ischemic stroke.

14. **What specific agents are used for treating patients with hypertensive emergencies?**
Table 52-1 reviews specific agents available for use.

15. **Are different agents more helpful for different clinical situations?**
Table 52-2 reviews specific agents recommended for specific situations.

TABLE 52-1. PARENTERAL AGENTS FOR USE IN HYPERTENSIVE EMERGENCIES							
Drug	Class/Mechanism	Usual Dose	Onset	Duration	Advantages	Disadvantages/Adverse Effects	Common Uses
Sodium nitroprusside	Direct arterial and venous vasodilator via cGMP	0.25-10 mcg/kg/min Average effective dose 3 mcg/kg/min	1-2 min	3-4 min after infusion stopped	Large amount of experience with use	Nausea, vomiting, muscle twitching, diaphoresis Cyanide toxicity, especially with renal insufficiency and prolonged infusions (>48 hr) Inactivated by light, needs to be given in light-protected delivery system Usually requires invasive intraarterial blood pressure monitoring Use cautiously with ↑ ICP as can worsen Use cautiously in ACS as can cause coronary steal	Has been used in all syndromes of hypertensive emergencies (HE)
Clevidipine	Ultra–short-acting dihydropyridine calcium channel blocker	2-16 mcg/kg/min or 1 mg/hour titrated to maximum of 21 mg/hour	1-5 min	T½ 1 min, effect lasts 5-10 min after infusion stopped	Ultra–short-acting with rapid onset, offset of effect Little to no reflex tachycardia Metabolism independent of renal and hepatic function Arterial line not required No special delivery system needed, used with peripheral IV access	Contraindicated in severe aortic stenosis due to possible decrease in myocardial oxygen delivery	Studied in postoperative hypertension, post–cardiac surgery, and emergency department treatment of HE Potentially useful for all types of HE syndromes

Drug	Mechanism	Dose	Onset	Offset	Effect	Adverse effects	Comments
Fenoldopam	Peripheral, dopamine-1 receptor agonist, causes vasodilation especially in renal, cardiac, splanchnic beds	0.1 mcg/kg/min to max 1.6 mcg/kg/min Titrate in 0.05-0.1 mcg/kg/min increments	10 min Max effect in 30 min	1 hr after infusion stopped	Increases renal blood flow, improving CrCl especially in setting of impaired renal function Used without invasive BP monitoring	Reflex tachycardia HA, dizziness, flushing, nausea Worsening angina Atrial fibrillation Tachyphylaxis after 48 hr Contraindicated in glaucoma as causes dose-related increase in IOP	Especially useful in HE syndromes complicated by renal insufficiency or failure
Nicardipine	Dihydropyridine calcium channel blocker Vasodilator	5 mg/hr, can ↑ by 2.5 mg/hr to max 15 mg/hr	≤10 min	2-6 hr after infusion stopped	Dilates coronary vessels, can use with known CAD Used without invasive BP monitoring	HA, flushing, dizziness, hypotension, digital dysesthesias Abrupt withdrawal can cause or worsen angina or hypertension Metabolized in liver, use with caution in cirrhotics	Has been used extensively in postoperative hypertension, especially after CT surgery
Nitroglycerin	Direct venous vasodilator	5 mcg/min to max 400 mcg/min	2-5 min	5-10 min	Dilates coronary vessels	Ineffective arterial vasodilator HA, hypotension, tachycardia	Not used for most HE, reserved for cardiac ischemia and cardiogenic pulmonary edema
Enalaprilat	ACE inhibitor	1.25 mg IV at 4-6 hr intervals, max 5 mg in 6 hr	15 min to 4 hr to peak effect	12-24 hr		BP response variable, unpredictable, and not dose-related May not peak for 4 hr Contraindicated in pregnancy	Not generally useful for HE syndromes
Hydralazine	Direct arterial vasodilator	10-20 mg IV	10-20 min	1-4 hr	Increases uterine blood flow	Flushing, HA, nausea Significant reflex tachycardia Has precipitated MI Use cautiously in CKD, CAD, CVD	Used only for eclampsia/preeclampsia

Continued

TABLE 52-1. PARENTERAL AGENTS FOR USE IN HYPERTENSIVE EMERGENCIES *(continued)*

Drug	Class/Mechanism	Usual Dose	Onset	Duration	Advantages	Disadvantages/Adverse Effects	Common Uses
Esmolol	Selective β_1-adrenoceptor blocker	Load 250-500 mcg/kg over 1-3 min Can infuse at 50-100 mcg/kg/min Titrate every 5 min with repeat bolus and ↑ drip by 50 mcg/kg/min to max dose 300 µg/kg/min	6-20 min after bolus Max effect 5 min	Effects last for 20 min after infusion stopped	Ultra-short-acting	Bradycardia Hypotension Bronchospasm Seizure Acute pulmonary edema Abrupt w/d can precipitate chest pain Requires central access, as extravasation can cause local tissue necrosis and can cause small vein phlebitis Use with caution in CKD	Often used in combination with vasodilators to reduce reflex tachycardia
Labetalol	Combined α- and β-adrenoceptor blocker	20 mg IV over 2 min Additional boluses every 10 min with escalating doses of 40, 80 mg to max, cumulative dose of 300 mg Can start infusion with 1-2 mg/min	2-5 min after bolus with peak in 5-15 min	2-4 hr after stopping infusion or last bolus	Decreases reflex tachycardia from other agents Does not affect cerebral blood flow Does not decrease cardiac blood flow or CO Does not affect renal function	Profound orthostasis Contraindicated in decompensated CHF, heart block, asthma, pheochromocytoma Can cause profound hypotension Dizziness, nausea, vomiting, paresthesias, scalp tingling, bronchospasm	Often used in combination with vasodilators to reduce reflex tachycardia associated with those agents

Phentolamine	Pure α-adrenergic antagonist	5-20 mg IV bolus every 5 min Can infuse at 0.2-0.5 mg/min	1-2 min	10-30 min	Used for catecholamine-induced HE	Significant tachycardia CAD, CVD, has caused or precipitated MI and stroke Contraindicated with history of significant arrhythmia Use cautiously in CKD Use cautiously or not at all if recent phosphodiesterase-5 inhibitor (sildenafil, tadalafil, vardenafil) use as can cause vasospasm	Used only for catecholamine-induced HE, such as cocaine-induced HE, pheochromocytoma, and MAOI tyramine–induced HE

ACS, Acute coronary syndrome; *BP*, blood pressure; *CAD*, coronary artery disease; *CHF*, congestive heart failure; *CKD*, chronic kidney disease; *CO*, cardiac output; *CrCl*, creatine clearance; *CT*, cardiothoracic; *CVD*, cardiovascular disease; *HA*, headache; *HE*, hypertensive emergency; *ICP*, intracranial pressure; *IOP*, intraocular pressure; *IV*, intravenous; *MAOI*, monoamine oxidase inhibitor; *max*, maximum; *MI*, myocardial infarction.

TABLE 52-2. SPECIFIC ANTIHYPERTENSIVE AGENTS SUGGESTED FOR SPECIFIC HYPERTENSIVE EMERGENCY SYNDROMES

Syndrome	Suggested Anti hypertensive Agents
Aortic dissection	Nitroprusside, often in combination with esmolol, labetalol Nicardipine with β-blocker β-Blocker alone
Acute pulmonary edema	Nitroglycerin preferred Fenoldopam Nicardipine Clevidipine
Acute coronary syndrome	β-Blocker Nitroglycerin Clevidipine
HE with acute or chronic renal failure	Labetalol Nicardipine Fenoldopam Clevidipine
Eclampsia	Labetalol Nicardipine Hydralazine (all in conjunction with magnesium sulfate)
Acute ischemic stroke or ICH (If expert guidance deems BP control necessary)	Nicardipine Labetalol Clevidipine
Hypertensive encephalopathy	Clevidipine Labetalol Esmolol Nicardipine Fenoldopam Nitroprusside
Adrenergic crisis with HE	Phentolamine Nitroprusside β-Blocker

β-Blocker, beta-adrenergic blocking agent; *BP*, blood pressure; *HE*, hypertensive emergency; *ICH*, intracerebral hemorrhage.

BIBLIOGRAPHY, SUGGESTED READINGS, AND WEBSITE

1. Adams HP Jr, DelZoppo G, Alberts MJ, et al: Guidelines for the early management of adults with ischemic stroke: a guideline from the American Heart Association/American Stroke Association Council, Clinical Cardiology Council, Cerebrovascular Radiology and Intervention Council, and the Atherosclerotic Peripheral Vascular Disease and Quality of Care Outcomes in Research Interdisciplinary Working Groups, *Stroke* 38:1655–1711, 2007.

2. Amin A: Parenteral medication for hypertension with symptoms, *Ann Em Med* 51:S1–S15, 2008.

3. Elliott WJ: Clinical features in the management of selected hypertensive emergencies, *Prog Cardiovasc Dis* 48:316–325, 2006.

4. Flanigan JS, Vitberg D: Hypertensive emergencies and severe hypertension: what to treat, who to treat, and how to treat, *Med Clin North Am* 90:439–451, 2006.

5. Gray RO: Hypertension. In Marx JA, Hockberger RS, Walls RM, editors: *Rosen's emergency medicine: concepts and clinical practice*, ed 6, Philadelphia, 2006, Mosby.

6. Haas AR, Marik PE: Current diagnosis and management of hypertensive emergency, *Semin Dial* 19:502–512, 2006.

7. Hebert CJ, Vitdt DG: Hypertensive crises, *Prim Care* 35:475–487, 2008.

8. Marik PE, Varon J: Hypertensive crisis: challenges and management, *Chest* 131:1949–1962, 2007.

9. National Heart, Lung, Blood Institute: *Seventh report of the Joint National Committee on Prevention, Detection, Evaluation, and Treatment of High Blood Pressure (JNC-7). Publication no. NIH 03-5233*, Bethesda, Md, 2003, NHLBI. pp 54–55.

10. Qureshi AI, Bliwise DL, Bliwise NG, et al: Rate of 24-hour blood pressure decline and mortality after spontaneous intracerebral hemorrhage: a retrospective analysis with a random effects regression model, *Crit Care Med* 27:480–485, 1999.

11. Stewart DL, Feinstein SE, Colgan R: Hypertensive urgencies and emergencies, *Prim Care* 33:613–623, 2006.

12. Strandgaard S, Olesen J, Skinhoj E, et al: Autoregulation of brain circulation in severe arterial hypertension, *Br Med J* 1:507–510, 1973.

13. Zampaglione B, Pascale C, Marchisio M, et al: Hypertensive urgencies and emergencies: prevalence and clinical presentation, *Hypertension* 27:144–147, 1996.

CHAPTER 53

ORAL ANTICOAGULATION

Sarah A. Spinler, PharmD, BCPS (AQ Cardiology)

1. How does warfarin work?

Warfarin (and related coumarin compounds) inhibit the activity of hepatic vitamin K-2,3 epoxide, which is used to recycle the *active* form of vitamin K, vitamin K hydroquinone. Without sufficient vitamin K hydroquinone, clotting factors II, VII, IX, and X fail to be carboxylated, leaving them in an inactive state. The onset of warfarin anticoagulation is gradual and related to the elimination half-lives of the already synthesized active forms of these procoagulation factors. In addition to inhibiting the formation of active factors II, VII, IX, and X, warfarin also inhibits the vitamin K–dependent formation of two coagulation inhibitors, proteins C and S, which may temporarily create a relative procoagulant state until full anticoagulation is achieved. Warfarin is a racemic mixture of *S* and *R* isomers. The *S* isomer has more inhibitory activity and is metabolized primarily by cytochrome P-450 (CYP) isoform 2C9 (CYP2C9), which is the major source of drug interactions with warfarin. The *R* isomer is metabolized primarily by CYP3A4 and CYP1A2, resulting in additional drug interactions.

2. What are the clinical situations in which warfarin is used and at what anticoagulation intensity?

The intensity of anticoagulation with warfarin depends primarily on the indication for anticoagulation. These are given in Table 53-1.

3. What is the role of warfarin in preventing transient ischemic attack and stroke in a patient with a history of ischemic stroke?

For most patients with noncardioembolic ischemic stroke, the underlying pathophysiology is similar to that of acute coronary syndromes—that is, arterial atherothrombosis. Therefore, antiplatelet drugs, either alone or in combination, have been slightly superior to warfarin in comparative trials for stroke prevention. In addition, despite no clinical advantage, the warfarin patients experience much more major and minor bleeding. Thus, warfarin has no role in the treatment of ischemic stroke (class Ia recommendation from American College of Chest Physicians [ACCP] 2012 guidelines for antiplatelet therapy rather than oral anticoagulation).

4. How should unfractionated heparin (UFH), low-molecular-weight heparin (LMWH), or fondaparinux be overlapped with warfarin for acute treatment of venous thromboembolism?

Regardless of the parenteral agent chosen for initial anticoagulation, warfarin should be initiated on day 1 of treatment. Choice of dose must be individualized based on patient-specific factors (age, concurrent medications, nutrition status, and comorbidities). However, for most patients, 5 mg daily is an adequate starting dose. According to the ACCP's Antithrombotic Therapy and Prevention of Thrombosis, 9th edition, for younger, "healthier" patients, consideration may be given for initiating warfarin at 10 mg daily. UFH, LMWH, or fondaparinux should be overlapped with warfarin for a minimum of 4 to 5 days and until the international normalized ratio (INR) is therapeutic (INR more than 2.5 for 1 day, or more than 2.0 for 2 consecutive days). Recommended procedures for switching between warfarin and the newer oral anticoagulants dabigatran etexilate, apixaban, and rivaroxaban are reviewed in Question 14.

TABLE 53-1. INDICATIONS FOR ANTICOAGULATION WITH WARFARIN AND RECOMMENDED INTERNATIONAL NORMALIZED RATIO INTENSITY

Indication	Class and Source of Recommendation	INR Intensity
Stroke prevention in atrial fibrillation	AHA/ASA 2012 Scientific Advisory on Oral Anticoagulants for Stroke Prevention in Nonvalvular Atrial Fibrillation: ■ Class Ia recommendation ACCP 2012 Atrial Fibrillation guidelines: ■ Class 2B recommendation as a second line agent to dabigatran etexilate	2.0-3.0
Post-MI or LV Thrombus	HFSA 2010 Guidelines: ■ Class B strength of evidence for 3 months if symptomatic or symptomatic ischemic cardiomyopathy and recent large anterior wall myocardial infarction or left ventricular thrombus	From ACCF/AHA 2013 ST segment elevation myocardial infarction guidelines: ■ With 75-81 mg aspirin and/or clopidogrel, 2.0-2.5 From HFSA 2010 guidelines: ■ 2.0-3.0
DVT or PE Treatment	ACCP 2012 VTE Treatment guidelines: ■ Grade 2B recommendation as second line to LMWH for patients with active cancer ■ Grade 2B recommendation as preferred over dabigatran or rivaroxaban	■ Target 2.5 (range 2.0-3.0) for 3 months: Grade 1B if provoked by surgery; Grade 1B if first unprovoked; Grade 1B if bleeding risk is high; Grade 2B if provoked by nonsurgical transient risk factor ■ Target 2.5 (range 2.0-3.0) for more than 3 months: Grade 1B for second unprovoked VTE and low bleeding risk
Mechanical heart valves	ACCP 2012 Antithrombotic Therapy in Valvular Heart Disease Guidelines: ■ Grade 1A recommendation in rheumatic mitral disease when left atrial diameter is >55 mm or when left atrial thrombus ■ Grade 1A recommendation for recurrent stroke/TIA and patent foramen ovale ■ Grade 2C recommendation for 3 months following bioprosthetic mitral valve placement ■ Grade 1B recommendation for all mechanical valves	■ Target 2.5 (range 2.0-3.0) for 3 months for bioprosthetic mitral valve ■ Target 2.5 (range 2.0-3.0) for all mechanical aortic heart valves ■ Target 3.0 (range 2.5-3.5) for all mechanical mitral valves ■ Adding low dose aspirin 50-100 mg to warfarin for all mechanical heart valves for patients at low-risk of bleeding (Grade B recommendation)

ACCF, American College of Cardiology Foundation; *ACCP*, American College of Chest Physicians; *AHA*, American Heart Association; *ASA*, American Stroke Association; *DVT*, deep vein thrombosis; *ESC*, European Society of Cardiology; *HFSA*, Heart Failure Society of America; *INR*, international normalized ratio; *LV*, left ventricular; *MI*, myocardial infarction; *PE*, pulmonary embolism; *TIA*, transient ischemic attack; *VTE*, venous thromboembolism.

5. **What is the role of pharmacogenomics in warfarin dosing?**

Warfarin dosing is challenging, in part, because of the varied response and the wide range of doses required to achieve a therapeutic INR in an individual patient. Contributors to this variability are polymorphisms in the CYP2C9 metabolizing enzyme responsible for the majority of warfarin metabolism, and in the target enzyme for warfarin, vitamin K epoxide reductase. Patients with either or both of these genetic polymorphisms tend to be more sensitive to warfarin and require lower doses. As genetic testing for these polymorphisms becomes less expensive and more accessible, pharmacogenetic dose selection may allow for a shorter time to a therapeutic INR and reduced bleeding complications. For these reasons, the 2012 ACCP Guidelines recommend against pharmacogenetic testing for patients initiating warfarin at this time.

6. **How should warfarin be managed in patients who need surgery?**

For patients who need INR normalized before surgery, warfarin should be stopped 5 days before the surgery. Depending on the reason for anticoagulation, bridging may be necessary. The most common indications for bridging therapy are patients with mechanical valves and recent deep vein thrombosis (DVT) and/or pulmonary embolism (PE). These patients should receive full-dose subcutaneous (subcut) LMWH during the bridging period. The last dose of LMWH should be given no later than 24 hours before the procedure. LMWH should be resumed 24 to 48 hours (the next evening) after the procedure, depending on bleeding and thrombotic risks of the patient. Warfarin should be restarted within 12 to 24 hours after (evening of or next morning) of the procedure with risk somewhat mitigated by delayed onset of effect. The reader should be aware that, as with many drugs, although LMWH is not *approved* for bridging, it is often used for this purpose. Different practitioners will have different thresholds of confidence for the use of LMWH as a bridging agent. The most caution in exercising decisions regarding outpatient LMWH bridging versus inpatient intravenous UFH bridging should be in patients with mechanical mitral valves (as the low pressure gradient between the left atrium and left ventricle during diastole may increase the risks of thrombosis compared with mechanical valves in the aortic position). A 2008 Guideline from the American College of Cardiology Foundation (ACCF) and American Heart Association (AHA) discusses bridging and the role of LMWH (see Suggested Readings).

For patients who need urgent surgery, it is recommended to give intravenous vitamin K, 5 to 10 mg. Fresh frozen plasma or other similar agents will give a more rapid (albeit temporary) reversal of anticoagulation therapy and can be combined with vitamin K. For patients with warfarin-associated major bleeding, prothrombin complex concentrates, rather than plasma are recommended for reversal, in combination with intravenous vitamin K.

Relatively minor surgeries, such as dental and dermatologic procedures, do not generally require the discontinuation of warfarin. Typically, any excess in bleeding related to those procedures can be managed with local hemostatic agents.

7. **What are some of the common drug interactions with warfarin?**

Because of its complex metabolism and relatively narrow therapeutic index, drug interactions involving warfarin are both common and clinically significant. The majority of the interactions occur at the level of CYP metabolism, although other mechanisms may be possible. Table 53-2 lists some of the more common interactions.

For the medications listed in Table 53-2, the strength of the clinical evidence is sufficient to expect a change in INR, requiring either adjusting the warfarin dose up or down by 25% to 50% in anticipation of the resulting change in INR, or frequent INR monitoring to determine the dose adjustment necessary.

Foods and supplements may also alter the INR. Foods that increase the INR include garlic, mango, ginseng, grapefruit juice, and possibly cranberry juice. Ginger and fish oil have additive antithrombotic effects. Foods and supplements that reduce the INR include high vitamin K–content foods, enteral feeds, and soy milk.

TABLE 53-2. COMMONLY ENCOUNTERED MEDICATIONS THAT INCREASE OR DECREASE WARFARIN'S INTERNATIONAL NORMALIZED RATIO

Medications that Increase INR	Proposed Mechanism	Medications that Decrease INR	Proposed Mechanism
Amiodarone	CYP3A4, CYP1A2 and CYP2C9 inhibitor	Carbamazepine	Induces CYP3A4
Cimetidine	CYP3A4 and CYP1A2 inhibitor	Methimazole	Unknown
Ciprofloxacin	CYP1A2 inhibitor	Nelfinavir	Unknown
Clarithromycin	CYP3A4 inhibitor	Nevirapine	CYP3A4 inducer
Cyclosporine	CYP3A4 substrate	Phenobarbital	Induces CYP3A4
Efavirenz	CYP2C9 inhibitor	Phenytoin	Induces CYP3A4
Erythromycin	CYP3A4 inhibitor	Rifampin	Induces CYP3A4 and CYP2C9
Fenofibric acid	CYP2C9 inhibitor	Ritonavir, Ritonavir/ lopinavir	CYP3A4 and CYP2C9 inducer
Fluconazole	CYP3A4 and CYP2C9 inhibitor		
Fluvastatin	CYP2C9 inhibitor		
Flourouracil	CYP2C9 inhibitor		
Fluvoxamine	CYP1A2 inhibitor		
Itraconazole	CYP3A4 inhibitor		
Ketoconazole	CYP3A4 inhibitor		
Levofloxacin	CYP1A2 inhibitor		
Lovastatin	CYP3A4 substrate		
Metronidazole	CYP3A4 inhibitor		
Miconazole	CYP3A4 inhibitor		
Nelfinavir	CYP3A4 inhibitor		
Phenytoin	CYP2C9 substrate		
Prednisone	CYP3A4 inhibitor		
Rosuvastatin	Unknown		
Saquinavir	CYP3A4 substrate and inhibitor		
Simvastatin	CYP3A4 substrate		
Sulfamethoxazole	CYP3A4 substrate		
Tamoxifen	CYP2C9 substrate		
Voriconazole	CYP3A4 and CYP2C9 inhibitor		

INR, International normalized ratio.

8. **How should warfarin be managed in patients with underlying chronic liver disease?**
Management of warfarin in patients with underlying significant liver disease can be difficult. In addition to elevated baseline INRs, these patients often have low protein stores, thrombocytopenia, and reduced hepatic clearance, making them especially sensitive to effects of warfarin and more likely to have significant bleeding issues. Recommendations include lower starting doses and more frequent laboratory and clinical monitoring.

9. **How should elevated INRs in patients taking warfarin be managed?**
If there is no overt evidence of bleeding and rapid reversal is not necessary, the 2012 ACCP guidelines recommend against routine vitamin K administration unless the INR is more than 10. For INRs less than 4.5 without bleeding, the guidelines recommend lowering the dose or holding the next dose with frequent INR monitoring until the INR is within the therapeutic range and then resuming a lower dose. For INRs 4.5 to 10 without bleeding, the 2012 ACCP guidelines recommend omitting 1 to 2 doses, frequent INR monitoring, and resuming a lower warfarin dose when the INR is within the therapeutic range. When the INR is greater than 10 without overt bleeding, the 2012 ACCP guidelines recommend low-dose (5 mg or less) oral vitamin K.

For patients experiencing minor bleeding with an elevated INR, oral vitamin K is recommended at a dose of 2.5 to 5 mg, repeated at 24 hour intervals until the INR is within the therapeutic range and then resuming a lower dose of warfarin.

10. **What are important patient counseling points for warfarin?**
A patient medication guide is mandated to be dispensed by pharmacists to patients receiving prescriptions for warfarin. Important counseling points are:
- Explain to patients the reason for warfarin therapy.
- Explain the meaning and significance of the INR.
- Identify each patient's warfarin prescriber, current INR, and date of next scheduled INR test.
- Explain the need for frequent INR testing and the target INR for each patient's medical condition(s).
- Explain the importance of compliance with therapy and related laboratory work (INR checks).
- Describe common sites and signs of bleeding and what to do if they occur. Explain that bleeding and bruising are more likely to occur and that common sites of bleeding include the gums, urinary tract, and nose. Patients should be aware of any changes in stool color and to report dark, tarry stools to the health care provider immediately. Patients should also report any uncontrolled bleeding to the health care provider.
- Counsel patients to avoid alcohol and activities or sports that may result in a fall or injury.
- Explain how consuming foods containing vitamin K may impact the effectiveness of warfarin therapy and that the most important thing concerning the diet is not to make any significant changes without talking to the health care provider.
- Explain to patients the importance of telling all health care providers that warfarin is being taken and that the health care provider prescribing warfarin needs to be informed of all scenarios where warfarin might need to be held (e.g., dental work, surgery, and other invasive procedures).
- Explain to patients the importance of contacting the pharmacy if the color of the warfarin tablet is different.
- Explain that warfarin should be taken at the same time each day and that if a dose is missed and it is within 12 hours of when the dose was supposed to be taken, it is okay to take the dose. Otherwise, the dose should be skipped and resumed the next day. The dose should not be doubled.
- Discuss potential drug interactions. Explain that patients should contact their warfarin prescriber before taking any over-the-counter medications (including herbal supplements) or if a different health care provider starts them on a new medication (especially antibiotics).
- Explain that women of child-bearing age must use birth control measures and notify their health care provider immediately if they become pregnant.
- Advise patients to carry identification noting that they are taking warfarin.
- Depending on the indication for warfarin, counsel patients on signs of clotting (e.g., calf pain, redness, swelling, shortness of breath, and stroke symptoms).
- Document that the patient education session has occurred.

11. **What are potential advantages of the newer oral anticoagulants dabigatran etexilate, apixaban, and rivaroxaban?**

Dabigatran etexilate, apixaban, and rivaroxaban are three newer oral anticoagulants which offer the following advantages over warfarin: quick onset of anticoagulant effects, no need for bridging, fewer drug interactions, and no routine anticoagulation monitoring. Dabigatran etexilate is an oral direct thrombin (factor IIa) inhibitor that is a prodrug hydrolyzed after absorption to form dabigatran, the active agent. Dabigatran is primarily eliminated renally (80%). Apixaban is a direct-acting factor Xa inhibitor that is renally excreted (27%) and hepatically metabolized (25% primarily by CYP3A4). Rivaroxaban is a direct-acting factor Xa inhibitor that is both metabolized (51% primarily by CYP3A4/5) and eliminated renally (36%). Dabigatran, apixaban, and rivaroxaban are substrates for the efflux transporter P-glycoprotein (P-gp), also known as multidrug resistance protein 1 (MDR1) or ATP-binding cassette subfamily B member 1 (ABCB1). As of this writing, dabigatran etexilate and rivaroxaban are U.S. Food and Drug Administration (FDA)-approved for stroke prevention in nonvalvular atrial fibrillation (NVAF) and rivaroxaban is FDA-approved for DVT prevention following hip and knee replacement surgery, for stroke prevention in NVAF, and treatment of DVT and pulmonary embolism. Dosing recommendations are described in Table 53-3. These newer anticoagulants should be avoided in patients with moderate to severe hepatic disease or in patients with hepatic disease showing signs of coagulopathy.

12. **What are current guideline recommendations for dabigatran etexilate, apixaban, and rivaroxaban in U.S. practice guidelines for stroke prevention in nonvalvular atrial fibrillation?**

Two current practice guidelines are available for management of stroke prevention in atrial fibrillation (AF), the 2012 ACCP guidelines and the 2012 AHA/American Stroke Association (ASA) guidelines. The 2012 ACCP guidelines do not include rivaroxaban or apixaban because they were not FDA-approved for stroke prevention in NVAF at the time of guideline writing. The 2012 ACCP guidelines recommend oral anticoagulation over aspirin in patients with a $CHADS_2$ score (see Fig. 34-1 and Table 34-1) of 2 or greater, and in particular, recommend dabigatran over warfarin anticoagulation. This recommendation is based on the results of a large randomized clinical trial showing that there are fewer strokes and intracranial hemorrhages with dabigatran, as well as similar rates of major bleeding and slightly higher gastrointestinal bleeding with dabigatran compared to warfarin. The 2012 AHA/ASA Science Advisory gives class I recommendations to warfarin, dabigatran, and apixaban for stroke prevention in AF in patients with at least one risk factor for stroke and to rivaroxaban for stroke prevention in AF in patients with at least two risk factors for stroke. The 2012 AHA/ASA Science Advisory recommends against using either dabigatran or rivaroxaban in patients with creatine clearance of less than 15 mL/min and against using apixaban in patients with creatinine clearance of less than 25 mL/min. Rivaroxaban was found to be noninferior to warfarin for both stroke prevention and major bleeding, but demonstrated a reduction in the frequency of intracranial hemorrhage in its large phase III randomized double-blind clinical trial in NVAF. Dabigatran 150 mg twice daily was superior to warfarin for stroke prevention (for both ischemic stroke and intracranial hemorrhage reduction) with similar major bleeding rates in its large Phase III open-label trial in NVAF. Apixaban demonstrated superiority in stroke prevention, reduction in intracranial hemorrhage risk and major bleeding, along with a reduction in total mortality in its Phase III randomized double blind trial compared to warfarin in NVAF. In another randomized, double-blind Phase III trial in patients with NVAF unsuitable for warfarin, apixaban reduced stroke with similar major bleeding compared to aspirin.

13. **What are some of the common drug interactions with dabigatran etexilate, apixaban, and rivaroxaban?**

Because dabigatran etexilate, apixaban, and rivaroxaban are P-glycoprotein 1 (P-gp) substrates, apixaban a substrate for CYP3A4, and rivaroxaban a substrate for CYP3A4/5, their serum concentrations may be increased by P-gp inhibitors, and apixaban and rivaroxaban concentrations increased by CYP3A4 inhibitors. Potential drug interactions and labeled warnings are listed in Table 53-4. Dabigatran etexilate should not be coadministered with P-gp inhibitors in patients with creatinine

TABLE 53–3. DOSING RECOMMENDATIONS FOR DABIGATRAN ETEXILATE AND RIVAROXABAN

Agent	Indication	Dose
Dabigatran etexilate	Stroke prevention in NVAF	CrCl > 30 mL/min: 150 mg po bid CrCl 15-30 mL/min: 75 mg po bid CrCl < 15 mL/min: avoid use Acute kidney injury: avoid use
	Can be crushed and administered via an oral nasogastric feeding tube	No
Rivaroxaban	Stroke prevention in NVAF	CrCl > 50 mL/min: 20 mg po daily with the evening meal CrCl 15-50 mL/min: 15 mg po daily with the evening meal CrCl < 15 mL/min: Avoid use
	Prophylaxis of DVT following hip or knee replacement surgery	10 mg po daily with or without food started at least 6 hr following surgery and once hemostasis has been achieved; patients with CrCl < 30 mL/min were excluded from clinical trials
	Treatment of DVT or PE and prevention of recurrence of DVT or PE	15 mg twice daily po with food for the first 21 days for initial treatment of acute DVT or PE followed by 20 mg po once daily with food for the duration of therapy CrCl < 30 mL/min: Avoid use
	Can be crushed and administered via an oral nasogastric feeding tube	Yes
Apixaban	Stroke prevention in NVAF	5 mg po bid Reduce dose to 2.5 mg PO bid if 2 of the following present: Either age ≥ 80 years, body weight ≤ 60 kg, or serum creatinine ≥ 1.5 mg/dL
	Can be crushed and administered via an oral nasogastric feeding tube	Yes

NVAF, Nonvalvular atrial fibrillation; *DVT*, deep vein thrombosis; *CrCl*, creatinine clearance; *PE*, pulmonary embolism.

clearance less than 30 mL/min. A dose reduction in dabigatran etexilate to 75 mg orally twice daily is recommended for patients with creatinine clearance less of 30 to 50 mL/min who are also taking dronedarone or systemic ketoconazole. Rifampin, a strong P-gp inducer should be avoided with dabigatran. Combined use of strong CYP3A4 inhibitors and P-gp inhibitors is contraindicated with rivaroxaban. The dose of apixaban should be reduced to 2.5 mg twice daily when it is coadministered with combined strong CYP3A4 and P-gp inhibitors such as ketoconaole, itraconazole, ritonavir, and clarithromycin. For patients initially prescribed apixaban 2.5 mg twice daily, combined use of strong dual CYP3A4 and P-gp inhibitors necessitates apixaban discontinuation and selection of another anticoagulant. Combined use of strong CYP3A4 inducers and P-gp inducers, such as rifampin, should be avoided with rivaroxaban and apixaban. Examples are provided in Table 53-4.

TABLE 53-4. **POTENTIAL DRUG INTERACTIONS WITH DABIGATRAN ETEXILATE, APIXABAN, AND RIVAROXABAN WHICH INCREASE OR DECREASE THEIR CONCENTRATIONS**

Apixaban and Rivaroxaban			
Strong CYP3A4 Inducers	**P-gp Inducers**	**Strong CYP3A4 Inhibitors**	**P-gp Inhibitors**
Carbamazepine	Carbamazepine	Clarithromycin	Amiodarone
Phenytoin	Phenytoin	Conivaptan	Conivaptan
Rifampin	Rifampin	Grapefruit juice (high-dose, double strength)	Clarithromycin
St. John's wort	Tipranavir/ritonavir	Indinavir	Cyclosporine
	St. John's wort	Itraconazole	Dronedarone
		Ketoconazole	Erythromycin
		Lopinavir/ritonavir	Indinavir/ritonavir
		Nefazodone	Lopinavir/ritonavir
		Nelfinavir	Itraconazole
		Posaconazole	Ketoconazole
		Ritonavir	Quinidine
		Saquinavir	Ritonavir
		Telaprevir	Verapamil
		Telithromycin	
		Voriconazole	
Dabigatran Etexilate			
	P-gp Inducers		**P-gp Inhibitors**
	Carbamazepine		Amiodarone
	Phenytoin		Conivaptan
	Rifampin		Clarithromycin
	Tipranavir/ritonavir		Cyclosporine
	St. John's wort		Dronedarone
			Erythromycin
			Indinavir/ritonavir
			Lopinavir/ritonavir
			Itraconazole
			Ketoconazole
			Quinidine
			Ritonavir
			Verapamil

P-gp, P-glycoprotein.

14. **How should patients taking dabigatran etexilate, apixiban, or rivaroxaban be transitioned to and from other anticoagulants?**

One of the major advantages of the newer oral anticoagulants is their rapid onset and offset of effect. The onset of anticoagulant effect with dabigatran etexilate, apixaban, and rivaroxaban is rapid. Peak concentration, and thus complete anticoagulant effect for dabigatran etexilate, is achieved in 1 hour in the fasting state and by 2 hours following a meal, in 2 to 3 hours following apixaban, and in 2 to 4 hours following rivaroxaban. Recommendations for switching between warfarin and either dabigatran, apixaban, or rivaroxaban as well as between an injectable anticoagulant are described in Table 53-5. For patients discontinuing dabigatran, these recommendations include monitoring renal function, as drug clearance (and thus clearance of anticoagulant effect) is delayed in patients with acute kidney injury or chronic kidney disease. Switching between rivaroxaban, apixaban, and dabigatran has not been studied, but practicality indicates that first doses may be administered at the time the dose of the discontinued agent would be administered.

15. **What is the effect of dabigatran etexilate, apixaban, and rivaroxaban on coagulation tests and can they be monitored?**

Dabigatran etexilate, apixaban, and rivaroxaban have predictable anticoagulation effects following fixed-dose administration, and therefore routine coagulation monitoring is not recommended at this time in any patient population.

Dabigatran etexilate, apixaban, and rivaroxaban affect several common coagulation tests. Unlike warfarin, which impacts the formation of clotting factors and therefore its effects are long-lasting, newer oral anticoagulant impact the coagulation tests in a concentration- and time-dependent manner, that is, peak effects on coagulation tests occur at the time of peak drug concentration and then diminish over time. Therefore, the degree of abnormality of the coagulation test depends on the time the test was drawn after the patient took their last dose. Following dabigatran etexilate administration, more than twofold prolongations in activated partial thromboplastin time (aPTT) may be observed. Dabigatran, apixaban, and rivaroxaban increase the prothrombin time (PT) with the PT being more sensitive to apixaban and rivaroxaban than dabigatran at concentrations achieved in vivo. INRs are not interpretable following apixaban, rivaroxaban, or dabigatran and its elevation cannot be interpreted as a risk factor for bleeding, as is the case with warfarin. Differences in effects are also observed between different brands of reagents for the different coagulation tests. Therefore, elevations in either aPTT or PT or INR above baseline (control) should be interpreted as indicating presence of drug, but the risk of bleeding cannot be assessed. Values within the normal range should *not* be interpreted as the patient having normal coagulation.

There is early research suggesting that the preferred coagulation test for determining accumulation of dabigatran concentrations may be the dilute thrombin time (dTT), with trough dTT concentrations of more than 200 ng/mL suggesting increased bleeding risk.

Because apixaban and rivaroxaban are factor Xa inhibitors, the preferred monitoring test measures anti–factor Xa activity levels, but tests are not readily available and there is no guidance on interpretation of their results at this time.

16. **Can the anticoagulant effect of dabigatran etexilate, apixaban, and rivaroxaban be reversed?**

At this time, there is insufficient data and experience to recommend any methods of reversing the anticoagulant effects of dabigatran etexilate, apixaban, or rivaroxaban. Administration of activated charcoal is recommended if less than 2 hours has passed since the anticoagulant has been ingested. Hemodialysis removes about 60% of dabigatran over a 2 to 3 hour dialysis session and should be initiated immediately for life-threatening bleeding in a patient with recent dabigatran exposure. Administration of fresh frozen plasma alone is ineffective and not recommended. A four-factor prothrombin complex concentrate (PCC) containing clotting factors II, VII, IX, and X, has shown reversal of prolonged PTs in healthy volunteers given rivaroxaban, and in animal models with dabigatran. However, the only available PCC in the U.S. at this time is a three-factor PCC, which has a lower concentration of factor VII. Recombinant factor VIIa (rVIIa) administration has demonstrated partial reversal of thrombin generation due to rivaroxaban in an in vitro

TABLE 53-5. CONVERTING FROM OR TO PARENTERAL ANTICOAGULANTS AND WARFARIN WITH DABIGATRAN ETEXILATE, APIXABAN, AND RIVAROXABAN

Switching From	Switching to	Recommendation
Unfractionated heparin	Dabigatran etexilate	Give first dose at time heparin is discontinued.
	Rivaroxaban	Give first dose at time heparin is discontinued.
	Apixaban	Give first dose at time heparin is discontinued.
LMWH	Dabigatran etexilate	Give first dose at time next LMWH dose is due.
	Rivaroxaban	Give first dose at time next LMWH dose is due.
	Apixaban	Give first dose at time next LMWH dose is due.
Warfarin	Dabigatran etexilate	Monitor INR; start dabigatran when INR < 2.0.
	Rivaroxaban	Monitor INR; start rivaroxaban when INR < 3.0.
	Apixaban	Monitor INR; start apixaban when INR < 2.0.
Dabigatran etexilate	Unfractionated heparin	For CrCl ≥ 30 mL/min start UFH 12 hours after last dose dabigatran. For CrCl < 30 mL/min, start UFH 24 hours after last dose of dabigatran.
	LMWH	For CrCl ≥ 30 mL/min give first injection 12 hours after last dose dabigatran. For CrCl < 30 mL/min, give first injection 24 hours after last dose of dabigatran.
	Warfarin	For CrCl ≥ 50 mL/min - start warfarin 3 days before discontinuing dabigatran. For CrCl 30-50 mL/min - start warfarin 2 days before discontinuing dabigatran. For CrCl 15-30 mL/min - start warfarin 1 day before discontinuing dabigatran.
	Rivaroxaban	Not studied; give first dose at the time of the next scheduled dabigatran dose.
	Apixaban	Give first dose at the time of the next scheduled dabigatran dose.
Rivaroxaban	Unfractionated heparin	Start UFH at time of the next scheduled rivaroxaban dose.
	LMWH	Give first injection at the time of the next scheduled rivaroxaban dose.
	Warfarin	Use parenteral anticoagulant bridge.
	Dabigatran etexilate	Give first dose at the time of the next scheduled rivaroxaban dose.
	Apixaban	Give first dose at the time of the next scheduled rivaroxaban dose.
Apixaban	Unfractionated heparin	Start UFH at the time of the next scheduled apixaban dose.
	LMWH	Give first injection at the time of the next scheduled apixaban dose.
	Warfarin	Use parenteral anticoagulation bridge.
	Dabigatran etexilate	Give first dose at the time of the next scheduled apixaban dose.
	Rivaroxaban	Give first dose at the time of the next scheduled apixaban dose.

CrCl, Creatinine clearance; *INR*, international normalized ratio; *LMWH*, low-molecular-weight heparin; *UFH*, unfractionated heparin.

model but does not reverse the effects of dabigatran. Low-dose anticoagulant inhibitor complex (factor VIII inhibitor bypassing activity FEIBA NF; Baxter Bioscience, Deerfield, Ill.) has demonstrated reversal of endogenous thrombin potential, maximum concentration, lag-time, and time to reach maximum concentration of thrombin after both dabigatran and rivaroxaban administration in an ex vivo healthy volunteer study. However, higher doses of FEIBA increased thrombin generation in this study, and administration of any clotting factor heightens all thromboembolic risk, so the best advice in the case of significant bleeding associated with any of the new oral anticoagulants is to discontinue the anticoagulant and consult with a hematology anticoagulation specialist.

17. **What are the important counseling points for patients taking dabigatran etexilate?**

The manufacturers of dabigatran etexilate, apixaban, and rivaroxaban have web sites with patient medication and disease state information, discount insurance co-pay cards, and options for improving medication adherence. A patient medication guide is mandated to be dispensed by pharmacists to patients receiving prescriptions for dabigatran etexilate. Important counseling points are:

- Explain to patients that dabigatran is being taken for stroke prevention in NVAF.
- Explain that dabigatran etexilate may cause gastrointestinal upset and that if it occurs, patients may take the medication with food to minimize effect.
- For patients with a prior history of taking warfarin, explain that dabigatran may affect the INR blood test, but that test is not used for monitoring the level of anticoagulation.
- Explain the importance of compliance with therapy.
- Describe common sites and signs of bleeding and what to do if they occur. Explain that bleeding and bruising are more likely to occur and that common sites of bleeding include the gums, urinary tract, and nose. Patients should be aware of any changes in stool color and to report dark, tarry stools to the health care provider immediately. Patients should also report any uncontrolled bleeding to the health care provider.
- Counsel patients to avoid alcohol and activities or sports that may result in a fall or injury.
- Explain to patients the importance of telling all health care providers that dabigatran etexilate is being taken and that the health care provider prescribing dabigatran needs to be informed of all scenarios where dabigatran might need to be held (e.g., dental work, surgery, and other invasive procedures).
- Explain that dabigatran should be taken at the same time each day and that if a dose is missed and it is within 6 hours of when the dose was supposed to be taken, it is okay to take the dose. Otherwise, the dose should be skipped. The dose should not be doubled.
- Discuss potential drug interactions. Explain that patients should contact their dabigatran prescriber before taking any over-the-counter medications (including herbal supplements) or if a different health care provider starts them on a new medication. Avoid taking nonsteroidal antiinflammatory drugs, including aspirin, with dabigatran.
- Discuss the need for periodic monitoring of blood tests for kidney function.
- Women of child-bearing age must notify their health care provider immediately if they become pregnant.
- Advise patients to carry identification noting that they are taking dabigatran etexilate.
- Advise each patient to date the bottle label when opening, and to discard any unused capsules after 4 months.
- Counsel patients on signs of stroke symptoms.
- Document that the patient education session has occurred.

18. **What are the important counseling points for patients taking apixaban and rivaroxaban?**

A patient medication guide is mandated to be dispensed by pharmacists to patients receiving prescriptions for apixaban and rivaroxaban. Important counseling points are:

- Explain to patients the reason that apixaban or rivaroxaban is being taken.

- For patients with a prior history of taking warfarin, explain that may affect the PT/INR blood test, but the test is not used for monitoring the level of anticoagulation.
- Explain the importance of compliance with therapy.
- Describe common sites and signs of bleeding and what to do if they occur. Explain that bleeding and bruising are more likely to occur and that common sites of bleeding include the gums, urinary tract, and nose. Patients should be aware of any changes in stool color and should report dark, tarry stools to the health care provider immediately. Patients should also report any uncontrolled bleeding to the health care provider.
- Counsel patients to avoid alcohol and activities or sports that may result in a fall or injury.
- Explain to patients the importance of telling all health care providers that apixaban or rivaroxaban is being taken and that the health care provider prescribing rivaroxaban needs to be informed of all scenarios where rivaroxaban might need to be held (e.g., dental work, surgery, and other invasive procedures).
- Explain that apixaban or rivaroxaban should be taken at the same time each day and that if a dose is missed it may be taken on the same day as soon as it is remembered, otherwise resume the medication the next day.
- Explain that doses of rivaroxaban 15 mg or 20 mg must be taken with a meal and that doses of 10 mg may be taken without regard to meals. Apixaban may be taken with or without food.
- Discuss potential drug interactions. Explain that patients should contact their apixaban or rivaroxaban prescriber before taking any over-the-counter medications (including herbal supplements) or if a different health care provider starts them on a new medication. Avoid taking nonsteroidal antiinflammatory drugs, including aspirin, with either apixaban or rivaroxaban.
- Discuss the need for periodic monitoring of blood tests for kidney function.
- Women of child-bearing age must notify their health care provider immediately if they become pregnant.
- Advise patients to carry identification noting that they are taking rivaroxaban.
- Depending on the indication apixaban or for rivaroxaban, counsel patients on signs of clotting (e.g., calf pain, redness, swelling, shortness of breath, or stroke symptoms).
- Document that the patient education session has occurred.
- For acute treatment of VTE, counsel the patient that the initial rivaroxaban dose of 15 mg twice daily will need to be reduced to 20 mg once daily after 21 days of treatment.
- Patient information and resources for the prescriber, including discount.

19. **What is the safety of using combination antiplatelet therapy in a patient requiring warfarin, dabigatran etexilate, apixaban, or rivaroxaban as well?**

The post–myocardial infarction (MI) patient and stented patient on combination antiplatelet therapy will often develop a clinical condition, such as atrial fibrillation, requiring the addition of warfarin therapy. Unfortunately, there are limited prospective data from clinical trials that accurately assess the bleeding risk of so-called "triple antithrombotic" with warfarin plus combination antiplatelet therapy. From the available data, it appears the risk for a major bleed exceeds the additive risk of the individual agents. Therefore, recommendations to reduce bleeding risk include (1) using the smallest dose of aspirin as soon as clinically feasible; (2) using warfarin plus clopidogrel and omitting aspirin (after initial triple therapy following stent placement); (3) considering the use of bare-metal stents to reduce the exposure time to combination antiplatelet therapy; (4) using a tighter INR range of 2.0 to 2.5; and (5) performing more frequent INR testing for these patients at high risk for bleeding complications. None of these recommendations has been validated in large prospective randomized studies.

Because of limited clinical experience with dabigatran plus dual antiplatelet therapy, and because of higher rates of bleeding and intracranial hemorrhage with either apixaban or rivaroxaban plus aspirin and clopidogrel, these combinations are not recommended at this time.

There is insufficient information on use of warfarin (as well as dabigatran etexilate, apixaban, and rivaroxaban) in patients taking aspirin plus either prasugrel or ticagrelor. Product labeling for these two newer oral $P2Y_{12}$-inhibitor antiplatelet agents specifically advise against their use with warfarin. Thus, clopidogrel is the preferred $P2Y_{12}$ inhibitor for use in a patient requiring aspirin plus anticoagulation with warfarin.

BIBLIOGRAPHY, SUGGESTED READINGS, AND WEBSITES

1. *Agency for Healthcare Research and Quality: Blood thinner pills: your guide to using them safely.* Available at: http://www. ahrq.gov/consumer/btpills.htm. Accessed Sep 10, 2012.

2. Bonow RO, Carabello BA, Chatterjee K, et al: 2008 Focused update incorporated into the ACC/AHA 2006 guidelines for the management of patients with valvular heart disease: a report of the American College of Cardiology/American Heart Association Task Force on Practice Guidelines (Writing Committee to Revise the 1998 Guidelines for the Management of Patients With Valvular Heart Disease): endorsed by the Society of Cardiovascular Anesthesiologists, Society for Cardiovascular Angiography and Interventions, and Society of Thoracic Surgeons, *Circulation* 118:e523–e661, 2008.

3. Dewilde WJM, Oirbans T, Verheugt FWA, et al: *Use of clopidogrel with or without aspirin in patients taking oral anticoagulant therapy and undergoing percutaneous coronary intervention: an open-label, randomised controlled trial, Lancet*, published online February 13, 2013. Available at: http://dx.doi.org/10.1016/S0140-6736(12)62177-1 Accessed March 4, 2013.

4. Douketis JD, Spyropoulos AC, Spencer FA, et al: Perioperative management of antithrombotic therapy: Antithrombotic Therapy and Prevention of Thrombosis, ed 9: American College of Chest Physicians Evidence-Based Clinical Practice Guidelines, *Chest* 141(Suppl 2):e326S–e350S, 2012. Erratum in: *Chest* 2012 141 1129.

5. Eerenberg ES, Kamphuisen PW, Sijpkens MK, et al: Reversal of rivaroxaban and dabigatran by prothrombin complex concentrate: a randomized, placebo-controlled, crossover study in healthy subjects, *Circulation* 124:1573–1579, 2011.

6. *Eliquis (apixaban) prescribing information*, Bristol-Myers Squibb Company, Princeton, NJ, December 2012.

7. *European Medicines Agency: Questions and answers on the review of bleeding risk with Pradaxa (dabigatran etexilate).* Available at: http://www.ema.europa.eu/docs/en_GB/document_library/Medicine_QA/2012/05/WC50012 7768.pdf. Accessed Sep 10, 2012.

8. Faxon DP, Eikelboom JW, Berger PB, et al: Antithrombotic therapy in patients with atrial fibrillation undergoing coronary stenting: a North American perspective: executive summary, *Circ Cardiovasc Interven* 4:522–534, 2011.

9. Furie KL, Goldstein LB, Albers GW, et al: Oral antithrombotic agents for prevention of stroke in nonvalvular atrial fibrillation: a science advisory for healthcare professionals from the American Heart Association/American Stroke Association, *Stroke* 43:3442–3453, 2012.

10. Guyatt GH, Akl EA, Crowther M, et al: Executive summary: Antithrombotic Therapy and Prevention of Thrombosis, ed 9: American College of Chest Physicians Evidence-Based Clinical Practice Guidelines, *Chest* 141(Suppl 2):7S–47S, 2012.

11. Kaatz M, Kouides PA, Garcia DA: Guidance on the emergent reversal of oral thrombin and factor Xa inhibitors, *Am J Hematol* 87:S141–S145, 2012.

12. Kearon C, Akl AL, Comorota AJ, et al: Antithrombotic therapy for VTE disease: Antithrombotic Therapy and Prevention of Thrombosis, ed 9: American College of Chest Physicians Evidence-Based Clinical Practice Guidelines, *Chest* 141(Suppl 2):e419S–e494S, 2012.

13. Lansberg MG, O'Donnell MJ, Khatri P, et al: Antithrombotic and thrombolytic therapy for ischemic stroke: Antithrombotic Therapy and Prevention of Thrombosis, ed 9: American College of Chest Physicians Evidence-Based Clinical Practice Guidelines, *Chest* 141(Suppl 2):e601–e636S, 2012.

14. Lindenfeld J, Albert NM, Boehmer JP, et al: HFSA 2010 comprehensive heart failure practice guideline, *J Card Fail* 16:e1–e194, 2010.

15. Marlu R, Enkelejda H, Paris A, et al: Effect of non-specific reversal agents on anticoagulant activity of dabigatran and rivaroxaban, *Thromb Haemost* 108:217–224, 2012.

16. O'Gara PT, Kushner FG, Ascheim DD, et al: 2013 ACCF/AHA Guideline for the Management of ST-elevation Myocardial Infarction: A report of the American College of Cardiology Foundation/American Heart Association Task Force on Practice Guidelines, *J Am Coll Cardiol* 61:e78–140, 2013.

17. Pradaxa (dabigatran etexilate) prescribing information. Boehringer Ingelheim Pharmaceuticals Inc., Ridgefield, CT; 2012.

18. Samama MM, Contact G, Spiro TE, et al: Evaluation of the anti-factor Xa chromogenic assay for the measurement of rivaroxaban plasma concentrations using calibrators and controls, *Thromb Haemostas* 107:379–387, 2012.

19. *U.S. Food and Drug Administration: Drug development and drug interactions: table of substrates, inhibitors and inducers.* Available at: http://www.fda.gov/drugs/developmentapprovalprocess/developmentresources/druginteractionslabeling/ucm 093664.htm#inhibitors. Accessed Sep 10, 2012.

20. Whitlock RP, Sun JC, Fremes SE, et al: Antithrombotic and thrombolytic therapy for valvular disease: Antithrombotic Therapy and Prevention of Thrombosis, ed 9: American College of Chest Physicians Evidence-Based Clinical Practice Guidelines, *Chest* 141(Suppl 2):e576S–e600S, 2012.

21. You JJ, Singer DE, Lane DA, et al: Antithrombotic therapy for atrial fibrillation: Antithrombotic Therapy and Prevention of Thrombosis, ed 9: American College of Chest Physicians Evidence-Based Clinical Practice Guidelines, *Chest* 141(Suppl 2):e531S–e575S, 2012.

22. *Xarelto (rivaroxaban) prescribing information*, Janssen Pharmaceuticals, Inc, Titusville, NJ, March, 2013.

CHAPTER 54

PERICARDITIS, PERICARDIAL CONSTRICTION, AND PERICARDIAL TAMPONADE

Brian D. Hoit, MD

1. **The pericardium is not necessary for life. What does it do? Why is it important?**
   The pericardium serves many important but subtle functions. It limits distension and facilitates interaction of the cardiac chambers, influences ventricular filling, prevents excessive torsion and displacement of the heart, minimizes friction with surrounding structures, prevents the spread of infection from contiguous structures, and equalizes gravitational, hydrostatic, and inertial forces over the surface of the heart. The pericardium also has immunologic, vasomotor, fibrinolytic, and metabolic activities. Therapeutically, the pericardial space can be used for drug delivery.

2. **What diseases affect the pericardium?**
   The pericardium is affected by virtually every category of disease (Box 54-1), including idiopathic, infectious, neoplastic, immune and inflammatory, metabolic, iatrogenic, traumatic, and congenital disease.

3. **What is pericarditis? What are the clinical manifestations? What are the causes?**
   Acute pericarditis is a syndrome of pericardial inflammation characterized by typical chest pain (sharp, retrosternal pain that radiates to the trapezius ridge, often aggravated by lying down and

---

Box 54-1 CAUSES OF PERICARDIAL HEART DISEASE

- **Idiopathic**
- **Infectious**
  Bacterial, viral, mycobacterial, fungal, protozoal, HIV-associated
- **Neoplastic**
  Metastatic (breast, lung, melanoma, lymphoma, leukemia)
  Primary (mesothelioma, fibrosarcoma)
- **Immune/inflammatory**
  Connective tissue disease, arteritis, acute myocardial infarction, post–pericardial injury syndrome
- **Metabolic**
  Nephrogenic, myxedema, amyloidosis, aortic dissection
- **Iatrogenic**
  Drugs, radiation therapy, device/instrumentation, cardiac resuscitation
- **Traumatic**
  Blunt, penetrating, surgical
- **Congenital**
  Pericardial cysts, congenital absence of pericardium, mulibrey nanism

HIV, Human immunodeficiency virus.
Modified from Hoit BD: Diseases of the pericardium. In Fuster V, O'Rourke RA, Walsh RA, et al, editors: *Hurst's the heart*, ed 12, New York, 2008, McGraw-Hill.

---

relieved by sitting up), a pathognomonic pericardial friction rub (characterized as superficial, *scratchy, crunchy*, and evanescent), and specific electrocardiographic changes (diffuse ST-T wave changes (Fig. 54-1) with characteristic evolutionary changes and PR segment depression). Causes include infection (viral, bacterial, fungal, mycobacterial, or human immunodeficiency virus [HIV] associated), neoplasia (usually metastatic from lung or breast; melanoma, lymphoma, or acute leukemia), myocardial infarction, injury (postpericardiotomy and traumatic), radiation, myxedema, and connective tissue disease.

4. **Should patients presenting with acute pericarditis be hospitalized? Why?**
   Hospitalization is warranted for high-risk patients with an initial episode of acute pericarditis, in order to determine a cause and to observe for the development of cardiac tamponade; close, early follow-up is critically important for the remainder of patients not hospitalized. Features indicative of high-risk pericarditis include fever greater than 38° C, subacute onset, an immunosuppressed state, trauma, oral anticoagulant therapy, myopericarditis, a moderate or large pericardial effusion, cardiac tamponade, and medical failure.

5. **What is the treatment for acute pericarditis?**
   Acute pericarditis usually responds to oral nonsteroidal antiinflammatory drugs (NSAIDs), such as aspirin (650 mg every 3 to 4 hours) or ibuprofen (300-800 mg every 6 hours). Colchicine (1 mg/day) may be used to supplement the NSAIDs as it may reduce symptoms and decrease the rate of recurrences. Chest pain is usually alleviated in 1 to 2 days, and the friction rub and ST segment elevation resolve shortly thereafter. Most mild cases of idiopathic and viral pericarditis are adequately treated within a week or two of treatment start, but the duration of therapy is variable and patients should be treated until inflammation or an effusion, if present, has resolved. If colchicine is used, it should be given for 3 months; this is based on the randomized, open label Colchicine for Acute Pericarditis (COPE) trial. The intensity of therapy is dictated by the distress of the patient, and narcotics may be required for severe pain. Corticosteroids should be avoided unless there is a specific indication (such as connective tissue disease or uremic pericarditis) because they enhance viral multiplication and may result in recurrences when the dosage is tapered. Although the European Society of Cardiology (ESC) recently published guidelines for the diagnosis and management of pericardial diseases, there are only a few randomized, placebo-controlled trials from which appropriate therapy may be selected.

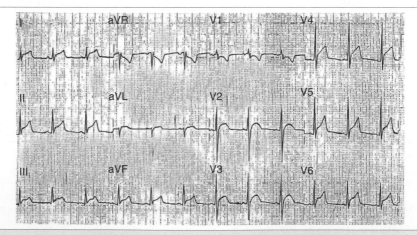

Figure 54-1. The diffuse ST segment elevations seen in pericarditis.

6. **What is recurrent pericarditis? How is it treated?**

Recurrences of pericarditis (with or without pericardial effusion) occur in up to one-third of patients, usually within 18 months of the acute attack, and may follow a course of many years. Although they may be spontaneous, occurring at varying intervals after discontinuation of drug treatment, they are more commonly associated with either discontinuation or tapering of antiinflammatory drugs. A poor initial response to therapy with NSAIDs and the use of corticosteroids predict recurrences. Two randomized placebo-controlled trials of colchicine for recurrent pericarditis (CORE and Colchicine for Recurrent Pericarditis [CORP] trials) reported marked and significant reductions in symptom persistence at 72 hours and recurrence at 18 months when colchicine was added to conventional therapy. Although painful recurrences of pericarditis may require corticosteroids (preferably at low to moderate doses with slow tapering), once administered, dependency and the development of steroid-induced abnormalities are potential perils. Pericardiectomy should be considered only when repeated attempts at medical treatment have clearly failed.

7. **What is post–cardiac injury syndrome?**

Post–cardiac injury syndrome (PCIS) refers to pericarditis or pericardial effusion that results from injury of the pericardium. The principal conditions considered under these headings include post–myocardial infarction syndrome, postpericardiotomy syndrome, and traumatic (blunt, sharp, or iatrogenic) pericarditis. Clinical features include the following:
- Prior injury of the pericardium, myocardium, or both
- A latent period between the injury and the development of pericarditis or pericardial effusion
- A tendency for recurrence
- Responsiveness to NSAIDs and corticosteroids
- Fever, leukocytosis, and elevated erythrocyte sedimentation rate (and other markers of inflammation)
- Pericardial and sometimes pleural effusion, with or without a pulmonary infiltrate
- Alterations in the populations of lymphocytes in peripheral blood

When the pericardial injury syndrome occurs after an acute myocardial infarction, it is also known as Dressler syndrome, which is now much less common than in the past. In the randomized multi-center Colchicine for the Prevention of Post-Pericardiotomy Syndrome (COPPS) study, prophylactically administered colchicine reduced the incidence of postpericardiotomy syndrome after cardiac surgery.

8. **What are the pericardial compressive syndromes? What are their variants?**

The complications of acute pericarditis include cardiac tamponade, constrictive pericarditis, and effusive constrictive pericarditis. *Cardiac tamponade* is characterized by the accumulation of pericardial fluid under pressure and may be acute, subacute, low pressure (occult), or regional. *Constrictive pericarditis* is the result of thickening, calcification, and loss of elasticity of the pericardial sac. Pericardial constriction is typically chronic but may be subacute, transient, and occult. *Effusive constrictive pericarditis* is characterized by constrictive physiology with a coexisting pericardial effusion, usually with tamponade. Elevation of the right atrial and pulmonary wedge pressures persists after drainage of the pericardial fluid.

9. **What are similarities between tamponade and constrictive pericarditis?**

Characteristic of both tamponade and constrictive pericarditis is greatly enhanced ventricular interaction (interdependence), in which the hemodynamics of the left and right heart chambers are directly influenced by each other to a much greater degree than normal. Other similarities include diastolic dysfunction and preserved ventricular ejection fraction; increased respiratory variation of ventricular inflow and outflow; equally elevated central venous, pulmonary venous, and ventricular diastolic pressures; and mild pulmonary hypertension.

10. **What are the differences between tamponade and constrictive pericarditis?**

In tamponade, the pericardial space is open and transmits the respiratory variation in thoracic pressure to the heart, whereas in constrictive pericarditis, the cavity is obliterated and the pericardium does not transmit these pressure changes. The dissociation of intrathoracic and intracardiac pressures (along with ventricular interaction) is the basis for the physical, hemodynamic, and echocardiographic findings of constriction.

In tamponade, systemic venous return increases with inspiration, enlarging the right side of the heart and encroaching on the left, whereas in constrictive pericarditis, systemic venous return does not increase with inspiration. The mechanism of diminished left ventricular and increased right ventricular volume in constrictive pericarditis is impaired left ventricular filling because of a lesser pressure gradient from the pulmonary veins.

In tamponade, early ventricular filling is impaired, whereas it is enhanced in constriction.

11. **What are the physical findings of tamponade?**
Cardiac tamponade is a hemodynamic condition characterized by equal elevation of atrial and pericardial pressures, an exaggerated inspiratory decrease in arterial systolic pressure (pulsus paradoxus), and arterial hypotension. The physical findings are dictated by both the severity of cardiac tamponade and the time course of its development. Inspection of the jugular venous pulse waveform reveals elevated venous pressure with a loss of the y descent (because of the decrease in intrapericardial pressure that occurs during ventricular ejection, the systolic atrial filling wave and the x descent are maintained). Pulsus paradoxus is an inspiratory decline of systolic arterial pressure exceeding 10 mm Hg, which is measured by subtracting the pressure at which the Korotkoff sounds are heard only during expiration from the pressure at which sounds are heard throughout the respiratory cycle. Tachycardia and tachypnea are usually present.

12. **What are the physical findings of constrictive pericarditis?**
Constrictive pericarditis resembles the congestive states caused by myocardial disease and chronic liver disease. Physical findings include ascites, hepatosplenomegaly, edema, and, in long-standing cases, severe wasting. The venous pressure is elevated and displays deep y and often deep x descents. The venous pressure fails to decrease with inspiration (the Kussmaul sign). A pericardial knock that is similar in timing to the third heart sound is pathognomonic but occurs infrequently. Except in severe cases, the arterial blood pressure is normal.

13. **What is the role of echocardiography in tamponade?**
Although tamponade is a clinical diagnosis, echocardiography plays major roles in the identification of pericardial effusion and in the assessment of its hemodynamic significance (Fig. 54-2). The use of echocardiography for the evaluation of all patients with suspected pericardial disease was given a class I recommendation by a 2003 task force of the American College of Cardiology (ACC), the American Heart Association (AHA), and the American Society of Echocardiography (ASE). Except in hyperacute cases, a moderate to large effusion is usually present and swinging of the heart within the effusion may be seen. Reciprocal changes in left and right ventricular volumes occur with respiration. Echocardiographic findings suggesting hemodynamic compromise (atrial and ventricular diastolic collapses) are the result of transiently reversed right atrial and right ventricular diastolic transmural pressures and typically occur before hemodynamic embarrassment. The respiratory variation of mitral and tricuspid flow velocities is greatly increased and out of phase, reflecting the increased ventricular interaction. Less than a 50% inspiratory reduction in the diameter of a dilated inferior vena cava reflects a marked elevation in central venous pressure, and abnormal right-sided venous flows (systolic predominance and expiratory diastolic reversal) are diagnostic. In patients who do not have tamponade on first assessment, repeat echocardiography during clinical follow-up was given a class IIa recommendation by the 2003 ACC/AHA/ASE task force.

14. **What is the role of echocardiography in constrictive pericarditis?**
Echocardiography is an essential adjunctive procedure in patients with suspected pericardial constriction. The use of echocardiography for the evaluation of all patients with suspected pericardial disease is a class I recommendation of the ACC/AHA/ASE task force. Echocardiography findings to be

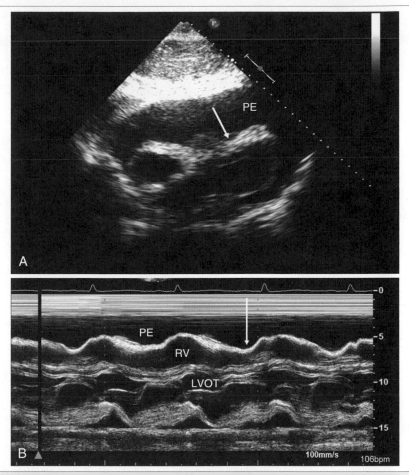

Figure 54-2. Echocardiography in cardiac tamponade. **A**, Subcostal two-dimensional echo. A large effusion *(PE)* with marked compression of the right ventricle *(arrow)* is seen. **B**, M-mode of the parasternal long axis. Note the right ventricular *(long arrow)* collapse. *LVOT*, Left ventricular outflow tract; *PE*, pericardial effusion; *RV*, right ventricular.

sought include increased pericardial thickness (best with transesophageal echocardiography), abrupt inspiratory posterior motion of the ventricular septum in early diastole, plethora of the inferior vena cava and hepatic veins, enlarged atria, and an abnormal contour between the posterior left ventricular the left atrial posterior walls. Although no sign or combination of signs on M-mode is diagnostic of constrictive pericarditis, a normal study virtually rules out the diagnosis. Doppler is particularly useful, showing a high *E* velocity of right and left ventricular inflow and rapid deceleration, a normal or increased tissue Doppler *E'*, and a 25% to 40% fall in transmitral flow and marked increase of tricuspid velocity in the first beat after inspiration. Increased respiratory variation of mitral inflow may be missing in patients with markedly elevated left atrial pressure, but may be brought out by preload reduction (e.g., head-up tilt). Hepatic vein flow reversals increase with expiration, reflecting the ventricular interaction and the dissociation of intracardiac and intrathoracic pressures, and pulmonary venous flow shows marked respiratory variation.

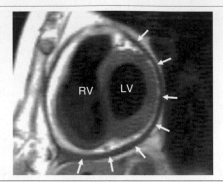

Figure 54-3. Magnetic resonance imaging demonstrating thickened pericardium encasing the heart *(arrows)*. (Reproduced with permission from Pennell D: Cardiovascular magnetic resonance. In Libby P, Bonow R, Mann D, Zipes DP, editors: *Braunwald's heart disease: a textbook of cardiovascular medicine*, ed 8, Philadelphia, 2008, Saunders, p. 405.) *LV*, Left ventricle; *RV*, right ventricle.

15. Are other imaging modalities useful in pericardial disease?

Other imaging techniques, such as computed tomography (CT) and cardiac magnetic resonance imaging (CMR) are not necessary if two-dimensional and Doppler echocardiography are available. However, pericardial effusion may be detected, quantified, and characterized by CT and CMR. CT scanning of the heart is extremely useful in the diagnosis of constrictive pericarditis; findings include increased pericardial thickness (greater than 4 mm) and calcification. CMR provides direct visualization of the normal pericardium, which is composed of fibrous tissue and has a low magnetic resonance imaging (MRI) signal intensity. CMR is claimed by some to be the diagnostic procedure of choice for the detection of constrictive pericarditis (Fig. 54-3). Late gadolinium enhancement of the pericardium may predict reversibility of transitory constrictive pericarditis (see later) following treatment with antiinflammatory agents.

16. Constrictive pericarditis is a surgical disease, except when very early or in severe, advanced disease. What is the role for medical therapy in constrictive pericarditis?

Medical therapy of constrictive pericarditis plays a small but important role. Diuretics and digoxin (in the presence of atrial fibrillation) are useful in patients who are not candidates for pericardiectomy because of their high surgical risk. Preoperative diuretics should be used sparingly with the goal of reducing, not eliminating, elevated jugular pressure, edema, and ascites. Postoperatively, diuretics should be given if spontaneous diuresis does not occur; the central venous pressure may take weeks to months to return to normal after pericardiectomy. In some patients, constrictive pericarditis resolves either spontaneously or in response to various combinations of NSAIDs, steroids, and antibiotics (transitory constriction). Therefore, before pericardiectomy is recommended, conservative management for 2 to 3 months in hemodynamically stable patients with subacute constrictive pericarditis is recommended.

BIBLIOGRAPHY, SUGGESTED READINGS, AND WEBSITES

1. Cheitlin MD, Armstrong WF, Aurigemma GP, et al: *ACC/AHA/ASE 2003 Guidelines for the Clinical Application of Echocardiography.* Available at: http://www.acc.org/qualityandscience/clinical/statements.htm. Accessed February 26, 2013.

2. Hoit BD: Diseases of the pericardium. In Fuster V, Walsh RA, editors: *Hurst's the heart*, ed 13, New York, 2011, McGraw-Hill. pp. 1917-39.

3. Hoit BD: Treatment of pericardial disease. In Antman E, Sabatine MS, editors: *Cardiovascular therapeutics. A companion to Braunwald's heart disease*, ed 4, Philadelphia, 2011, Elsevier. pp. 667-675.

4. Hoit BD: Management of effusive and constrictive pericardial heart disease, *Circulation* 105:2939–2942, 2002.

5. Little WC, Freeman GL: Pericardial disease, *Circulation* 113:1622–1632, 2006.

6. Maisch B, Seferovic PM, Ristic AD, et al: Guidelines on the diagnosis and management of pericardial diseases executive summary; The Task Force on the Diagnosis and Management of Pericardial Diseases of the European Society of Cardiology, *Eur Heart J* 25:587–610, 2004.

7. Shabetai R: *The pericardium*, Norwell, Mass, 2003, Kluwer Academic Publishers.

CHAPTER 55

PERIPHERAL ARTERIAL DISEASE

Panos Kougias, MD, FACS, and Carlos F. Bechara, MD, MS

1. **What are the key components of the vascular physical examination?**
   According to the American College of Cardiology/American Heart Association (ACC/AHA) guidelines on peripheral arterial disease (PAD), the key components of the vascular physical examination include the following:
   - Blood pressure measurements in both arms
   - Carotid pulse palpation for upstroke and amplitude, and auscultation for bruits
   - Auscultation of the abdomen and flank for bruits
   - Palpation of the abdomen for aortic pulsation and its maximal diameter
   - Palpation of brachial, radial, ulnar, femoral, popliteal, dorsalis pedis, and posterior tibial pulses; pulse intensity is scored as follows: 0, absent; 1, diminished; 2, normal; 3, bounding
   - Performance of the Allen test when knowledge of hand perfusion is needed
   - Auscultation of the femoral arteries for the presence of bruits
   - Inspection of the feet for color, temperature, and integrity of the skin, and for ulcers
   - Observation of other findings suggestive of severe PAD, including distal hair loss, trophic skin changes, and hypertrophic nails

2. **Can the location of the patient's lower extremity claudication help to localize the site of occlusive disease?**
   The answer is a qualified yes. Because the pathophysiology of claudication is complex, there is not a perfect correlation between anatomic site of disease and location of symptoms. However, in general, the following statements can be made:
   - Occlusive iliac artery disease may produce hip, buttock, and thigh pain, as well as calf pain.
   - Occlusive femoral and popliteal artery disease usually produces calf pain.
   - Occlusive disease in the tibial arteries may produce calf pain or, more rarely, foot pain and numbness.

3. **What noninvasive tests are used in the assessment of lower limb claudication?**
   - **Ankle-brachial index (ABI):** The ankle-brachial index is the ankle systolic pressure (as determined by Doppler) divided by the brachial systolic pressure. An abnormal index is less than 0.90. The sensitivity is approximately 90% for diagnosis of PAD. (See Question 4 for further details.)
   - **Pulse volume recordings (PVRs):** Pulse volume recordings measure changes in volume of toes, fingers, or parts of limbs that occur with each pulse beat as blood flows into or out of the extremity. A toe-to-brachial index of less than 0.6 is abnormal, and values of less than 0.15 are seen in patients with rest pain (toe pressures of less than 20 mm Hg).
   - **Duplex ultrasonography:** Duplex ultrasonography is a noninvasive method of evaluating arterial stenosis and blood flow. This method can localize and quantify the degree of stenosis. Ultrasonography is dependent on operator skill.
   - **Transcutaneous oxygen tension measurements:** These measurements are useful in assessing tissue viability for wound healing. Measurements greater than 55 mm Hg are considered normal and less than 20 mm Hg are associated with nonhealing ulcers.
   - **Exercise testing:** This testing determines treadmill walking time and preexercise and postexercise ABI. In those without significant PAD, the ABI is unchanged after exercise. In patients with PAD, the ABI falls after exercise. This test is more sensitive for detecting disease than a resting ABI alone.

4. **What is the ABI?**

The ABI is the ratio of systolic blood pressure at the level of the ankle to the systolic blood pressure measured at the level of the brachial artery. More specifically, blood pressure is measured in both brachial arteries (with the higher systolic blood pressure being used) and is measured using a Doppler instrument with a blood pressure cuff on the lower calf, in both posterior tibial and dorsalis pedis arteries. Pulse wave reflections in healthy persons should result in higher blood pressures in the ankle vessel pressure (10-15 mm Hg higher than in the brachial arteries), and thus a normal ABI should be greater than 1.00. Using a diagnostic threshold of 0.90 to 0.91, several studies have found the sensitivity of the ABI to be 79% to 95% and the specificity to be 96% to 100% to detect stenosis of 50% or more reduction in lumen diameter.

Experts emphasize that the ABI is a continuous variable below 0.90. Values of 0.41 to 0.90 are considered to be mildly to moderately diminished; values of 0.40 or less are considered to be severely decreased. An ABI of 0.40 or less is associated with an increased risk of rest pain, ischemic ulceration, or gangrene. Patients with long-standing diabetes or end-stage renal disease on dialysis and elderly patients may have noncompressible leg arterial segments caused by medial calcification, precluding assessment of the ABI. These patients are best evaluated using digital pressures and with assessment of the quality of the arterial waveform in the PVR studies. A system for interpretation of the ABI is given in Table 55-1.

5. **What are the recommended medical therapies and lifestyle interventions in patients with lower extremity PAD?**

A supervised exercise regimen is recommended as the initial treatment modality for patients with intermittent claudication. Supervised exercise training is recommended over unsupervised exercise training. Cilostazol treatment can lead to a modest increase in exercise capacity. Because agents with similar biologic effects have been shown to increase mortality in patients with heart failure, this drug should not be used in patients with heart failure. Smoking cessation must be strongly emphasized to the patient. Other measures include general secondary prevention interventions. Recommended medical therapies and lifestyle interventions in patients with lower extremity PAD are summarized in Box 55-1. An algorithm for the management of patients with suspected peripheral arterial disease is presented in Figure 55-1.

6. **What are the interventional treatment options for patients with claudication?**

Claudication that severely interferes with quality of life or employment should be treated. Endovascular and open surgical reconstruction have both been extensively used for this purpose. Endovascular options are less invasive, typically performed on an outpatient basis, and are associated with lower complication rates. Open surgical options are more durable and best suited for good risk or young patients. Outcomes of either type of intervention are vascular-bed dependent. Iliac stenting has been

TABLE 55-1.	INTERPRETATION OF THE ANKLE-BRACHIAL INDEX
ABI	**Interpretation**
>1.30	Noncompressible
1.00-1.29	Normal
0.91-0.99	Borderline (equivocal)
0.41-0.90	Mild to moderate PAD
0.00-0.40	Severe PAD

Modified from Hiatt WR: Medical treatment of peripheral arterial disease and claudication, *N Engl J Med* 344:1608-1621, 2001.
ABI, Ankle-brachial index; *PAD*, peripheral arterial disease.

associated with 5-year patency rates that in most cases are only slightly inferior to that of their open counterparts. Endovascular intervention in the infrainguinal segment, however, is associated with inferior patency, particularly when compared to open bypass using venous conduit.

7. **What is critical limb ischemia (CLI) and how is it graded clinically?**
Whereas claudication is produced by decreased perfusion to the muscles upon increased demand, CLI refers to inadequate tissue perfusion at rest and is manifested as rest pain or tissue loss. Patients with CLI have multilevel disease that typically involves iliac, femoral, and tibial arteries. Due to extent of the disease and the coexistent comorbidities, the management of the patient with CLI involves substantial judgment. Hybrid procedures that include simultaneous open and endovascular components, multiple debridements, and extensive rehabilitation therapy programs are fairly typical. Best results are achieved with multidisciplinary approaches that involve interventionalists, surgeons, internists, podiatrists, and infectious disease and endocrine specialists, among others. Isolated vessel-based intervention in the absence of a grand plan for overall patient management should be discouraged, as most of these patients benefit from coordinated treatment in centers familiar with the intricacies and the issues surrounding the management of CLI. One widely used scheme for classifying limb ischemia is given in Table 55-2.

8. **What are the main complications of open and endovascular infrainguinal interventions?**
Complications of open interventions include cardiac events, respiratory complications, bleeding, wound infection, hernias, and graft failure. Complications associated with endovascular procedures include access site hematoma, bleeding or pseudoaneurysm, vessel rupture, contrast-induced nephropathy or anaphylactic reactions, recurrent stenosis or occlusion, and radiation-related patient injury. Thrombolytic treatment in particular is associated with increased risk of intracavitary, extremity, or intracranial bleeding, which is heavily dependent on the thrombolytic dose and duration of administration.

Box 55-1 RECOMMENDED MEDICAL THERAPIES AND LIFESTYLE INTERVENTIONS IN PATIENTS WITH LOWER EXTREMITY PERIPHERAL ARTERIAL DISEASE

- Statin treatment to lower LDL level to <70-100 mg/dL
- Antihypertensive therapy to lower blood pressure to <140/90 mm Hg (<130/80 mm Hg in patients with diabetes or those with chronic kidney disease)
  - β-Blockers are not contraindicated in patients with PAD.
  - The use of ACE inhibitors is reasonable in symptomatic lower extremity PAD patients to reduce the risk of adverse cardiovascular events.
- Patients with PAD should be offered smoking cessation interventions.
- Antiplatelet therapy is indicated to reduce the risk of MI, stroke, or vascular death.
  - Aspirin in doses of 75-325 mg is recommended.
  - Clopidogrel can be used as an alternate therapy to aspirin.
- Supervised exercise training is the recommended initial treatment modality for intermittent claudication.
  - Exercise should be for a minimum of 30-45 minutes at least three times per week.
- Cilostazol (100 mg orally twice a day) is recommended to improve symptoms and increase walking distance in patients with intermittent claudication. (Cilostazol should not be used in patients with heart failure.)

Modified from Hirsch AT, Haskal ZJ, Hertzer NR, et al: ACC/AHA guidelines for the management of patients with peripheral arterial disease, *J Am Coll Cardiol* 47(6):1239-1312, 2006.
ACE, Angiotensin-converting enzyme; *β-blocker*, beta-adrenergic blocking agent; *LDL*, low-density lipoprotein; *MI*, myocardial infarction; *PAD*, peripheral arterial disease.

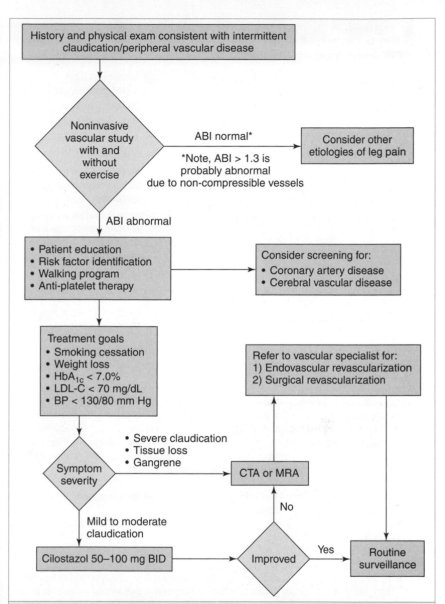

Figure 55-1. Algorithm for the evaluation and management of patients with suspected lower extremity peripheral artery disease. (From Toth PP, Shammas NW, Dippel EJ, et al: Cardiovascular disease. In Rakel RE, editor: *Textbook of family medicine*, ed 7, Philadelphia, 2007, Saunders.) *ABI*, Ankle-brachial index; *BP*, blood pressure; *CTA*, computed tomographic angiography; *Hg*, glycated hemoglobin; *LDL*, low-density lipoprotein; *MRA*, magnetic resonance angiography.

TABLE 55-2. CLINICAL CATEGORIES OF CHRONIC LIMB ISCHEMIA

Grade	Category	Clinical Description
	0	Asymptomatic, not hemodynamically correct
I	1	Mild claudication
	2	Moderate claudication
	3	Severe claudication
II	4	Ischemic rest pain
	5	Minor tissue loss: nonhealing ulcer, focal gangrene with diffuse pedal ulcer
III	6	Major tissue loss extending above transmetatarsal level, functional foot no longer salvageable

From Rutherford RB, Baker JD, Ernst C, et al: Recommended standards for reports dealing with lower extremity ischemia: revised version, *J Vasc Surg* 26:517, 1997.

9. **What are the causes of renal artery stenosis (RAS)?**

Approximately 90% of all renal arterial lesions are due to atherosclerosis. Atherosclerotic-related lesions usually affect the ostium and the proximal 1 cm of the main renal artery.

Fibromuscular dysplasia (FMD) is the next most common cause. Although it classically occurs in young women, it can affect both genders at any age. Less common causes of renovascular hypertension include renal artery aneurysms, Takayasu arteritis, atheroemboli, thromboemboli, William syndrome, neurofibromatosis, spontaneous renal artery dissection, arteriovenous malformations (AVMs) or fistulas, retroperitoneal fibrosis, and prior abdominal radiation therapy.

10. **What are ACC/AHA class I indications for the referral for diagnostic study to identify clinically significant RAS?**

Clinical scenarios that are recognized as class I indications for the performance of a diagnostic study to identify RAS include the following:

- Onset of hypertension before age 30
- Onset of hypertension after age 55
- Accelerated hypertension (sudden and persistent worsening of previously controlled hypertension), resistant hypertension (failure to achieve blood pressure goal with full adherences to full doses of an appropriate three-drug regimen that includes a diuretic), and malignant hypertension (hypertension with acute end-organ damage)
- New azotemia or worsening renal function after angiotensin-converting enzyme (ACE) inhibitor or angiotensin-receptor blocker (ARB) treatment
- Unexplained atrophic kidney or discrepancy in size between the two kidneys of more than 1.5 cm
- Sudden, unexplained pulmonary edema (especially in azotemic patients)

11. **What are the main indications for RAS percutaneous revascularization?**

Most ACC/AHA indications for percutaneous revascularization are class IIa recommendations, meaning the procedure is reasonable.

Class I (Indicated):
- Hemodynamically significant RAS and recurrent, unexplained congestive heart failure or sudden, unexplained pulmonary edema

Class IIa (Reasonable):
- Hemodynamically significant RAS and accelerated hypertension, resistant hypertension, malignant hypertension, hypertension with an unexplained unilateral small kidney, and hypertension with intolerance to medication
- Hemodynamically significant RAS and unstable angina
- RAS and progressive chronic kidney disease with bilateral RAS or a RAS to a solitary functioning kidney
- Although percutaneous intervention is generally the procedure of choice for lesions and disease involving the proximal and main renal artery, surgical revascularization is generally recommended for those cases with complex disease involving branching or segmental arteries or when aortic surgery is also indicated.

12. **What are the most common types of visceral artery aneurysms?**
Visceral artery aneurysms are an uncommon form of vascular disease whose pathogenesis and natural history remain incompletely characterized. Their typical presentation involves rupture or erosion into an adjacent viscus, resulting in life-threatening hemorrhage. Nearly 22% of reported visceral artery aneurysms present with rupture, resulting in an 8.5% mortality rate. The distribution of aneurysms among the visceral vessels includes the splenic artery (60%), hepatic artery (20%), superior mesenteric artery (5.5%), celiac artery (4%), gastric and gastroepiploic arteries (4%), jejunal, ileal, colic (3%), pancreaticoduodenal and pancreatic arteries (2%), gastroduodenal artery (1.5%), and inferior mesenteric artery (<1%). Typical indication for treatment include size more than 2 cm and childbearing age in a female patient, because rupture is common during pregnancy and is associated with very high maternal and fetal mortality

13. **In general, when should patients with an infrarenal or juxtarenal abdominal aortic aneurysm (AAA) undergo repair?**
Current recommendations are that patients with an infrarenal or juxtarenal AAA should undergo repair when the aneurysm measures 5.5 cm or greater (although it is also a class IIa recommendation that it can be beneficial to repair aneurysms 5.0 to 5.4 cm in diameter). Patients with infrarenal or juxtarenal AAA measuring 4.0 to 5.4 cm in diameter should be monitored by ultrasound or computed tomography (CT) scans every 6 to 12 months. In those with AAA smaller than 4.0 cm, ultrasound examination every 2 to 3 years is felt to be reasonable.

14. **What are the relative pros and cons of the treatment options for patients with infrarenal AAA that meets size criteria for repair?**
The traditional open AAA repair has been compared to endovascular infrarenal AAA repair (EVAR) extensively with three large multicenter trials, two in Europe and one in the US. EVAR is associated with lower perioperative mortality and complication rates, particular respiratory complications. However, it also implies the need for long-term follow-up with serial CT scans to assess the endograft and confirm the absence of endoleak or migration. The impact of this follow-up protocol in terms of impact on renal function and radiation-related injury is unclear at present. The survival benefit of EVAR disappeared in all studies after 2 to 3 years of follow-up. Open AAA repair has the additional issue of postoperative late ventral hernia development, which appears to occur in approximately 15% to 20% of patients.

15. **What are the anatomic eligibility criteria for endovascular infrarenal AAA repair?**
These include the following:
- Proximal aortic neck of at least 15 mm in length and no more than 32 mm in diameter
- Angulation of aortic neck less than 60 degrees
- Iliac vessels of adequate diameter to accommodate the delivery device

As device platforms evolve, more challenging anatomies are routinely treated today with endovascular means. In addition, fenestrated and branched devices, and advanced "snorkel" techniques have enabled physicians to successfully treat juxtarenal and thoracoabdominal aneurysms in high-risk patients with endovascular means.

16. **What are the primary indications for treatment of extracranial carotid artery occlusive disease?**

    In very general terms, indications for intervention are as follows:
    - Symptomatic stenosis 50% to 99% diameter if the risk of perioperative stroke or death is less than 6%
    - Asymptomatic stenosis greater than 60% in diameter if the expected perioperative stroke rate is less than 3% and if life expectancy is greater than 2 years

    Controversy surrounds the overall topic of interventional treatment of asymptomatic carotid artery occlusive disease. The notion that maximizing medical treatment can be as good as intervention with respect to stroke prevention has been gaining acceptance; however, high-quality data to support it are scarce.

17. **What are the relative indications for carotid endarterectomy (CEA) and carotid artery stenting (CAS)?**

    Carotid stenting indications include the following:
    - High carotid lesion not approachable via neck incision using standard techniques
    - Redo neck surgery
    - History of radiation in the neck
    - Presence of tracheostomy
    - High physiologic risk for open CEA

    CEA and CAS have been compared in four large randomized controlled trials that are listed in the references section and the reader is encouraged to review their results. CAS appears to be associated with higher stroke but lower myocardial event rates, and no extracranial nerve damage. The topic of first-line treatment in the management of symptomatic carotid artery occlusive disease is somewhat controversial at present, with two slightly conflicting society guideline statements. There is agreement that in the treatment of asymptomatic carotid artery occlusive disease, CEA should be the treatment of choice.

18. **What are possible causes of lower limb arterial disease and ischemia or claudication in young patients?**

    Atherosclerosis tends to primarily affect older persons; however, it can manifest in younger patients who have familial hyperlipidemic syndromes, Buerger disease (thromboangiitis obliterans), or hypercoagulable disorders. Popliteal entrapment syndrome is an anatomic abnormality in which the popliteal artery gets compressed, either by an abnormal muscle band or because it has taken an abnormal (medial) course behind the knee and is compressed by a normal gastrocnemius muscle. Popliteal adventitial cystic disease is also in the differential diagnosis of claudication in young patients; it produces a popliteal stenosis that gives a classic "scimitar sign" on angiography. Exercise-induced compartment syndrome may produce similar symptoms of leg pain with exercise that is relieved by rest.

19. **What is fibromuscular dysplasia (FMD)?**

    Fibromuscular dysplasia (FMD), formerly called fibromuscular fibroplasia, is a group of nonatherosclerotic, noninflammatory arterial diseases that can affect almost any artery but most commonly involves the renal arteries. Histologic classification discriminates three main subtypes: intimal, medial, and perimedial, which may be found in a single patient. Angiographic classification includes the following:
    - Multifocal type, with multiple stenoses and the "string-of-beads" appearance that is classic for medial fibroplasias
    - Focal type, which is more suggestive of intimal fibroplasia

20. What is Buerger disease?

Buerger disease, more appropriately called thromboangiitis obliterans, is a disease of small- and medium-sized arteries, as well as veins and nerves. Buerger disease is a nonatherosclerotic disease, instead caused by inflammatory processes and thrombosis.

Clinically, it presents most commonly with ischemia of the digits and hand, arm, feet, or calf claudication. Ischemic ulcers may also occur. It occurs almost exclusively in tobacco users, and the only true "treatment" is smoking cessation. The presence of "corkscrew" collaterals is a pathognomonic angiographic finding.

21. What is Takayasu arteritis?

Takayasu arteritis is a vasculitis of unknown cause, primarily affecting the aorta and its primary branches. It is more common in Asian populations and predominantly affects women. Over time, it can lead to narrowing or occlusion of the aorta and its branches, such as the subclavian artery. Clinically, patients most commonly manifest upper arm claudication but may also develop neurologic symptoms as a result of vertebrobasilar ischemia.

22. What is May-Thurner syndrome?

Iliocaval compression, or May-Thurner syndrome (MTS), was initially described as the development of spurs in the left iliac vein as a consequence of compression from the contralateral right common iliac artery against the lumbar vertebra. The pathogenesis of MTS is not completely understood, but it is theorized that it may be a combination of both mechanical compression and arterial pulsations by the right iliac artery that leads to the development of intimal hypertrophy within the wall of the left common iliac vein. This can lead to potential endothelial changes and thrombus formation. Patients with MTS tend to be young women in the second to fourth decade of life who develop the syndrome after periods of prolonged immobilization or pregnancy. Patients may have a history of several days or more of persistent, unexplained pain and swelling of the left thigh and calf. Duplex ultrasound characteristically may reveal left common iliac vein thrombosis. Management of symptomatic MTS in association with deep vein thrombosis may involve catheter-directed thrombolysis, anticoagulation, and potentially iliocaval stenting.

BIBLIOGRAPHY, SUGGESTED READINGS, AND WEBSITES

1. Blankensteijn JD, de Jong SE, Prinssen M, et al: Two-year outcomes after conventional or endovascular repair of abdominal aortic aneurysms, *N Engl J Med* 352:2398–2405, 2005.

2. Brott TG, Halperin JL, Abbara S, et al: JASA/ACCF/AHA/AANN/AANS/ACR/ASNR/CNS/SAIP/SCAI/SIR/SNIS/SVM/SVS guideline on the management of patients with extracranial carotid and vertebral artery disease: executive summary, *Circulation* 124:489–532, 2011. *Stroke* 42:e420-e463, 2011; and *J Am Coll Cardiol* 57:1002-1044, 2011.

3. Brott TG, Hobson RW 2nd, Howard G, et al: Stenting versus endarterectomy for treatment of carotid-artery stenosis, *New Engl J Med* 363:11–23, 2010.

4. Eckstein HH, Ringleb P, Allenberg JR, et al: Results of the stent-protected angioplasty versus carotid endarterectomy (space) study to treat symptomatic stenoses at 2 years: a multinational, prospective, randomised trial, *Lancet Neurol* 7:893–902, 2008.

5. Greenhalgh RM, Brown LC, Kwong GP, Powell JT, Thompson SG: Comparison of endovascular aneurysm repair with open repair in patients with abdominal aortic aneurysm (EVAR trial 1), 30-day operative mortality results: Randomised controlled trial, *Lancet* 364:843–848, 2004.

6. Hiatt WR: Medical treatment of peripheral arterial disease and claudication, *N Engl J Med* 344:1608–1621, 2001.

7. Hirsch AT, Haskal ZJ, Hertzer NR, et al: ACC/AHA guidelines for the management of patients with peripheral arterial disease, *J Am Coll Cardiol* 47:1239–1312, 2006.

8. Norgren L, Hiatt WR, Dormandy JA, et al: Inter-society consensus for the management of peripheral arterial disease (tasc ii), *Eur J Vasc Endovasc Surg* 33 (Suppl 1):S1-75, 2007.

9. Lederle FA, Freischlag JA, Kyriakides TC, et al: Outcomes following endovascular vs open repair of abdominal aortic aneurysm: A randomized trial, *JAMA* 302:1535–1542, 2009.

10. Mas JL, Trinquart L, Leys D, et al: Endarterectomy Versus Angioplasty in Patients with Symptomatic Severe Carotid Stenosis (EVA-3S) trial: results up to 4 years from a randomised, multicentre trial, *Lancet Neurol* 7:885–892, 2008.

11. Murad MH, Shahrour A, Shah ND, et al: A systematic review and meta-analysis of randomized trials of carotid endarterectomy vs stenting, *J Vasc Surg* 53:792–797, 2011.

12. Norgren L, Hiatt WR, Dormandy JA, et al: Inter-Society Consensus for the Management of Peripheral Arterial Disease (TASC II), *Eur J Vasc Endovasc Surg* 33(Suppl 1):S1–S75, 2007.

13. Ricotta J, AbuRahma A, Ascher E, et al: Updated Society for Vascular Surgery guidelines for management of extracranial carotid disease, *J Vasc Surg* 54:832–836, 2011.

14. Ringleb PA, Allenberg J, Bruckmann H, et al: 30 day results from the space trial of stent-protected angioplasty versus carotid endarterectomy in symptomatic patients: a randomised non-inferiority trial, *Lancet* 368:1239–1247, 2006.

15. Sacco RL, Adams R, Albers G, et al: AHA/ASA guidelines for prevention of stroke in patients with ischemic stroke or transient ischemic attack, *Stroke* 37:577–617, 2006.

16. White CJ, Jaff MR, Haskal ZJ, et al: Indications for renal arteriography at the time of coronary arteriography: a science advisory from the American Heart Association Committee on Diagnostic and Interventional Cardiac Catheterization, Council on Clinical Cardiology, and the Councils on Cardiovascular Radiology and Intervention and on Kidney in Cardiovascular Disease, *Circulation* 114:1892–1895, 2006.

17. Yadav JS, Wholey MH, Kuntz RE, et al: Protected carotid-artery stenting versus endarterectomy in high-risk patients, *New Engl J Med* 351:1493–1501, 2004.

CHAPTER 56

PREOPERATIVE CARDIAC EVALUATION

Lee A. Fleisher, MD, FACC, FAHA

1. What is the natural history of perioperative cardiac morbidity?

Perioperative cardiac morbidity occurs most commonly during the first 3 postoperative days and includes perioperative myocardial infarction (MI), unstable angina, cardiac death, and nonfatal cardiac arrests. Previously, the peak incidence of perioperative MI was thought to occur during postoperative day 3, although recent studies have suggested it occurs earlier and may arise most commonly in the first 48 hours. Additionally, the mortality from a perioperative cardiac MI has decreased from previous rates of 30% to 50% to approximately 12%. A large number of patients also demonstrate isolated biomarker elevations, which are predictive of worse long-term, but not short-term, survival.

2. What is the cause of perioperative cardiac morbidity?

The cause of perioperative MI is multifactorial. The postoperative period is associated with a stress response, which includes the release of catecholamines and cortisol, resulting in tachycardia and hypertension. The tachycardia can lead to supply/demand mismatches distal to a critical coronary stenosis, causing myocardial ischemia, and, if prolonged, can lead to perioperative MI. Tissue injury, tachycardia, and the hypercoagulable state also leads to plaque rupture and acute thrombosis, potentially resulting in a perioperative MI. Therefore, many perioperative events will not be predicted by identifying critical stenoses or by preoperative imaging. Additionally, perioperative strategies to reduce cardiac morbidity require a multimodal approach of both reducing supply/demand mismatches and reducing the risk of acute thrombosis.

3. What are the strongest predictors of perioperative cardiac events?

For some specific patients, surgery represents a very high risk of cardiac complications and either therapy should be initiated preoperatively or the benefits of surgery must significantly outweigh the risks if the decision is to proceed to surgery. According to the 2009 American College of Cardiology Foundation/American Heart Association (ACCF/AHA) Guidelines on Perioperative Cardiovascular Evaluation, active cardiac conditions for which the patient should undergo evaluation and treatment before noncardiac surgery include unstable coronary syndromes, active heart failure, severe valvular disease, and severe arrhythmias. Specific conditions within these general categories are shown in Table 56-1. Analysis of administrative data suggests that the elevated risk of a recent MI continues for at least the first 60 days.

4. What is the revised cardiac risk index (RCRI) and how is it used clinically?

Cardiac risk indices for perioperative risk stratification have been used in clinical practice for more than 30 years. These indices do not inform clinicians on how to modify perioperative care specifically, but they do provide a baseline assessment of risk and the value of different intervention strategies. Calculation of an index is not a substitute for providing detailed information of the underlying heart disease, its stability, and ventricular function. The RCRI was developed by studying more than 5000 patients and identifying six risk factors, including the following:

- High-risk surgery
- Ischemic heart disease
- History of congestive heart failure
- History of cerebrovascular disease
- Preoperative treatment with insulin
- Preoperative serum creatinine greater than 2 mg/dL

TABLE 56-1. ACTIVE CARDIAC CONDITIONS FOR WHICH THE PATIENT SHOULD UNDERGO EVALUATION AND TREATMENT BEFORE NONCARDIAC SURGERY (CLASS I, LEVEL OF EVIDENCE B)

CONDITION	EXAMPLES
Unstable coronary syndromes	Unstable or severe angina* (CCS class III or IV)[†]
	Recent MI[‡]
	Decompensated HF (NYHA functional class IV; worsening or new-onset HF)
Significant arrhythmias	High-grade atrioventricular block
	Mobitz II atrioventricular block
	Third-degree atrioventricular heart block
	Symptomatic ventricular arrhythmias
	Supraventricular arrhythmias (including atrial fibrillation) with uncontrolled ventricular rate (HR > 100 beats/min at rest)
	Symptomatic bradycardia
	Newly recognized ventricular tachycardia
Severe valvular disease	Severe aortic stenosis (mean pressure gradient >40 mm Hg, aortic valve area <1.0 cm^2, or symptomatic)
	Symptomatic mitral stenosis (progressive dyspnea on exertion, exertional presyncope, or HF)

Modified from Fleisher LA, Beckman JA, Brown KA, et al: ACC/AHA guidelines on perioperative cardiovascular evaluation and care for noncardiac surgery: executive summary, *J Am Coll Cardiol* 50:1716, 2007.
CCS, Canadian Cardiovascular Society; *HF*, heart failure; *HR*, heart rate; *MI*, myocardial infarction; *NYHA*, New York Heart Association.
*According to Campeau L: Grading of angina pectoris [letter]. *Circulation* 54:522-523.
[†]May include *stable* angina in patients who are unusually sedentary.
[‡]The American College of Cardiology National Database Library defines recent MI as more than 7 days but less than or equal to 1 month (within 30 days).

In determining the need and value of preoperative testing and interventions, the ACCF/AHA guidelines incorporate the number of risk factors from the RCRI, other than high-risk surgery, which is incorporated elsewhere. Importantly, diabetes (without regard to type of treatment) is considered one of the risk factors, as opposed to insulin treatment.

5. **What is the importance of exercise capacity?**
Numerous studies have demonstrated the importance of exercise capacity on overall perioperative morbidity and mortality. Based on several of these studies, patients can be dichotomized into poor functional capacity (less than 4 metabolic equivalents [METS]) versus moderate or excellent exercise capacity. Patients with moderate to excellent exercise capacity rarely need further testing before noncardiac surgery.

6. **What is the influence of the surgical procedure on the decision to perform further diagnostic testing?**
In all patients, regardless of the type of surgery, determination of the presence of active cardiac conditions is first and foremost, because proceeding to surgery should only be done after assessing and potentially treating these conditions. Low-risk surgeries (those associated with a perioperative

cardiac morbidity and mortality less than 1%) rarely, if ever, require a change in management based on the results of a diagnostic test. The most common such procedures are those performed on an outpatient basis. Multiple studies have focused on patients undergoing vascular surgery, particularly open aortic and lower extremity revascularization. Therefore, these patients are treated uniquely in the assessment of the need to perform diagnostic testing, based on the extensive evidence and the high perioperative cardiac morbidity and mortality, often in the range of 5% or greater. In the intermediate group of procedures, a gradation of risk is based on the specific surgical procedures and the institution-specific risk is critical to determine if further diagnostic testing would add value. For example, increased surgical volume is associated with lower perioperative risk, and preoperative testing may not lead to changes in management in such institutions.

7. **How do the ACCF/AHA guidelines suggest an approach to preoperative evaluation?**

The algorithm from the 2009 guidelines can be found in Figure 56-1. Importantly, any decision to perform diagnostic testing based on the algorithm must incorporate the value of the information to change perioperative management. Changes in management can include the decision to undergo coronary revascularization, but may also include decisions by the patient to forego surgery and decisions by the surgeon to change the type of procedure. The algorithm incorporates the urgency of surgery, clinical risk factors, and functional status. For patients with risk factors, who are undergoing vascular surgery, the studies demonstrate no difference in outcomes between coronary revascularization before noncardiac surgery and proceeding directly to the noncardiac surgery, incorporating heart rate control perioperatively. The class of recommendation and strength of evidence, based on the ACCF/AHA criteria, is shown on the algorithm.

8. **What is the value of coronary revascularization before noncardiac surgery?**

Previously it was thought that patients who had undergone prior coronary artery bypass grafting (CABG) had a lower rate of perioperative cardiac morbidity compared with patients with a similar extent of coronary disease who had not undergone revascularization. However, several randomized trials have questioned the value of acute revascularization before noncardiac surgery. In the Coronary Artery Revascularization Prophylaxis (CARP) trial, 500 patients were randomized to coronary revascularization versus medical therapy and followed for up to 6 years. Importantly, patients with left main coronary artery (LMCA) disease, severe triple vessel disease with depressed ejection fraction, and severe comorbidities were excluded. Two-thirds of the patients who underwent coronary revascularization had percutaneous coronary interventions (PCI). There was no difference in either perioperative or long-term morbidity and mortality. In the Dutch Echocardiographic Cardiac Risk Evaluation Applying Stress Echocardiography II (DECREASE-II) trial, patients with one to two clinical risk factors were randomized to preoperative testing and revascularization or proceeded directly to vascular surgery with tight heart rate control; again no difference in outcome was detected. In the DECREASE-V pilot study of 101 patients with extensive coronary artery disease, no difference in perioperative cardiac morbidity and mortality was seen between the revascularization and medical therapy arms of the trial, although the authors were able to demonstrate better short- and long-term outcomes in the subset of patients for whom revascularization was successful. However, the quality of the data from the DECREASE trials has recently been questioned. Similarly, analysis of the nonrandomized patients in the CARP database demonstrated improved perioperative outcomes in the subset of patients with LMCA disease who underwent coronary revascularization. Therefore, current high-quality evidence suggests that coronary revascularization before major noncardiac surgery is of limited or no benefit in stable patients and in those with only 1 or 2 risk factors; however, there may be benefit to coronary artery bypass grafting in patients with LMCA or severe triple vessel disease.

9. **What is the concern regarding surgery in patients with a previous PCI?**

Patients who have previously undergone PCI have not been shown to have a significant difference in perioperative outcomes compared with case-matched controls. Importantly, the risk of thrombosis after PCI is high and the hypercoagulable perioperative state increases the probability of this occurring. Multiple cohort studies and case reports have reported the occurrence of acute thrombosis and

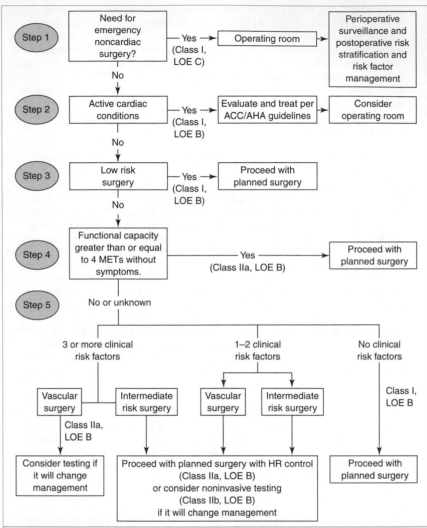

Figure 56-1. Algorithm from the American College of Cardiology Foundation/American Heart Association *(ACCF/AHA)* for the decision for preoperative cardiovascular testing in patients undergoing noncardiac surgery. (Modified from Fleisher LA, Beckman JA, Brown KA, et al: 2009 ACCF/AHA focused update on perioperative beta blockade incorporated into the ACC/AHA 2007 guidelines on perioperative cardiovascular evaluation and care for noncardiac surgery. *J Am Coll Cardiol* 54:e13-e118, 2009.) *HR*, Heart rate; *LOE*, level of evidence; *MET*, metabolic equivalent.

perioperative MI at the site of coronary stents. In patients with bare metal stents, this most commonly occurs in patients who have undergone noncardiac surgery within 30 days. In patients with drug-eluting stents, the higher rate of acute thrombosis can be seen for at least 1 year, and there are data to suggest it continues after this period. Therefore, the current recommendation is to delay elective surgery for at least 14 days after balloon angioplasty (without stenting), at least 30 days after placement of bare metal stents, and until 1 year after placement of drug-eluting stents.

10. **How should antiplatelet agents be managed in the perioperative period?**
The consensus statement from the ACCF/AHA in 2007, as well as the perioperative guidelines, advocate continuing aspirin in all patients who have had a previous PCI. In patients currently taking a P2Y12 inhibitor particularly those within 30 days of placement of a bare metal stent or 1 year for drug-eluting stents, the agent should either be continued, or discontinued for a short period and restarted as quickly as possible in the postoperative period. The critical period may be 5 days for the P2Y12 inhibitor.

11. **How should beta-adrenergic blocking agents (β-blockers) be managed in the perioperative period?**
Based on cohort studies and consensus opinion, patients who are receiving chronic β-blocker therapy at the time of surgery should be continued on these agents to avoid the risk of β-blocker withdrawal, which is associated with tachycardia and an increased incidence of perioperative MI. Currently, controversy exists regarding the acute administration of β-blocker therapy for those patients at high risk of perioperative event but not currently taking these agents. The DECREASE trial and subsequent cohort studies from the Erasmus group have demonstrated improved outcome in patients with known coronary heart disease with the administration of bisoprolol at lower doses, started a minimum of 7 days prior to surgery and titrated to a heart rate less than 80 beats/min, although there is currently controversy regarding the quality of the study data published by Poldermans. In the Perioperative Ischemic Evaluation (POISE) study, 8351 patients were randomized to high-dose metoprolol succinate, a long-acting agent, which was compared with placebo. Although nonfatal perioperative MIs were reduced, the incidence of death and stroke was significantly increased, and was associated with higher rates of hypotension. Therefore, initiating high-dose β-blocker therapy in the perioperative period without titration to heart rate and blood pressure could lead to greater harm than benefit and should not be considered. However, heart rate control remains a critical approach to reducing perioperative cardiac morbidity and initial treatment should focus on treating the cause of tachycardia, including pain management, after which, careful titration of β-blockers is appropriate. In patients who should be taking β-blockers (independent of noncardiac surgery) for underlying coronary artery disease, initiation and titration a week or more in advance of surgery has been advocated based on data by some authors, but the safest protocol is controversial. There is also nonrandomized data to suggest that atenolol is associated with improved outcome compared to metoprolol.

12. **How should statins be managed in the perioperative period?**
Previously there was concern that continuation of statins in the perioperative period could lead to an increased incidence of rhabdomyolysis, and most clinicians discontinued these agents before surgery. However, evidence has accumulated that statin therapy is protective and that withdrawal is harmful. There is randomized data to suggest that starting statin therapy at least 7 days in advance in high-risk patients is associated with improved outcome. In the 2009 perioperative guidelines, the committee advocated continuing statins in all patients currently taking these agents.

BIBLIOGRAPHY, SUGGESTED READINGS, AND WEBSITES

1. Devereaux PJ, Xavier D, Pogue J, et al: Characteristics and short-term prognosis of perioperative myocardial infarction in patients undergoing noncardiac surgery: a cohort study, *Ann Intern Med* 154:523–528, 2011.

2. Devereaux PJ, Yang H, Yusuf S, et al: Effects of extended-release metoprolol succinate in patients undergoing non-cardiac surgery (POISE trial): a randomised controlled trial, *Lancet* 371:1839–1847, 2008.

3. Fleisher LA, Beckman JA, Brown KA, et al: 2009 ACCF/AHA focused update on perioperative beta blockade incorporated into the ACC/AHA 2007 guidelines on perioperative cardiovascular evaluation and care for noncardiac surgery, *J Am Coll Cardiol* 54:e13–e118, 2009.

4. McFalls EO, Ward HB, Moritz TE, et al: Coronary-artery revascularization before elective major vascular surgery, *N Engl J Med* 351:2795–2804, 2004.

5. Poldermans D, Bax JJ, Boersma E, et al: Guidelines for pre-operative cardiac risk assessment and perioperative cardiac management in non-cardiac surgery: the Task Force for Preoperative Cardiac Risk Assessment and Perioperative Cardiac Management in Non-cardiac Surgery of the European Society of Cardiology (ESC) and endorsed by the European Society of Anaesthesiology (ESA), *Eur Heart J* 30:2769–2812, 2009.

6. Poldermans D, Bax JJ, Schouten O, et al: Should major vascular surgery be delayed because of preoperative cardiac testing in intermediate-risk patients receiving beta-blocker therapy with tight heart rate control? *J Am Coll Cardiol* 48:964–969, 2006.

7. Poldermans D, Boersma E, Bax JJ, et al: The effect of bisoprolol on perioperative mortality and myocardial infarction in high-risk patients undergoing vascular surgery. Dutch Echocardiographic Cardiac Risk Evaluation Applying Stress Echocardiography Study Group [see comments], *N Engl J Med* 341:1789–1794, 1999.

CHAPTER 57

PULMONARY EMBOLISM

Talal Dahhan, MD, Christian Castillo, MD, and Victor F. Tapson, MD

1. Who first described pulmonary embolism?

Pulmonary embolism (PE) was probably first reported in the early 1800s clinically, but Rudolf Virchow elucidated the mechanism by describing the connection between venous thrombosis and PE in the late 1800s. He also coined the term *embolism*.

2. What is Virchow's triad?

Virchow's triad comprises the three broad categories of risk factors that contribute to thrombosis, including:
- Endothelial injury
- Stasis or turbulence of blood flow
- Blood hypercoagulability

3. What percentage of patients with acute PE have clinical evidence of lower extremity deep vein thrombosis (DVT)?

In the Prospective Investigation of Pulmonary Embolism Diagnosis (PIOPED) II study of 192 patients with angiographically documented PE, 47% had evidence of DVT by physical examination. The majority of patients with proven PE do have residual DVT present proven by imaging. More than 90% of emboli originate in the deep veins of the legs and thighs.

4. What percentage of patients with proximal DVT will develop PE?

Approximately 50% of patients with proximal DVT will develop PE.

5. What is the usual cause of death in subjects with PE?

It is well established that right ventricular (RV) failure is the cause of cardiovascular collapse and death in acute massive PE. Registry data have also suggested that patients with RV dysfunction on echocardiogram are at increased risk of all-cause mortality at 3 months.

6. What are the major risk factors for venous thromboembolism (VTE)?

Risk factors are crucial in raising suspicion for acute VTE, although the disease may be idiopathic. Previous thromboembolism, immobility, cancer, advanced age, major surgery, trauma, acute medical illness, and certain thrombophilias impart significant risk. A list of risk factors for VTE is shown in Box 57-1.

7. How commonly are recommended VTE prevention measures used?

Recent data suggest that worldwide, prophylaxis is underused. A recent study including more than 67,000 patients, the Epidemiologic International Day for the Evaluation of Patients at Risk for Venous Thromboembolism in the Acute Hospital Care Setting (ENDORSE) registry, indicated that in many countries less than half of patients deemed appropriate candidates for prophylaxis measures actually received them.

8. How should a patient with suspected DVT be initially evaluated?

The symptoms and signs of DVT are nonspecific, and although clinical prediction rules can be useful, there should be a low threshold to proceed to compression ultrasonography. D-dimer testing may be useful; the diagnosis of DVT can be excluded without the need for ultrasound if the patient has a combination of a low or moderate clinical probability estimate and a negative D-dimer result. If the patient falls into the moderate or high clinical pretest probability or has a positive D-dimer test,

Box 57-1 RISK FACTORS FOR VENOUS THROMBOEMBOLISM*

Hereditary
- Antithrombin deficiency
- Protein C deficiency
- Protein S deficiency
- Factor V Leiden
- Activated protein C resistance without factor V Leiden
- Prothrombin gene mutation
- Dysfibrinogenemia
- Plasminogen deficiency
- Elevated factor VIII level

Acquired
- Reduced mobility
- Advanced age
- Active cancer
- Acute medical illness
- Nephrotic syndrome
- Major surgery
- Trauma
- Spinal cord injury
- Pregnancy and postpartum period
- Myeloproliferative disorders: polycythemia vera
- Antiphospholipid antibody syndrome
- Oral contraceptives
- Hormonal replacement therapy
- Chemotherapy
- Obesity
- Central venous catheters
- Immobilizer or cast

Possible/probable but not certain risk factors
- Low tissue factor pathway inhibitor levels
- Elevated levels of the following:
  1. Homocysteine
  2. Factors VIII, IX, XI
  3. Fibrinogen
  4. Thrombin-activatable fibrinolysis inhibitor
  5. Lipoprotein (a)

*The hereditary versus acquired nature of some disorders listed remains unclear and causes may involve both genetic and environmental factors.

further evaluation with ultrasound is advised. The enzyme-linked immunosorbent assay (ELISA)–based D-dimer tests have superior sensitivity (96% to 98%). DVT is discussed further in Chapter 50.

9. **What are the symptoms and signs of acute PE?**
   The symptoms and signs of PE are generally nonspecific but most commonly include dyspnea and chest pain, and may include the following:
   - Dyspnea (either sudden in onset or evolving over days)
   - Chest pain, often pleuritic (such chest pain may be associated with chest wall tenderness and generally occurs with pulmonary infarct)

- Hemoptysis (generally occurs with pulmonary infarct)
- Palpitations
- Light headedness
- Syncope
- Tachypnea
- Tachycardia
- Pleural rub
- Fever
- Wheezing
- Rales

If PE is associated with pulmonary hypertension, then elevated neck veins, a loud P2, RV heave, or a right-sided gallop may be noted.

10. **What are four clinical syndromes seen with acute PE?**
    - **Massive PE with acute cor pulmonale:** Not all patients with acute cor pulmonale will go on to develop hypotension (which defines massive PE), but such a presentation should raise concern.
    - **Submassive PE:** This is defined as acute PE which causes RV dysfunction. Of note, based upon the Pulmonary Embolism Severity Index (see Question 19), low-risk and intermediate-risk categories have been referred to as "nonmassive PE."
    - **Pulmonary infarction and/or pulmonary hemorrhage:** Because of dual blood supply and free anastomosis between the pulmonary capillaries, emboli usually don't cause infarction in a healthy lung. Pulmonary infarction is uncommon when emboli obstruct central arteries but much more common when distal arteries are occluded. Obstruction of distal arteries can result in pulmonary hemorrhage as a result of an influx of bronchial arterial blood at systemic pressure. Hemorrhage causes symptoms and radiographic changes usually attributed to pulmonary infarction.
    - **Acute unexplained dyspnea:** A diagnosis of PE should be considered in patients with dyspnea of unclear cause and may merit consideration even when there is another potential explanation.

11. **What is the Wells score for suspected acute PE?**
    First described in 1998, the Wells score is a clinical prediction score based on simple, noninvasive clinical parameters. It has evolved over the years, has been validated, and is useful in determining pretest probability for suspected acute PE. Pretest probability can be defined based on the calculated score from the modified Wells score (Table 57-1). PE has ultimately been classified as "unlikely" if the clinical decision score was 4 or less, and "likely" with a score of more than 4 points. This cutoff was chosen because it has been shown to give an acceptable VTE diagnostic failure rate of 1.7% to 2.2% when in combination with a normal D-dimer test result. Moreover, with a score of 4 or less and a negative D-dimer test, no further testing appears to be necessary. A score greater than 4 requires further evaluation, and computed tomographic angiography (CTA) is usually performed. High clinical suspicion, however, should always take precedence, even if the Wells score is low.

12. **What are the most common findings on electrocardiography (ECG) in acute PE?**
    Sinus tachycardia is commonly present in acute PE. The "classic" $S_1Q_3T_3$ pattern (Fig. 57-1) is seen in a minority of patients. Other ECG findings include the following:
    - Arrhythmias (premature atrial and ventricular beats)
    - First-degree atrioventricular block
    - Supraventricular tachycardia
    - RV strain (right axis deviation)
    - RV hypertrophy
    - Right bundle branch block
    - Depression, elevation, or inversion of ST segments and T waves

    ST-T changes, when present, are often most marked in the right precordial leads. Although the ECG may be suggestive of PE, it cannot diagnose or rule out acute PE.

TABLE 57-1. THE MODIFIED WELLS PRETEST PROBABILITY SCORING OF PULMONARY EMBOLISM POINT SCORE

Score Assignment

VARIABLE	SCORE
PE is likely or more likely than alternate diagnosis	3.0
Clinical signs or symptoms of DVT	3.0
Heart rate ≥ 100 beats/min	1.5
Prior DVT or PE	1.5
Immobilization, limited to bed rest for >3 days	1.5
Surgery within the last 4 weeks	1.5
Hemoptysis	1.0
Active malignancy	1.0

Modified Wells Pretest Probability Assessment (Used with $\dot{V}/\dot{Q}$)

Score < 2:	Score 2 TO 6:	Score > 6:
Low probability	Intermediate probability	High probability

Dichotomized Wells Pretest Probability Assessment* (Used with CTA)

Score ≤ 4:	Score > 4:
PE unlikely	PE likely

CTA, Computed tomographic angiography; DVT, deep vein thrombosis; PE, pulmonary embolism; $\dot{V}/\dot{Q}$, ventilation-perfusion.
*Wells PS, Anderson DR, Rodger M, et al: Excluding pulmonary embolism at the bedside without diagnostic imaging: management of patients with suspected pulmonary embolism presenting to the emergency department by using a simple clinical model and D-dimer. Ann Intern Med 135:98-107, 2001.

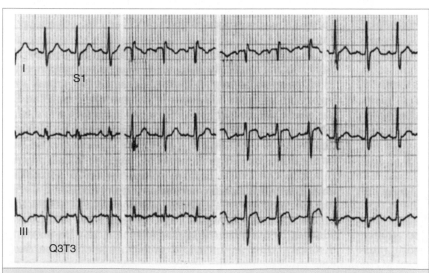

Figure 57-1. An electrocardiogram in a patient with acute pulmonary embolism (PE). Sinus tachycardia, the most common ECG finding in PE, is present. In addition, there is an S1Q3T3 pattern present, with an S wave in lead I and a Q and T wave in lead III. The S1Q3T3 pattern finding is an uncommon finding in PE, but its presence in the appropriate clinical context should raise suspicion for PE.

13. **What are the common chest radiographic findings in patients with acute PE?**
The chest radiograph is commonly abnormal in acute PE, although a significant minority of patients have a normal film. When it is abnormal, however, the findings are nonspecific and include an elevated hemidiaphragm, focal or multifocal infiltrates, pleural effusion, platelike atelectasis, enlarged pulmonary arteries, focal oligemia (the Westermark sign), and RV enlargement.

Hampton and Castleman described in detail the radiographic findings in PE and pulmonary infarction in 1940, having assembled 370 cases of PE and infarction. In pulmonary infarction, they suggested that the cardiac margin of the opacity of a pulmonary infarction on a chest radiograph is rounded or *hump*-shaped (i.e., the Hampton hump).

14. **What are typical arterial blood gas (ABG) findings in patients with PE?**
Low Pa_{O_2}, low Pa_{CO_2}, high alveolar-arterial oxygen difference. Although nonspecific, one of these findings is likely to be present in up to 97% of cases. A normal ABG does not absolutely exclude PE.

15. **When should a ventilation-perfusion ($\dot{V}/\dot{Q}$) scan be performed?**
The $\dot{V}/\dot{Q}$ scan is most useful when the chest radiograph is normal and there is no cardiopulmonary disease. In this setting, it has the highest likelihood of being either normal or high probability. Diagnostic tests (especially those for PE) must be interpreted in light of the patient's pretest probability score. It is crucial to remember that commonly the $\dot{V}/\dot{Q}$ scan is low or intermediate probability, even when PE is present.

$\dot{V}/\dot{Q}$ scanning may also be useful in patients with abnormal renal function, in which a CTA using iodinated contrast agent may be contraindicated.

16. **Does a negative CTA indicate that PE is not present with certainty?**
No, but a good quality CTA is extremely sensitive. We learned from the PIOPED II study, published in 2006, that clinical probability is extremely important when considering CTA results. Approximately 60% (9/15) of patients who had high clinical pretest probability but a negative CTA were ultimately diagnosed with PE. Similarly, 42% (16/38) of patients with a low clinical pretest probability and a positive CTA did not have PE. A recent study of more than 3000 patients with suspected acute PE by the Christopher Investigators suggested that if CTA is negative, outcome at 3 months is excellent without therapy. Nonetheless, it is prudent to consider additional imaging when a negative CTA is accompanied by high clinical suspicion; furthermore, imaging quality is not uniformly high in all clinical settings. Finally, computed tomographic (CT) scanning has evolved such that modern day multislice scanners are more sensitive than their predecessors. A large PE, documented by CTA, is shown in Figure 57-2. A diagnostic algorithm, which can be used as a guide, is offered in Figure 57-3.

17. **How does echocardiography aid in the diagnosis of PE?**
Transthoracic echocardiography can detect RV strain and dilation. Risk stratification should be strongly considered in patients diagnosed with PE. The McConnell sign, a normally contracting right ventricular apex associated with severe hypokinesis of the mid–free wall, is an echocardiographic pattern that suggests, but is *not* diagnostic of, acute PE.

18. **What is the most appropriate initial therapy for patients with documented acute PE?**
In patients with acute PE, a therapeutic level of anticoagulation should ideally be achieved within 24 hours, because this reduces the risk of recurrence. The 9th American College of Chest Physicians Evidence-Based Clinical Practice Guidelines (ACCP-9) from February 2012, recommend initiation of treatment while awaiting diagnostic tests if clinical suspicion is deemed high. Initial treatment with low-molecular-weight heparin (LMWH), unfractionated heparin (UFH), or fondaparinux for at least 5 days, together with initiation of oral anticoagulant therapy until the international normalized ratio (INR) is 2.0 or more for at least 24 hours, is recommended. Warfarin should be started on the first treatment day. ACCP-9 also recommends that in patients with acute nonmassive PE, initial treatment

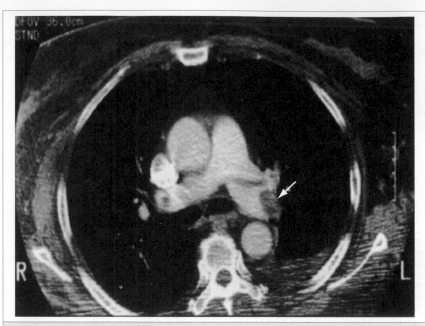

Figure 57-2. A large embolism *(arrow)* in the left pulmonary artery is shown by computed tomographic arteriography.

with LMWH rather than intravenous UFH be used, if feasible, based on advantages of LMWH, including subcutaneous rather than intravenous delivery, much less need for monitoring, and a lower rate of heparin-induced thrombocytopenia. The LMWH preparations are also more bioavailable and thus, more predictable than standard UFH in terms of degree of anticoagulation. Anticoagulation clearly improves survival in patients with acute symptomatic PE.

Rivaroxaban, a new oral anticoagulant approved for the treatment of DVT/PE, is discussed in Question 27 below.

19. **How should one stratify patient risk with acute PE?**
    Outcomes of PE depend on a number of factors. The Pulmonary Embolism Severity Index (PESI) allows stratification on a clinical basis. Several therapeutic implications exist for patients with PE. High-risk patients (who represent about 5% of all symptomatic patients, with about a 15% short-term mortality) should be considered for aggressive treatment with thrombolytic therapy or surgical or catheter embolectomy. Low-risk patients (most patients with PE, with a short-term mortality of about 1%) benefit from anticoagulation therapy, and can sometimes be monitored and followed as outpatients. Intermediate-risk patients (who represent about 30% of all symptomatic patients) should be admitted to the hospital, anticoagulated, and be considered for thrombolytic therapy if indicated. Low-risk and intermediate-risk categories can be referred to as nonmassive PE. The PESI has been simplified (Table 57-2) to ease clinical application. The 305 of 995 patients (30.7%) who were classified as low risk by the simplified PESI had a 30-day mortality of 1.0% (95% confidence interval [CI] of 0.0% to 2.1%) compared with 10.9% (95% CI of 8.5% to 13.2%) in the high-risk group.

20. **Are there any laboratory investigations that may help in the prognosis of patients with PE?**
    B-type natriuretic peptide (BNP) and N-terminal of B-type natriuretic peptide (NT-proBNP) levels and cardiac biomarkers such as troponin T or I may help to identify severity of PE. Elevated troponin has

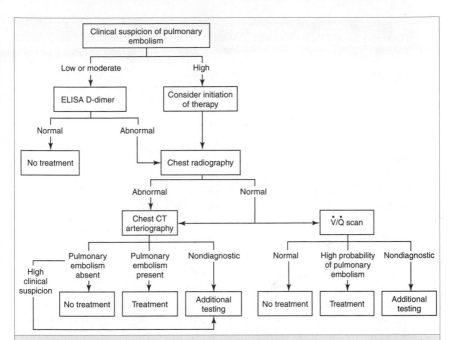

Figure 57-3. A diagnostic strategy for suspected acute pulmonary embolism (PE). The use of a clinical prediction score and D-dimer testing may reduce the need for imaging. If suspicion for acute PE is high and the bleeding risk deemed low, initiation of anticoagulant therapy should be considered. The V̇/Q̇ scan is most useful when the chest radiograph is normal or minimally abnormal. When significant renal insufficiency is present, computed tomographic arteriography (CTA) is contraindicated and the V̇/Q̇ scan may be useful. Finally, when chest CTA is nondiagnostic, V̇/Q̇ scanning can be considered; a negative V̇/Q̇ scan is highly sensitive and a high-probability scan is quite sensitive. However, V̇/Q̇ scans are often nondiagnostic particularly when underlying lung disease is present. When the V̇/Q̇ scan is nondiagnostic, and CTA cannot be done, ultrasound of the legs or magnetic resonance imaging of the legs and/or lungs can be considered. A *negative* leg study, does not, however, rule out PE. (Modified from Tapson VF: Acute pulmonary embolism. *N Engl J Med* 358:1037-1052, 2008.) *CT*, Computed tomography; *ELISA*, enzyme-linked immunosorbent assay; *V̇/Q̇*, ventilation-perfusion.

been correlated with increased mortality in acute PE. Neither of these tests, however, is sensitive or specific.

21. **What is the primary indication for thrombolytic therapy?**
    Proven PE with cardiogenic shock is the clearest indication. ACCP-9 also notes that in selected high-risk patients without hypotension who are judged to have a low risk of bleeding, thrombolytic therapy can be considered. This received a grade 2C recommendation—that is, a decision made based on limited data and expert opinion to support the suggestion. An example would be in submassive PE (RV dilation and hypokinesis without hypotension). The decision to use thrombolytic therapy depends on the clinician's assessment of PE severity, prognosis, and risk of bleeding. Thus, it is often considered in patients with hypotension but without shock. Box 57-2 summarizes recommendations with regard to thrombolytic therapy in PE.

22. **What are some complications and contraindications of thrombolytic therapy?**
    Intracranial hemorrhage is the most devastating complication of thrombolytic therapy and has been reported in approximately 1% of patients in clinical trials, but in about 3% of patients from the International Cooperative Pulmonary Embolism Registry (ICOPER) representing a more "real world" patient population. Other complications include retroperitoneal and gastrointestinal bleeding and bleeding

TABLE 57-2.   ORIGINAL AND SIMPLIFIED PULMONARY EMBOLISM SEVERITY INDEX

Variable	Original PESI*	Simplified PESI†
Age > 80 years	Age in years	+1
Male sex	+10	
History of cancer	+30	+1
History of heart failure‡	+10‡	+1‡
History of chronic lung disease‡	+10‡	
Heart rate ≥ 110 beats per min	+20	+1
Systolic blood pressure < 100 mm Hg	+30	+1
Respiratory rate ≥ 30 breaths per min	+20	
Temperature < 36° C	+20	
Altered mental status	+60	
Arterial oxygen saturation < 90%	+20	+1

Patients classified as low risk by the simplified pulmonary embolism severity index *(PESI)* had a 30-day mortality of 1.0% (95% confidence interval [CI], 0.0%-2.1%) compared with 10.9% (95% CI, 8.5%-13.2%) in the high-risk group.
*For the original index, the total point score is reached by adding the total points plus the patient's age in years: Class 1 = ≤65 points; class 2 = 66-85; class 3 = 86-105; class 4 = 106-125; class 5 = >125. (Classes 1 and 2 are considered low risk, and classes 3-5 high risk.)
†For the simplified index, the total points are added: 0 = low risk, ≥1 = high risk. Empty cells imply that the variable is not included.
‡For the simplified index, history of heart failure and of chronic lung disease are combined as cardiopulmonary disease for 1 point.

from surgical wounds or from sites of recent invasive procedures. Contraindications to thrombolytic therapy are divided into major and relative contraindications and are listed in Box 57-3.

23. **Has thrombolytic therapy been shown to improve mortality from PE?**
No. Thrombolytic therapy has never been shown to improve mortality from PE in a clinical trial. It has been shown to improve hemodynamics and lung scans with a suggestion that younger (less than 50 years old) patients, and patients with new emboli (less than 48 hours old) and larger emboli respond better. However, based upon a review of the available medical literature, the standard of care in the absence of absolute contraindications is to administer thrombolytic therapy in the setting of massive PE.

24. **What are the indications for inferior vena caval (IVC) filter placement?**
ACCP-9 states that the primary indications for placement of an IVC filter include contraindications to anticoagulation, major bleeding complications during anticoagulation, and recurrent PE despite adequate anticoagulation. Although there are no firm trial data, some experts suggest filter placement in the case of massive PE when it is believed that additional emboli might be lethal, particularly if thrombolytic therapy is contraindicated.

25. **What are some complications of IVC filter placement?**
IVC filters increase the subsequent incidence of DVT (in about 20% of patients) and have not been shown to increase overall survival. Other complications of IVC filters include procedural-related insertion-site thrombosis (8%), pneumothorax, air embolism, or hematoma, and late complications of IVC thrombosis (2% to 10%), postthrombotic syndrome, IVC penetration, and filter migration. Most models of IVC filters are retrievable, typically within several months of insertion. While this may alleviate some of the late complications of IVC filter placement, complications may also occur with

> **Box 57-2 SYNOPSIS OF KEY THROMBOLYTIC THERAPY RECOMMENDATIONS FROM THE 9TH AMERICAN COLLEGE OF CHEST PHYSICIANS CONSENSUS**
>
> 1. All pulmonary embolism (PE) patients should undergo rapid risk stratification (Grade 1C).
> 2. When there is hypotension, thrombolytic therapy is recommended, unless there are major contraindications owing to bleeding risk (Grade 2C).
> 3. Thrombolysis in patients with hypotension should not be delayed, because irreversible cardiogenic shock may ensue.
> 4. In selected patients with acute PE not associated with hypotension and with a low bleeding risk whose initial clinical presentation, or clinical course after starting anticoagulant therapy, suggests a high risk of developing hypotension, thrombolytic therapy is suggested (Grade 2C).
> 5. The decision to use thrombolytic therapy depends on the clinician's assessment of PE severity, prognosis, and risk of bleeding.
> 6. In patients with acute PE, when a thrombolytic agent is used, short infusion times (e.g., a 2-hour infusion) over prolonged infusion times (e.g., a 24-hour infusion) are suggested (Grade 2C).
> 7. In patients with acute PE, when a thrombolytic agent is used, peripheral vein administration rather than direct pulmonary artery infusion is recommended (Grade 2C).
> 8. In patients with acute PE associated with hypotension and who have contraindications to thrombolysis, failed thrombolysis, or shock that is likely to cause death before systemic thrombolysis can take effect (e.g., within hours), if appropriate expertise and resources are available, catheter-assisted thrombus removal (over no such intervention) is suggested (Grade 2C).
>
> Recommendations are graded based on the evidence. Grade 1 indicates that benefit appears to outweigh potential harm, whereas with Grade 2, this is less certain. The lettered recommendation indicates the quality of the methodology used to make the recommendation. "*A*" recommendations are the strongest and are based on data from very good-quality prospective, randomized trials. Most of these recommendations are Grade 2C, that is, there are inadequate prospective, randomized, double-bind data to make a recommendation. Grade 2C indicates that the data are from uncontrolled, observational studies. Level 2 is considered a "suggestion" and not a recommendation.
>
> Modified from Kearon C, Akl EA, Comerota AJ, et al: Antithrombotic therapy for VTE disease: Antithrombotic Therapy and Prevention of Thrombosis, 9th ed: American College of Chest Physicians Evidence-Based Clinical Practice Guidelines. Chest 141:e419S-e494S, 2012.

retrieval. Clearly, more data are needed examining the indications for IVC filter placement and the pros and cons of retrieval. At present, the evidence base is inadequate to recommend either retrieval or leaving an IVC filter in place.

26. Can PE be treated as an outpatient?

Although the use of LMWH as outpatient therapy for DVT is well established, the data for outpatient treatment of acute PE are less robust. Recent data suggest that early discharge in acute PE can be done safely if patients are carefully screened. Initial admission, even if brief, is clearly the most common practice today.

27. Are there any advances in oral anticoagulation therapy for PE?

Several new oral anticoagulant drugs have been developed. These direct (i.e., antithrombin-independent) inhibitors of factor Xa (e.g., rivaroxaban, apixaban) or thrombin (e.g., dabigatran) avoid most of the drawbacks of heparin and could replace vitamin K antagonists and heparins in many patients. These drugs

> ### Box 57-3 MAJOR AND RELATIVE CONTRAINDICATIONS TO THROMBOLYTIC THERAPY
>
> **Major contraindications include:**
> - Structural intracranial disease
> - Previous intracranial hemorrhage
> - Ischemic stroke within 3 months
> - Active bleeding
> - Recent brain or spinal surgery
> - Recent head trauma with fracture or brain injury
> - Bleeding diathesis
>
> **Relative contraindications include:**
> - Systolic blood pressure above or equal to 180 mm Hg
> - Diastolic blood pressure above or equal to 110 mm Hg
> - Recent bleeding (non-intracranial)
> - Recent surgery
> - Recent invasive procedure
> - Ischemic stroke more than 3 months previously
> - Traumatic cardiopulmonary resuscitation
> - Pericarditis or pericardial fluid
> - Diabetic retinopathy
> - Pregnancy
> - Age 75 years or above

are administered in fixed doses, do not need coagulation monitoring in the laboratory, and have very few drug–drug or drug–food interactions. Dabigatran and rivaroxaban are U.S. Food and Drug Administration (FDA)-approved for treatment of nonvalvular atrial fibrillation. Rivaroxaban is also approved for prophylaxis for both total hip and total knee replacement. Both drugs have proven noninferior to warfarin in acute treatment of DVT and PE, after a short period of bridging with LMWH. Oral rivaroxaban was FDA-approved for the treatment of acute DVT and/or PE based upon the EINSTEIN-DVT and EINSTEIN-PE studies. In EINSTEIN-PE, oral rivaroxaban was noninferior to the standard approach of parenteral antico-agulation together with warfarin therapy with regard to recurrent VTE events. Importantly, major bleeding rates were significantly less with rivaroxaban.

BIBLIOGRAPHY, SUGGESTED READINGS, AND WEBSITES

1. Christopher Study Investigators: Effectiveness of managing suspected pulmonary embolism using an algorithm combining clinical probability, D-dimer testing, and computed tomography, *JAMA* 295:172–179, 2006.

2. Chunilal SD, Eikelboom JW, Attia J, et al: Does this patient have pulmonary embolism? *JAMA* 290:2849–2858, 2003.

3. Cohen AT, Tapson VF, Bergmann JF, et al: Venous thromboembolism risk and prophylaxis in the acute hospital care setting (ENDORSE study): a multinational cross-sectional study, *Lancet* 371:387–394, 2008.

4. Dalen JE: Pulmonary embolism: what have we learned since Virchow? Natural history, pathophysiology, and diagnosis, *Chest* 122:1440–1456, 2002.

5. Dalen JE: Pulmonary embolism: what have we learned since Virchow? Treatment and prevention, *Chest* 122:1801–1817, 2002.

6. Dong B, Jirong Y, Liu G, Wang Q, Wu T: Thrombolytic therapy for pulmonary embolism, *Cochrane Database Syst Rev* 2:CD004437, 2006.

7. Goldhaber S, Bounameaux H, et al: Pulmonary embolism and deep vein thrombosis, *Lancet* 379:1835–1846, 2012.

8. Goldhaber SZ, Visani L, De Rosa M: Acute pulmonary embolism: clinical outcomes in the International Cooperative Pulmonary Embolism Registry (ICOPER), *Lancet* 353:1386–1389, 1999.

9. Hanna CL, Michael B, Streiff MB: The role of vena caval filters in the management of venous thromboembolism, *Blood Rev* 19:179–202, 2005.

10. Jiménez D, Aujesky D, Moores L, et al: Simplification of the pulmonary embolism severity index for prognostication in patients with acute symptomatic PE, *Arch Intern Med* 170:1383–1389, 2010.

11. Kearon C, Akl EA, Comerota AJ, et al: Antithrombotic therapy for VTE disease: Antithrombotic therapy and prevention of thrombosis, 9th ed: American College of Chest Physicians Evidence-Based Clinical Practice Guidelines, *Chest* 141:e419S–e494S, 2012.

12. Kurzyna M, Torbicki A, Pruszczyk P: Disturbed right ventricular ejection pattern as a new Doppler echocardiographic sign of acute pulmonary embolism, *Am J Cardiol* 90:507–511, 2002.

13. Piazza G, Goldhaber S: Fibrinolysis for acute pulmonary embolism, *Vasc Med* 15:419–428, 2010.

14. PIOPED Investigators: Value of the ventilation/perfusion scan in acute pulmonary embolism, *JAMA* 263:2753–2759, 1990.

15. Simonneau G, Sors H, Charbonnier B, et al: A comparison of low-molecular weight heparin with unfractionated heparin for acute pulmonary embolism, *N Engl J Med* 337:663–669, 1997.

16. Stein PD, Alnas M, Skaf E, et al: Outcomes and complications of retrievable inferior vena cava filters, *Am J Cardiol* 94:1090–1093, 2004.

17. Stein PD, Fowler SE, Goodman LR, et al: Multidetector computed tomography for acute pulmonary embolism (PIOPED II), *N Engl J Med* 354:2317–2327, 2006.

18. Tapson VF: Acute pulmonary embolism, *N Engl J Med* 358:1037–1052, 2008.

CHAPTER 58

PULMONARY HYPERTENSION

Zeenat Safdar, MD, FCCP, FACP, FPVRI

1. **What is the hemodynamic criteria used to define pulmonary arterial hypertension?**

   At the Fourth World Symposium on Pulmonary Hypertension, the definition of pulmonary arterial hypertension (PAH) was updated as the mean pulmonary arterial pressure equal to or more than 25 mm Hg at rest, with a pulmonary arterial wedge or left atrial pressure equal to or less than 15 mm Hg. The exercise and pulmonary vascular resistance criteria were removed from this updated definition due to the poor availability of evidence. Right-sided heart catheterization (RHC) is the diagnostic gold standard to confirm PAH diagnosis. During the RHC, pulmonary artery pressures, right atrial pressure, right ventricle (RV) pressure, cardiac output, cardiac index, and pulmonary artery wedge pressures are measured; and vasodilator testing and shunt calculation (if indicated) are undertaken.

2. **What are the usual physical findings in patients with pulmonary hypertension?**

   The most common findings on physical examination include the following:
   - Loud pulmonic valve closure sound (P_2)
   - Right ventricular heave
   - Murmur of tricuspid regurgitation (a systolic murmur over the left lower sternal border)
   - Murmur of pulmonic insufficiency (a diastolic murmur over the left sternal border)
   - Jugular venous distension (indicating elevated central venous pressures)
   - Peripheral edema
   - Hepatomegaly
   - Hepatojugular reflux
   - Ascites
   - Cyanosis

3. **How is PAH classified?**

   At the Fourth World Conference on Pulmonary Hypertension (held in Dana Point, Calif., in 2008), the term *familial PAH* was replaced by *hereditary PAH*, and schistosomiasis and chronic hemolytic anemia were added to Group 1 PAH. Current classification is outlined in Box 58-1. Pulmonary hypertension is classified as pulmonary arterial hypertension (Group 1), pulmonary hypertension resulting from left heart disease (Group 2), pulmonary hypertension resulting from lung diseases and/or hypoxia (Group 3), chronic thromboembolic pulmonary hypertension (CTEPH) (Group 4), and pulmonary hypertension with unclear multifactorial mechanisms (Group 5).

4. **Is pulmonary hypertension a genetic disease?**

   About 6% of patients with PAH have hereditary PAH. Mutations in the gene encoding bone morphogenetic receptor 2 (BMPR2) were found in approximately 70% of families with hereditary PAH and in 20% to 30% of patients with idiopathic PAH. Due to incomplete penetrance, most patients with this mutation never develop the disease. A subject with a mutation has a 10% to 20% estimated lifetime risk of acquiring PAH.

Box 58-1 UPDATED PULMONARY HYPERTENSION CLASSIFICATION

Group 1. Pulmonary Arterial Hypertension (PAH)
- Idiopathic PAH
- Heritable: BMPR2, Alk1, unknown
- Drug- and toxin-induced
- PAH associated with:
  - Collagen vascular disease
  - Congenital heart disease
  - Human immunodeficiency virus (HIV)
  - Schistosomiasis
  - Portal hypertension
  - Chronic hemolytic anemia
- Persistent pulmonary hypertension of newborn
- 1′ Pulmonary venoocclusive disease and/or pulmonary capillary hemangiomatosis

Group 2. Pulmonary Hypertension Resulting from Left Heart Disease
- Systolic dysfunction
- Diastolic dysfunction
- Valvular disease

Group 3. Pulmonary Hypertension Resulting from Lung Disease and/or Hypoxia
- COPD
- Interstitial lung disease
- Other pulmonary disease with mixed restrictive and obstructive pattern
- Sleep-disordered breathing
- Alveolar hypoventilation disorders
- Chronic exposure to high altitude
- Developmental abnormalities

Group 4. Chronic Thromboembolic Pulmonary Hypertension (CTEPH)

Group 5. Pulmonary Hypertension with Unclear Multifactorial Mechanisms
- Hematological disorders: myeloproliferative disorders, splenectomy
- Systemic disorders: sarcoidosis, pulmonary Langerhans cell histiocytosis, lymphangioleiomyomatosis, neurofibromatosis, vasculitis
- Metabolic disorders: glycogen storage disease, Gaucher disease, thyroid disorders
- Others: tumoral obstruction, fibrosing mediastinitis, chronic renal failure on dialysis

From Dana Point, 2008. Simonneau G, Robbins I M, Beghetti M, et al: Updated clinical classification of pulmonary hypertension, *J Am Coll Cardiol* 54:S43–S54, 2009.

5. **What should the clinical evaluation for possible pulmonary hypertension include?**

Evaluation should begin with a thorough history and physical examination. Possible causes of PAH should be addressed in the history. In addition, travel to or residence in an area endemic for schistosomiasis should be considered. All patients should receive a basic initial screening evaluation, consisting of collagen vascular disease serologic testing, human immunodeficiency virus (HIV) testing, hepatitis panel, chest radiograph, pulmonary function testing, ventilation-perfusion (V̇/Q̇) scan, hypercoagulable work-up (if indicated), electrocardiogram, and echocardiogram.

Patients with no clues to the cause on history or physical examination should be given a broad, *detailed* evaluation; patients with a suspected secondary cause should receive a *focused* evaluation to verify that cause, followed by the broad evaluation if necessary. In addition to these tests, arterial

TABLE 58-1. CONDITIONS AND SYMPTOMS ASSOCIATED WITH PULMONARY HYPERTENSION	
CATEGORY	**CONDITIONS OR SYMPTOMS**
Heart Failure (Systolic or Diastolic)	Dyspnea, exercise intolerance, angina, prior myocardial infarctions, systemic hypertension, valvular heart disease
Current Smoking	Shortness of breath, "smokers cough", hypoxia
Obstructive Sleep Apnea	Snoring, excessive somnolence, witnessed apneic episodes
Autoimmune Diseases	History of skin changes, arthritis, gastrointestinal problems, and renal disease
Chronic Thromboembolic Disease	Prior history of pulmonary embolism, deep vein thrombosis, and genetic or acquired hypercoagulable conditions
Drug History	Illicit drug abuse, prior anorexiant use, and herbal products
Chronic Liver Disease	History of jaundice, ascites, chronic viral hepatitis, and alcohol abuse. Symptoms of portal hypertension, including abdominal distention and gastrointestinal bleed
HIV Infection	Risky sexual behavior, intravenous drug abuse and needle sharing
Congenital Diseases	History of congenital heart disease and intracardiac shunts, family history of sickle cell disease

HIV, Human immunodeficiency virus.

blood gases and pulmonary angiography may be indicated. If undertaken, pulmonary angiography should be performed by a radiologist experienced in working with pulmonary hypertension patients. Conditions and symptoms associated with pulmonary hypertension are listed in Table 58-1.

An assessment of the patient's functional status and six-minute walk test should also be performed. Table 58-2 lists the World Health Organization (WHO) classification of functional status of patients with pulmonary hypertension.

6. **Which connective tissue diseases most commonly cause pulmonary hypertension?**
   - Systemic sclerosis (especially CREST syndrome)
   - Mixed connective tissue disease
   - Systemic lupus erythematosus
   - Rheumatoid arthritis
   - Dermatomyositis and polymyositis
   - Sjögren syndrome

7. **What population group is most commonly affected by PAH?**
   Although PAH occurs in both genders and virtually all age groups, it has a tendency to affect females. The modern U.S. PAH patient population is older (mean age at diagnosis is 47 years) and has a female preponderance. According to a French registry, female-to-male predominance is 1.7:1, whereas according to the Registry to Evaluate Early and Long-term Pulmonary Arterial Hypertension Disease Management (REVEAL) data, the female-to-male ratio is 3.6:1. REVEAL registry is a multicenter, observational U.S. based registry of PAH patients initiated in 2006 and data from this registry shows that factors associated with increased mortality include men older than 60 years of age, hereditary PAH, pulmonary vascular resistance (PVR) greater than 32 Woods units, portopulmonary hypertension, and New York Heart Association (NYHA)/WHO functional class IV (Table 58-3).

TABLE 58-2. WORLD HEALTH ORGANIZATION CLASSIFICATION OF FUNCTIONAL STATUS OF PATIENTS WITH PULMONARY HYPERTENSION

CLASS	DESCRIPTION
I	Patients with pulmonary hypertension but without resulting limitation of physical activity. Ordinary physical activity does not cause undue dyspnea or fatigue, chest pain, or near syncope.
II	Patients with pulmonary hypertension resulting in slight limitation of physical activity. They are comfortable at rest. Ordinary physical activity causes undue dyspnea or fatigue, chest pain, or near syncope.
III	Patients with pulmonary hypertension resulting in marked limitation of physical activity. They are comfortable at rest. Less than ordinary activity causes undue dyspnea or fatigue, chest pain, or near syncope.
IV	Patients with pulmonary hypertension with inability to carry out any physical activity without symptoms. These patients manifest signs of right-sided heart failure. Dyspnea or fatigue may even be present at rest. Discomfort is increased by any physical activity.

Modified from Rubin LJ: Diagnosis and management of pulmonary arterial hypertension: ACCP evidence-based clinical practice guidelines, *Chest* 126:7S-10S, 2004.

TABLE 58-3. HEMODYNAMIC DEFINITION OF PULMONARY HYPERTENSION

PULMONARY HYPERTENSION	MEAN PAP ≥ 25 mm Hg	PH Group
Precapillary pulmonary hypertension	Mean PAP ≥ 25 mm Hg PCWP ≤ 15 mm Hg Cardiac output normal or reduced	Group 1. PAH Group 3. PH due to lung disease Group 4. CTEPH Group 5. PH multifactorial etiology
Postcapillary pulmonary hypertension	Mean PAP ≥ 25 mm Hg PCWP > 15 mm Hg Cardiac output normal or reduced or increased	Group 2. PH due to left heart disease

CTEPH, chronic thromboembolic pulmonary hypertension; *PAH*, pulmonary arterial hypertension; *PAP*, pulmonary artery pressure; *PCWP*, pulmonary capillary wedge pressure; *PH*, pulmonary hypertension.

8. **Is surgical therapy now an option for patients with pulmonary hypertension secondary to chronic recurrent thromboembolism?**
A patient with PAH and a V̇/Q̇ scan suggestive of CTEPH must have a pulmonary angiogram for accurate diagnosis and assessment of resectability of the thrombi. It is now possible to surgically remove an organized thrombus from the proximal pulmonary arteries of such patients. Operative mortality is low in most experienced centers, and lifelong anticoagulation and inferior vena cava (IVC) filter placement are essential for such patients.

9. **What is the average survival outlook for a PAH patient?**
According to the National Institutes of Health Registry on Primary Pulmonary Hypertension, in the past, the median survival was approximately 2.8 years from the date of diagnosis. With the availability of

new therapeutic modalities, survival has improved. According to the French registry, the 1-year survival is 88% and according to REVEAL registry, the 1-year survival is 85% and 5-year survival is 57%.

10. **What is considered conventional therapy for patients with PAH?**
   Conventional therapy for patients with PAH includes the following:
   - *Supplemental oxygen* as needed to maintain an oxygen saturation of at least 91%
   - *Diuretics* if the patient has clinically significant edema or ascites
   - *Anticoagulation* in the absence of contraindications
   - *Digoxin* is used occasionally to improve RV function

11. **Are calcium channel blockers used in the treatment of PAH?**
   Calcium channel blockers (CCBs) are only used in patients with a documented vasodilator response to a short-acting vasodilator at the time of an RHC. This comprises 6% of all PAH patients; of these patients, 50% continue to be sustained responders. CCBs should not be empirically used in patients without the demonstration of vasoreactivity. If patients have a favorable response to acutely administered vasodilators, this predicts a response to CCBs. The 1-, 3-, and 5-year survival in patients on a CCB was 94% for all three time periods, as compared with 68%, 47%, and 38%, respectively, in those classified as nonresponders. If patients do not have a favorable response to acutely administered vasodilators, consider treatment with an endothelin receptor antagonist, a phostodiesterase-5 inhibitor, or prostacyclin therapy.

12. **What is considered a favorable response to acutely administered vasodilators?**
   A positive vasodilator response is defined as a fall in mean pulmonary artery pressure of at least 10 mm Hg to 40 mm Hg or less with an increased or unchanged cardiac output. Approximately 6% to 10% of PAH patients will have an acute positive response; however, only half of these patients will have a sustained response to CCBs. Only patients with a positive response should be considered candidates for a trial of an oral CCB. The agents used to determine vasoreactivity include intravenous epoprostenol and inhaled nitric oxide.

13. **What are the approved therapies to treat PAH?**
   Currently nine U.S. Food and Drug Administration (FDA)-approved therapies target the three identified pathways involved in the pathogenesis of PAH. Table 58-4 lists the FDA-approved drugs to treat pulmonary arterial hypertension.
   - *Endothelin receptor antagonists.* Endothelin-1, a potent vasoconstrictor, acts as a mitogen, induces fibrosis, and leads to the proliferation of vascular smooth muscle cells. The effects of endothelin-1 are mediated through the activation of ET_A and ET_B receptors. Differential activation of ET_A and ET_B receptors leads to the vasoconstricting and vascular proliferative actions of endothelin-1. Bosentan is a dual endothelin receptor blocker, whereas ambrisentan is an ET_A blocker.
   - *Prostacyclins.* Prostacyclin is the main product of arachidonic acid in the vascular endothelium. By the production of cyclic adenosine monophosphate (cAMP), prostacyclin promotes pulmonary vascular relaxation and inhibits growth of smooth muscle cells. In addition, prostacyclin is a powerful inhibitor of platelet aggregation. There are three prostacyclins approved for therapy; these include intravenous, subcutaneous, and inhaled treprostinil, intravenous epoprostenol, and inhaled iloprost.
   - *Phosphodiestersae-5 (PDE-5) inhibitors.* Phosphodiestersae-5 (PDE-5) inhibitors block the breakdown of cyclic guanosine monophosphate (cGMP) in the vascular endothelium, resulting in increased activity of endogenous nitric oxide that enhances pulmonary vasodilation. Sildenafil and tadalafil are the PDE-5 inhibitors approved to treat PAH in U.S.

14. **What are the complications associated with prostanoid therapy?**
   Because prostanoids are nonselective vasodilators, a common complication is systemic hypotension. Other commonly reported side effects include flushing, headaches, nausea, diarrhea, leg pain, and jaw pain. Because intravenous administration of prostacyclin requires central venous access, line infections (especially gram negative sepsis related to treprostinil use) and catheter-associated

TABLE 58-4. FDA-APPROVED DRUGS TO TREAT PULMONARY ARTERIAL HYPERTENSION

CLASS	PDE-5 INHIBITORS		ENDOTHELIN RECEPTOR ANTAGONISTS		PROSTACYCLINS			
Mode of action	Block degradation of cGMP		Competitive antagonists of endothelin receptor		Provide exogenous prostacyclin			
Individual Drugs	Tadalafil	Sildenafil	Ambrisentan	Bosentan	Epoprostenol	Treprostinil	Iloprost	Tyvaso
Individual dose	40 mg	20 mg	5-10 mg	62.5-125 mg	0.5>100 mg/kg/min	0.5>100 mg/kg/min	2.5 or 5 mcg	9-12 breaths
Frequency of administration	Daily	tid	Daily	bid	Continuous infusion	Continuous infusion	Every 2 hr	4 times daily
Elimination half-life	17.5 h	3-5 h	15 h	5.4 h	2-3 min	3-4 h	20-30 min	3-4 h
Route of administration	Oral	Oral	Oral	Oral	IV	IV, SC	INH	INH
Side-effects	Headache, myalgia, back pain, flushing, dyspepsia, diarrhea, nausea, pain in extremities	Headache, myalgia, back pain, flushing, dyspepsia, diarrhea	Peripheral edema, headaches, dizziness, nasal congestion	Peripheral edema, headaches, dizziness, cough, syncope, abnormal hepatic function	Headache, flushing, jaw pain, anxiety, nervousness, diarrhea, flu-like symptoms, nausea and vomiting	Headache, diarrhea, nausea, jaw pain, flu-like symptoms; SC infusion: site pain, reactions, and bleeding	Headache, flushing, flu-like symptoms, nausea and vomiting, jaw muscle spasm, cough, tongue pain, and syncope	Cough, headache, pharyngolaryngeal pain, throat irritation, nausea, flushing, and syncope

cGMP, Cyclic guanosine monophosphate; FDA, U.S. Food and Drug Administration; INH, inhalation treatment; IV, intravenous infusion; PDE-5, phosphodiesterase 5; SC, subcutaneous infusion.

thrombosis are common. Proper care of the catheter and anticoagulation help lessen these risks, but there is still the chance for significant and life-threatening complications.

15. **How do I treat the pulmonary hypertension associated with CREST syndrome?**
    Pulmonary hypertension is a common, life-threatening complication of CREST syndrome and accounts for the significant morbidity and mortality of this disease. Orally available vasodilators have been notoriously ineffective in the treatment of pulmonary hypertension associated with CREST. Recently, infused prostacyclin has been shown to improve the functional status of patients with CREST and pulmonary hypertension and is being used in the clinical setting more commonly.

16. **Is transplantation possible in patients with PAH?**
    Yes. Lung transplantation is an option in carefully selected patients, especially those who do not respond to aggressive PAH treatment. A combined heart and lung transplant is no longer believed to be required, because the right ventricle appears to recover function after lung transplantation. Occasionally, heart-lung transplantation is required in patients with uncorrectable congenital heart defects (e.g., Eisenmenger syndrome).

BIBLIOGRAPHY, SUGGESTED READINGS, AND WEBSITES

1. Barst RJ, Rubin LJ, Long WA, et al: A comparison of continuous intravenous epoprostenol (prostacyclin) with conventional therapy for primary pulmonary hypertension. The Primary Pulmonary Hypertension Study Group, *N Engl J Med* 334:296–302, 1996.

2. Benza RL, Miller DP, Gomberg-Maitland M, et al: Predicting survival in pulmonary arterial hypertension: insights from the Registry to Evaluate Early and Long-Term Pulmonary Arterial Hypertension Disease Management (REVEAL). *Circulation* 122:164–172.

3. Channick RN, Simonneau G, Sitbon O, et al: Effects of the dual endothelin-receptor antagonist bosentan in patients with pulmonary hypertension: a randomised placebo-controlled study, *Lancet* 358:1119–1123, 2001.

4. Galiè N, Brundage BH, Ghofrani HA, et al: Tadalafil therapy for pulmonary arterial hypertension, *Circulation* 119:2894–2903, 2009.

5. Galiè N, Ghofrani HA, Torbicki A, et al: Sildenafil citrate therapy for pulmonary arterial hypertension, *N Engl J Med* 353:2148–2157, 2005.

6. Galiè N, Olschewski H, Oudiz RJ, et al: Ambrisentan for the treatment of pulmonary arterial hypertension: results of the ambrisentan in pulmonary arterial hypertension, randomized, double-blind, placebo-controlled, multicenter, efficacy (ARIES) study 1 and 2, *Circulation* 117:2966–2968, 2008.

7. Humbert M, Sitbon O, Chaouat A, et al: Pulmonary Arterial Hypertension in France: results from a National Registry, *Am J Respir Crit Care Med* 173:1023–1030, 2006.

8. McGoon M, Gutterman M, Steen V, et al: Screening, early detection, and diagnosis of pulmonary arterial hypertension: ACCP evidence-based clinical practice guidelines, *Chest* 126:14S–34S, 2004.

9. McLaughlin VV, Archer SL, Badesch DB, et al: ACCF/AHA 2009 expert consensus document on pulmonary hypertension a report of the American College of Cardiology Foundation Task Force on Expert Consensus Documents and the American Heart Association developed in collaboration with the American College of Chest Physicians; American Thoracic Society, Inc.; and the Pulmonary Hypertension Association, *J Am Coll Cardiol* 53:1573–1619, 2009.

10. Miyamoto S, Nagaya N, Satoh T, et al: Clinical correlates and prognostic significance of six-minute walk test in patients with primary pulmonary hypertension. Comparison with cardiopulmonary exercise testing, *Am J Respir Crit Care Med* 161:487–492, 2000.

11. Oudiz RJ: *Primary Pulmonary Hypertension.* Available at: http://emedicine.medscape.com/article/301450-overview. Accessed March 26, 2013.

12. Simonneau G, Barst RJ, Galiè N, et al: Continuous subcutaneous infusion of treprostinil, a prostacyclin analogue, in patients with pulmonary arterial hypertension: a double-blind, randomized, placebo-controlled trial, *Am J Respir Crit Care Med* 165:800–804, 2002.

13. Simonneau G, Robbins IM, Beghetti M, et al: Updated clinical classification of pulmonary hypertension, *J Am Coll Cardiol* 54:S43–S54, 2009.

14. Sitbon O, Humbert M, Jais X, et al: Long-term response to calcium channel blockers in idiopathic pulmonary arterial hypertension, *Circulation* 111:3105–3111, 2005.

15. Sitbon O, Humbert M, Nunes H, et al: Long-term intravenous epoprostenol infusion in primary pulmonary hypertension: prognostic factors and survival, *J Am Coll Cardiol* 40:780–788, 2002.

CHAPTER 59

STROKE AND TRANSIENT ISCHEMIC ATTACK

Sharyl R. Martini, MD, PhD, and Thomas A. Kent, MD

1. **What is stroke? How common is stroke? How common is it in the setting of cardiac disease?**

   Stroke is a focal disturbance of blood flow to the brain. Stroke is not a single disease but the end result of many different pathophysiologies leading to cerebrovascular occlusion or rupture. It can be classified as either primarily ischemic (80%) or hemorrhagic (20%). Ischemic strokes can develop a hemorrhagic component, termed hemorrhagic conversion, especially if the stroke is large. There are approximately 700,000 strokes per year in the United States, and it is the leading cause of disability. The biggest risk factor for stroke is prior stroke, and the second biggest risk factor is age. Risk factors common to both stroke and atherosclerotic cardiac disease include hypertension, diabetes, and smoking. In addition, cardiac diseases such as atrial fibrillation and valvular disease are risk factors for stroke. Strokes occur after cardiac procedures at a rate of 0.7% to 7%, depending on the procedure, and may be due to intrinsic disease or emboli or micro-emboli from the procedure itself.

2. **What is a transient ischemic attack, and why is the clinical recognition of it important?**

   Transient ischemic attack (TIA) is a neurologic deficit that, by definition, resolves within 24 hours, although most resolve within 5 to 15 minutes. It is important to identify TIAs because they represent an opportunity to intervene with appropriate strategies to prevent future strokes and permanent disability. Ninety-day stroke rates for patients with TIA are in excess of 10% in some series, with the greatest risk within the 48 hours to first week after the TIA. Longer duration, a lesion on diffusion-weighted magnetic resonance imaging (MRI), and the presence of large cerebral artery stenosis (seen on carotid duplex, computed tomographic [CT], or magnetic resonance [MR] angiography) are all associated with a higher risk of stroke following TIA.

3. **What are the major causes of stroke and TIA?**

   The major etiologies of ischemic stroke are cardioembolism, small vessel vasculopathy leading to lacunar stroke, and large vessel atherosclerosis (including intracranial atherosclerotic plaque rupture, as well as embolization from large arteries, such as the carotid, vertebral, and basilar arteries, to cerebral arteries [Fig. 59-1 and Table 59-1]). Hemorrhagic strokes include subarachnoid hemorrhage (usually due to aneurysm rupture) and intraparenchymal hemorrhage. Intraparenchymal hemorrhages are classified by their location: subcortical (associated with uncontrolled hypertension in 60% of cases) versus cortical (more concerning for underlying mass, arteriovenous malformation, or cerebral amyloid angiopathy; see Fig. 59-1). Figure 59-2 summarizes the major causes of stroke and their relative frequency.

   Among the other potential causes of stroke, dissection of the blood vessels needs to be considered, especially if there is face or neck pain or a history of trauma. Illicit drug use is a possible cause of either ischemic stroke (cocaine-, stimulants-, or "bath salts"–induced spasm) or hemorrhagic stroke (as a result of vascular injury or sudden massive increase in blood pressure). Patent foramen ovale (PFO) remains a controversial cause of stroke (see Question 18). Other, rarer, causes of stroke include hypercoagulable states (e.g., lupus and antiphospholipid antibody syndrome) and genetic disorders, such as homocystinuria and fibromuscular dysplasia.

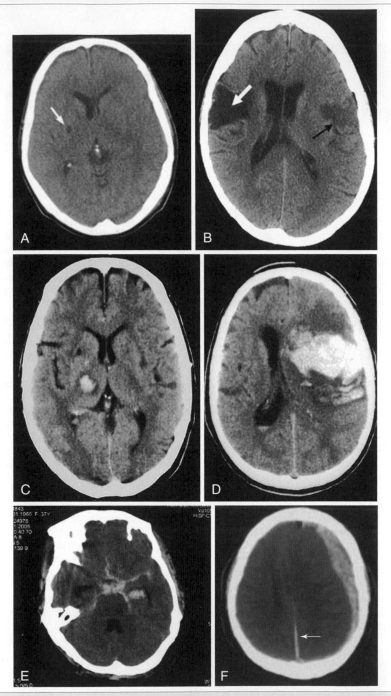

Figure 59-1. The computed tomographic findings of strokes and stroke mimics. **A,** Lacunar ischemic stroke, typical of small vessel disease; **B,** multiple ischemic strokes of different ages, typical of cardioembolism; **C,** Subcortical intraparenchymal hemorrhage; **D,** cortical intraparenchymal hemorrhage; **E,** subarachnoid hemorrhage; **F,** subdural hematoma, with a small amount of subarachnoid hemorrhage along the falx *(arrow).*

TABLE 59-1.	CLINICAL FEATURES OF THE THREE MOST COMMON TYPES OF STROKE	
Type	**Clinical Features**	**Classic Syndromes**
Large Vessel Atherosclerosis	■ Often occur on waking; may have history of TIAs in same vascular distribution, symptoms may fluctuate. ■ Caused either by large artery thrombosis or artery-to-artery thromboembolism. ■ Associated trauma suggests dissection as source of artery-to-artery embolism (may see ipsilateral Horner's syndrome with carotid injury).	■ Anterior circulation: contralateral arm and face > leg weakness, sensory loss, visual field cut, plus word finding difficulty and difficulty understanding commands (left), or contralateral neglect (right). ■ Posterior circulation: cerebellar or cranial nerve abnormalities predominate, but can present with coma and blindness (top of the basilar syndrome). Vertigo common.
Cardioembolic	■ Associated history or clinical features of heart disease. ■ Stroke symptoms are maximal at onset because the clot is pre-formed. ■ TIA symptoms are usually different from one another, representing emboli to different vascular distributions. ■ Often occur during waking hours; can be associated with Valsalva maneuvers. ■ Caused by embolism, usually from left atrial appendage (in setting of atrial fibrillation) or left ventricle (in case of akinetic segment). ■ Emboli from infected valves (septic emboli) are likely to bleed and should not be treated with tPA.	■ Symptoms depend on area of embolization; may have strokes of different ages in different vascular territories.
Small Vessel Lacunar	■ Strong association with hypertension and microbleeds; occur in subcortical regions such as basal ganglia or brainstem. ■ Never see cortical findings of language disturbance or neglect. ■ May have TIAs with similar symptoms. ■ These small strokes can also be due to large vessel atherosclerosis or small emboli.	■ Pure motor: contralateral face/arm/leg weakness ■ Pure sensory: contralateral face/arm/leg sensory loss ■ Sensorimotor: loss of face/arm/leg motor and sensory ■ Ataxic hemiparesis: contralateral ataxia out of proportion to mild weakness ■ Clumsy hand dysarthria: weak face and clumsy ipsilateral hand, dysarthria and dysphagia

TIA, transient ischemic attack; *tPA*, tissue plasminogen activator.

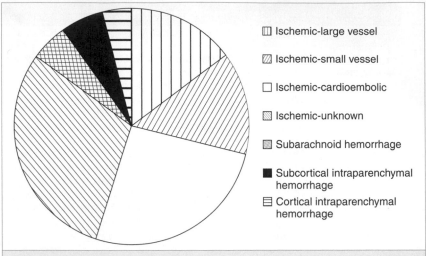

Figure 59-2. Relative frequencies of different types of stroke. (Compiled using data from the Greater Cincinnati Northern Kentucky Stroke Study.)

4. **How are stroke and TIA diagnosed?**
   Stroke and TIA are diagnosed clinically, and no imaging correlation is usually required for the diagnosis, although imaging procedures are performed to rule out other causes, such as tumor. Focal neurologic deficits with sudden onset should be considered as a vascular event until proven otherwise because of the possibility of recurrence or progression of the deficit. Focal weakness, numbness, facial asymmetry, or speech difficulties are classic presentations. Altered level of consciousness, vertigo, and cranial nerve deficits are often seen with vertebrobasilar-brainstem strokes. See Table 59-1 for lists of the clinical signs and symptoms of the major subtypes of stroke: large vessel atherosclerosis and thrombosis, cardioembolic stroke, and small vessel stroke.

5. **What should be done in cases of suspected stroke or TIA?**
   A head CT must be performed immediately to distinguish ischemic from hemorrhagic strokes (see Fig. 59-1) because these are managed very differently. The CT itself does not diagnose stroke; it is primarily used to rule out causes other than ischemic stroke, including hemorrhagic infarction, tumor, subdural hematoma, and other causes. Figure 59-1 demonstrates the CT findings of strokes and stroke mimics.

   In cases of suspected stroke, one should page the stroke team (when one exists) or the service responsible to rapidly address stroke—every minute counts. Immediately check blood glucose because hypoglycemia or hyperglycemia can cause focal neurologic deficits mimicking stroke. Also obtain an electrocardiogram (ECG) and basic blood analysis (complete blood cell count, coagulation studies, and renal/electrolyte panel). The ECG and cardiac workup initially can reveal atrial fibrillation or the surprisingly common coexistence of various kinds of acute cardiac syndromes with stroke.

6. **How are ischemic acute strokes treated?**
   Three possible treatments are now suggested to improve outcomes after acute ischemic stroke: (1) intravenous tissue plasminogen activator (tPA); (2) aspirin; and, in the case of large strokes, (3) hemicraniectomy performed before clinical herniation.

tPA

The only medication approved by the U.S. Food and Drug Administration (FDA) for acute ischemic strokes is intravenous (IV) tPA, administered within 3 hours of symptom onset. Based on

BOX 59-1   CONTRAINDICATIONS TO INTRAVENOUS tPA FOR THE TREATMENT OF STROKE.

- Presentation more than 3 hours (4.5 hours in select cases) from the time the patient was last seen normal
- Any history of spontaneous intracerebral hemorrhage
- Intracranial neoplasm or arteriovenous malformation
- Minor or rapidly resolving deficits (including transient ischemic attack [TIA])
- Uncontrolled hypertension greater than 185/110 mm Hg despite antihypertensive treatment
- Major surgery in the previous 2 weeks
- Gastrointestinal (GI) or urinary hemorrhage in the previous 3 weeks
- Stroke, head trauma, intracranial/intraspinal surgery, or myocardial infarction within 3 months
- Current bacterial endocarditis
- International normalized ratio (INR) > 1.7
- Platelet count < 100,000
- Elevated partial thromboplastin time (PTT)
- Clinical picture concerning for subarachnoid hemorrhage or aortic dissection

the European Cooperative Acute Stroke Study III (ECASS III), American Heart Association (AHA) guidelines recommend treatment with IV tPA in selected patients out to 4.5 hours after symptom onset, but this is not yet approved by the FDA. *Note, however, that the earlier tPA is given, the better the clinical outcome.* The greatest benefit of tPA occurs at earlier time points. It is critical to give tPA as soon as possible if head CT does not reveal signs of hemorrhage or hypodensity. Only tPA is approved for acute stroke thrombolysis. Only eight stroke patients need to be treated with IV tPA to result in one patient with complete or near-complete recovery, and this number needed to treat (NNT) takes into account the increased risk of hemorrhage after tPA administration. Patients of any age benefit from tPA. Contraindications to IV tPA for the treatment of stroke are given in Box 59-1. Although tPA administration is not contraindicated in the setting of moderately elevated international normalized ratios (INR of 1.3-1.7), recent studies suggest an increased risk of brain hemorrhage compared to tPA administraton with a normal INR. Importantly, patients who have their strokes after cardiac catheterization and who meet these criteria may still benefit from tPA, despite the recent administration of heparin and glycoprotein IIb/IIIa inhibitors, although this is outside the usual protocols and should be done only with expert help. In this situation, various treatments have been reported, including intraarterial therapy or IV abciximab, but these uses remain investigational.

After tPA administration, frequent clinical examinations are crucial and blood pressure must be controlled to less than 180/105 mm Hg. Subcutaneous heparin and antiplatelet agents are held for 24 hours, until follow-up imaging confirms absence of hemorrhagic conversion.

In patients with ischemic stroke who are not candidates for tPA, optimal blood pressure is not known but is often permitted to run high (up to 220/120 mm Hg), as long as there are no signs of hypertensive end-organ damage. This is theoretically designed to increase perfusion of brain tissue at continued risk for ischemia, but it is unknown if outcome is improved. Cautious control of blood pressure is recommended to avoid sudden drops or rises. Any hypotension or relative hypotension associated with neurologic worsening should be treated with intravenous fluids and, if necessary, pressors until clinical examination improves or upper limits specified earlier are reached.

Endovascular devices for cerebral clot disruption/retrieval are FDA approved, although their efficacy for improving outcome has yet to be demonstrated. The Interventional Management of Stroke 3 trial did not show a benefit of combined IV tPA plus endovascular treatment over IV tPA alone. At this time, endovascular treatment of acute stroke is often suggested in patients who present early but are ineligible for IV tPA because of anticoagulation or another condition posing an unacceptably high risk of systemic bleeding, but ongoing randomized trials may clarify their exact role.

Aspirin

In patients not already treated with thrombolytic therapy, aspirin is given (orally or rectally) as soon as possible and reduces the chances of recurrent stroke when given within 48 hours of presentation.

Hemicraniectomy

Patients with malignant middle cerebral artery occlusion are at risk of death from cerebral edema and herniation. Removal of the overlying skull has been shown to improve mortality with an NNT of 2. It is also often suggested for strokes within the cerebellar hemisphere, but this is largely anecdotal. Early consultation with neurosurgery is suggested.

7. **How are hemorrhagic strokes managed?**
Hemorrhagic strokes are managed by reversing any coagulopathy and withholding administration of subcutaneous heparin and antiplatelet agents. Controlling blood pressure is a focus of interest because high blood pressure is associated with hematoma expansion and rebleeding. It is considered safe to decrease blood pressure by up to 25% in the first 2 to 6 hours, as long as findings on neurologic examination do not worsen.

8. **What other measures are important in the management of all strokes?**
In patients not treated with thrombolytic therapy, subcutaneous heparin or low-molecular-weight heparinoids for deep vein thrombosis (DVT) prophylaxis should be started as soon as possible in nonambulatory patients unless contraindicated. Keep patients nil per os (NPO) until safe swallowing can be confirmed, to prevent aspiration. Physiological variables are maintained as close to the patient's normal as possible, but there is no evidence yet for aggressive management of blood sugar, in particular, although hyperglycemia is associated with a worse outcome.

9. **Is the presence of atrial fibrillation in patients with stroke or TIA an important consideration for future management?**
Yes. Any patient with atrial fibrillation who has had a stroke or TIA is considered at high risk for future strokes without anticoagulation (see Question 11). As such, all patients should be monitored with telemetry to optimize identification of intermittent (paroxysmal) atrial fibrillation, because intermittent atrial fibrillation is as much of a risk factor for stroke as persistent atrial fibrillation. A single ECG (unless it reveals atrial fibrillation) is inadequate for detection of this important risk factor. Prolonged event monitors reveal subclinical atrial fibrillation in a substantial proportion of patients with cryptogenic stroke, and are warranted in cases where clinical suspicion is high.

10. **What is the utility of echocardiogram for workup of acute stroke?**
In stroke patients with a suspected cardioembolic cause, echocardiogram is indicated (see also Chapter 5 on echocardiography). Transesophageal echocardiogram is often performed in patients with suspected embolic stroke and a nondiagnostic transthoracic echocardiogram. An echocardiogram is not needed to determine secondary stroke prevention strategies for stroke patients with known atrial fibrillation, because these patients should be anticoagulated; however, identification of a cardiac thrombus would affect timing of anticoagulation initiation and may have some prognostic value.

11. **Which patients with atrial fibrillation merit anticoagulation therapy for the prevention of stroke?**
All patients with history of stroke *and* atrial fibrillation merit consideration for anticoagulation, because the risk of subsequent stroke in these patients is 2% to 15% per year and anticoagulation results in a greater than 60% reduction in ischemic strokes. Other high-risk groups include those over the age of 75 (especially women) and those with the following risk factors: poorly controlled hypertension, diabetes, and poor left ventricular function or recent heart failure. A number of risk stratification schemes can help determine which patients should be anticoagulated to prevent stroke. These include

CHADS$_2$ (see Fig. 34-1), Stroke Prevention in Atrial Fibrillation (SPAF), Atrial Fibrillation Investigators (AFI), and Framingham, among others. These schemes integrate risk factors to assist in the decision for anticoagulation therapy: The greater the number of risk factors, the higher the risk of stroke. It is important to note that these schemes relate to *primary* prevention in atrial fibrillation; a stroke or TIA automatically places a patient in the high-risk category for each of these schemes. As such, secondary prevention of stroke in patients with atrial fibrillation should involve anticoagulation unless there is a contraindication. The elderly also appear to benefit from anticoagulation for secondary stroke prevention; thus, age alone is not a contraindication, although elderly patients are at higher risk for bleeding.

Contraindications to preventive anticoagulant therapy include history of severe gastrointestinal (GI) bleeding and history of falls or an extremely high fall risk. The HAS-BLED score is a simple method for assessing bleeding risk, although this score was validated in a group that had already been considered safe for anticoagulation, which is a serious limitation of its applicability. After stroke, many patients are at risk for falls. As they improve, their fall risk status may also improve, so it is important to reconsider anticoagulation at future visits. Goal INR for secondary stroke prevention is 2 to 3; studies have demonstrated that many stroke prevention *failures* are the result of subtherapeutic INRs. The most serious bleeding risk associated with anticoagulation is intraparenchymal hemorrhage. This risk is probably higher for patients with extensive small vessel disease or cortical microhemorrhages than for those with healthier brain parenchyma. Many centers will perform a susceptibility-sensitive MRI (e.g., gradient echo) to assess the presence of microhemorrhages, particularly in the cortex. The decision for anticoagulation in particular patients should be a collaborative one, with the risks, benefits, and monitoring schedule clearly explained so that the patient can make an informed decision.

12. **What are the benefits and risks of the newer anticoagulants for stroke prevention in the setting of atrial fibrillation?**
New oral anticoagulants include the direct thrombin inhibitor dabigatran and the factor Xa inhibitors apixaban and rivaroxaban (Fig. 59-3). Dabigatran and apixaban were superior to warfarin in preventing vascular events and death in large randomized controlled trials of subjects with atrial fibrillation; rivaroxaban was noninferior to warfarin. The benefit of these agents over warfarin is due to better efficacy for stroke prevention, as well as lower overall bleeding risk (Table 59-2). The most serious complication of anticoagulation is intracerebral hemorrhage, which was reduced substantially with these agents. Subgroup analysis of the dabigatran trial found that concomitant aspirin use increased risk of intracerebral hemorrhage 1.6-fold. Dabigatran and rivaroxaban had a higher rate of GI bleeding relative to warfarin; apixaban showed no such trend. Dabigatran has shown a small but consistent increase in myocardial infarction (MI) compared to warfarin, although it decreases overall vascular events and mortality.

13. **Are there options other than anticoagulation for secondary stroke prevention in the setting of atrial fibrillation?**
Treatments aimed at reducing stroke risk in atrial fibrillation (and thus the need for anticoagulation) include restoring sinus rhythm, resecting the left atrial appendage, and transcatheter closure of the left atrial appendage opening. Unfortunately, no studies have thus far demonstrated a sufficient reduction of stroke risk to warrant anticoagulation discontinuation. The Atrial Fibrillation Follow-up Investigation of Rhythm Management (AFFIRM) study found that restoring sinus rhythm did not reduce stroke risk. The Watchman trial, which studied the efficacy of device closure of the left atrial appendage, similarly did not find a reduction in stroke risk; additional device trials are ongoing. The Left Atrial Appendage Occlusion Study II is an ongoing phase 3 trial comparing surgical excision of the left atrial appendage with best medical therapy. At this time, anticoagulation is the only intervention that has been demonstrated to reduce stroke in the setting of atrial fibrillation.

14. **Which patients merit antiplatelet therapy for prevention of stroke? What is the benefit? What are the risks?**
All patients who do not meet criteria for anticoagulation after stroke should receive antiplatelet therapy with either (a) aspirin, (b) clopidogrel, or (c) aspirin plus extended release dipyridamole. These

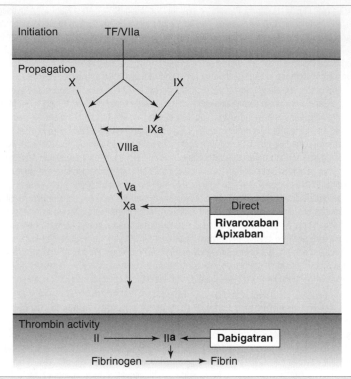

Figure 59-3. Targets of Novel Anticoagulants for Long-Term Use. Dabigatran etexilate is a prodrug that generates active compounds able to bind directly to the catalytic site of thrombin (factor II); rivaroxaban and apixaban are direct FXa inhibitors. Warfarin inhibits synthesis of factor II, factor VII , factor IX and factor X. Unfractionated heparin, low molecular weight heparin, and fondaparinux indirectly inhibit factor II and/or factor Xa. (Adapted from De Caterina R, Husted S, Wallentin L, et al: New oral anticoagulants in atrial fibrillation and acute coronary syndromes: ESC Working Group on Thrombosis-Task Force on Anticoagulants in Heart Disease position paper. *J Am Coll Cardiol* 59(16): 1413–25, 2012.)

three agents are similarly efficacious for stroke prevention, decreasing risk of second stroke by 14% to 18%. Ensuring optimal compliance with antiplatelet therapy is more important than the individual agent used, so the choice of agent should be guided by comorbidities, tolerability, and cost. Clopidogrel may be preferred in patients with history of significant GI bleeding, peripheral vascular disease, or drug-eluting cardiac stents. Aspirin plus dipyridamole can cause headaches initially and so may be difficult to tolerate for patients with chronic headache. The Prevention Regimen for Effectively Avoiding Second Strokes (PROFESS) trial comparing clopidogrel with aspirin plus extended release dipyridamole found that neither regimen was superior; each regimen had a somewhat different side-effect profile. Aspirin alone may be a good choice when not contraindicated, particularly when cost of the alternative agents would hinder compliance.

Aspirin should not be used in combination with clopidogrel *for long-term secondary stroke prevention,* as the combination showed an unacceptably high bleeding risk without additional protection from strokes, compared with either aspirin alone (in lacunar stroke patients) or clopidogrel alone (in all stroke patients), particularly after 90 days. However, the Stenting and Aggressive Medical Management for Preventing Recurrent Stroke in Intracranial Stenosis (SAMMPRIS) trial used aspirin plus clopidogrel for 90 days followed by aspirin alone in their management of high-risk intracranial stenosis patients with better-than-expected outcomes, although this regimen was not compared to a single-agent regimen. Patients may require both aspirin and clopidogrel for cardiac conditions such

TABLE 59-2.   SUMMARY OF MECHANISM AND CLINICAL TRIALS OF THE NEWER ANTICOAGULANTS USED FOR STROKE PREVENTION IN ATRIAL FIBRILLATION

Agent	Apixaban	Dabigatran	Rivaroxaban
Mechanism of action	Direct Xa inhibitor	Direct IIa inhibitor	Direct Xa inhibitor
Half-life	8-15 h	12-17 h	5-13 h
Time to maximum inhibition	1-4 h	0.5-2 h	1-4 h
Renal elimination	27%	85%	66%
Reversal agent	Possibly FFP, PCCs, or VIIa	Possibly hemodialysis, PCCs, or VIIa	Possibly FFP, PCCs, or VIIa
Contraindications	CrCl < 15; strong inhibitors of CYP3A4 and P-gp (azole antimycotics, HIV protease inhibitors)	CrCl < 30; dronedarone; potent P-gp inducers (rifampicin, St. John's wort, carbamazepine, and phenytoin)	CrCl < 15; strong inhibitors of CYP3A4 and P-gp (azole antimycotics, HIV protease inhibitors)
Cautions	CrCl 15-29; strong CYP3A4 and P-gp inducers (rifampicin, phenytoin, carbamazepine, phenobarbital)	CrCl 30-50; verapamil	CrCl 15-29; strong CYP3A4 and P-gp inducers (rifampicin, phenytoin, carbamazepine, phenobarbital)
Trial	ARISTOTLE	RE-LY	ROCKET AF
Dose	5 mg bid*	150 mg bid†	20 mg daily‡
Mean CHADS score	2.1 ± 1.1	2.2 ± 1.2	3.5 ± 0.94
Stroke or systemic embolism	0.79 (0.66-0.95)	0.65 (0.52-0.81)	0.88 (0.75-1.03)
Myocardial infarction	0.88 (0.66-1.17)	1.27 (0.94-1.71)	0.81 (0.63-1.06)
All-cause mortality	0.89 (0.80-0.998)	0.88 (0.77-1.00)	0.85 (0.70-1.02)
Major bleeding	0.69 (0.60-0.80)	0.93 (0.81-1.07)	1.04 (0.90-1.20)
Intracranial hemorrhage	0.51 (0.35-0.75)	0.26 (0.14-0.49)	0.59 (0.37-0.93)
GI bleeding	0.89 (0.70-1.15)	1.50 (1.19-1.89)	Not reported

All odds ratios (95% confidence intervals) are reproduced from the corresponding clinical trial; the comparator for each trial was Coumadin with international normalized ratio (INR) goal of 2 to 3.
CrCl, Creatinine clearance (mL/min); *FFP*, fresh frozen plasma; *GI*, gastrointestinal; *PCCs*, prothrombin complex concentrates; *P-gp*, P-glycoprotein 1.
*2.5 mg dose in subjects >80 years, body weight ≤ 60 kg, or serum creatinine ≥ 1.5 mg/dL.
†Subjects were also randomized to 110 mg dose.
‡15 mg daily in subjects with CrCl 30-49 mL/min.

as drug-eluting stents, and such patients may be continued on this combination regimen after stroke, with an understanding that bleeding risk may be elevated.

15. **How soon after a stroke or TIA should anticoagulation or antiplatelet therapy be initiated?**
In general, antiplatelet therapy can be initiated immediately in patients who are not candidates for tPA and do not have any indication of hemorrhagic component, and after 24 hours in patients who

received tPA once lack of hemorrhage has been confirmed by imaging. Timing of anticoagulation is highly case-specific. Larger strokes are more likely to bleed than small strokes, especially early on. The risk of a second stroke in the 2 weeks after initial stroke in patients with atrial fibrillation is only 0.5% (in the absence of a known cardiac thrombus). The risk of bleeding from full dose heparinization of 1 week duration has been estimated at 5% based on the Trial of ORG 10172 in Acute Stroke Treatment (TOAST) trial. Because of this, it is common practice to wait 1 month after a large stroke before initiating anticoagulation, although such a strategy has not been prospectively studied in a large trial. Patients with very small strokes may be started on anticoagulation within 1 or 2 days of stroke. The decision is much more difficult in patients with large strokes at higher risk for embolization, such as those with mechanical valves or demonstrated cardiac thrombus. In such cases, oral anticoagulation may be started cautiously after 5 to 15 days, depending on the individual situation. Retrospective data suggest bridging with heparin or low-molecular-weight heparin causes higher bleeding risk. In the absence of clinical or laboratory evidence of a hypercoagulable state, it is probably acceptable to start warfarin at low doses to achieve therapeutic anticoagulation slowly. Some clinicians suggest use of aspirin until an INR of 2 is achieved.

16. How should patients with carotid stenosis be managed?

Patients with symptomatic carotid stenosis greater than 70% should be treated with carotid endarterectomy within 2 weeks of a TIA or non-disabling stroke because their risk of recurrent stroke is 15% per year over 5 years, and carotid endarterectomy CEA cuts this rate in half. Patients with symptomatic stenosis 50% to 69% benefit less from CEA but have the same up-front surgical risk, so good perioperative results are critical to their management. Asymptomatic patients, especially those with 60% stenosis or greater, have a 2% to 4% annual stroke rate, which is also cut in half after CEA. However, because up-front risk of death or stroke from the procedure is 3% to 6%, overall benefit is less than with symptomatic carotid stenosis, and a longer duration of survival is needed to benefit from the procedure.

The Carotid Revascularization Endarterectomy versus Stenting Trial (CREST) comparing CEA with carotid stenting showed higher stroke and death rates in the carotid stenting group, but higher MI rates with CEA: overall rates of the combined endpoint were not different between groups. Older patients fared better with CEA than with carotid stenting and quality of life was better in those with MI than those with stroke.

17. How should patients with intracranial stenosis be managed?

In the SAMMPRIS trial, subjects with a recent mild stroke or TIA in the territory of a major cerebral artery with 70% to 99% stenosis were randomized to receive stenting within 3 days plus protocol-guided aggressive medical management, versus medical management alone. All subjects received aspirin plus clopidogrel for 90 days, followed by aspirin alone. In addition to blood pressure and lipid goals, lifestyle coaches developed goals for weight loss, regular exercise, and smoking cessation with each participant. The trial was stopped early because 14.7% of subjects in the stenting arm had a stroke within 30 days (the majority within 1 day of stenting) compared with 5.8% in the medical management group; 1-year stroke rates were 20% and 12.2% respectively. Based on these data, stroke due to intracranial atherosclerosis is now managed with aggressive medical management.

18. How should patients with stroke and patent foramen ovale be managed?

The CLOSURE I trial compared PFO closure to best medical management in subjects with cryptogenic stroke, and did not find a benefit of PFO closure after 2 years of follow up. More than 75% of subjects in each group with recurrent stroke had evidence of a mechanism other than paradoxical embolism.

BIBLIOGRAPHY, SUGGESTED READINGS, AND WEBSITES

1. Adams HP Jr, Bendixen BH, Kappelle LJ, et al: Classification of subtype of acute ischemic stroke. Definitions for use in a multicenter clinical trial. TOAST: Trial of Org 10172 in Acute Stroke Treatment, *Stroke* 24:35–41, 1993.
2. Archives of Internal Medicine [No authors listed] Risk factors for stroke and efficacy of antithrombotic therapy in atrial fibrillation. Analysis of pooled data from five randomized controlled trials, *Arch Intern Med* 154:1449–1457, 1994.

3. Furie KL, Kasner SE, Adams RJ, et al: American Heart Association Stroke Council, Council on Cardiovascular Nursing, Council on Clinical Cardiology, and Interdisciplinary Council on Quality of Care and Outcomes Research: Guidelines for the prevention of stroke in patients with stroke or transient ischemic attack: a guideline for healthcare professionals from the American Heart Association/American Stroke Association, *Stroke* 42(1):227-76, 2011.

4. Giraldo EA: *Stroke (CVA)*. Available at: http://www.merckmanuals.com/professional/neurologic_disorders/stroke_cva/overview_of_stroke.html. Accessed March 26, 2013.

5. Jauch EC, Kissela B, Stettler B: *Acute Management of Stroke*. Available at: http://emedicine.medscape.com/article/1159752-overview. Accessed March 26, 2013.

6. Jauch EC, Saver JL, Adams HP Jr, et al: American Heart Association Stroke Council, Council on Cardiovascular Nursing, Council on Peripheral Vascular Disease, and Council on Clinical Cardiology: Guidelines for the early management of patients with acute ischemic stroke: a guideline for healthcare professionals from the American Heart Association/American Stroke Association, *Stroke* j4(3):870-947, 2013.

7. Morgenstern LB, Hemphill JC 3rd, Anderson C, et al: American Heart Association Stroke Council and Council on Cardiovascular Nursing: Guidelines for the management of spontaneous intracerebral hemorrhage: a guideline for healthcare professionals from the American Heart Association/American Stroke Association, *Stroke* 41(9):2108-29, 2010.

8. Khatri P, Taylor RA, Palumbo V, et al: The safety and efficacy of thrombolysis for strokes after cardiac catheterization, *J Am Coll Cardiol* 51:906–911, 2008.

9. National Heart, Lung and Blood Institute and Boston University: *The Framingham Heart Study risk score profiles*. Available at: www.framinghamheartstudy.org/risk. Accessed March 26, 2013.

10. The National Institute of Neurological Disorders and Stroke rt-PA Stroke Study Group: Tissue plasminogen activator for acute ischemic stroke, *N Engl J Med* 333:1581–1587, 1995.

11. Schneck MJ, Xu L: *Cardioembolic Stroke*. Available at: http://emedicine.medscape.com/article/1160370-overview. Accessed March 26, 2013.

CHAPTER 60

SYNCOPE

Glenn N. Levine, MD, FACC, FAHA

1. **What is the word syncope derived from?**

   According to text in the European Society of Cardiology (ESC) Guidelines on the Management of Syncope, the word *syncope* is derived from the Greek words *syn*, meaning "with," and the verb *kopto*, meaning "I cut" or "I interrupt."

2. **What is the underlying mechanism causing syncope?**

   Transient global cerebral hypoperfusion. Note that other conditions that do not cause transient global cerebral hypoperfusion can cause a transient loss of consciousness, and some experts believe these conditions should be referred to as *transient loss of consciousness* instead of syncope.

3. **Cessation of cerebral blood flow of what duration causes syncope?**

   Cessation of cerebral blood flow for as short a period as 6 to 8 seconds can precipitate syncope.

4. **What is the most common cause of syncope in the general population?**

   Neurocardiogenic syncope is the most common cause of syncope in the general population. This is also variably referred to in the literature as *vasovagal syncope, neurally mediated syncope,* and *vasodepressor syncope.*

5. **What are the most common causes of syncope in pediatric and young patients?**

   According to the scientific statement on syncope from the 2006 American Heart Association/American College of Cardiology Foundation (AHA/ACCF), the most common causes of syncope in pediatric and young patients are neurocardiogenic syncope, conversion reactions (psychiatric causes), and primary arrhythmic causes (e.g., long QT syndrome, Wolff-Parkinson-White syndrome). In contrast, elderly patients have a higher frequency of syncope caused by obstructions to cardiac output (e.g., aortic stenosis, pulmonary embolism) and by arrhythmias resulting from underlying heart disease.

6. **What is the most common cause of sudden cardiac death in young athletes?**

   Hypertrophic cardiomyopathy, followed by anomalous origin of a coronary artery. Other causes of sudden cardiac death in younger persons, in general, include long QT syndrome, Brugada syndrome, and arrhythmogenic right ventricular dysplasia (ARVD), as well as pulmonary embolism.

7. **What are the common causes of syncope?**

   - **Neurocardiogenic:** This is the most common cause of syncope in otherwise healthy persons, particularly younger persons. It is often precipitated by fear, anxiety, or other types of emotional distress. Its course is usually benign.
   - **Orthostatic hypotension:** Orthostatic hypotension results from venous pooling and decreased cardiac output and fall in blood pressure. It may be due to volume depletion, anemia or acute bleeding, peripheral vasodilators (most notoriously the α-adrenoceptor blockers used to treat benign prostatic hypertrophy), or autonomic dysfunction (e.g., diabetic neuropathy, dysautonomia caused by central nervous system [CNS] disease).
   - **Carotid sinus hypersensitivity:** This condition is suggested by syncope precipitated by neck movement, or by tight collars or ties. The diagnosis is made by carotid sinus massage (see Question 12).

- **Cerebrovascular disease:** Carotid artery stenosis usually leads to focal neurologic deficits rather that frank syncope (except perhaps in the very rare case of severe bilateral carotid artery disease, in which global cerebral hypoperfusion can occur). Vertebrobasilar disease is more likely to lead to syncope, although this is a rare cause of syncope in the general population.
- **Tachyarrhythmias:** Ventricular tachycardia (VT) and torsades de pointes are the most ominous cause of syncope. In patients with a history of prior myocardial infarction or those with significantly depressed left ventricular (LV) ejection fraction (less than 30% to 35%), the presumptive cause of syncope is VT until proven otherwise. Polymorphic VT and torsades de pointes is the presumptive cause of syncope in those with prolonged QT intervals because of drugs or congenital long QT syndrome, and in those with Brugada syndrome (see Question 17). Supraventricular tachycardia (SVT) may produce presyncope but does not usually produce overt syncope.
- **Bradyarrhythmias:** Syncope may be caused by intermittent complete heart block. *Sick sinus syndrome* is a general term covering multiple disorders of the conduction system. *Tachy-Brady syndrome* is the more appropriate term used to describe patients with intermittent atrial fibrillation who, when the atrial fibrillation terminates, then have a several or more second period of asystole before normal sinus rhythm and ventricular depolarization resume.
- **Structural-functional:** Aortic stenosis is the most common structural cause of syncope in older patients. The dynamic obstruction that occurs in hypertrophic cardiomyopathy (see Chapter 27) is the most common cause of structural-functional–mediated syncope in younger patients. Left atrial myxoma, causing functional mitral stenosis, is an extremely rare cause of syncope. Syncope can also occur with massive pulmonary embolism, which obstructs the pulmonary artery to such an extent that it compromises blood flow to the LV.

Box 60-1 lists the causes of syncope and loss of consciousness.

8. **What are the important causes of ventricular tachyarrhythmias (VTs)?**
   - Coronary artery disease (CAD). Acute ischemia or myocardial infarction (MI) may cause VT.
   - Depressed LV ejection fraction (EF). Whether due to CAD or nonischemic, cardiomyopathy with depressed EF (<30%-35%) predisposes to VT.
   - Hypertrophic cardiomyopathy (HCM). Patients with HCM are at increased risk of VT, particularly if there is a history of syncope, familial history of sudden cardiac death, or markedly thickened ventricular septum (>30 mm).
   - Prolonged QT interval. The QT interval may be prolonged due to drugs or may be seen in congenital QT prolongation (see Question 16). A prolonged QT interval predisposes to torsades de pointes.
   - Brugada syndrome. Discussed later (see Question 17), this condition predisposes to polymorphic VT.
   - Arrhythmogenic right ventricular dysplasia (ARVD). A rare condition in which there is fatty and fibrotic infiltration of the right ventricle.
   - Right ventricular outflow tract (RVOT) VT. VT may originate from the RVOT. VT in this condition less commonly leads to death.

9. **What is the approach to the patient with syncope?**
   The goals of the evaluation of patients with syncope are not only to identify the cause of syncope but also to determine if the cause is cardiac or noncardiac. Noncardiac causes of syncope generally have a relatively benign course (overall 1-year mortality rates of 0% to 12% and an approximately 0% mortality rate with neurally mediated syncope). Unexplained and undiagnosed causes have an intermediate 1-year mortality rate of 5% to 6%. Cardiac causes, in contrast, are associated with 1-year mortality risk of 18.5% to 33%. Thus, there is a premium on excluding a cardiac cause of syncope, even if the exact cause of syncope cannot be determined.

   A detailed history and physical examination, along with electrocardiogram (ECG) examination, can identify the presumptive cause of syncope in 40% to 50% of cases. Premonitory symptoms such as nausea or diaphoresis, especially in a younger person, or symptoms caused by anxiety, pain, or emotional distress, suggest neurocardiogenic syncope. Syncope during or immediately after urination, defecation, or certain other activities suggests situational syncope. Recent initiation of certain blood pressure–lowering medications, particularly α-adrenoceptor blockers (such as those used to treat

---

Box 60-1 CAUSES OF SYNCOPE AND LOSS OF CONSCIOUSNESS

I. Cardiac Syncope
A. Structural-functional
 1. Aortic stenosis
 2. Hypertrophic cardiomyopathy
 3. Left atrial myxoma
 4. Pulmonary embolism
B. Arrhythmic
 1. Bradyarrhythmic
  a. Profound (sinus) bradycardia
  b. Sick sinus syndrome or brady-tachy syndrome
  c. Heart block
  d. Pacemaker malfunction
 2. Tachyarrhythmia
  a. Ventricular tachycardia
   i. Coronary artery disease, ischemia, myocardial infarction
   ii. Hypertrophic cardiomyopathy
   iii. Dilated cardiomyopathy and/or depressed LV systolic function
   iv. Brugada syndrome
   v. Arrhythmogenic right ventricular dysplasia
  b. Torsades de pointes
   i. Drug-induced QT prolongation
   ii. Congenital QT prolongation

II. Noncardiac Syncope
 ■ Neurocardiogenic
 ■ Carotid sinus hypersensitivity
 ■ Situational (e.g., micturition, defecation, cough, swallowing)
 ■ Orthostatic hypotension (volume depletion, anemia or bleeding, drugs, autonomic dysfunction)
 ■ Subclavian steal
 ■ Vertebrobasilar disease (very rarely severe bilateral carotid disease)

III. Nonsyncope "Loss of Consciousness"
 ■ Seizures
 ■ Hypoglycemia
 ■ Hypoxemia
 ■ Psychogenic

LV, Left ventricular.

---

benign prostatic hypertrophy), raise suspicion for orthostatic hypotension, which can be confirmed on examination. A history of prior MI or depressed EF raises the concern for VT. Cardiac systolic murmurs suggest aortic stenosis or HCM. Table 60-1 gives the factors on history, physical examination, and ECG that may suggest a specific cause for the patient's syncope.

10. **How does one properly test for orthostatic hypotension?**
Recommendations vary, but according to the ESC Guidelines on the Management of Syncope, one first has the patient lie supine for 5 minutes. Blood pressure is then measured 3 minutes after the patient stands, with subsequent blood pressure measurements each minute thereafter if the blood pressure falls and continues to fall compared with supine values. Orthostatic hypotension is defined as a 20 mm Hg or greater drop in systolic blood pressure or systolic blood pressure falling to less than 90 mm Hg. Some other experts also consider falls of diastolic blood pressure of 10 mm Hg or more or increases in heart rate of 20 beats/min or more as criteria to diagnose orthostatic hypotension.

TABLE 60-1. SYMPTOMS AND FINDINGS OBTAINED ON THE HISTORY, PHYSICAL DIAGNOSIS, AND ELECTROCARDIOGRAM, AND THE ETIOLOGY FOR SYNCOPE THAT THEY SUGGEST

SYMPTOMS/FINDINGS	SUGGESTED ETIOLOGY
History	
Post-episode fatigue or weakness	Suggests neurocardiogenic syncope
Syncope precipitated by anxiety, pain, or emotional distress	Suggests neurocardiogenic syncope
Auras, postictal confusion, focal neurological signs/symptoms	Favors a neurological cause
History of MI, depressed EF, or repaired congenital heart disease	Raises concern of a ventricular arrhythmia
Syncope precipitated by neck turning	Suggests carotid sinus hypersensitivity
Sudden onset shortness of breath and/or chest pain	Suggests pulmonary embolism or arrhythmia
Syncope related to micturition, coughing, swallowing, or defecation	Suggests "situational syncope"
Arm movement and use precipitate syncope	Suggests subclavian steal
Palpitations	Suggests cardiac tachyarrhythmia
Family history of sudden cardiac death	Suggests hypertrophic cardiomyopathy, long QT syndrome, or Brugada syndrome
Physical Exam	
Orthostatic changes	Suggests orthostatic hypotension due to dehydration, drugs, or autonomic dysfunction
Carotid sinus hypersensitivity	Suggests carotid sinus hypersensitivity
Carotid bruit	Suggests underlying coronary artery disease, as well as possible carotid stenosis
Systolic ejection murmur	Suggests aortic stenosis or hypertrophic cardiomyopathy
Unequal blood pressures, bruit over subclavian area	Suggests subclavian steal
Electrocardiogram	
Prolonged PR interval +/- bundle branch block	Suggests heart block as cause
Marked sinus bradycardia	Raises the possibility of sick sinus syndrome
Prolonged QT interval	Raises the possibility of torsades de pointes due to congenital long QT syndrome or drugs
Marked left ventricular hypertrophy	Raises possibility of hypertrophic cardiomyopathy
Q waves	Suggests old myocardial infarction and the possibility of ventricular tachycardia
Unusual ST segment elevation in V1 to V2	Suggests Brugada syndrome and polymorphic VT

EF, Ejection fraction; *MI*, myocardial infarction; *VT*, ventricular tachycardia.

11. **What other testing can be performed when the cause of syncope remains unclear?**

When the diagnosis is still not clear, echocardiography can be obtained, looking for unsuspected depressed LV ejection fraction or right ventricular dysfunction, HCM (which may predispose to VT), or obstructive heart disease (aortic stenosis, HCM, rare left atrial myxoma). Note that although echocardiography has become part of the *shotgun* evaluation of syncope for many practitioners, and is recommended as a diagnostic test to consider by both the AHA/ACCF and the ESC, its yield in patients with unremarkable cardiac histories, physical examination, and ECGs is low. In cases in which neurocardiogenic syncope is suspected and further testing is desired, a tilt table test can be obtained. Exercise stress testing has been suggested by some to assess for cardiac ischemia or exercise-induced arrhythmias in appropriately selected patients. In patients in whom a bradyarrhythmia or tachyarrhythmia is suspected, a Holter monitor, event monitor, or implantable loop recorder can be considered or, under certain circumstances, electrophysiologic testing can be performed.

12. **During carotid sinus massage, what is considered a diagnostic response?**

According to the ESC Guidelines on Management of Syncope, a ventricular pause lasting 3 seconds or longer, or a fall in systolic blood pressure of 50 mm Hg or more, is considered abnormal and defines carotid sinus hypersensitivity. Note that carotid sinus massage should not be performed in patients with a recent transient ischemic attack (TIA) or stroke, or those with carotid bruits.

13. **What is a tilt table test?**

Tilt table testing is most commonly performed on patients with neurally mediated syncope (e.g., neurocardiogenic syncope). The patient first lies supine on a board with a foot support. The table is then rotated to a tilt angle of 60 to 80 degrees, so that the patient is almost in the standing position. This maneuver leads to venous pooling and later loss of plasma volume as a result of movement into interstitial spaces. Overall, there is an approximate 15% to 20% (700 mL) decrease of plasma volume. The normal neuroregulatory mechanisms of the body will usually compensate for this, maintaining blood pressure. Vasovagal reactions can occur during monitoring, leading to decrease in heart rate and blood pressure. In a typical protocol, the patient is tilted for 30 minutes, and if no loss of consciousness has occurred, isoproterenol infusion is started and the patient retilted. Other protocols may administer different provocative agents, such as nitroglycerin or adenosine. Criteria have been established to classify the patient responses as cardioinhibitory, vasodepressor, or mixed, based on falls in heart rate, blood pressure, and the occurrence of syncope.

14. **How should one decide between ordering a Holter monitor, an event or ambulatory monitor, or an implantable loop monitor?**

A Holter monitor, which is usually worn for 24 to 48 hours, is useful if the patient experiences syncope or presyncope at least once a day. An event or ambulatory monitor, which most commonly is ordered for approximately 4 weeks, is useful if the patient experiences symptoms at least once or several times a month. An implantable loop monitor is reasonable to consider in a patient with occasional symptoms that occur less than once per month.

15. **Should a *shotgun* neurologic evaluation, including computed tomography (CT) scan, carotid ultrasound, and electroencephalogram, be ordered in all patients with syncope?**

No. True syncope (or loss of consciousness) is an unusual manifestation of neurologic syncope (excluding causes such as reflex, situational, or neurocardiogenic syncope and dysautonomia). In one report, electroencephalogram provided diagnostic information in less than 2% of cases of syncope, and almost all those patients had a history of seizures or symptoms suggesting seizure. Neurologic workup should only be undertaken if a neurologic cause is suggested by the history or physical examination. TIAs usually do not cause syncope. Carotid disease and stroke more likely lead to focal neurologic deficits than to *global* neurologic ischemia and syncope (the rare exception being severe bilateral carotid artery disease). Severe bilateral vertebrobasilar disease can cause syncope, but is

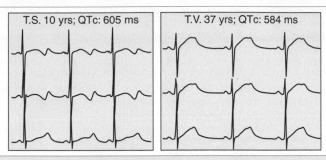

Figure 60-1. Typical electrocardiogram of two long QT syndrome patients showing QT interval prolongation and T wave morphologic abnormalities. (From Libby P, Bonow RO, Mann DL, Zipes DP: *Braunwald's heart disease: a textbook of cardiovascular medicine*, ed 8, Philadelphia, 2008, Saunders.) *QTc*, Corrected QT interval.

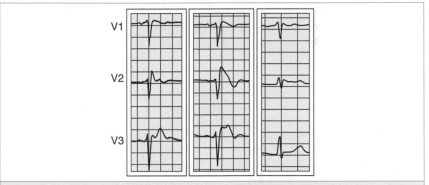

Figure 60-2. Example of the ST segment elevations in leads V1 through V3 seen in patients with Brugada syndrome. (From Libby P, Bonow RO, Mann DL, Zipes DP: *Braunwald's heart disease: a textbook of cardiovascular medicine*, ed 8, Philadelphia, 2008, Saunders.)

not easily diagnosed by screening studies. Importantly, cerebral hypoperfusion caused by ventricular tachycardia can result in seizure-like activity, and the report by family members or other witnesses of the event of "seizure-like" activity in the patient should not cause one to be misled toward a search for neurologic causes based on this alone.

16. **What is long QT syndrome?**

    Long QT syndrome is characterized by a corrected QT interval (QTc) of greater than 450 ms (Fig. 60-1). The QT interval is prolonged because of delayed repolarization as a result of a genetic defect in either potassium or sodium channels. Syncope in patients in long QT syndrome likely is due to torsade des pointes. The onset of symptoms most commonly occurs during the first two decades of life. The risk of developing syncope or sudden cardiac death increases with QTc, with lifetime risks of approximately 5% in those with QTc less than 440 ms, but 50% in those with QTc more than 500 ms. Patients with long QT syndrome should be referred to electrophysiologists for further evaluation and treatment, which may include medicines or placement of an implantable cardioverter defibrillator (ICD).

17. **What is Brugada syndrome?**

    Brugada syndrome is a disorder of sodium channels, resulting in sometimes intermittent unusual ST segment elevation in leads V1 through V3, as well as a right bundle branch block–like pattern (Fig. 60-2). Such patients are susceptible to developing polymorphic VT. Patients with suspected Brugada syndrome should be referred for specialized cardiac evaluation and a probable placement of an ICD.

BIBLIOGRAPHY, SUGGESTED READINGS, AND WEBSITES

1. Brignole M, Alboni P, Benditt DG, et al: Guidelines on management (diagnosis and treatment) of syncope-update. Executive summary, *Eur Heart J* 25:2054–2072, 2004.

2. Calkins H, Zipes DP: Hypotension and syncope. In Libby P, Bonow RO, Mann DL, Zipes DP, editors: *Braunwald's Heart Disease: A Textbook of Cardiovascular Medicine*, ed 8, Philadelphia, 2008, Saunders. pp. 975-984.

3. Morag R: *Syncope*. Available at: http://emedicine.medscape.com/article/811669-overview. Accessed March 26, 2013.

4. Fogel RI, Varma J: Approach to the patient with syncope. In Levine GN, Mann DL, editors: *Primary care provider's guide to cardiology*, Philadelphia, 2000, Lippincott Williams & Wilkins.

5. Higginson LA: *Syncope*. Available at: http://www.merckmanuals.com/professional/cardiovascular_disorders/symptoms_of_cardiovascular_disorders/syncope.html. Accessed March 26, 2013.

6. Kapoor WP: Syncope, *Eur Heart J* 25:2054–2072, 2004.

7. Priori SG, Napolitano C, Schwartz PJ: Genetics of cardiac arrhythmias. In Libby P, Bonow RO, Mann DL, Zipes DP, editors: *Braunwald's Heart Disease: A Textbook of Cardiovascular Medicine*, ed 8, Philadelphia, 2008, Saunders. pp. 101-110.

8. Strickberger SA, Benson DW, Biaggioni I, et al: AHA/ACCF scientific statement on the evaluation of syncope, *J Am Coll Cardiol* 47:473–484, 2006.

CHAPTER 61

TRAUMATIC HEART DISEASE

Fernando Boccalandro, MD, FACC, FSCAI

1. What is the most common cause of cardiac injury?
Motor vehicle accidents are the most common cause of cardiac injury.

2. List the physical mechanisms of injury in cardiac trauma.
Physical mechanisms of injury include penetrating trauma (i.e., ribs, foreign bodies, sternum); nonpenetrating trauma (or blunt cardiac injury); massive chest compression (or crush injury); deceleration, traction, or torsion of the heart or vascular structures; and sudden rise in blood pressure caused by acute abdominal compression.

3. What is myocardial contusion?
Myocardial contusion is a common form of blunt cardiac injury; it is considered a reversible insult and is the consequence of a nonpenetrating myocardial trauma. It is detected by elevations of specific cardiac enzymes with no evidence of coronary occlusion, and by reversible wall motion abnormalities detected by echocardiography. It can manifest in the electrocardiogram (ECG) by ST-T wave changes or by arrhythmias. Myocardial contusion is pathologically characterized by areas of myocardial necrosis and hemorrhagic infiltrates that can be recognized on autopsy.

4. Which major cardiovascular structures are most commonly involved in cardiac trauma?
Cardiac trauma most commonly involves traumatic contusion or rupture of the right ventricle (RV), aortic valve tear, left ventricle (LV) or left atrial rupture, innominate artery avulsion, aortic isthmus rupture (Fig. 61-1), left subclavian artery traumatic occlusion, and tricuspid valve tear.

5. What bedside findings can be detected in patients with suspected major cardiovascular trauma?
Obvious clinical signs in patients with nonpenetrating trauma are rare. However, a bedside evaluation by an astute clinician to detect possible life-threatening cardiovascular and thoracic complications can reveal important signs in just a few minutes (Table 61-1).

6. Can an acute myocardial infarction complicate cardiac trauma?
Myocardial infarction is an unusual complication in patients with chest trauma. Chest trauma can injure a coronary artery, leading to myocardial infarction due to coronary spasm, thrombosis, laceration, or dissection of the arterial wall. Patients with underlying coronary artery disease have favorable pathophysiologic conditions to suffer an acute coronary syndrome during trauma, as a result of limited coronary flow reserve, excess of circulating catecholamines, hypoxia, blood loss, and hypotension. It may be relevant in the appropriate clinical scenario to consider the possibility of cardiac syncope as the primary cause resulting in a traumatic event due to ventricular arrhythmias in a patient with an acute myocardial infarction and concomitant trauma. Chest trauma can elevate cardiac-specific enzymes without significant coronary stenosis; therefore, careful interpretation of these indicators in a trauma victim is warranted.

7. What is the most common type of myocardial infarction suffered in trauma victims?
According to the universal definition of myocardial infarction, patients who have myocardial necrosis during trauma usually suffer a type 2 myocardial infarction. This type of myocardial necrosis is

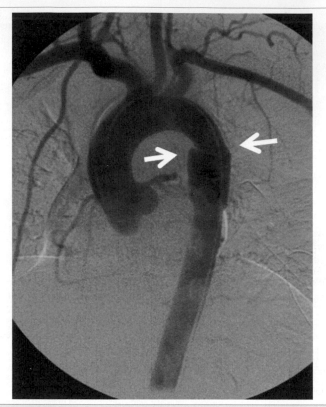

Figure 61-1. Traumatic rupture of the descending thoracic aorta *(arrows)* at the aortic isthmus. Modified from Valji K: *Vascular and Interventional Radiology,* ed 2, Philadelphia, 2006, Saunders.

secondary to direct trauma or ischemia, and is a result of a relative imbalance of either increased myocardial oxygen demand or decreased myocardial oxygen supply (e.g., coronary artery spasm, coronary embolism, anemia, arrhythmias, hypertension, anemia, or hypotension), rather than coronary occlusion caused by advanced atherosclerosis or an acute coronary thrombotic event (type 1 myocardial infarction), and is characterized by a variable increase in cardiac biomarkers with no ischemic symptoms or ECG changes.

8. **What is the preferred treatment for an ST elevation acute myocardial infarction in the event of chest trauma?**
The treatment of choice is emergent coronary angiography. Thrombolytic therapy caries with it a high risk of bleeding complications. The withholding of nitrates, angiotensin-converting enzyme (ACE) inhibitors, and beta-adrenergic blocking agents (β-blockers) should be considered until it is established that the patient is hemodynamically stable. Aspirin can be used in patients with no evidence of severe bleeding. Aortic balloon counterpulsation is contraindicated in patients with acute myocardial infarction, and in patients in cardiogenic shock with acute traumatic aortic regurgitation or any suspected aortic lesions. If a coronary intervention is needed, percutaneous thrombectomy and balloon angioplasty without stenting are preferred, if the patient is not a candidate for dual antiplatelet therapy due to concomitant trauma.

TABLE 61-1. IMPORTANT SIGNS OF CARDIOVASCULAR AND THORACIC TRAUMA

Finding	Suggested Lesions
Pale skin color, conjunctiva, palms, and oral mucosa	Suggests important blood loss
Decreased blood pressure in the left arm	Seen in patients with traumatic rupture of the aortic isthmus, pseudocoarctation, or traumatic thrombosis of the left subclavian artery
Decreased blood pressure in the right arm	Consider innominate artery avulsion
Subcutaneous emphysema and tracheal deviation	Consider pneumothorax
Elevated jugular venous pulse with inspiratory raise (i.e., the Kussmaul sign)	Suggests cardiac tamponade or tension pneumothorax
Prominent systolic V wave in the venous pulse examination	Suggests tricuspid insufficiency as a result of tricuspid valve tear
Nonpalpable apex or distant heart sounds	Suspect cardiac tamponade
Pericardial rub	Diagnostic for pericarditis
Pulsus paradoxus	Seen in patients with cardiac tamponade, massive pulmonary embolism, or tension pneumothorax
Continuous murmurs or thrills	Consider traumatic arteriovenous fistula or rupture of the sinus of Valsalva
Harsh holosystolic murmurs	Suspect traumatic ventricular septal defect
Early diastolic murmur and widened pulse pressure	Suspect aortic valve injury
Cervical and supraclavicular hematomas	Seen in traumatic carotid rupture
New focal neurological symptoms	Traumatic carotid, aortic, or great vessel dissection

9. **List the causes of shock in patients with cardiac trauma.**
   The first cause to address is always hypovolemic shock caused by acute blood loss, usually from an abdominal source. If the shock persists despite fluid resuscitation or the degree of hemodynamic compromise is not in proportion to the degree of blood loss, consider cardiogenic causes or tension pneumothorax. The three main cardiac causes of cardiogenic shock are cardiac tamponade, acute valvular dysfunction, and ventricular akinesia or hypokinesia. Rupture of any intrapericardial vessel or cardiac structure (e.g., coronary arteries, proximal aorta, great veins, ventricle) can produce a rapid state of shock because of cardiac tamponade, unless there is a concomitant pericardial tear. Acute valvular dysfunction due to mechanical disruption of the valvular apparatus can lead to acute valvular regurgitation leading to shock, and is usually associated with the presence of a new murmur in physical examination. Cardiac akinesia or severe hypokinesia with temporary myocardial stunning could be a consequence of cardiac trauma and could lead to cardiogenic shock or acute heart failure. Cardiac akinesia or severe hypokinesia requires volume resuscitation to increase the cardiac preload and inotropic support until contractile recovery is achieved.

10. **What workup should be considered in a patient with suspected cardiac trauma?**
    - **Laboratory testing:** Hemoglobin, hematocrit, chemistries, blood typing, and coagulation panel are routine.

- **Chest radiograph:** Radiographs are used to evaluate the cardiac silhouette, mediastinum, and lung fields.
- **Electrocardiogram:** ECG is not a sensitive or specific test, but it may reveal nonspecific ST or T changes, conduction abnormalities, sinus tachycardia, premature atrial contractions, ventricular premature beats, or more complex arrhythmias suggestive of myocardial contusion. Low voltage is suggestive of pericardial effusion, whereas electrical alternans is suspicious for impending cardiac tamponade.
- **Bedside ultrasound:** A focused assessment with sonography in trauma victims (or FAST) is encouraged, because it is an accurate screening tool for pericardial tamponade and hemo-pericardium, allowing timely management of life-threatening conditions, and identifying those patients at risk for complications.

If the patient is stable from the cardiovascular standpoint, no further workup may be required. Routine use of cardiac biomarkers does not appear to improve the management of patients with blunt chest trauma. However, in patients older than 60 years, with ischemic symptoms or new ECG ischemic changes, cardiac biomarkers and serial ECGs may be appropriate. If more complex heart lesions are suspected, complete echocardiography with color and spectral Doppler imaging is the test of choice. This test is fast, inexpensive, and readily available to provide information regarding the pericardial space, wall motion, valvular function, myocardium, and proximal aorta. Special attention to the RV is warranted, because its anterior location close to the sternum makes it prone to myocardial contusion and to the development of RV thrombus. Transthoracic echocardiography may have important limitations in patients with complicated trauma (e.g., unstable chest, ventilated patients, chest tube drainages) because of limited echocardiographic windows. Echocardiography contrast agents and transesophageal echocardiography (TEE) could play an important role in this group of patients. TEE may not be possible in those with an unstable neck or facial trauma. In suspected aortic involvement, and in patients who are not candidates for TEE, contrast computed tomography (CT) is the test of choice.

11. **What are the signs of cardiac tamponade?**
Classical signs for cardiac tamponade include three signs, known as the *Beck triad:* hypotension caused by decreased stroke volume, jugular-venous distension as a result of impaired venous return to the heart, and muffled heart sounds caused by fluid inside the pericardial sac. Other signs of tamponade include pulsus paradoxus and general signs of shock, such as tachycardia, tachypnea, and decreasing level of consciousness.

12. **Can a patient suffering from traumatic cardiac tamponade have a normal jugular venous pulse?**
In hypovolemic patients, the jugular-venous distension may be difficult to interpret even in the presence of cardiac tamponade. Thus, attention to the volume status is important while examining the venous pulse in trauma victims.

13. **How can one confirm the diagnosis in a patient with suspected pericardial tamponade?**
A large cardiac silhouette by chest radiograph and low-voltage QRS complexes or electrical alternans in the ECG can suggest the presence of cardiac tamponade. CT can identify the size of an effusion, but cannot confirm the diagnosis. Echocardiography can confirm the diagnosis of tamponade and is the test of choice. If cardiac tamponade is suspected, an echocardiogram (with respirometry) should be ordered promptly. Echocardiography can assess the amount and localization of the pericardial effusion, and identify signs of elevated intrapericardial pressure suggesting a tamponade physiology (i.e., right atrial and RV collapse, left atrial collapse). Respirometry is a very simple technique that can be performed during the echocardiographic examination, allowing timing of the respiratory cycle with the mitral and tricuspid inflow. It is used to assess the hemodynamic effect of the pericardial effusion in the ventricular filling (using spectral Doppler analysis) and can confirm the presence of cardiac tamponade.

14. **How can one treat a patient with pericardial tamponade?**
Pericardial tamponade requires immediate treatment with either a surgical subxiphoid approach (pericardial window) or with a percutaneous approach using bedside echocardiography or fluoroscopic guidance.

15. **What interventions during resuscitation and management of an unstable trauma patient can precipitate cardiac tamponade in a patient with a pericardial effusion?**
In a patient with a moderate to large effusion, cardiac tamponade can be precipitated by hypovolemia or positive-pressure ventilation during trauma management. Therefore, meticulous attention to the patient's hemodynamics is needed in these circumstances to avoid hemodynamic collapse.

16. **What are the mechanisms of injury of the thoracic great vessels?**
Deceleration and traction are the most common mechanisms of injury of the thoracic arteries. Sudden horizontal deceleration creates marked shearing stress at the aortic isthmus (i.e., the junction between the mobile aortic arch and the fixed descending aorta), whereas vertical deceleration displaces the heart caudally and pulls the ascending aorta and the innominate artery. Rapid extension of the neck or traction on the shoulder can also overstretch the arch vessels and produce tears of the intima, disruption of the media, or complete rupture of the vessel wall, leading to bleeding, dissection, thrombosis, or pseudoaneurysm formation. Aortic rupture leads to immediate hypovolemic shock and death in the vast majority of cases.

17. **Describe the management of thoracic arterial lesions.**
Usually, all arterial lesions require surgical repair, except benign ones like wall hematomas and limited dissections. An effort should be made to control the blood pressure with β-blockers in all arterial lesions if the patient is hemodynamically stable. Venous lesions usually do not lead to a rapid hemodynamic compromise unless the implicated vessel drains to the pericardium, possibly leading to cardiac tamponade. Thoracic aortic lesions such as limited traumatic dissections are increasingly being managed using thoracic endovascular aortic repair (TEVAR), with thoracic stent graft placement because of reduced perioperative mortality and morbidity in comparison with open surgical repair.

18. **What are potential late complications of heart trauma?**
Late complications can include fistulas between different structures, constrictive pericarditis as a late consequence of hemopericardium, embolization from a mural thrombus, ventricular aneurysm formation, valvular insufficiency, and postpericardiotomy syndrome.

19. **What is commotio cordis?**
Sudden death after a blunt chest trauma is a rare phenomenon known as *commotio cordis*. It is theorized that commotio cordis is caused by ventricular fibrillation secondary to an impact-induced energy transmission via the chest wall to the myocardium during the vulnerable repolarization period. This can cause lethal arrhythmias resulting in sudden death.

20. **Describe the cardiac complications of electrical or lightning injuries.**
Patients in whom an electric current has a vertical pathway are at high risk for cardiac injury. Arrhythmias are frequently seen. Damage to the myocardium is uncommon and occurs mainly because of heat injury or coronary spasm causing myocardial ischemia. Direct current (DC) and high-tension alternate current (AC) are more likely to cause ventricular asystole, whereas low-tension AC produces ventricular fibrillation. The most common ECG abnormalities are sinus tachycardia and nonspecific ST-T wave changes.

The effect of lightning on the heart has been called *cosmic cardioversion* and results in ventricular standstill and, in some reports, ventricular fibrillation. Standstill usually returns to sinus rhythm, but often the patient has a persistent respiratory arrest that causes deterioration of the rhythm. If initial ECG changes are not seen, it is unlikely that significant arrhythmias will occur later.

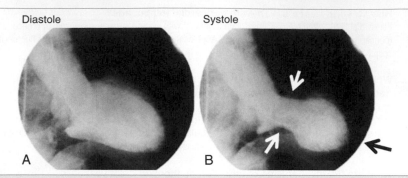

Figure 61-2. Left ventriculography of a patient who developed a tako-tsubo cardiomyopathy following a crush injury, showing the classic apical ballooning of the left ventricle. **A** is during diastole; **B** is during systole. There is systolic contraction of the base of the heart *(white arrows)* but apical ballooning of the left ventricular apex *(black arrow)*. Modified from Daroff R, Fenichel G, Jankovic J, et al: *Bradley's Neurology in Clinical Practice*, ed 6, Edinburgh, 2012, Saunders.

21. **Can a patient develop a trauma-related cardiomyopathy?**

    Tako-tsubo cardiomyopathy, also known as *transient apical ballooning, stress-induced cardiomyopathy,* and simply *stress cardiomyopathy,* is a nonischemic cardiomyopathy in which there is sudden temporary LV systolic dysfunction. The cause is debated and appears to involve high circulating levels of catecholamines and is not specific for mechanical trauma, but can be seen in patients after both emotional and physical trauma. Because this finding is associated with emotional stress, this condition is also known as *broken heart syndrome.* The typical presentation of someone with tako-tsubo cardiomyopathy is a sudden onset of congestive heart failure or chest pain associated with ECG changes suggestive of an anterior wall myocardial ischemia (which may be indistinguishable initially from an acute coronary syndrome) after a major trauma. During the course of evaluation, dilation of the LV apex with a hyper-contractile base of the LV is often noted by echocardiography or angiography (Fig. 61-2). It is this finding that earned the syndrome its name *tako-tsubo,* or "octopus trap," in Japan, where it was first described. Evaluation of individuals with tako-tsubo cardiomyopathy may include coronary angiography, which generally does not reveal any significant coronary artery disease. Provided that the individual survives the initial presentation, the LV function usually improves within several months with medical therapy.

BIBLIOGRAPHY, SUGGESTED READINGS, AND WEBSITES

1. Bansal MK, Maraj S, Chewaproug D, et al: Myocardial contusion injury: redefining the diagnostic algorithm, *Emerg Med J* 22:465–469, 2005.

2. Chockalingam A, Mehra A, Dorairajan S, et al: Acute left ventricular dysfunction in the critically ill, *Chest* 138:198–207, 2010.

3. Cook CC, Gleason TG: Great vessel and cardiac trauma, *Surg Clin North Am* 89:797–820, 2009.

4. Gianni M, Dentali F, Grandi AM, et al: Apical ballooning syndrome or takotsubo cardiomyopathy: a systematic review, *Eur Heart J* 27:1523–1529, 2006.

5. Holanda MS, Domínguez MJ, López-Espadas F, et al: Cardiac contusion following blunt chest trauma, *Eur J Emerg Med* 13:373–376, 2006.

6. Kapoor D, Bybee KA: Stress cardiomyopathy syndrome: a contemporary review, *Curr Heart Fail Rep* 6:265–271, 2009.

7. Karmy-Jones R, Jurkovich GJ: Blunt chest trauma, *Curr Probl Surg* 41:211–380, 2004.

8. Khandhar SJ, Johnson SB, Calhoon JH: Overview of thoracic trauma in the United States, *Thorac Surg Clin* 17:1–9, 2007.

9. Madias C, Maron BJ, Weinstock J, et al: Commotio cordis—sudden cardiac death with chest wall impact, *J Cardiovasc Electrophysiol* 18:115–122, 2007.

10. Mandavia DP, Joseph A: Bedside echocardiography in chest trauma, *Emerg Med Clin North Am* 22:601–619, 2004.

11. McGillicuddy D, Rosen P: Diagnostic dilemmas and current controversies in blunt chest trauma, *Emerg Med Clin North Am* 25:695–711, 2007.

12. Moore EE, Malangoni MA, Cogbill TH, et al: Organ injury scaling. IV: Thoracic vascular, lung, cardiac, and diaphragm, *J Trauma* 36:299–300, 1994.

13. Reissig A, Copetti R, Kroegel C: Current role of emergency ultrasound of the chest, *Crit Care Med* 39:839–845, 2011.

14. Ritenour AE, Morton MJ, McManus JG, et al: Lightning injury: a review, *Burns* 34:585–594, 2008.

15. Thygesen K, Alpert JS, White HD: Joint ESC/ACCF/AHA/WHF Task Force for the Redefinition of Myocardial Infarction. Universal definition of myocardial infarction, *J Am Coll Cardiol* 50:2173–2195, 2007.

16. Wolf SJ, Bebarta VS, Bonnett CJ, et al: Blast injuries, *Lancet* 374:405–415, 2009.

INDEX

Note: Page numbers followed by *f* indicate figures; *t,* tables; and *b,* boxes.

A

A wave, 90–91

A-B-C (airway, breathing, compression), 290

Abacavir, 340

Abdominal aortic aneurysm (AAA), 405

Abrupt vessel closure, 152

Accelerated atherosclerosis
   HIV patients and, 338–339

Ace inhibitor. *See* Angiotensin-converting enzyme (ACE)
      inhibitor

Acquired immune deficiency syndrome (AIDS)
   cardiac complications of, 8

Acquired lipodystrophy, 339

Acute antibody-mediated rejection (AMR), 223, 224t
   risk factors and treatment of, 225

Acute cellular rejection (ACR), 223, 224t
   incidence, risk factors, treatment of, 225, 227t

Acute coronary syndrome (ACS). *See also* Non-ST
      segment elevation acute coronary
      syndrome (NSTE-ACS)
   chest pain and, 110–114
   tropin elevations and, 124, 126t

Acute decompensated heart failure (ADHF), 4
   cardiorenal syndrome and, 170
   definition of, 166
   diuretics and, 169
   high risk for, 167–168, 168b, 168f
   inotropes and, 170
   invasive hemodynamic monitoring and, 170
   patient discharge and, 170–171, 171b
   role of biomarkers in, 167, 167f
   subcategories of, 166
   therapy goals for, 169, 169b

Acute myocardial infarction (AMI)
   cardiac trauma and, 451–452
   chest pain and, 113t
   cocaine ingestion and, 353–354
   exercise stress testing and, 50
   pregnancy and, 369
   Swan-Ganz placement for, 94–96

Acute pericarditis, 7

Acute pulmonary embolism
   chest radiographic findings for, 419
   electrocardiography findings and, 417
   lower extremity deep vein thrombosis and, 415
   risk stratification for, 420
   symptoms of, 416–417

Acute pulmonary embolism *(Continued)*
   syndromes of, 417
   therapy for, 419–420
   Wells score and, 417

Acute ST segment elevation myocardial infarction
   treatment for chest trauma and, 452

Acute viral myocarditis, 192

Adenosine
   dosing regimen for, 296
   narrow complex tachyarrhythmia and, 294
   supraventricular tachycardia and, 271

Advanced heart failure, 166

Aerobic interval training (AIT), 327

African American, hypertension and, 304

Airway obstruction, causes of, 290

Alcohol septal ablation (ASA), 209

Alcohol-induced cardiomyopathy, 199

Aldosterone antagonist
   adverse effects of, 178
   discussion of, 177
   indications of, 177–178, 179t
   safety of, 178

Allergic reaction, iodine based contrast agents and,
      108

Allograft
   definition of, 247–248
   rejection
      clinical signs of, 223
      diagnosis of, 224
      types of, 223

Allotransplantation, 218

Alpha-adrenergic blocking agent (α-blocker), 303–304

Ambulatory electrocardiography (AECG) monitoring
   abnormalities found during, 63
   indications for, 60, 60b
   ischemic heart disease and, 64–65
   stroke and, 66
   types of, 61–62
   ventricular arrhythmia and, 63

Ambulatory real-time continuous cardiac monitoring, 61–62

Ambulatory telemetry, 61–62

American College of Cardiology Foundation/American Heart
      Association (ACCF/AHA)
   guidelines for unstable angina/non-ST elevation MI
      by, 409
   guidelines on preoperative cardiovascular evaluation
      by, 409, 411, 412f